DRUGS AFFECTING LIPID METABOLISM

Medical Science Symposia Series

Volume 2

The titles published in this series are listed at the end of this volume.

DRUGS AFFECTING LIPID METABOLISM

Edited by

A.L. Catapano
Institute of Pharmacological Sciences,
University of Milan, Milan, Italy

A.M. Gotto, Jr.
Baylor College of Medicine and The Methodist Hospital,
Houston, Texas, U.S.A.

L.C. Smith
Department of Experimental Medicine, The Methodist Hospital,
Houston, Texas, U.S.A.

and

R. Paoletti
Institute of Pharmacological Sciences,
University of Milan, Milan, Italy

SPRINGER SCIENCE+BUSINESS MEDIA, B.V.

Library of Congress Cataloging-in-Publication Data

Drugs affecting lipid metabolism / edited by A.L. Catapano ... [et
al.].
        p.   cm. -- (Medical science symposia series ; v. 2)
    Proceedings of the 11th International Symposium on Drugs Affecting
Lipid Metabolism, held in 1992 in Florence, Italy.
    Includes index.
    ISBN 978-94-010-4746-3   ISBN 978-94-011-1703-6 (eBook)
    DOI 10.1007/978-94-011-1703-6
    1. Antilipemic agents--Congresses.   2. Hyperlipidemia-
-Chemotherapy--Congresses.   3. Atherosclerosis--Chemotherapy-
-Congresses.   4. Coronary heart disease--Chemotherapy--Congresses.
I. Catapano, Alberico L.   II. International Symposium on Drugs
Affecting Lipid Metabolism, (11th : 1992 : Florence, Italy)
III. Series.
    [DNLM: 1. Antilipemic Agents--congresses.   2. Lipids--metabolism-
-congresses.   3. Lipoproteins--metabolism--congresses.
4. Metabolism--drug effects--congresses.   W1 ME46RD v.2 1993 / QU
85]
RC632.H87D78   1993
615'.739--dc20
DNLM/DLC
for Library of Congress   93-5111

ISBN 978-94-010-4746-3

Printed on acid-free paper

CONTENTS

VII: LP(A)

VIII: ANTIOXIDANTS, LIPOPROTEINS AND ATHEROSCLEROSISX

IX: DRUGS AFFECTING ATHEROSCLEROSIS AND THROMBOSIS

SYMPOSIA

E: HDL, PHOSPHOLIPIDS AND ATHEROSCLEROSIS

PREFACE

The recent Symposium on Drugs Affecting Lipid Metabolism took place at a very peculiar time for the development in this field.

Many experimental, clinical and epidemiological data have been gathered to confirm the strict and causal correlation between plasma lipoproteins and coronary heart desease. However, as it usually happens in research, many more interesting issues are being studied opening new fields of research for the future. The highlights of these concepts are presented in this book that reports the proceedings of the meeting held in Florence.

In our opinion special attention should be paid to new areas such as a) the involvement of dysfuction of the coagulation and fibrinolytic system in the development of coronary artery disease, b) direct effect of hypolipidemic drugs on the arterial wall, c) development of new drugs that can modulate the reaction of cells within the arterial wall to stress (hyperlipidemia, hypertension, etc.).

These new advances, together with the combined efforts of cell biologists and lipoprotein chemists, have set the pace for an exciting period of research and clinical applications of diets and drugs affecting plasma and cell lipids. This volume, which includes the work of many of the leading world laboratories, represents an authoritative and up-to-date appraisal of the status of the art and a stimulus to future research at the laboratory and clinical level in a fascinating area for clinical and preventive medicine.

The Editor

LIST OF FIRST AUTHORS

Gerd ASSMANN
Institut f. Klinische
Chemie
u. Laboratoriumsmedizin
der WWu
Albert-Schweitzer Str. 33
DW-4400 MÜNSTER
Germany

Pietro AVOGARO
Primario
Divisione Medica II
Ospedali Civili Riuniti
I-30100 VENEZIA
Italy

Kåre BERG
Chairman and Director
Institute of Medical
Genetics
University of Oslo
P.O.B. 1036 BLINDERN
N-0315 OSLO-3
Norway

David H. BLANKENHORN
Director
Atherosclerosis Research
Institute
University of Southern
California
2025 Zonal Avenue
LOS ANGELES, CA 90033
USA

C.T. CAMPOS
Box 290 UMHC
420 Delaware St. SE
MINNEAPOLIS, MN 55455
USA

Antonio CAPURSO
Cattedra di Gerontologia
Istituto di Clinica
Medica
Università di Bari
Policlinico
P. Giulio Cesare
I-70100 BARI
Italy

A.L. CATAPANO
Istituto di Scienze
Farmacologiche
Università di Milano
Via Balzaretti 9
I-20133 MILANO
Italy

Lawrence CHAN
Director Lab. Molecular
Biology
Dept. of Cell Biology
Rm12A
Baylor College of
Medicine
One Baylor Plaza
HOUSTON, TX 77030
USA

John Y.L. CHIANG
Dept. of Biochemistry
Northeastern Ohio
Universities
College of Medicine
ROOTSTOWN, OH 44272
USA

Gaetano CREPALDI
Istituto di Medicina
Interna
Catt. di Patologia Med.
II
Università di Padova
Via Giustiniani 2
I-35128 PADOVA
Italy

Roger A. DAVIS
Hepatobiliary Research
Center
University of Colorado
Health Sciences Center
Box B158 - 4200 E. Ninth
Av.
DENVER, CO 80262
USA

Shlomo EISENBERG
Department of Medicine B
Hadassah University
Hospital
P.O.Box 12000
JERUSALEM
Israel

Frederick H. EPSTEIN
Professor of Preventive
Medicine
University of Zürich
Sumatrastrasse 30
CH-8006 ZURICH
Switzerland

Guido FRANCESCHINI
Istituto di Scienze
Farmacologiche
Università di Milano
Via Balzaretti 9
I-20133 MILANO
Italy

J.C. FRUCHART
Institut Pasteur
1, rue Calmette
F-59019 LILLE
France

C. GALLI
Istituto di Scienze
Farmacologiche
Via Balzaretti 9
I-20133 MILANO
Italy

Giovanni GALLI
Istituto di Scienze
Farmacologiche
Univ. di Milano
Via Balzaretti 9
I-20133 MILANO
Italy

Sandra H. GIANTURCO
Lipoprotein Metabolism
Department of Medicine
ARU
University of Alabama at
Birmingham
690 Diabetes Hospital-UBA
Station
BIRMINGHAM, AL 35294
USA

A.M. GOTTO, Jr.
Chairman
Department of Medicine
Baylor College of
Medicine
One Baylor Plaza
Houston, TX 77030
USA

H.W. HAHMANN
Institut f. Praventive
Kardiologie
a. d. Universitätsklinik
Homburg
Gebaude 51
DW-6650 HOMBURG/SAAR
Germany

M. Daria HAUST
Health Sciences Centre
Dept. of Pathology
The University of Western
Ontario
University Drive
LONDON, ONTARIO
Canada N6A 5CI

Michael R. HAYDEN
Department of Medical
Genetics
Univ. Hospital-UBC Site
Rm.F168-Wesbrook Mall
The University of British
Columbia
VANCOUVER B.C.
Canada V6T 2B5

Richard L. JACKSON
Marion Merrell Dow
Research Institute
2110 E. Galbraith Road
CINCINNATI, OH 45215
USA

L.A. JOKUBAITIS
Sandoz Research Institute
Bldg. 501/1
59 Route 10 East
EAST HANOVER, NJ 07936
USA

Herbert J. KAYDEN
Department of Medicine
New York University
550 First Avenue
NEW YORK, NY 10016
USA

G.M. KOSTNER
Head
Dept. of Medical
Biochemistry
University of Graz
A-8010 GRAZ
Austria

John C. LaROSA
Dean of Research
George Washington
University
Medical Center
Suite 713
2300 Eye Street Northwest
WASHINGTON, DC 20037
USA

Matthias LESCHKE
Medizinische Klinik B
Abteilung f. Kardiologie
Pneumologie u. Angiologie
Heinrich-Heine
Universität Düsseldorf
Moorenstrasse 5
DW-4000 DÜSSELDORF 1
Germany

Beatriz LEVY-WILSON
Dept. of Pharmaceutical
Chemistry
The Gladstone Foundation
Labs.
University of California
2550-23rd Street
P.O.B. 40608
SAN FRANCISCO, CA 94140
USA

Barry LEWIS
4 Sutclife Close
LONDON NW11 6NT
UK

Timothy J. LYONS
Assistent Professor of
Medicine
Division of Endocrinology
Medical University of
South Carolina
1711 Ashley Avenue
CHARLESTON, SC
USA

Mario MANCINI
Istituto di Medicina
Interna
e Malattie Dismetaboliche
II Fac. di Med. e
Chirurgia
Nuovo Policlinico- Univ.
di Napoli
Via Pansini 5
I-80131 NAPOLI
Italy

V. MANNINEN
National Public Health
Institute
Mannerheinzinttie 166
F-00280 HELSINKI
Finland

Joel D. MORRISETT
Department of Medicine
Division of
Atherosclerosis and
Lipoprotein Research
Baylor College of
Medicine
One Baylor Plaza
HOUSTON, TX 77030
USA

A. NOTARBARTOLO
Cattedra di Patologia
Medica
Università di Palermo
Via del Vespro
I-90127 PALERMO
Italy

Anders G. OLSSON
Dept. of Internal
Medicine
University Hospital
S-581 85 LINKOPING
Sweden

Rodolfo PAOLETTI
Direttore
Istituto di Scienze
Farmacologiche
Università di Milano
Via Balzaretti 9
I-20133 MILANO
Italy

Josef R. PATSCH
Dept. of Medicine
University of Innsbruck
Annraen 52
A-6020 INNSBRUCK
Austria

Kenneth B. POMERANTZ
Department of Pathology
A-626
Cornell Univ. Medical
College
1300 York Avenue
NEW YORK, NY 10021
USA

Henry J. POWNALL
Scientific Director
Division of
Atherosclerosis
The Methodist Hospital
Baylor College of
Medicine
6565 Fannin St. M.S.
A-601
HOUSTON, TX 77030
USA

J. RAPACZ
Department of Genetics
Department of Meat &
Animal Science
Univerisity of Wisconsin-
Madison
MADISON, WI 53706
USA

Paola ROMA
Istituto di Scienze
Farmacologiche
Università di Milano
Via Balzaretti 9
I-20133 MILANO
Italy

M. ROSSENEU
A Z St-Jan
Labo. Chemie
Ruddershove 10
B-8000 BRUGGE
Belgium

George ROTHBLAT
Medical College Penn
Dept. Physiology and
Biochemistry
PHILADELPHIA, PA 19129
USA

G. SALVIOLI
Università di Modena
Viale Vittorio Veneto 9
I-41100 MODENA
Italy

Angelo M. SCANU
Dept. of Medicine
Biochemistry and
Molecular Biology
The University of Chicago
5841 South Mayland Avenue
Box 231
CHICAGO, IL 60637
USA

Ernst J. SCHAEFER
Chief Lipid Metabolism
Lab.
Human Nutrition Res.
Center on Aging
at Tufts University
711 Washington Street
BOSTON, MA 02111
USA

G. SCHMITZ
Institut f. Klinische
Chemie
u. Laboratoriumsmedizin
Zentral. u. Blutbank-
Univ. Rogensburg
Franz-Josef-Strauss
Allee 1
Postfach 10 06 62
DW-8400 ROGENSBURG
Germany

Peter SCHWANDT
Klinikum Großhadern
Medizinische Klinik II
University of München
Marchioninistrasse 15
DW-8000 MUNICH 70
Germany

Colin J. SCHWARTZ
Department of Pathology
UTHSC
7703 Floyd Curl Drive
SAN ANTONIO
TX 78284-7750
USA

James SHEPHERD
Reader in Pathological
Biochemistry
Univerisity of Glasgow
Royal Infirmary
GLASGOW G4 OSF
UK

Cesare R. SIRTORI
Istituto di Scienze
Farmacologiche
Univ. di Milano
Via Balzaretti 9
I-20133 MILANO
Italy

Louis C. SMITH
Professor of Experimental
Medicine
The Methodist Hospital
Department of Medicine
6565 Fannin M.S. A601
HOUSTON, TX 77030-2797
USA

Daniel STEINBERG
Univ. of California-San
Diego
Division of Endocrinology
and
Metabolism - Dept. of
Medicine
Basic Science Building -
Room 1080
LA JOLLA, CA 92093
USA

M.R. TASKINEN
Third Department of
Medicine
University of Helsinki
Haartmaninkatu 4
F-00290 HELSINKI
Finland

Elena TREMOLI
Istituto di Scienze
Farmacologiche
Univ. di Milano
Via Balzaretti 9
I-20133 MILANO
Italy

Akira YAMAMOTO
Vice Director of the
Research Institute
National Cardiovascular
Center
Research Institute
5-7-1 Fujishiro-dai-Suita
OSAKA 565
Japan

REGRESSION OF HUMAN AORTIC FATTY STREAKS OF EARLY LIFE

M. DARIA HAUST

ABSTRACT.   The fatty streaks of ascending aorta (AA) of infancy
disappear gradually from the surface as similar lesions increasingly
involve the descending thoracic and abdominal aorta with age.   To
"monitor" the fate of these lesions, 85 aortae obtained at post mortem
of patients ranging in age from birth to 20 years were treated with
Sudan IV and the stained areas recorded on diagrams. Tissues from four
standard areas were examined by light and electron microscopy.
Sudanophilic areas showed either diffusely dispersed, extracellular
fine lipid particles, or fat droplets in smooth muscle cells.   The
former appeared at times a few days after birth, the latter at 17-18
months of life.   Whereas gross sudanophilia was absent in most AA of
second decade, morphologically these areas showed the presence of
deeply-seated cholesterol crystals with no accompanying tissue
necrosis.   The superficial layers represented a new intima probably
constituted in the process of repair when the previously present fatty
streaks regressed.

INTRODUCTION

In individuals with no known genetic disease, atherosclerotic lesions
observed in infancy and childhood are those considered to represent
early forms or "lesions of inception", i.e., (a) fatty dots and
streaks; (b) gelatinous elevations; and (c) microthrombi [1,2].
   Of the above lesions the most commonly present in early age are
the fatty dots and streaks.   It was recognized already in the past
century that these lesions occur in the aortic intima of very young
children but at that time it was not acknowledged generally that these
represented precursors of atherosclerotic plaques of adult life.   Jores
discussed this problem at the turn of the century [3], and later
Schmidtmann, a student of Anitschkow, reviewed the available literature
pertaining to the occurrence of fatty dots and streaks in children when
reporting her important morphological studies conducted at the post
mortem of 44 patients who ranged in age from 14 days to 16 years [4].

A. L. Catapano et al. (eds.), Drugs Affecting Lipid Metabolism, 1–8.
© 1993 Kluwer Academic Publishers and Fondazione Giovanni Lorenzini.

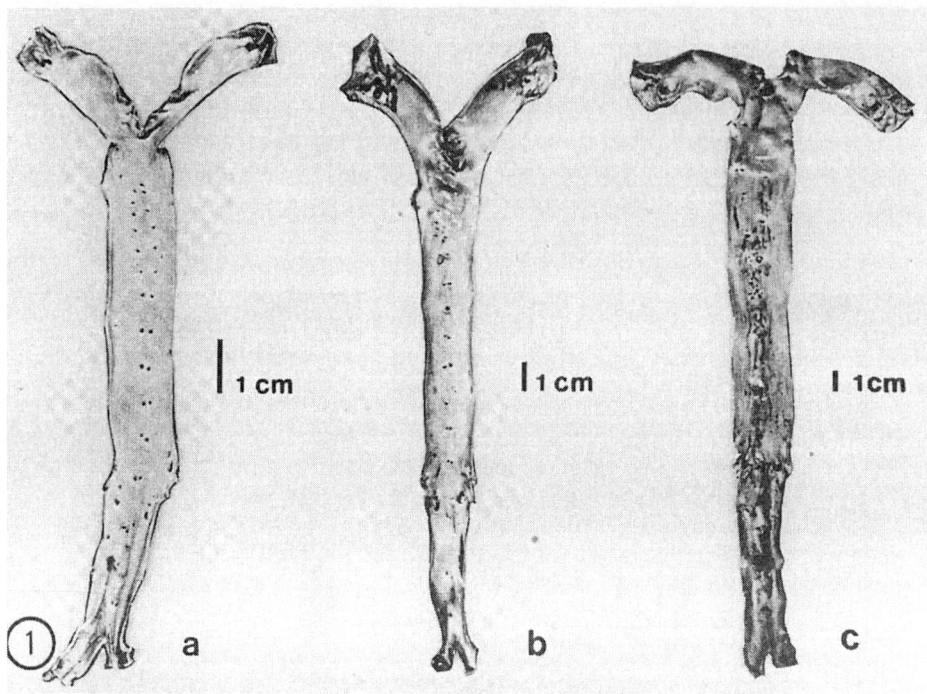

Figure 1. Aortae stained in toto with Sudan IV. A small surface is
stained in a one-day-old baby (1a), extensive areas in a 9-year-old
child (1b) and almost none in a 20-year-old patient (1c). Sudanophilia
is indicated in black (see TEXT).

Similar studies were undertaken subsequently by a number of
investigators, and there has been a considerable agreement that these
lesions are present in the aorta in early life. In some series, the
aortic surface of many children under the age of three years showed
fatty streaking which was present in all individuals older than that
age [5,6]. Other data indicate that by one year all children displayed
some degree of streaking [1,2,7,8], and the localization and extent of
aortic intimal involvement was similar in different geographical areas,
and various races, and did not seem to be related to dietary habits and
socio-economic status [9].
      Whereas the early fatty lesions are present in the aorta
throughout life, the pattern of distribution "shifts" with age. They
first appear above the aortic valve, increasing in number with age in
the ascending segment and arch, appear later in childhood in the
descending thoracic and finally in the abdominal aorta, where large
surfaces may be involved by the end of the second decade. The latter
are usually also the site of the most severe atherosclerotic plaques of
adult and old age and therefore here the fatty streaks may be plausibly

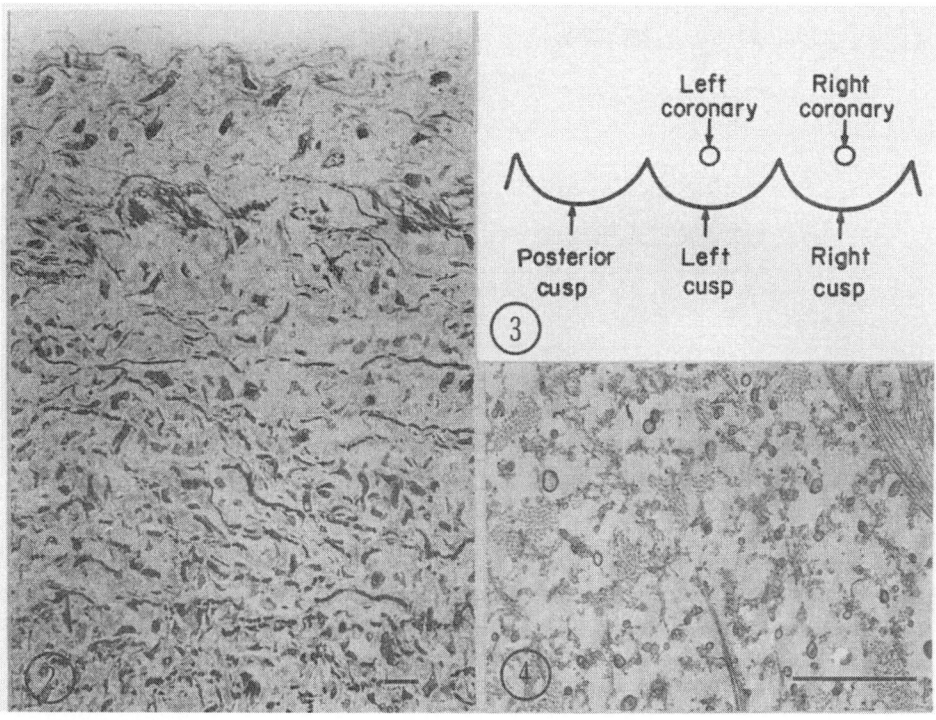

Figure 2. Small sudanophilic area is reflected in a focal intimal edema (top) in a 4-day-old infant. No cellular changes are evident. Plastic-embedded; one-micron-thick, toluidine blue-stained. Bar = 10 μm.
Figure 3. Schematic representation of sudanophilic affinity-areas at aortic origin: periorifices of coronary arteries and endocardial surface of left ventricle adjacent to leaflets of the valves.
Figure 4. Electron micrograph of an area shown in Figure 2. Small round profiles of finely dispersed lipids between connective tissues of the intima. Plastic embedded; ultrathin section stained with uranyl acetate and lead citrate. Bar = 1 μm.

considered to be the precursor lesions of advanced atherosclerosis. This role of the fatty streaks has been questioned however by numerous investigators who point out that were this the case, these lesions would progress to similar atherosclerotic plaques in the proximal aorta, a site where they made the appearance at the earliest age. To explain this puzzling phenomenon, some workers proposed that there are actually two forms of fatty streaks: these that remain innocuous and "arrested" throughout life and those that progress to the prominent atherosclerotic plaques.

There are neither morphological nor biochemical data to support the view that in fact two different distinct forms of fatty streaks

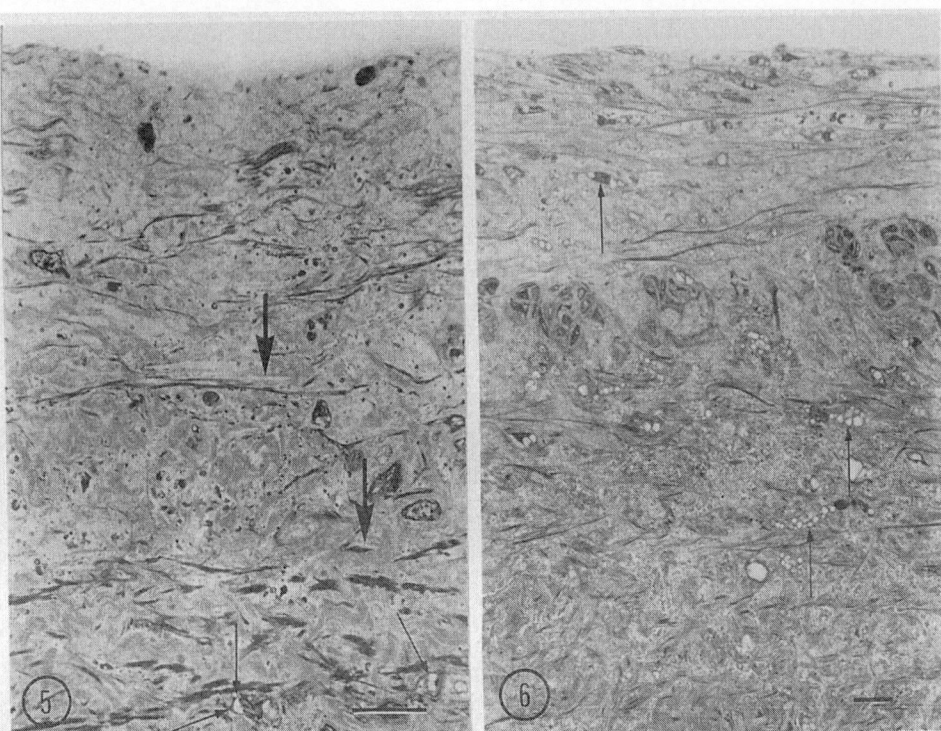

Figure 5. Sudanophilic flat area in an 18-month-old child contains numerous tiny (black) extracellular lipids and several slender cholesterol crystals (thick arrows), and a few lipid-droplets containing SMC's (thin arrows). Preparation as in Figure 2. Bar = 10 μm.

Figure 6. A well developed, fatty streak in a 3-year-old child contains many SMC's with fat droplets (arrows). Preparation as in Figure 2. Bar = 10 μm.

exist in man or experimental animals. If not, could the above phenomenon be explained on a different basis, e.g., that at certain aortic sites fatty dots and streaks at a certain stage of development may have the potential for regression?

The purpose of this communication is to report the preliminary results of a study undertaken to assess whether on morphological grounds there is sufficient evidence in support of the contention that the fatty streaks of the proximal aorta in infancy and childhood, do regress. Some aspects of these studies were reported briefly previously [10].

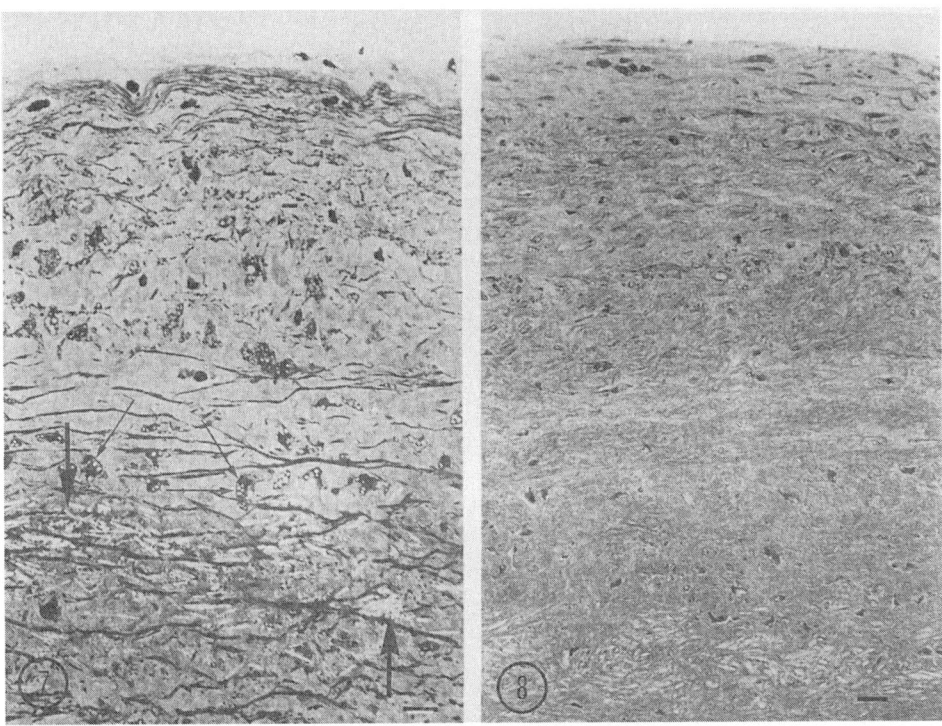

Figure 7. Prominent sudanophilic area in a 9-year-old child with edema in superficial intimal layers, SMC's containing lipid droplets in mid-zone and a pool of many slender cholesterol crystals at the intimal-medial interphase (thick arrows). Note that some of the lipid-containing SMC's appear to be necrotic (thin arrows). Preparation as in Figure 2. Bar = 10 μm.

Figure 8. This area in AA of a 20-year-old man was not sudanophilic and appeared normal. It shows a thick intima consisting of several layers, the most superficial containing the "youngest" tissues. A large pool of cholesterol crystals is deeply-seated (bottom). Lipids are not observed elsewhere in intima. Paraffin-embedded tissue; Masson Trichrome stain. Bar = 10 μm.

MATERIALS AND METHODS

Aortae obtained at necropsy of 85 patients whose age ranged from one day to 20 years were stained in toto with Sudan IV stain for neutral lipids. All specimens were photographed, and the stained areas were recorded on a diagram and described. Tissues removed from four standard sites of the ascending aortic segment and arch (AA) were processed for light and electron microscopic examination. Details of methods, including those of fixation, gross staining, mapping out sudanophilic areas on standard diagrams, processing for light and electron microscopy and staining, and data pertaining to patients are provided elsewhere [11] because of limitation of the allowable space for this presentation.

RESULTS

Sudanophilia was present on gross examination in the AA as early as one day after birth in some instances (Fig. 1a), and increased in intensity and extend up to the end of the first decade when usually small foci of staining began appearing at distal "lips" of orifices of intercostal arteries (Fig. 1b). With advancing age and extension of sudanophilic staining to larger areas of the posterior wall of the descending thoracic aorta and to the abdominal aortic segment, there was a gradual disappearance of the gross staining from the AA (Fig. 1c).

Microscopically, in the early months of life the sudanophilic areas in the AA showed a slight to moderate, focal, superficial intimal edema (Fig. 2). When present, the gross staining was detectable earliest in the most proximal aortic segment (around the orifices of either one or both coronary arteries), but at times on the endocardial surface immediately adjacent to the aortic valve cusps (Fig. 3). In routine paraffin-, and plastic- (Fig. 2) embedded tissues no cellular changes were apparent. Frozen-cut sections stained for neutral fat showed only the presence of increased amounts of finely dispersed extracellular lipids similar to those observed in normal intimas [12]. Electron microscopic examination confirmed the nature of these extracellular lipids (Fig. 4).

At the age of 17-18 months two additional features of grossly sudanophilic areas became apparent microscopically in the intima: the presence of thin, short or elongated cholesterol crystals "free" in the intercellular space, and localized areas of smooth muscle cells (SMC's) containing lipid droplets (= myogenic foam cells, MFC's). These features were only detectable in sections from plastic- (Fig. 5) but not from paraffin-embedded tissues. The appearance of the MFC's heralded the development of fatty streaks. By 3 years of age the fatty streaks were well developed (Fig. 6) in eleven of the 13 AA examined, and after that age they were present in all children.

With the beginning of "shifting" of gross sudanophilia to distal aorta (see above), the microscopic appearance of the lesions in the AA underwent a gradual transformation. The amount of extracellular lipids in the superficial layers of intima decreased as did the number of MFC's. The latter were still present in the deeper intimal layers for some years, but almost none were found towards the end of second decade. The most striking feature of the "transformation" process was the increasing accumulation of cholesterol crystals in the deep intimal layers, forming pools even prior to the end of the first decade of life (Fig. 7). With increasing age, when the sudanophilia was either entirely absent or of insignificant extent in the AA (Fig. 1), the now considerably thickened intima, appeared entirely fat-free with the exception of the deep-seated accumulations of small size cholesterol crystals. No cellular or connective tissue necrosis was apparent in the vicinity of these foci (Fig. 8).

COMMENTS AND CONCLUSIONS

Since the accumulations of focal, intimal, extracellular, finely dispersed lipids that correspond to the earliest gross sudanophilia in the AA, precedes the appearance of both, the cholesterol crystals and the fatty streaks, it seems reasonable to postulate that the crystals may be formed from both, i.e., the "insuded" lipids and those released later from the MFC's. The considerably thickened intima in the older age group consists of several layers of connective tissues and SMC's with features of a relatively recent proliferation. This phenomenon may be regarded as an outcome of repair process possibly induced by disintegration of the MFC's of fatty streaks. Lipids released from these cells may contribute to the basal pool of cholesterol crystals which appear sequestered and inert without associated areas of necrosis. The thick layer of the "new" intima would easily explain why in the presence of such deep-seated cholesterol crystal pools these AA-regions were not sudanophilic towards the end and beyond the second decade of life.

The presence of cholesterol crystal pools in deep layers of the intima may be thus considered to be a hallmark of the once present fatty streaks in the AA. Whether the process involved may represent a "regression" in a true sense of the definition or is rather the outcome of repair is a matter for dispute.

ACKNOWLEDGEMENTS

The author wishes to express her appreciation to Ms. Wojewodzka, Mr. Roger Dewar, Mrs. Renate Feulgen, Mrs. Susan Coulson and Mrs. Wendy Thomas for their skilful technical assistance, to Ms. Kris Milne for her expert gross photography and artwork, and to Mrs. Betty Gardiner for the competent and patient typing of the manuscript.

This work was supported by a grant-in-aid T.3-11 from the Heart and Stroke Foundation of Ontario, Toronto, Ontario, Canada.

REFERENCES

1. Haust, M.D. (1978) 'Atherosclerosis in childhood', in H. Rosenberg and R. Bolande (eds.), Perspectives in Pediatric Pathology, Vol. 4, Year Book Medical Publishers, Inc., Chicago, pp. 155-216.
2. Haust, M.D. (1990) The genesis of atherosclerosis in pediatric age-group, Ped. Pathol. 10, 253-271.
3. Jores, L. (1903) Wesen und Entwicklung der Arteriosklerose. J.F. Bergmann, Wiesbaden.
4. Schmidtmann, M. (1925) Das Vorkommen der Arteriosklerose bei Jugendlichen und seine Bedeutung für die Ätiologie des Leidens, Virchows Archiv (Pathol. Anat.) 255, 206-272.

5. Holman, R.L. (1961) Atherosclerosis - a pediatric nutrition problem? Am. J. Clin. Nutr. 9, 565-569.
6. Holman, R.L., McGill, H.C. Jr., Strong, J.P., and Geer, J.C. (1958) The natural history of atherosclerosis. The early aortic lesions as seen in New Orleans in the middle of the 20th Century, Am. J. Pathol. 34, 209-235.
7. Eggen, D.A., and Solberg, L.A. (1968) Variation of atherosclerosis with age, Lab. Invest. 18, 571-579.
8. Schwartz, C.J., Ardlie, N.G., Carter, R.F., and Paterson, J.C. (1967) Gross sudanophilia and hemosiderin deposition. A study on infants, children, and young adults, Arch. Pathol. 83, 325-332.
9. McGill, H.C. Jr. (1977) 'The lesion in children', in G.W. Manning, and M.D. Haust (eds.), Atherosclerosis: Metabolic, Morphologic and Clinical Aspects, Plenum Press, New York, pp. 509-513.
10. Haust, M.D. (1988) 'The fate of early atherosclerotic lesions of childhood', in H. Morl, C. Diehm, and G. Heusel (eds.), 45 Jahre Herzinfarkt- und Fettstoffwechselforschung, Springer-Verlag, Berlin Heidelberg, pp. 69-76.
11. Haust, M.D., Wojewodzka, I., Schwartz, C.J., and Huber, J. (1992) Morphological studies of gross sudanophilic areas of human aorta in the first two decades of life, and their relevance to regression of early atherosclerotic lesions. Part I. Ascending aorta and arch, in preparation.
12. Movat, H.Z., Haust, M.D., and More, R.H. (1959) The morphologic elements in the early lesions of arteriosclerosis, Am. J. Pathol. 35, 93-101.

SERUM CHOLESTEROL AS A RISK FACTOR: EFFECTS OF GENDER AND AGE.

Frederick H. Epstein

Abstract

Prior to the age of 65 years, in "middle age", the relation between coronary heart disease (CHD) and total serum cholesterol (TC) is at least as strong in women as in men in terms of relative risk, indicating that elevated levels carry similar atherogenicity in the two genders. Attributable risk, on the other hand, is less in women than men because their absolute CHD risk is lower. Thus, preventive measures in middle age will benefit relatively fewer women than men during this period of life. Elderly women show an increase in relative risk due to elevated TC less consistently than men but their attributable risk is higher than for men beyond the age of 65 years. Therefore, older women potentially derive much benefit from prevention. Low-density lipoprotein cholesterol (LDL-C) is no more predictive for CHD than TC but HDL-C has independent predictive value in elderly women and men. The TC/HDL-C ratio is more strongly related to CHD risk than TC in either gender and at any age. However, TC remains significantly predictive in elderly men and, if allowance is made for competing risks, in elderly women so that there would be no scientific basis for putting an age limit on TC reduction in either men or women, taking additionally the large attributable risks into account.

Introduction

Proper planning of strategies for the prevention of coronary heart disease (CHD) requires, amongst others, answers to 2 questions: (1) is the relation between serum cholesterol and CHD similar for men and women, and (2) is this relation maintained as age advances? It is still being asked sometimes whether women need preventive treatment as much as men and whether elderly women and men require lipid-lowering therapy at all. Answers to the 2 questions raised will provide the scientific evidence for making these decisions.

Serum cholesterol and CHD risk by gender and age

A review of 25 prospective studies in men and 14 such studies in women below 65 years of age indicates that the relative CHD risk is, if anything, higher in women than in men [1]; comparing risk at total serum cholesterol levels of 6.20 mmol/L or higher with the risk below 5.17 mmol/L, the pooled relative risk ratio is 2.44 for women and 1.73 for

A. L. Catapano et al. (eds.), Drugs Affecting Lipid Metabolism, 9–13.
© 1993 Kluwer Academic Publishers and Fondazione Giovanni Lorenzini.

men, both being significant. A recent report from Scotland provides similar findings, the risk ratio, comparing the top and bottom quintiles of serum cholesterol, being 1.77 for women and 1.56 for men [2]. The Scandinavian NORA project, comprising 44,900 women from 5 prospective studies, shows a gradual gradient of risk from the bottom to the top quintile, the risk ratio between them being about 3 [3]; the gradient for cholesterol is as steep as the gradient for blood pressure.

These findings leave no doubt that CHD risk is at least as strongly related to serum cholesterol in women as it is in men below the age of 65 years. In contrast to the relative risk which measures the strength of the association, the attributable risk pertaining to cholesterol is lower in women than men. The attributable risk is the excess risk above a certain threshold level, e.g. 6.2 mmol/L, as compared with the risk within the optimal range of serum cholesterol, i.e. below 5.2 mmol/L. The difference in attributable risk between men and women is due to the fact that women carry a lower absolute CHD risk than men, owing to the presence of protective factors. This difference has been the source of much confusion and unnecessary controversy. In order to assess the benefit which might accrue from cholesterol reduction, the attributable risk is the measure which counts. For assessing the cause-and-effect relationship between cholesterol level and CHD risk, i.e. obtaining a measure for the aetiological role of cholesterol in causing coronary atherosclerosis, the relative risk is the appropriate guide. It is proper to conclude that women require low or lower serum cholesterol levels as much as men for the prevention of coronary heart disease but that they will benefit from preventive therapy less than men in absolute terms. The benefit nevertheless remains substantial and there is no justification for excluding women from it.

It has become customary to draw the arbitrary dividing line between middle-age and older ages at 65 years. Beyond the age of 65 years, relative CHD risks, defined as above, decline, being 1.12 (barely reaching significance) for women, pooled for 16 studies, and 1.32 (still significant) for men, pooled for 24 studies [1]. Denke and Grundy argue plausibly that the main reason for the decline of predictive power with age is the rising prevalence of competing diseases and competing risk factors which tend to obscure the impact of lipid risk factors [4]. With respect to competing risk factors, this view is supported by data from the Framingham Study which show that the impact of serum cholesterol on CHD risk does not diminish with age amongst women and men with low levels of other risk factors [5]. Another consideration relates to the time at which serum cholesterol is being measured. It would stand to reason that the most predictive cholesterol measurement, as far as atherogenesis as opposed to thrombogenesis is concerned, is not the most recent measurement, in Framingham within the last 2 years, but a measurement further back in time. In fact, in Framingham, earlier measurements predict slightly better [6] and, in the Whitehall Study in London [7] much better. On the other hand, in the Honolulu Heart Study, among men of Japanese descent, a more recent measurement predicted as well as a more remote measurement [8]. In this connection, a further confounding factor may be the trend of serum cholesterol with age which rises in women up to age 65 years and then stays flat, whereas in men, levels rise up to age 50-55 years and then decline continuously [6].

Until the influence these cross-currents on the apparent decline of relative risk with advancing age can be understood better, it should not be taken for granted that that this ratio necessarily declines with age in all persons. Instead, it would seem reasonable to assume that relative risk remains substantial as age advances.

With regard to attributable risk, there is no question that it increases with rising age in men and even more in women. This happens because absolute CHD risk gets larger with aging so that even a comparably modest elevation in relative risk causes a marked excess in CHD morbidity and mortality. The high attributable risk in elderly men and women has been commented on [4, 6, 9]. In general, relative risk declines and attributable risk increases with age [10]. On account of the high excess risk attributable to elevated serum cholesterol levels, the need for preventive treatment of the elderly, regardless of relative risk, is evident.

Triglycerides as a CHD risk factor are not part of this assigned topic. Nevertheless, a brief mention of their role is desirable. Pooled relative risks, comparing levels of 1.47 mmol/L with levels under 1.13 mmol/L, are significantly elevated for younger (based on 7 studies) and older (based on 10 studies) men; relative risks are also significantly elevated for younger and older women (based on 6 and 8 studies, respectively) [1]. However, on multivariate analysis, triglycerides are an independent risk factor only in younger and older women but not men in Framingham [5] while, in the Rancho Bernardo Study in California, the reverse holds, relative hazards being significantly higher in men only [11]; however, even in men, the ratio is very low (1.03). Yet, in a later publication from Rancho Bernardo, triglycerides are stated to be risk factors in both men and women over age 70 years [12]. It would seem that the role of triglycerides as independent CHD risk factors in the elderly remains to be more clearly defined.

The role of lipoproteins as risk factors in women and the elderly

Does the cholesterol contained in LDL and HDL predict CHD as well or better than total serum cholesterol? In men and women under 65 years of age, both LDL-C and HDL-C are significantly related in most studies with available measurements [1]. In elderly men, LDL-C is nearly always and significantly predictive, but, in several studies, a low HDL-C fails to be associated with CHD risk [1]; in elderly women, the situation is reversed, with HDL-C almost always being predictive while LDL-C is not consistently related to risk which would have been expected from the relationship with total serum cholesterol [1]. In the Bronx Aging Study, LDL-C is associated with myocardial infarction risk in women but not in men while HDL-C low HDL-C is predictive only in men, mean age at entry being 79 years; however, in this study, lipoproteins were measured in terms of change between the initial and final examination, unlike in all the other studies [13].

The most detailed and informative data on lipoprotein relationships come from the Framingham Study. Allowing for other risk factors, the multivariate CHD risk is significantly related to total, LDL and HDL cholesterol in women under the age of 65 years; in younger men, the association is significant for LDL-C and HDL-C but, surprisingly, not for total cholesterol [5]. Among the elderly, the only significant associations are for LDL-C and HDL-C in women [5]. Apparently, these results, as far as statistical significance is concerned, very much depend on the method of analysis. The data just summarized are based on multivariate regression coefficients while a somewhat more recent analysis uses the Cox multivariate hazard ratio, comparing the top and bottom quintiles of the various lipid parameters [6]. In the latter analysis, referring to persons aged 50 to 80 years, the Q_5/Q_1 multivariate hazard ratios for total cholesterol (TC), LDL-C and HDL-C are, respectively 2.2, 2.5 and 0.3 for men and 4.2, 4.9 and 0.3 for women; the ratios are slightly higher for LDL-C than TC and higher for women than men

[6]. The TC/HDL-C hazard ratios are 3.4 for men and 4.6 for women. All the above ratios are highly significant (p less than .001). The LDL-C/HDL-C ratio is similar to the TC/HDL-C ratio in both men and women so that it offers no additional advantage. It is of decisive importance to note that the risk attached to total cholesterol is lower than the risk in terms of the TC/HDL-C ratio but it is still high. Therefore, it would be incorrect to dismiss total cholesterol and, by implication, LDL-C, as a risk factor in the elderly because it is less predictive than the TC/HDL-C ratio. It is still highly predictive and thus remains highly important in the elderly from the pathogenetic point of view.

Practical implications

A summary view of the evidence presented indicates that total serum cholesterol remains a CHD risk factor in terms of relative and, particularly, attributable risk in both women and men as age advances. While relative risk decreases with increasing age, it stays markedly elevated, the decrease being more than counterbalanced by the excess risk attributable to serum cholesterol levels beyond the optimal range. Needless to say, elevated total serum cholesterol levels may be due to high levels of HDL-C. Therefore, in order to assess individual risk for the purpose of the high-risk strategy of prevention, it is necessary or, at least, desirable, to measure HDL. However, in general, preventive treatment by diet and, if needed, drugs must aim at lowering LDL-C because, if there is less LDL, less HDL is needed for its disposal. Presumably, a low TC/HDL-C ratio not only predicts low CHD risk but lowering the ratio by lowering TC, increasing HDL or both, will reduce CHD risk. All this applies to women and men of all ages, including the elderly, though not with the same intensity and urgency. All this applies to both the population and the high risk strategy because, since serum cholesterol remains a risk factor with advancing age, preventing the progression of coronary atherosclerosis should also have no age limit.

Direct evidence that serum cholesterol reduction, with or without raising HDL-C, will reduce CHD risk can only come from preventive trials, possibly supported by regression studies. Three trials which included primarily middle-aged men, suggest that the benefit extended to the oldest participants [14]. However there is a need for more definitive intervention studies.

The questions concerning prevention which have been discussed should cease to exist as a new generation grows up, provided that the messages advocating healthier life styles will take root in the population at large. In such a new world, carriers of high risk will have been detected long before they become elderly and received treatment beyond the preventive measure inherent in the improved habits of everyday living for everyone. The population and high-risk strategies will then have become a reality in a society where the risk is reduced for all women and men and high risk has become less prevalent. Until this time has arrived, it is imperative that the growing number of elderly people be protected and that criteria be defined which give high-risk women of all ages the same protection afforded to men.

References

1. Manolio, T.A., Pearson, T.A., Wenger, N.K. et al. (1992) Cholesterol and heart disease in older persons and women: review of an NHLBI Workshop. Ann Epidemiol 2, 161-176.

2. Isles, C.G., Hole, D.J., Hawthorne, V.M. and Lever, A.F. (1992) Relation between coronary risk and coronary mortality in women of the Renfrew and Paisley survey: comparison with men. Lancet 1, 702-706.

3. Wedel, H. (Coordinator) The NORA Project, including the North Karelia Project, the Tromsø Heart Study, the National Norwegian Screening Service, The Glostrup Study and the Swedish Primary Prevention Study. In preparation.

4. Denke, M.A. and Grundy, S.M. (1990) Hypercholesterolemia in elderly persons: resolving the treatment dilemma. Ann Int Med 112, 780-792.

5. Castelli, W.P., Anderson, K., Wilson P.W.F. and Levy, D. (1992) Lipids and coronary heart disease: The Framingham Study. Ann Epidemiol 2, 23-28.

6. Kannel, W.B., Anderson K. and Evans, J.C. (1992) Relevance of blood lipids in the elderly: The Framingham Study. Cardiovascular Risk Factors, 2, No. 3 (in press).

7. Shipley, M.J., Pocock, S.J. and Marmot, M.G. (1991) Does plasma cholesterol concentration predict mortality from coronary heart disease in elderly people? 18 year follow up in Whitehall Study. Brit med J, 2, 89-92.

8. Reed, D. and Benfante, R. (1992) Lipid and lipoprotein predictors of coronary heart disease in elderly men in the Honolulu Heart Program. Ann Epidemiol, 2, 29-34.

9. Menotti, A. (1992) The relationship of total serum cholesterol to coronary heart disease in older men: the Italian rural areas of the Seven Countries Study. Ann Epidemiol, 2, 107-112.

10. Malenka, D.J. and Baron, J.A. (1988) Cholesterol and coronary heart disease: the importance of patient-specific attributable risk. Arch Int Med, 148, 2247-52.

11. Barrett-Connor, E. (1992) Hypercholesterolemia predicts early death from coronary heart disease in elderly men but not women: the Rancho Bernardo Study. Ann Epidemiol 2, 77-84.

12. Langer, R.D., Barrett-Connor, E., Criqui, M.H. and Klauber, M.R. (1992) Contrasts in risk factors at older ages. Circulation, 85, 875.

13. Zimetbaum, P., Frishman, W.H., Ooi, W.L. et al. (1992) Plasma lipids and lipoproteins and the incidence of cardiovascular disease in the very elderly: the Bronx Aging Study. Arteriosclerosis and Thrombosis 12, 416-423.

14. Einhorn, P.T. and Rifkind, B.M. (1991) Cholesterol lowering in the elderly. Heartbeat (J of the Int Soc Fed Cardiol), No. 3, September 1991, 2-3.

INFLUENCE OF ATHEROGENIC LIPOPROTEINS ON THE THROMBOTIC POTENTIAL OF ENDOTHELIAL CELLS

Elena Tremoli, Marina Camera, Susanna Colli, Luigi Sironi, Livia Prati, Cristina Banfi and Luciana Mussoni

Abstract

In this article the relationship between atherogenic lipoproteins, i.e. VLDL LDL and modified LDL, and "endothelial cell perturbation" is discussed. Data in the literature indicate that LDL as well as modified LDL influence a variety of functional aspects of endothelial cells, that include adhesive properties for monocytes/macrophages and regulation of vascular tone. In addition these lipoproteins influence the capacity of endothelial cells both to generate and to remove fibrin. The data so far available indicate that atherogenic lipoproteins influence both tissue factor expression and the release of plasminogen activator inhibitor type 1 by endothelial cells, thus increasing the prothrombotic potential of vascular endothelium.

Introduction

Vascular endothelium is known to play a fundamental role in the initiation and even in the progression of atherosclerotic lesions. This single cell-thick lining is known to constitute a dynamic interfaces between blood cells, plasma and the vessel wall (Gimbrone M.A. Jr. 1981). The appreciation that vascular endothelium may undergo phenotypic modulation in response to pathophysiological stimuli has lead to the development of the concept of "endothelial dysfunction" in the context of the pathogenesis of thrombosis and atherosclerosis (Gimbrone M.A.Jr. 1980). This concept includes the loss of specific biochemical properties of vascular endothelial cells coupled to the acquisition of new prothrombotic or proinflammatory functions. A number of pathophysiological conditions as well as a multiplicity of agents are known to be capable of inducing "endothelial cell dysfunction". Among agents, known to influence functional or biochemical aspects of endothelial cells, are atherogenic lipoproteins and in particular very low (VLDL) and low (LDL) density lipoproteins as well as modified LDL. In this article the possibility that atherogenic lipoproteins may directly influence specific properties of vascular endothelial cells, thus inducing endothelial cell perturbation and increasing the prothrombotic and atherogenic potential of the vascular wall, will be considered and discussed.

Atherogenic lipoproteins and endothelial cell perturbation

The interaction between atherogenic lipoproteins and functional or biochemical properties of endothelial cells (EC) have been extensively investigated. Initial studies

A. L. Catapano et al. (eds.), Drugs Affecting Lipid Metabolism, 15–22.
© 1993 Kluwer Academic Publishers and Fondazione Giovanni Lorenzini.

have shown that LDL and, to a greater extent, oxidized LDL induce toxicity of EC (Hessler J.R. et al 1979, Steinberg D. et al. 1989) at concentrations that do not impair cell viability nor induce cell toxicity. On the other hand, oxidized LDL have been shown to influence monocyte adherence to EC, to induce monocyte recruitment as well as their differentiation within the vascular wall (Berliner J.A. et al. 1990). Recently, it has been demonstrated that minimally modified LDL (mm-LDL), i.e. partially oxidized LDL, increase the adhesion properties of EC for monocyte/macrophages (Cushing S.D. et al. 1990). Indeed, mm-LDL induce the expression of mRNA for colony stimulating factors (CSFs) in EC (Cushing S.D. et al.1990 and Rajavashisth T.B. et al. 1990). This effect is of importance also in regard to vessel wall lipid accumulation and the development of the atherosclerotic lesions. In fact, CSFs are known to induce smooth muscle cell proliferation and M-CSF has been shown to increase the uptake and degradation of acetyl-LDL and the accumulation of cholesterol esters in macrophages (Ishibashi S. et al. 1990).

In addition to their influence on the adhesion properties of EC, atherogenic lipoproteins have been shown to interfere in a complex manner with the capacity of these cells to control vascular tone. EC tightly regulate vascular tone through the release of factors with both vasodilatory and vasoconstrictory properties. Among factors with vasodilatory properties are PGI_2 and the more recently discovered, "endothelial cell relaxing factor", that has been demonstrated to be nitric oxide (endothelial cell-derived nitric oxide, EDNO) (Furghott R.F. and Vanhoutte P.M. 1989 and Flavahan N.A. 1991). Both PGI_2 and EDNO induce smooth muscle cell relaxation and modulate the reactivity of blood circulating cells, thus influencing platelet aggregation and leukocyte adhesion. In addition EDNO potentiates the inhibitory effect of PGI_2 on platelet aggregation, thus influencing the formation of platelet thrombi.

A number of data indicate that in experimentally induced hypercholesterolemia as well as in the hyperlipidemic condition a reduction in vascular production of relaxing factors occurs (Flavahan N.A. 1991). Oxidized LDL have been shown, in fact, to impair the release of EDNO in response to acetylcholine by isolated arteries and/or EC in culture.

As previously mentioned, EC have the capacity to synthesize substances with vasoconstrictory properties as the arachidonate products PGH_2/TXA_2 and endothelin-1 (Yanagisawa M. et al. 1988). It is interesting to note that oxidized LDL increase the release of endothelin-1 by aortic EC in culture and that this effect is due to the interaction of the lipoprotein with the scavenger receptor present on the cells (Boulanger C.M. 1992). This observation coupled to the previously discussed effect of oxidized LDL on the release of EDNO by EC, indicates that atherogenic lipoproteins may impair the control of vascular control through different mechanisms and that this effect may be of importance in the pathogenesis of vasospastic events.

Atherogenic lipoproteins and the control of fibrin deposition and removal by endothelial cells

EC play a fundamental role in the regulation both of the coagulation and of the fibrinolytic systems. Under normal conditions, these cells do not promote fibrin formation but in the presence of "endothelial cell perturbation" they may express procoagulant activity. Recent studies have shown that atherogenic lipoproteins may affect both the procoagulant activity and the fibrinolytic capacities of EC.

Atherogenic lipoproteins and endothelial cell procoagulant activity

EC, under normal conditions, are not capable to initiate blood coagulation cascade, they, however, may express procoagulant activity in response to a variety of stimuli, as the bacterial lipopolysaccharide, thrombin, interleukin 1 etc.. EC procoagulant activity has been identified as "tissue factor", a transmembrane cell surface protein that in the presence of Factor VII, calcium and phospholipids directly activates factor IX and X of the coagulation system thus inducing thrombin generation and ultimately fibrin (fig. 1).

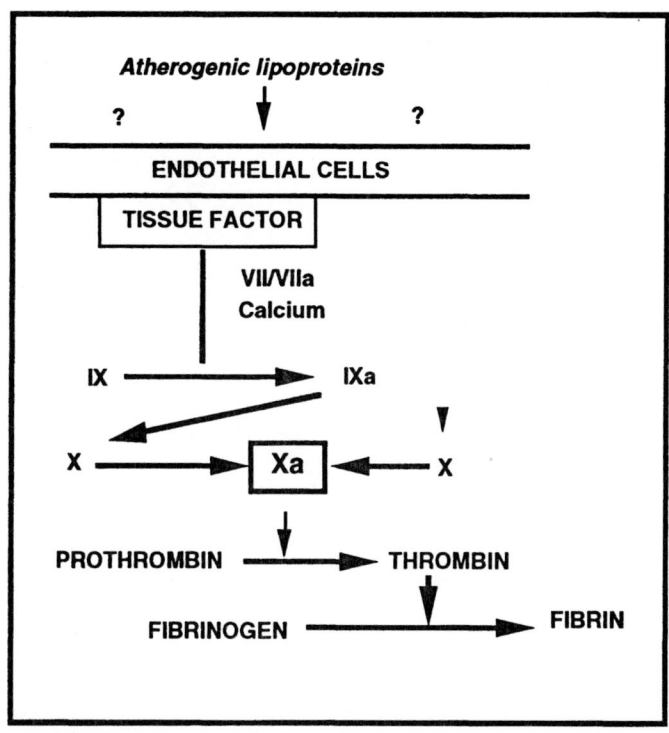

FIG. 1 Vascular endothelial cells regulate the plasma coagulation system through the expression of Tissue Factor that in the presence of Factor VII/VIIa induces the activation of Factor IX and factor X of the coagulation system. Atherogenic lipoproteins may influence the endothelial cell tissue factor expression.

The potential activity of normal and modified LDL on tissue factor expression by EC has been recently investigated. Although normal LDL do not influence tissue factor expression by these cells (Weis J.R. 1991, Drake T.A. 1991 and Tremoli E. 1993), mm-LDL increase the expression of tissue factor by human EC in culture (Drake T.A. 1991). Studies, carried out incubating human umbilical vein EC with normal or chemically oxidized lipoproteins, indicate that the oxidized LDL is capable to stimulate tissue factor activity by these cells (fig. 2). These data are in agreement with those previously published by Weiss J.R. et al. (1991). Interestingly, the effect is specific for the oxidized LDL because other modified lipoproteins, as the acetyl-LDL, do not influence tissue factor activity of EC. On the basis of the above described studies it is possible to conclude that oxidized LDL, increasing the capacity of vascular endothelium to generate fibrin, may exert, under appropriate conditions, a prothrombotic effect.

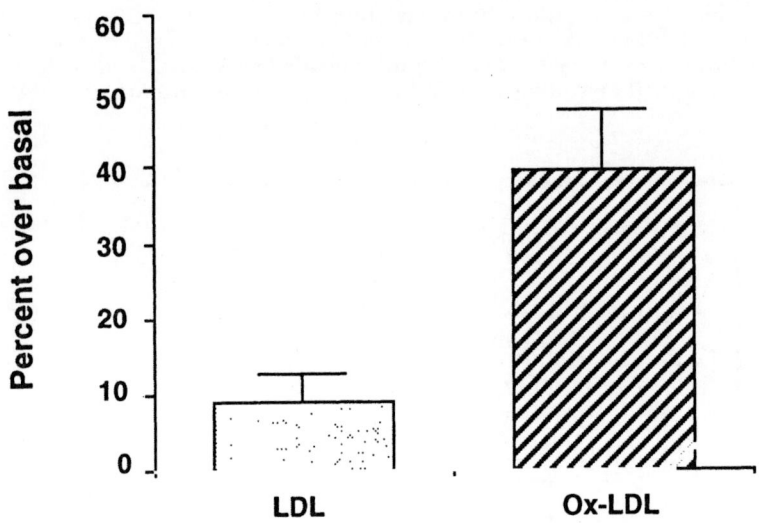

FIG. 2 Effect of Native and oxidized (cupric sulphate) LDL on Tissue factor activity by human umbilical vein endothelial cells. Confluent human umbilical vein endothelial cells between the second and the 4th passages were incubated for 14-16 hours in Medium 199 or medium 199 supplemented with 50 μg protein/ml LDL or oxidized LDL. At the end of the incubation the medium was discarded and cells scraped and subjected to five cycles of freezing and thawing. Tissue factor activity was determined on cell lysates by one stage clotting assay. Values are the means±SEM of eight experiments performed with cells obtained from single cords and with individual lipoprotein preparations.

Atherogenic lipoproteins and endothelial cell fibrinolytic system

Vascular endothelium is known to tightly regulate the fibrinolytic system through the release of activators, i.e. the tissue type plasminogen activator (t-PA) and urokinase, and inhibitors, i.e. the plasminogen activator inhibitor type 1 (PAI-1), of the fibrinolytic system (Van Hinsberg V.W.M.1988a, Van Hinsberg V.W.M.1988b) (fig. 1). On the other hand several clinical studies have indicated the existence of a direct relationship between the fibrinolytic system and plasma lipids, in particular triglycerides (Andersen P. et al 1981, Brommer E.J.P. et al 1982, Mussoni L. et al 1992). Studies, carried out in patients survivors of myocardial infarction and with ischemic heart disease, have shown that a direct correlation between triglyceride levels and plasma levels of PAI-1 exists (Aznar J. et al. 1988, Hamsten A. et al. 1985 Mussoni L. et al. 1992). These observations have drawn the attention toward the relationship between alterations of plasma lipids and/or lipoprotein levels and modifications in the plasma fibrinolytic capacity. Moreover, they have suggested that atherogenic lipoproteins may directly influence the fibrinolytic capacity of vascular endothelium (fig. 3). Indeed, in a number of studies, it has been shown that atherogenic lipoproteins may "regulate" the synthesis and/or release of PAI-1 by EC, thus increasing the antifibrinolytic potential of the vessel wall.

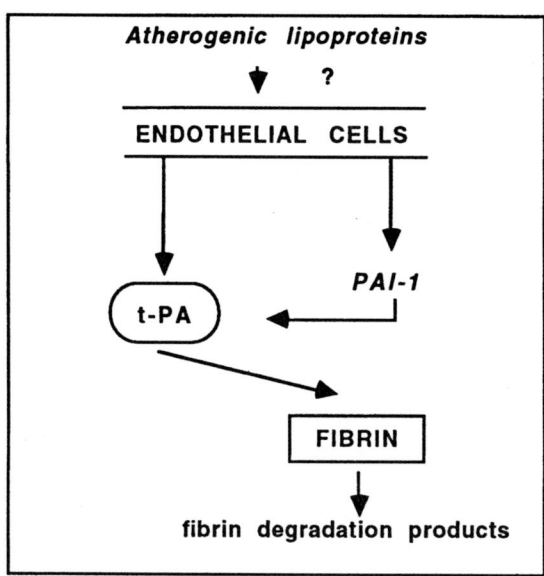

FIG. 3. Vascular endothelial cells regulate the plasma fibrinolytic system through the release of t-PA and PAI-1. Atherogenic lipoproteins may influence the endothelial cell fibrinolytic potential through an effect on the synthesis of t-PA and/or PAI-1.

Initial studies were carried out incubating very low density lipoproteins (VLDL) with human umbilical vein endothelial cells (Mussoni L. et al. 1990). The results indicate that VLDL, added *in vitro* to EC, concentration-dependently, in the range between 25 - 100 μg protein/ml, increase the amounts of PAI-1 released in conditioned medium of cells. These data are in agreement with those published by Stiko-Rahm et al. (Stiko-Rahm A., 1990), demonstrating that the effect of VLDL on the release of PAI-1 by EC is dependent on the interaction of the lipoproteins with the apoB/E receptor on EC.
In an attempt to investigate whether not only triglyceride rich, but also cholesterol rich lipoproteins, as normal or chemically modified LDL, influenced the release of either t-PA or PAI-1 by EC, a series of studies was performed in our laboratory. Both LDL and acetyl-LDL, at the concentration of 100 μg protein/ml, increased the synthesis and release of PAI-1 by the cells (fig. 4). The effect of both lipoproteins was shown to be concentration-dependent and specific for PAI-1. In fact, both LDL and acetyl-LDL did not influence the release of t-PA by cells nor they induced the expression of procoagulant activity (see above). In addition, at variance to what demonstrated for the VLDL-EC interaction, the effect of LDL on PAI-1 release by EC was shown to be not dependent on the interaction of LDL with the LDL-receptor on EC (Tremoli E. et al. 1993). Indeed, the observation that acetyl-LDL, that interacts with the scavenger receptor on EC, behaved in a similar fashion as normal LDL tended to exclude the possibility that the stimulatory effect of LDL on PAI-1 release was due to an interaction of the lipoprotein with the LDL receptor. On the other hand, preincubation of cells with an antibody directed against the LDL receptor present on endothelial cells failed to reverse the stimulatory effect of LDL on PAI-1 release by cells. Another set of data, obtained using binding-defective LDL, further ruled out the possibility that the increases of PAI-1, as induced by LDL, were due to a receptor-dependent mechanism.

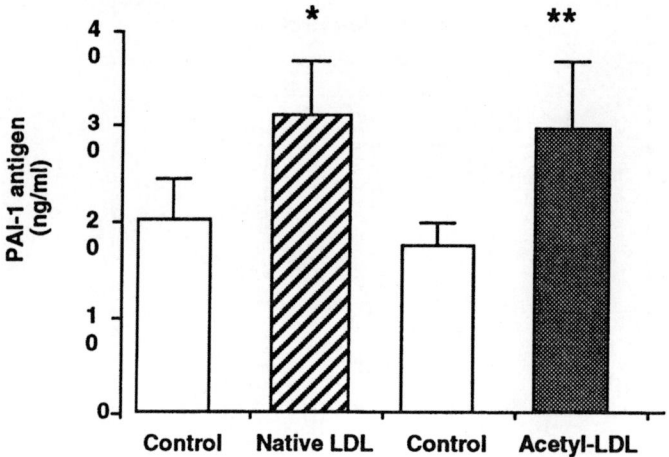

FIG. 4 Effect of Native and Acetylated LDL on PAI-1 release by EC. Confluent human umbilical vein endothelial cells between the second and the 4th passages were incubated for 14-16 hours in Medium 199 or medium 199 supplemented with 100 μg protein/ml LDL or acetyl-LDL. At the end of the incubation the medium was removed and PAI-1 antigen levels determined by a specific ELISA. Values are the means±SEM of seven experiments performed with cells obtained from single cords and with individual lipoprotein preparations. * p<0.05 and ** p<0.001 versus appropriate control.

Other groups (Latron Y. 1991), have shown that ultraviolet-oxidized LDL (2 hours), a procedure that results in mild oxidation of the lipoprotein, are also capable to stimulate PAI-1 release by human EC. In addition it has been proposed that stimulation of PAI-1, as induced by ox-LDL is mediated by a phospholipase, probably phospholipase A, acting on phosphatidylinositol (Chautan M. 1993). The presence of lipid peroxides in oxidized LDL has been proposed to be responsible for such effects on PAI-1 release by EC. The degree of oxidation of the LDL appears to be critical for such phoenomenon to occur; in fact, LDL exposed to ultraviolet light for time periods longer than 2 hours failed to induce PAI-1 release by the cells (Latron Y. 1991). In addition, extensively oxidized LDL, i.e. LDL exposed to cupric sulphate inhibited PAI-1 release by EC. This latter effect was observed at concentrations of ox-LDL ranging between 25-100 μg protein LDL, in the absence of measurable cell toxicity (Tremoli E. 1993).
The interaction of atherogenic lipoproteins with the fibrinolytic system at the level of vascular endothelium is even more complex than that initially expected. Indeed, another lipoprotein, the atherogenic Lp(a) has been shown to interact at different levels with the pro/antifibrinolytic properties of EC. Lp(a), in fact, interferes in vitro with the binding of plasminogen to EC, thus reducing the fibrinolytic capacity of the cells (Hajjar K.A. 1989). On the other hand Lp(a) has been shown to induce the synthesis of PAI-1 by EC, with an effect that involves an increase in PAI-1 mRNA accumulation (Etingin O.R. 1991).
The evidence above described strongly indicates that atherogenic lipoproteins, increase the antifibrinolytic potential of vascular endothelium. What is surprising is the fact that different lipoprotein classes, as the VLDL, the LDL and the chemically modified LDL, i.e. acetyl and oxidized LDL, all possibly acting through different mechanisms,

share the capacity to induce the synthesis and/or release of the inhibitor of tissue plasminogen activator, thus providing a common effect for reducing locally the potential of endothelial cells to remove fibrin.

References

Andersen, P., Arnesen, H., Hierman, I. (1981). Hyperlipoproteinaemia and reduced fibrinolytic activity in healthy coronary high-risk men. Acta Medica Scand. 209,199-202

Aznar,J., Estelles, A., Tormo, G., Sapena, P., Tormo, C., Blanch, S., Espana, F. (1988). Plasminogen activator inhibitor activity and other fibrinolytic variables in patients with coronary artery disease. Br. Heart J. 59, 535-541.

Berliner, J.A., Territo, M.C., Sevanian, A., Rammin, S., Kim, J.A, Bamsnad, B., Esterson, M., Fogelman, A.M. (1990). Minimally modified low density lipoprotein stimulates monocyte endothelial interactions. J. Clin. Invest. 85, 1260-1266.

Boulanger, C.M., Tanner, F.C., Béa, M.L., Hahn, A.W.A., Werner, A., Luscher, T.F. (1992). Oxidized low density lipoproteins induce mRNA expression and release of endothelin from human and porcine endothelium. Circulation Res. 70, 1191-1197.

Brommer, E.J.P., Gevers-Leuven, J.A., Barrett-Bergshoeff, M.M., Schouten, J.A. (1982). Responses of fibrinolytic activity and factor VII related antigen to stimulation with desmopressin in hyperlipoproteinemia. J. Lab. Clin. Med. 100,105-114.

Chautan,M., Latron, Y., Anfosso, F., Alessi, M.C., Lafont, H., Juhan-Vague, I., Nalbone, G. (1993). Phosphatidylinositol turnover during stimulation of plasminogen activator inhibitor-1 secretion induced by oxidized low density lipoproteins in human endothelial cells. J. Lipid Res. 34,101-110.

Cushing, S.D., Berliner, J.A., Valente, A.J., Territo, M.C., Navab, M., Parhami, F., Gerrity, R., Schwartz, C.J., Fogelman, A.M. (1990). Minimally modified low density lipoprotein induce monocityc chemotactic protein I in human endothelial cells and smooth muscle cells. Proc. Natl. Acad. Sci. USA 87, 5134-5138.

Etingin,O.R., Hajjar, D.P., Harpel, P.C., Nachman, R.L.(1991). Lipoprotein(a) regulates plasminogen activator inhibitor-1 expression in endothelial cells. A potential mechanism in thrombogenesis. J. Biol. Chem. 266, 2459-2465.

Flavahan, N.A. (1991). Atherosclerosis or lipoprotein-induced endothelial dysfunction. Potential mechanisms underlying reduction in EDRF/nitric oxide activity. Circulation 85, 1927-1938.

Furghott, R.F., Vanhoutte, P.M. (1989). Endothelium-derived relaxing and contracting factors. FASEB J. 3, 2007-2018.

Gimbrone, M.A. Jr (1980). Endothelial dysfunction and the pathogenesis of atherosclerosis. In "Gotto et al. (eds) Atherosclerosis V; Proceedings of the Vth International symposium on atherosclerosis, Springer Verlag, New York, pp. 415-425.

Gimbrone, M.A. Jr (1981). Vascular endothelium and atherosclerosis. In Moore S. (ed) Vascular Injury and atherosclerosis. Marcel Dekker, New York, ch 2,pp. 25-52.

Hajjar, K.A., Gavish, D., Breslow, J.L., Nachman, R.L. (1989). Lipoprotein(a) modulation of endothelial cells surface fibrinolysis and its potential role in atherosclerosis. Nature (Lond) 330,113-114.

Hamsten, A., Wiman,B., de Faire, U., Blomback, M. (1985). Increased plasma levels of a rapid inhibitor of tissue plasminogen activator in young survivors of myocardial infarction. N. Engl. J. Med. 313,1557-1563.

Hessler, J.R., Robertson, A.L. Jr, Chisolm, G.M. (1979). LDL-induced cytotoxicity and its inhibition by HDL in human vascular smooth muscle and endothelial cells in culture. Atherosclerosis 32, 213-229.

Ishibashi, S., Inaba, T.., Shimano, H., Harada, K., Inoue, I., Mokuno, H., Mori, N., Gotoda, T., Takaku, F., Yamada, N. (1990). Monocyte colony-stimulating factor enhances uptake and degradation of acetylated low density lipoproteins and cholesterol esterification in human monocyte-derived macrophages. J. Biol. Chem. 265,1409-1417.

Latron, Y., Chautan, M., Anfosso, F., Alessi, C., Nalbone, G., Lafont, H., Juhan-Vague, I. (1991). Stimulating effect of oxidized low density lipoproteins on plasminogen activator inhibitor-1 synthesis by endothelial cells. Arterioscler. Thromb. 11, 1821-1829.

Mussoni , L., Maderna, P., Camera, M., Bernini, F., Sironi, L., Sirtori, M., Tremoli, E. (1990). Atherogenic lipoproteins and the release of plasminogen activator inhibitor (PAI-1) by endothelial cells. Fibrinolysis 4 (suppl 2), 79-81.

Mussoni, L., Mannucci, L., Sirtori, M., Camera, M., Maderna, P., Sironi, L., Tremoli, E. (1992). Hypertriglyceridemia and regulation of fibrinolytic activity. Arterioscler. and Thromb. 12,19-27.

Rajavashisth T.B., Andalibi A., Territo, M.C., Berliner J.A., Navab, M., Fogelman, A.M., Luis, A.J. (1990). Induction of endothelial cell expression of granulocyte and macrophage colony-stimulating factors by modified low-density lipoproteins. Nature 334, 254-257.

Steinberg, D., Parthasarathy, S., Carew, T.E., Khoo, J.C., Witzum, J.L. (1989). Beyond cholesterol. Modification of low density lipoprotein that increase its atherogenicity. N. Engl. J. Med. 320, 915-924.

Stiko-Rahm, A., Wiman, B., Hamsten, A., Nilsson, J. (1990). Secretion of plasminogen activator inhibitor-1 from cultured human umbilical vein endothelial cells is induced by very low density lipoprotein. Arterioscler. and Thromb. 10, 1067-1073.

Tremoli, E., Camera, M., Maderna, P., Sironi, L., Prati, L., Colli, S., Bernini, F., Corsini, A., Mussoni, L. (1993). Increased synthesis of plasminogen activator inhibitor-1 by cultured human endothelial cells exposed to native and modified low density lipoproteins. Arterioscler. and Thromb. (in press).

Van Hisberg, V.W.M. (1988a). Synthesis and secretion of plasminogen activator and plasminogen activator inhibitor by endothelial cells. In C. Kluft (ed.)tissue-type plasminogen activator (t-PA):Physiological and Clinical aspects. Vol 2 Boca Raton Florida, CRC press, pp. 3-20

Van Hinsberg, V.W.M. (1988b). Regulation of the synthesis and secretion of plasminogen activator by endothelial cells. Hemostasis 18, 307-327.

Weis, J.R., Pitas, R.E., Wilson, B.D., Rodgers, G.M. (1991). Oxidized low-density lipoprotein increases cultured human endothelial cell tissue factor activity and reduces protein C activation. FASEB J. 5, 2459-2465.

Yanagisawa, M., Kurihara, H, Kimura, S., Tomobe, Y. (1988). A novel potent vasoconstrictor peptide produced by vascular endothelial cells. Nature (Lond) 332, 411-415.

PLURIMETABOLIC SYNDROME OR SYNDROME X. IS IT A REAL SYNDROME?

GAETANO CREPALDI, ENZO MANZATO, ROMANO NOSADINI

At the first annual meeting of the European Association for the Study of Diabetes we presented a paper entitled "Essential hyperlipemia, obesity and diabetes" (1). From the observations made in our patients we concluded for the existence of "a plurimetabolic syndrome including hyperlipemia, obesity and diabetes". Moreover, we stated that "the development of ischemic heart disease and, less frequently, of arterial hypertension is often found in these patients".

Interestingly enough, this early description of the association of clinical and metabolic abnormalities, highlightened the tenet of the heterogeneity of these patients with regard to hypertension. Indeed only about 50% of the patients with altered patterns of circulating lipids and glucose had also elevated blood pressure levels.

Our conclusion came from an exclusively clinical background, i.e. from the observation of the patients affected by an association of several metabolic disorders namely hyperlipidemia, diabetes or impaired glucose tolerance, obesity, hyperuricemia. We were far from considering hypertension as a metabolic disease at that time, as it would be now by some Authors.

Since then several Autors recognized the frequent association of the above mentioned diseases and each Author stressed some aspect of the syndrome.

In 1986 W.P. Castelli from the Framingham data observed that "a new syndrome, characterized by a high triglyceride level, a normal cholesterol level, and a low HDL level, appears to exist" (2). Overweight, diabetes mellitus, and often elevated serum uric acid levels were considered part of this syndrome. In this study the accent was on triglycerides.

In 1987 Ferrannini et al. (3) reported an association between impaired insulin induced extrahepatic carbohydrate utilization and hypertension in

A. L. Catapano et al. (eds.), Drugs Affecting Lipid Metabolism, 23–27.
© 1993 Kluwer Academic Publishers and Fondazione Giovanni Lorenzini.

lean patients with essential hypertension. These findings were in accord with the view that hyperinsulinemia contributes to the development of hypertension (5,6,7).

In June, 1988, R.R. Williams and coworkers published the results of a population study performed in Utah (U.S.A.) where they observed a syndrome consisting of hypertension, mixed lipid abnormalities (high triglycerides, high LDL, low HDL cholesterol), moderate obesity (4). In this study the accent was on hypertension.

In December, 1988, G.R. Reaven revisited the role of insulin resistance in human disease (4). In this review data are presented to support the hypothesis that resistance to insulin-stimulated glucose uptake, glucose intolerance, hyperinsulinemia, increased VLDL triglyceride, decreased HDL cholesterol, hypertension tends to occur in the same patient. This syndrome was called "syndrome X" and the basic point was related to hyperinsulinemia (8).

All these observations contributed greatly to a better understanding of the vascular risk in many patients and gave important hints to the research of the physiopathological mechanisms linking such different metabolic diseases as hypertriglyceridemia, obesity, diabetes, and, why not?, hypertension.

However, the definition of "Sindrome X" appeared slightly puzzling since this term had been already used for years to identify patients with chest pain normal coronary arteriograms, in whom symptoms are due to myocardial ischemia with reduced coronary perfusion reserve (9). Incidentally this latter group of patients also exhibit stimulated hyperinsulinemia (10). However, a more thorough drawback related to the use of the term "Syndrome X" in order to define the above mentioned constellation of symptoms, is the possible clouding of our understanding of the putative nature of the pathogenetic mechanisms, underlying the development of these clinical and metabolic abnormalities.

Beyond any question concerning how to indicate this syndrome which still seems to wait a clear definition, and for (question which we are now proposing our "plurimetabolic syndrome") we do believe that all the observations made in the patients must be put together to obtain the best complete description of this nosographic entity.

In our opinion as part of the "plurimetabolic syndrome" we must include a lipoprotein disorder (which could be hypertriglyceridemia and/or low HDL cholesterol with or without high LDL cholesterol), a carbohydrate disorder (which could be insulin resistance or impaired glucose tolerance or type 2 diabetes), a purine metabolism alteration and overweight or obesity.

Namely with the definition "Syndrome" we usually indicate a group of symptoms and signs of disordered function, related to one another by means of some anatomic, physiologic or biochemical peculiarity. It also embodies a hypothesis, concerning the deranged function of an organ, organ system or tissue (11).

The definition of "Syndrome X" as originally formulated by Reaven (8) and subsequently modified by De Fronzo et al. (12) as "Insulin Resistance Syndrome" maintains that impaired insulin sensitive is the common denominator accounting for the association among obesity, hypertension, insulin resistance and dyslipidemia in all patients, exhibiting the "Syndrome X". At odds with this view it appears to us crucial in order to gain further insights into the pathogenesis of these clinical disorders to point out the tenet that the association among hypertension insulin resistance, obesity and dyslipidemia is not mandatory and that on the contrary these individual clinical features can occur in vivo independently one from each other. In agreement with this concept is our original report on the association of hypertension with diabetes and hyperlipemia in some but not all patients with the "so called" Plurimetabolic Syndrome (1).

More recently we found an association between hypertension and impaired insulin sensitivity at extrahepatic level in non insulin-dependent diabetes (13) but not in essential hypertension (14). Familial genetic traits (4) and racial differences (15) have been shown to play a role in determining an heterogeneous association among abnormalities in blood pressure levels and carbohydrate and lipid metabolism. Although the reasons accounting for this heterogeneous association do not appear at the moment immediately understable, it seems to us important to bear in mind that the link among hypertension, dyslipidemia and insulin resistance is not mandatory. All together these findings speak against the contention that hyperinsulinemia itself, leads to hypertension. Conversely insulin resistance and blood pressure may be linked indirectly, through different mechanisms.

The question arises on the nature of these hypothetical, inherited or acquired mechanisms. Overweight does not appear to be the major determinant of the association between hypertension and insulin resistance, as several reports show a stronger relation between insulin sensitivity and abnormalities in cellular ion handling (16) (17) (18).

Preliminary results from our laboratory indicate that in non-insulin-dependent diabetes (13) in like manner, as previously observed in essential hypertension, a constellation of clinical and biochemical abnormalities such as hypertension, extrahepatic rather than hepatic insulin resistance, dyslipidemia, obesity, microalbuminuria and abnormalities in ion handling tend to cluster in the same cohort of patients. The identification of such cohort of patients will be certainly useful to gain further insights on the pathogenesis of these clinical disorders possibly confirming the hypothesis that a common genetic defects leads to the development of different phenotypic abnormalities (Fig. 1).

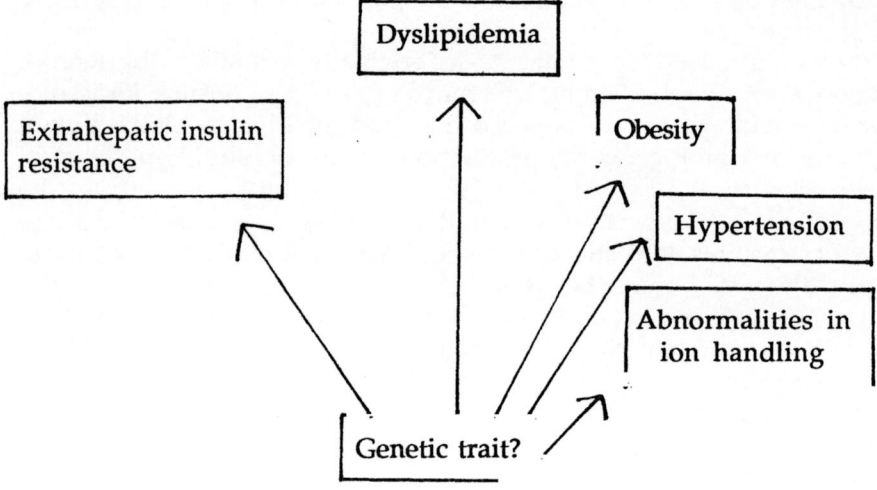

Figure 1. Hypothesis on the mechanistic link among the constellation of clinical disorders of the plurimetabolic syndrome.

References

1) Avogaro, P. and Crepaldi, G. (1965) 'Essential hyperlipemia, obesity and diabetes' EASD Meeting Montecatini, Italy 20-22 April.
2) Castelli, W.P. (1986) 'The triglyceride issue: a view from Framingham', Am. Heart J. 112, 432-437.
3) Ferrannini, E., Buzzigoli, G., Bonadonna, E. et al. (1987) 'Insulin resistance in essential hypertension', N. Engl. J. Med. 317, 350-357.
4) Williams, R.R., Hunt, S.C., Hopkins, P.N., Stults, B.M., Lily, L., Hassetedt, S.J., Barlow, G.K., Stephenson, S.H., Lalonel, J.M., and Kuida, H. (1988) 'Familial dyslipidemic hypertension', JAMA 259, 3579-3586.
5) Reaven, G.M. and Hoffman R.B. (1981) 'A role for insulin in the aetiology and course of hypertension?', Lancet 2, 435-7.
6) Sinager, P., Jodicke, W., Voigt, S., Hajdu, I., and Weiss, M. (1985) 'Post prandial hyperinsulinemia in patients with mild essential hypertension', Hypertension 7, 182-186.
7) Welborn, T.A., Breckenridge, A., Rubinstein, A.H., Dollery, C.T., and Fraser, T.R. (1966) 'Serum-insulin in essential hypertension and in peripheral vascular disease', Lancet 1, 1336-1337.
8) Reaven, G.M. (1988) 'Banting Lecture 1988: role of insulin resistance in human disease', Diabetes 37, 1595-1607.

9) Anou. (1987) 'Syndrome X', Lancet ii, 1247-1248.

10) Dean, J.D., Jones, C.J.H., Hutchison, S.J., Peters, J.R., and Henderson, A.H. (1991) 'Hyperinsulinemia and microvascular angina (Syndrome X)', Lancet 337, 456-457.

11) Harrison's Principles of Internal Medicine (1987) 11th Edition Mc Graw Hill, p. 3.

12) De Fronzo, R.A. and Ferrannini, E. (1991) 'Insulin resistance: a multifaceted syndrome responsible for NIDDM, obesity, hypertension, dyslipidemia and atherosclerotic cardiovascular disease', Diabetes Care 14, 173-194.

13) Solini, A., Sambataro, M., Piarulli, F., Milan, D., de Kreutzenberg, V., Muollo, B., Velussi, M., Morocutti, A., Barzon, I., and Nosadini, R. (1991) 'Type 2 diabetics with hypertension and microalbuminuria are more insulin resistant than normotensive type 2 diabetics', Diabetologia 34, 519-635.

14) Doria, A., Fioretto, P., Avogaro, A., Carraro, A., Morocutti, A., Trevisan, R., Frigato, F., Crepaldi, G., Viberti, G.C., and Nosadini, R. (1991) 'Insulin resistance is associated with high sodium-lithium countertransport in essential hypertension', Am. J. Physiol. 261, E684-E691.

15) Saad, M.F., Lilloja, S., Nyomba, B.L., and et al. (1991) 'Racial differences in the relation between blood pressure and insulin resistance', N. Engl. J. Med. 324, 733-739.

16) Nosadini, R., Fioretto, P., Trevisan, R., and Crepaldi, G. (1991) 'Insulin dependent diabetes mellitus and hypertension', Diabetes Care 14, 210-219.

17) Resnick, L.M., Gupta, R.K., Bhargava, K.K., and et al. (1991) 'Cellular ions in hypertension diabetes and obesity. A nuclear magnetic resonance spectroscopic study', Hypertension 17, 951-957.

18) Draznin, B., Sussman, K., Kao, M., Lewis, D., and Sherman N. (1987) 'The existence of an optimal range of cytosolic free calcium for insulin stimulated glucose transport in rat adipocytes', J. Biol. Chem. 161, 14385-88.

THREE LIVER-ENRICHED TRANSCRIPTION FACTORS: HNF-1, C/EBP, AND PROTEIN II ARE REQUIRED TO ENHANCE TRANSCRIPTION OF THE HUMAN APOLIPOPROTEIN B GENE

BEATRIZ LEVY-WILSON   AND ALAN R. BROOKS

ABSTRACT. The tissue-specific transcriptional enhancer of the human apolipoprotein B gene contains multiple protein-binding sites. Most of the enhancer activity is found in a 443 base pair (bp) fragment (+621 to +1064) that is located entirely within the second intron of the gene. Within this fragment, a 147-bp region (+806 to +952) containing a single 97-bp DNaseI footprint exhibits significant enhancer activity. We now report that this footprint contains four distinct protein binding sites that have the potential to bind nine distinct liver nuclear proteins. One of these proteins was identified as HNF-1 which binds to the 5' end of the large footprint. A binding site for C/EBP (or one of the related proteins that recognize similar sequences) was identified in the center of the 97-bp footprint. This binding site is coincident or overlaps with the binding sites for five other proteins, two of which appear to be distinct from the C/EBP-related family of proteins. The binding site for a nuclear factor designated protein I is located between the HNF-1 and C/EBP binding sites. Finally, the 3'-most 15 bp of the footprinted sequence contain a binding site for another nuclear protein, which we have called protein II. Mutations that abolish the binding of either HNF-1, protein II, or the C/EBP-related proteins severely reduce enhancer activity. However, deletion experiments demonstrated that neither the HNF-1 binding site alone, nor the combination of binding sites for HNF-1, protein I and C/EBP, nor the C/EBP binding site plus the protein II binding site is sufficient to enhance transcription from a strong apoB promoter. Rather, HNF-1 and C/EBP act synergistically with protein II to enhance transcription of the apolipoprotein B gene.

Introduction

Apolipoprotein (apo) B is the sole protein component of low density lipoprotein (LDL) and is the ligand for the recognition of LDL by the LDL receptor (for a review, see [15]). Elevated levels of LDL cholesterol and plasma apoB have been correlated with an increased risk of developing atherosclerosis [5,32], while moderately decreased levels of LDL cholesterol and hypobetalipoproteinemia [33,36] are generally associated with decreased risk of atherosclerosis. Therefore, it is important to understand the mechanisms that control the expression of the apoB gene.

We recently identified a tissue-specific transcriptional enhancer located mainly in the second

A. L. Catapano et al. (eds.), Drugs Affecting Lipid Metabolism, 29–44.
© 1993 Kluwer Academic Publishers and Fondazione Giovanni Lorenzini.

intron of the human apoB gene [3]. A 718-bp PvuII fragment including sequences from the first and second introns enhanced expression not only of the apoB promoter but also of the heterologous thymidine kinase promoter in transcriptionally active HepG2 and CaCo-2 cells but not in HeLa cells, in which the apoB gene is not transcribed. Most of the enhancer activity was contained within a 443-bp segment [3] situated entirely within the second intron. A 147-bp fragment, which we have designated as the "core enhancer," accounted for some 75% of the enhancer activity of the 443-bp segment [3].

Here we report that the 147-bp core enhancer contains a contiguous array of binding sites for at least nine distinct liver nuclear proteins spanning a region of 97 bp. One of these proteins is the liver-enriched transcription factor HNF-1 (LFB-1) (for a review see [25]), which has been implicated in the transcriptional activation of several liver-specific genes. A binding site for another important liver-enriched transcription factor, C/EBP [18,20] (or one of the related proteins that recognize similar sequences), was also identified within this 147-bp enhancer segment. These two protein-binding sites are necessary for maximal activation of transcription. Moreover, our results indicate that HNF-1 and C/EBP must interact synergistically with a novel protein factor (designated protein II), which recognizes the 3' end of the core enhancer in order to achieve maximal enhancement of transcription.

Materials and Methods

PLASMID CONSTRUCTION

The plasmid Pvu443F contains the 443-bp SmaI-PvuII enhancer region from the second intron of the human apoB gene [3] inserted immediately upstream of the apoB promoter (–898 to +121) fused to the reporter chloramphenicol acetyltransferase (CAT) gene. Plasmid Pvu147F (referred to as Xba7/1 in [3]) contains a 147-bp fragment spanning nucleotides +806 to +952 of the apoB gene inserted at an XbaI site immediately upstream of the apoB promoter (–898 to +121) fused to the CAT gene. To disrupt the 20-bp palindrome within footprint E of the enhancer, plasmids Pvu443F and Pvu147F were linearized at a unique SpeI site that lies at the center of the palindrome. After the removal of 5' overhangs with mung bean nuclease, the plasmids were ligated to KpnI linkers (5' GGGTACCC 3'), digested with KpnI to remove excess linkers, and re-ligated. The number of linkers introduced was determined by dideoxynucleotide sequencing [30] of double-stranded plasmid DNA [37].

To create deletions within the 147-bp core enhancer, four oligonucleotides complementary to 18-nucleotide stretches within the 147-bp core enhancer were synthesized. In addition, each oligonucleotide contained a tail incorporating the recognition site for the restriction enzyme XbaI. The polymerase chain reaction (PCR) was then used to amplify the DNA between the pairs of oligonucleotides Xba7/1(5') and X-TAS, Xba7/1(3') and T/XS, and XbaCore(3') and XbaCore(5'), using the plasmid TKCAT6-1 [3] as a template (see [4]).

To create mutations in the putative binding site for C/EBP, we synthesized an oligonucleotide, designated SPE854, spanning nucleotides +853 to +902 of the apoB gene and containing the desired point mutations. The PCR was then used to amplify the DNA between this oligonucleotide and a second oligonucleotide, designated vector which is complementary to vector sequences adjacent to the HindIII site of plasmid Pvu147R, which was used as the template. The amplified DNA was digested with SpeI and HindIII and used to replace the corresponding SpeI-HindIII fragment in Pvu147R to generate the plasmid designated Pvu147mutA. The integrity of the apoB DNA within this plasmid and the introduction of the desired mutations were verified by dideoxynucle-otide sequencing [30] of double-stranded plasmid DNA [37]. The *Xba*I insert from Pvu147mutA was subsequently inserted at the *Xba*I site of the plasmid –85CAT [27].

Mutations in the putative binding site for protein II were made by amplifying the DNA between oligonucleotides Xba7/1 5' and TXMUT. The amplified DNA was digested with *Xba*I and inserted in the forward orientation at the *Xba*I site of the plasmids pPVUCAT and –85CAT and the resulting clones were designated 147FmutII. The integrity of the apoB DNA within these plasmids and the introduction of the desired mutations were verified by DNA sequencing [37].

CELL CULTURE AND TRANSIENT EXPRESSION ASSAYS

These procedures were performed as described by Brooks and Levy-Wilson [3]

PREPARATION OF NUCLEAR EXTRACTS AND GEL MOBILITY SHIFT ASSAYS

Nuclear extracts from mouse liver were prepared essentially as described by Gorski et al. [16], except that the extract was dialyzed against 20 mM HEPES (N-2-hydroxyethyl)-1-pipera-zineethanesulfonic acid, pH 7.6), 0.5 mM EDTA, 0.1 mM dithiothreitol (DTT), 0.1 mM phenylmethylsulfonyl fluoride for 12 h at 4°C. The extract was then lyophilized and dissolved in 25 mM HEPES (pH 7.6), 40 mM KCl, 0.1 mM EDTA, 10% glycerol, 1 mM DTT.

Gel mobility shift assays were performed as previously described [3]. Proteins synthesized in rabbit reticulocyte lysates were added directly to the binding reaction. Antiserum was added to the binding reaction immediately after addition of the nuclear extract.

SYNTHESIS OF OLIGONUCLEOTIDES

Oligonucleotides were synthesized on an Applied Biosystems model 380B DNA synthesizer and purified on OPC columns (Applied Biosystems, Foster City, CA) as described by the manufac-turer.

Results and Discussion

THE CORE ENHANCER CONTAINS A BINDING SITE FOR HNF-1

We have previously localized a significant portion of the activity of the apoB second intron enhancer to a 147-bp fragment (the core enhancer), which contains a single 97-bp DNaseI footprint [3]. The base sequence of this footprint is 80% conserved between the human and the mouse genes [23]. Gel mobility shift assays suggested that the 5' end of this footprint may contain a binding site for the transcription factor HNF-1 [3].

To demonstrate that the core enhancer contained a binding site for HNF-1, we first carried out a series of gel mobility shift assays using a nuclear extract from mouse liver that had been enriched in the content of HNF-1 (a kind gift of D. Mendel and G. Crabtree). As illustrated in panel I of Fig-ure 1, this extract gave rise to a specific retarded complex when incubated with the double-stranded 28-mer oligonucleotide β-28 that contains the strong HNF-1 binding site from the β-fibrinogen pro-moter [11]. Formation of this complex was entirely eliminated by inclusion of a 150-fold molar excess of unlabeled β-28 oligomer in the binding reaction (lane 3). A retarded complex of similar mobility was generated when the nuclear extract was incubated with an XbaI-TaqI restriction fragment that encompasses the 5'-most 65 bp of the apoB core enhancer and contains the putative HNF-1 binding site (lane 5). A map showing the location of this probe is shown in panel II of Figure 1. Furthermore, the complex between the XbaI-TaqI DNA and the nuclear extract was specifically competed for by a 150-fold molar excess of the β-28 oligomer (lane 6), but not by an equivalent molar excess of an oligonucleotide containing the binding site for the transcription factor C/EBP (lane 7) (transthyretin oligomer 2 in [17]). The fact that PAL20, a 20-bp double-stranded oligonucleotide corresponding to the 20-bp palindrome from the apoB core enhancer and containing the putative HNF-1 binding site, failed to compete for the formation of this complex (Fig. 1, panel I, lane 8) suggests that additional sequences are required for HNF-1 binding. These results indicate that the XbaI-TaqI probe forms a specific complex with a nuclear protein similar or identical to HNF-1, but also strongly suggest that the binding site for this protein is situated partly outside of the palindrome.

To investigate the importance of the palindrome in the formation of the HNF-1-like complex, we took advantage of a unique SpeI site situated at the exact center of the palindrome. After digestion with SpeI, the 5' overhanging nucleotides were removed with mung bean nuclease, thereby deleting 4 bp from the sequence that is homologous to the consensus HNF-1 recognition site. The palindrome was further disrupted by the insertion of one or two KpnI linkers. In one of the selected clones, designated ∇16∆4, an additional 4 bp were deleted from the 3' end of the SpeI site. The sequence of this clone around the site of the mutation is shown in panel II of Figure 1. The XbaI-TaqI fragment was isolated from this clone, end-labeled, and used as a probe in a gel mobility shift assay with the HNF-1-enriched mouse liver nuclear extract (Fig. 1, panel I, lane 10). This mutated form of the XbaI-TaqI fragment was incapable of forming a HNF-1-like complex, suggesting that the binding site for the protein responsible for this complex lies at least partly within the palindrome.

To confirm that HNF-1 is responsible for the major retarded complex seen with the XbaI-TaqI probe, a polyclonal antibody [24] raised against a portion of the recombinant mouse HNF-1 protein was employed. This antibody does not block binding of HNF-1 to its recognition sequence, but does cause an alteration in the mobility of the retarded complex observed in a gel mobility shift assay [24,38]. Panel III of Figure 1 illustrates the effect of the HNF-1 antibody upon the binding of HNF-1-enriched mouse liver nuclear extract to the β-28 oligomer (lanes 1-3) and the XbaI-TaqI fragment (lanes 4-6). The presence of the antibody results in a small but significant shift in the mobility of the retarded complexes formed with both probes. This result confirms that HNF-1 binds to the XbaI-TaqI fragment of the core enhancer. Addition of antibody also results in the formation of a new retarded band of higher mobility (designated as X in Fig. 1, panel III) with the XbaI-TaqI probe, but not with the β-28 probe. The identity of this second complex and the reason for its formation remain unclear.

BINDING OF HNF-1 IS NECESSARY FOR FULL ACTIVITY OF THE APOB ENHANCER IN HEPG2 CELLS

To test the functional importance of the HNF-1 binding site within the core enhancer, the 20-bp palindrome harboring the likely recognition site for this protein was disrupted by insertion of KpnI linkers at a unique SpeI site that lies at the center of the palindrome. Linker insertion mutations were made in both the 443-bp enhancer fragment and the 147-bp core enhancer (Fig. 2). Four clones containing either one or two KpnI linkers inserted at the SpeI site were selected. These mutated variants of the enhancer were initially placed in the forward orientation immediately upstream of apoB

FIG. 1. Binding of mouse liver nuclear proteins to the XbaI-TaqI fragment of the core enhancer in gel mobility shift assays. Panel I, The 67-bp XbaI-TaqI fragment was isolated from the plasmid Pvu147F or from the plasmid 147∇16∆4, and end-labeled using [α-32 P]dCTP and Klenow DNA polymerase. The double-stranded β-28 oligomer was end-labeled with [γ-32 P]ATP and polynucleotide kinase. In each case an equal amount of HNF-1-enriched mouse liver nuclear extract was used. The additions of extract and the fold molar excess of unlabeled competitor DNA are indicated above each lane. Panel II, Diagram of the core enhancer showing the locations of the restriction fragments used as probes in gel mobility shift assays. The shaded box represents the location of the 97-bp footprint. The nucleotide sequence of the 20-bp palindrome (w.t.) that spans positions +850 to +869, and the corresponding sequence of the clone ∇16∆4 are shown at the bottom of panel II. The arrows indicate the two halves of the palindrome. Panel III, End-labeled XbaI-TaqI fragment (lanes 4-6) or β-28 oligomer (lanes 1-3) were incubated with HNF-1-enriched mouse liver nuclear extract in the presence or absence of 1 μl of rabbit polyclonal antiserum raised against recombinant mHNF-1α, under the same conditions used for the gel mobility shift assay. The binding reactions were then fractionated on a 5% native acrylamide gel. BSA, 2 μg of bovine serum albumin in place of nuclear extract.

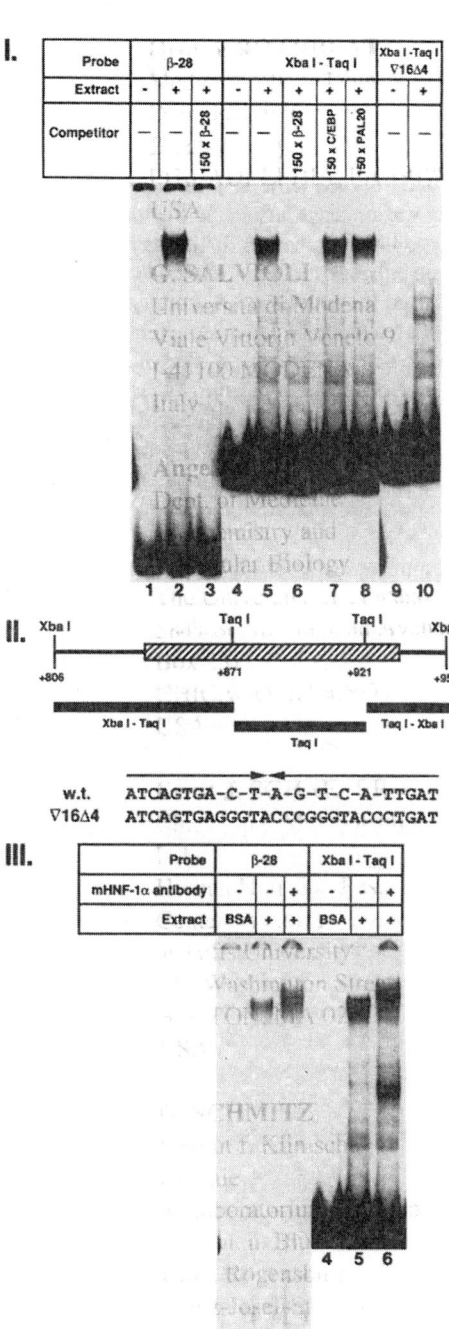

promoter sequences spanning nucleotides −898 to +121 fused to the CAT reporter gene. The ability of the wild-type and mutated variants of the enhancer to increase expression from the apoB promoter was then tested by transient transfection of HepG2 cells. In agreement with our previous results [3], the wild-type 443-bp enhancer increased CAT activity by 3.4-fold. The introduction of one linker at the *Spe*I site (443∇8) reduced the activity of the enhancer to 1.9-fold, which is 38% of the activity seen with the wild-type sequence. When two linkers were inserted (443∇16), CAT activity was reduced further, so that the enhancer activity was only 16% of that observed with the wild-type 443-bp enhancer. In this series of experiments the 147-bp core enhancer (147F) exhibited the same enhancer activity as the 443-bp fragment. Insertion of two linkers at the *Spe*I site (147∇16) reduced the activity of the core enhancer to 20% of that exhibited by the wild-type sequence. A similar reduction of enhancer activity was observed with the clone 147∇16Δ4, in which an extra 4 bp were deleted from the 3′ side of the *Spe*I site. Gel mobility shift assays using the *Xba*I-*Taq*I fragment isolated from plasmid 147∇16Δ4 demonstrated that this mutant form of the enhancer is unable to bind HNF-1 (Fig. 1, panel I, lane 10).

Thus, loss of HNF-1 binding results in an 80% reduction in the activity of both the core enhancer and the 443-bp enhancer. The core enhancer, the 443-bp enhancer, and one mutant variant of each were also placed in the forward orientation immediately upstream of a minimal apoB promoter (−85) containing just 85 bp of 5′-flanking sequence, linked to the CAT gene. This minimal apoB promoter has only 23% of the activity of the −898 promoter in HepG2 cells [27]. The results of transient transfection assays of these minimal promoter constructs in HepG2 cells are also presented in Figure 4. In this minimal promoter the 443-bp enhancer increased CAT activity by some 16-fold. This marked increase in the magnitude of the enhancer effect compared with its activity in the larger apoB promoter could have two explanations. First, increasing the proximity of the enhancer to the transcriptional start site might enable trans-acting factors bound to the enhancer to interact more readily with the basal transcription complex. Alternatively, the enhancer may exert a larger influence upon the weaker −85 promoter, where the basal transcription complex is more responsive to additional positive influences. Evidence from our laboratory supports the second possibility [28]. Disruption of the palindrome by insertion of two linkers reduced the effect of the 443-bp enhancer upon the −85 promoter to 6.5-fold, which is 36% of that observed with the wild-type sequence. Thus, in contrast to the −898 promoter, mutation of the HNF-1 binding site in the context of the −85 promoter leaves significant residual enhancer activity. This may reflect a difference in the mechanism of action of the enhancer at a distance. The 147-bp core enhancer increased transcription from the −85 promoter by 36-fold, which is 2-fold greater than the effect observed with the 443-bp fragment. Mutation of the HNF-1 site as in the 147∇16 mutant reduced enhancer activity to 40%. Thus, the loss of HNF-1 binding had a less pronounced effect upon the ability of the core enhancer to increase expression from the minimal apoB promoter (−85) than from the −898 promoter. These results demonstrate that the HNF-1 binding site detected in the gel retention studies is functional and necessary for full enhancer activity.

IN ADDITION TO HNF-1, THE CORE ENHANCER CONTAINS A BINDING SITE FOR C/EBP WHICH IS REQUIRED FOR THE ACTIVITY OF THE ENHANCER

The 97-bp DNaseI footprint within the core enhancer is presumably composed of the binding sites for several trans-acting factors. The 5′ end of this footprint binds HNF-1. To investigate DNA-protein interactions in the remainder of this footprint, the 147-bp core enhancer was digested with *Taq*I that yields, in addition to the 5′ *Xba*I-*Taq*I fragment, a 50-bp *Taq*I fragment containing the central portion of the footprint and a 31-bp *Taq*I-*Xba*I fragment containing the 3′-most 14 bp of the

	-898				-85			
	Relative CAT Activity	S.D.	N	Enhancer Activity %	Relative CAT Activity	S.D.	N	Enhancer Activity %
443 F	3.4	±0.4	6	100	16.3	±1.3	4	100
443 ∇8	1.9	±0.2	8	38	—			
443 ∇16	1.4	±0.1	4	16	6.5	±0.1	4	36
147 F	3.5	±0.8	10	100	36.3	±0.7	4	100
147 ∇16	1.5	±0.1	6	20	15.9	±1.6	4	42
147 ∇16Δ4	1.4	±0.2	6	16	—			

```
                        HNF-1
                    Consensus:  G T T A  A T N A T  T A A C
                                | |  | |  |  | |  | |
              W.T. Apo-B:  A T C A G T G A - C - T - A - G - T C A T T G A T T C G A


                 443 ∇8    A T C A G T G A [GGGTACCC] T C A T T G A T

                 443 ∇16
                 147 ∇16   A T C A G T G A|GGGTACCCGGGTACCC|T C A T T G A T

               147 ∇16Δ4   A T C A G T G A|GGGTACCCGGGTACCC|T G A T T C G A
```

FIG. 2. *Effect of disrupting the HNF-1 binding site upon enhancer activity in transiently transfected HepG2 cells. The left portion of the figure illustrates the apoB enhancer regions and their mutations that were cloned upstream of apoB promoter sequences –898 to +121 (–898) or –85 to +121 (–85) linked to the CAT gene. Chloramphenicol acetyltransferase activity is expressed relative to that of the promoter alone, whose activity was set to 1.0. S.D. is the standard deviation, and N is the number of independent transfection experiments performed. The results are also expressed as percentage of the activity of the wild-type enhancer (either 443 or 147) in the % columns. The lower part of the figure shows the nucleotide sequence of the 20-bp palindrome from the apoB enhancer and the corresponding sequences of the four linker insertion mutants shown above. The horizontal arrows indicate the two halves of the palindrome. Above the wild-type sequence is shown the homology to the HNF-1 consensus recognition sequence. The boxed nucleotides represent KpnI linkers.*

footprint (see Fig. 1, panel II). The binding of mouse liver nuclear proteins to the *Taq*I and *Taq*I-*Xba*I fragments was investigated using the gel mobility shift assay. Panel I of Figure 3 illustrates the results obtained when the *Taq*I fragment was used as a probe. At least six distinct complexes were formed, designated a to f (lane 2), each of which represents the binding of one or more nuclear proteins to the *Taq*I fragment. A 25-fold molar excess of unlabeled *Taq*I fragment (lane 3) efficiently competed for formation of all six retarded complexes. Furthermore, a 100-fold molar excess of the oligonucleotide containing the binding site for C/EBP from the transthyretin enhancer (lane 3) did efficiently compete for the major retarded complex d, and also for complexes a and b. The C/EBP oligomer also partially competed for complex e, but did not affect the formation of complexes c and f. This result suggested that one or more of the proteins binding to the *Taq*I fragment was C/EBP or one of the related proteins that recognize the same sequence as C/EBP

[1,6,8,12,26,29,34].

Analysis of the DNA sequence within the *Taq*I fragment revealed three regions with homology to the proposed consensus sequence (TCNTACTC) for C/EBP [9], and these are indicated by the arrows above the sequence in Figure 3. Two of these motifs are separated by 2 bp and arranged as an inverted repeat. The third segment homologous to the C/EBP consensus partly overlaps with one of the others. No other significant similarities to the C/EBP consensus exist within the core enhancer. To test the hypothesis that this was indeed the binding site for C/EBP, six point mutations were created within this sequence as described in Materials and Methods. The point mutations were designed to cause maximal disruption of the homology to the C/EBP consensus sequence and are shown below the wild-type sequence in Figure 3. These mutations were made in the context of the 147-bp core enhancer, and the resultant clone was designated mutA. The 50-bp *Taq*I fragment was

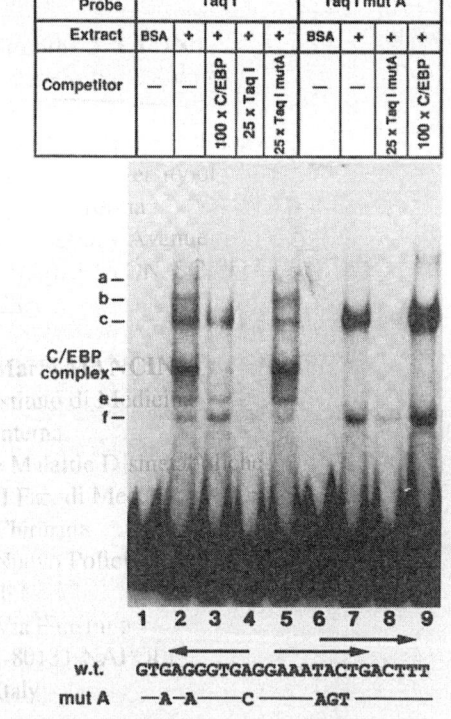

FIG. 3. Effect of mutations in the C/EBP site upon binding of nuclear proteins and enhancer activity. Panel I, The TaqI fragment of the core enhancer was isolated from the clone Pvu147F or from the clone Pvu147mutA (TaqI mutA), and end-labeled with [α- 32 P]dCTP and Klenow enzyme. Binding of unfractionated mouse liver nuclear extract (2 μg per reaction) was assayed using the gel mobility shift assay. Unlabeled competitor DNA was included in some binding reactions at the molar excess indicated. The bottom of panel I shows the sequence (+879 to +903) of the core enhancer in the vicinity of the C/EBP binding site. The arrows denote the three regions with homology to the consensus C/EBP recognition sequence. Also shown are the point mutations made in the clone mutA. Panel II, Results of transient transfections of HepG2 cells with plasmids containing the core enhancer (147) or the core enhancer containing mutations in the C/EBP site (147mutA) inserted upstream of the –898 apoB promoter segment or the –85 promoter segment. Chloramphenicol acetyltransferase activity is expressed relative to that of the promoter alone, whose activity was set to 1.0, and is the average of four independent transfections. S.D., standard deviation; N, number of independent transfections.

Panel I table:

Probe	Taq I				Taq I mut A			
Extract	BSA	+	+	+	+	BSA	+	+	+
Competitor	—	—	100 x C/EBP	25 x Taq I	25 x Taq I mutA	—	—	25 x Taq I mutA	100 x C/EBP

a —
b —
c —
C/EBP complex —
e —
f —

1 2 3 4 5 6 7 8 9

w.t.   GTGAGGGTGAGGAAATACTGACTTT
mut A   —A–A——C———AGT———

Panel II:

	Relative CAT Activity			
Promoter:	-898		-85	
		S.D.	N		S.D.	N
147	1.7	±0.2	4	36.3	±0.7	4
147 mut A	1.0	±0.1	4	18.3	±0.3	4

isolated from this clone and tested for binding to mouse liver nuclear proteins, in parallel with the wild-type *Taq*I fragment, as illustrated in panel I of Figure 3. An excess of the *Taq*I fragment from mutA partially competed for the formation of complexes c and f, but not for any of the other complexes (lane 5). When the *Taq*I fragment from mutA was used as a probe in the gel mobility shift assay only two retarded complexes with mobilities similar to complexes c and f were observed (lane 7). Thus point mutations within the putative C/EBP binding site abolished the binding of C/EBP (complex d), confirming the location of the binding site, and also prevented the binding of proteins responsible for complexes a, b, and e. This suggests that the binding sites for the proteins responsible for complexes a, b, and e overlap with the C/EBP binding site. The idea that the retarded complexes seen with the mutant *Taq*I fragment are caused by the same proteins responsible for the formation complexes c and f with the wild-type probe is supported by the fact that unlabeled mutant *Taq*I DNA competed for complexes c and f (lane 5 of Fig. 3). These two complexes formed with the mutant *Taq*I probe reflect specific interactions, because they were competed for by a 25-fold excess of unlabeled mutant *Taq*I DNA (lane 8), but not by a 100-fold molar excess of the oligomer containing the C/EBP binding site (lane 9). From these results it seemed likely that the binding sites for the proteins generating complexes c and f may lie outside of the C/EBP binding site. Alternatively, since the formation of complexes c and f was strengthened with the mutA clone, it is possible that these two proteins may also bind in the vicinity of the C/EBP site. In summary, the *Taq*I fragment from the core enhancer binds six proteins, one of which is C/EBP or one of the related proteins that recognize similar sequences. The binding sites for three of the remaining proteins (complexes a, b, and e), one of which (e) is heat-stable (Fig. 6, panel I), appear to overlap with that of C/EBP.

To test the functional importance of the C/EBP binding site, mutA was tested for its ability to increase the activity of both the –898 apoB promoter and the minimal (–85) apoB promoter when transiently transfected in to HepG2 cells. The mutant and wild-type core enhancer fragments were both placed in the reverse orientation upstream of the –898 promoter, and in the forward orientation upstream of the –85 promoter. The results are presented in panel II of Figure 3. The wildtype core enhancer increased transcription from the –898 apoB promoter by 1.7-fold, whereas the core enhancer containing the C/EBP mutation had the same activity as the promoter alone. Thus, at least in the reverse orientation, where the core enhancer consistently exhibits a rather low activation potential, binding of C/EBP is essential for the enhancer to function. In the context of the minimal apoB promoter, containing just 85 bp of 5'-flanking sequence, the C/EBP mutation reduced the activity of the core enhancer from 36-fold to 18-fold. So in this context the C/EBP binding site contributes 50% of the activation potential of the core enhancer. Because of the low activity of the core enhancer in the reverse orientation in the –898 promoter, it is difficult to be sure that the magnitude of the effect of the mutation is significantly different when assayed in the two promoters. Nevertheless, it is clear from these results that the C/EBP binding site constitutes an important cis-acting element of the core enhancer.

THE 3' END OF THE FOOTPRINT BINDS PROTEIN II, WHICH IS ALSO ESSENTIAL FOR THE ACTIVITY OF THE ENHANCER

The 31-bp *Taq*I-*Xba*I fragment formed only a single retarded complex when incubated with mouse liver nuclear extract (Fig. 4, Panel I, lane 1) that was heat labile (data not shown). Formation of this complex was efficiently competed for by a 100-fold molar excess of the unlabeled *Taq*I-*Xba*I fragment (lane 2). In an attempt to identify the protein generating this retarded complex, a series of unlabeled oligonucleotides containing known binding sites for a number of transcription factors were used as competitors. Only an oligonucleotide containing the binding site for AP2 displayed

FIG. 4. Effect of mutations in the binding site for protein II upon binding of nuclear proteins and enhancer activity. Panel I, the TaqI-XbaI fragment of the core enhancer was isolated from the clone Pvu147F or from the clone 147FmutII (TaqI-XbaI mutII) and end-labeled with [α- 32 P]dCTP. Binding of unfractionated mouse liver nuclear extract to these probes was assayed using the gel mobility shift assay. Some reactions contained unlabeled competitor DNA as indicated. The bottom of panel I shows the sequence (+921 to +953) of the wild-type TaqI-XbaI fragment together with the point mutations and one nucleotide deletion made in the clone mutII. Panel II, results of transient transfections of HepG2 cells with plasmids containing the core enhancer (147F) or the core enhancer containing mutations in the binding site for protein II (147FmutII) inserted upstream of the −898 apoB promoter segment or the −85 promoter segment. Chloramphenicol acetyltransferase activity is expressed relative to that of the promoter alone, whose activity was set to 1.0. S.D., standard deviation; N, number of independent transfections.

I.

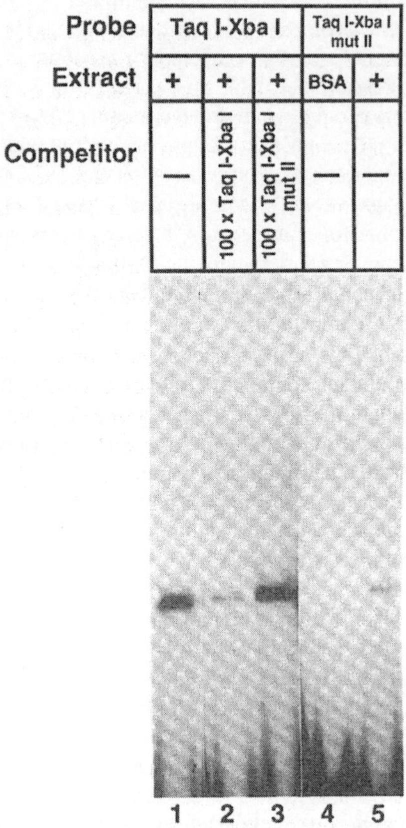

Probe	Taq I-Xba I			Taq I-Xba I mut II	
Extract	+	+	+	BSA	+
Competitor	—	100 x Taq I-Xba I	100 x Taq I-Xba I mut II	—	—

1 2 3 4 5

WT CGAACCTCCACCCCCCTTCCTATTTACCTGACCT
mut II ———GA——— G-A-△—————————

II.

Promoter	-898			-85		
	Relative CAT Activity	S.D.	N	Relative CAT Activity	S.D.	N
147 F	2.6	±0.3	8	37.5	±5.5	4
147 F mut II	1.5	±0.1	6	17.6	±2.5	4

any effect upon complex formation, and only at a rather high molar excess (data not shown). Thus, the identity of the protein binding to the *Taq*I-*Xba*I probe which we will refer to as protein II, remains obscure.

To localize the binding site for protein II, we made four nucleotide substitutions and a one nucleotide deletion in the 3′ end of the footprint. The resulting clone was designated mutII, and the sequence of the *Taq*I-*Xba*I fragment of this clone is shown together with the wild-type sequence in Figure 4, panel I. Binding of protein II to the *Taq*I-*Xba*I fragment from mutII was reduced by more than 10-fold (Fig. 4, lanes 1 and 5). Furthermore, this mutant *Taq*I-*Xba*I fragment was unable to compete for the binding of protein II to the wild type *Taq*I-*Xba*I fragment (Fig. 4, lane 3).

The effect of disrupting the protein II binding site upon the activity of the 147-bp core enhancer was tested by transient transfection of HepG2 cells (Fig. 4, panel II). In the context of the strong −898 apoB promoter, enhancer activity was reduced by 70%, while in the context of the −85 apoB promoter, disruption of protein II binding reduced the activity of the core enhancer by 50%. These results demonstrate that binding of protein II to the apoB core enhancer is essential for its activity. Furthermore, taken together with our previous results showing that disruption of HNF-1 and/or C/EBP binding also impaired enhancer activity, these data strongly suggest that protein II is the third component required for the full activity of the core enhancer.

HNF-1, C/EBP, AND PROTEIN II ACT SYNERGISTICALLY TO ENHANCE TRANSCRIPTION

Mutagenesis of the HNF-1, C/EBP, and protein II binding sites showed that binding of each of these factors is essential for full activity of the core enhancer. To investigate further the minimal sequence elements required for the function of the core enhancer, three deletions of the core enhancer were made using the PCR. These deletions were cloned upstream of both the −898 apoB promoter and the −85 apoB promoter and assayed for enhancer activity in transient transfections of HepG2 cells (Fig. 5). The Xba-Taq clone, which corresponds almost exactly to the *Xba*I-*Taq*I fragment of the core enhancer and contains only the HNF-1 binding site, exhibited no enhancer activity in the context of the −898 promoter. The Taq-Xba clone, which contains the 3′ half of the core enhancer and includes the C/EBP binding site and the protein II binding site, also failed to augment expression from the −898 promoter. Even when the HNF-1, protein I, and C/EBP binding sites were present together, as in the clone XbaCore, no enhancer activity was detected. From these results it is clear that neither HNF-1 nor C/EBP, alone or in combination with protein I, can enhance expression from the −898 promoter. This implicates the binding site for protein II as an essential component of the core enhancer.

Use of the −85 apoB promoter allowed a more sensitive assay for cis-acting elements within the core enhancer. However, since the DNA fragments being tested were placed only 85 bp upstream of the transcription start site, this cannot be considered a true measure of enhancer strength. The Xba-Taq clone that contained the binding site for HNF-1 increased CAT activity by 7-fold in the forward orientation. This result demonstrates that this region acts as an independent positive element in the context of a weak promoter. However, the positive effect of the Xba-Taq clone was only 18% of that of the intact core enhancer. The Taq-Xba clone exhibited 15-fold higher CAT activity than the control, which corresponds to 39% of the activity of the 147-bp core fragment. Thus, in the context of the −85 promoter, the combination of protein-binding sites within the Taq-Xba clone, which includes the C/EBP binding site and the binding site for protein II, exerted a 2-fold stronger effect upon transcription than the HNF-1 binding site (clone Xba-Taq). Surprisingly, the XbaCore clone that includes the binding sites for HNF-1, C/EBP, and protein I showed only a 6.4-fold enhancement of CAT activity in the forward orientation, which is less than that

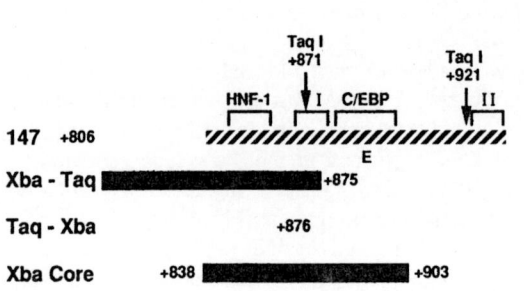

	Relative CAT Activity (HepG2)			
	-898 CAT		**-85 CAT**	
		S.D. N		S.D. N
147	F 2.6 ±0.3 4		F 36.3 ±0.7 4	
	R 1.7 ±0.2 4			
Xba - Taq	F 1.1 ±0.2 4		F 7.2 ±1.4 4	
	R 1.0 ±0.1 4			
Taq - Xba	R 1.1 ±0.1 4		* 14.7 ±0.9 4	
Xba Core	F 0.9 ±0.1 4		F 6.4 ±0.6 4	
			R 10.5 ±1.4 4	

FIG. 5. Deletion analysis of the apoB core enhancer in HepG2 cells. The left side of the figure shows a map of the core enhancer (147) in which the location of the 97-bp footprint "E" is shaded. Locations of the HNF-1 and C/EBP binding sites are indicated. Below this are illustrated the three deletion clones of the core enhancer. Each deletion was cloned in either the forward (F) or reverse (R) orientations upstream of either the –898 or the –85 apoB promoter CAT plasmids, and transiently transfected into HepG2 cells. The results are presented as CAT activity relative to that of the promoter alone, whose activity was set to 1.0. N and S.D. have already been defined. *, the orientation of this clone was not determined.

observed with the Xba-Taq clone that contains only the HNF-1 binding site. In the reverse orientation the positive effect of the XbaCore clone was slightly stronger (10.5-fold). This suggests that protein I does not contribute significantly to the activity of the enhancer, at least in the context of the –85 promoter.

From these results it may be concluded that combining the C/EBP binding site with the binding sites for HNF-1 and protein I does not significantly augment the level of transcriptional activation obtained with the HNF-1 binding site alone. A corollary of this conclusion is that the binding site for protein II must contribute significantly to the activation potential of the core enhancer. This deduction is in agreement with the observation that the Taq-Xba clone exhibited the strongest positive effect upon transcription from the –85 promoter. When two tandem copies of the enhancer region contained within XbaCore were inserted in reverse orientation upstream of the –898 promoter, CAT activity was increased by 1.8-fold (data not shown). In contrast five copies of the enhancer segment contained within the Xba-Taq clone exhibited almost no enhancer activity upon the –898 promoter (data not shown). Thus, the HNF-1 site alone cannot act as an enhancer even when multimerized, but it can do so when multimerized in combination with the binding sites for C/EBP and protein I. Five tandem copies of the enhancer sequences contained within the Taq-Xba clone increased CAT activity by 5.4-fold when placed upstream of the –898 promoter (data not shown), emphasizing the importance of cis-acting elements within this region of the core enhancer.

Thus, the core enhancer contains a number of positive cis-acting elements, which can act independently when placed close to the transcription start site of a weak apoB promoter. However, all these elements are necessary to obtain the full positive effect of the core enhancer in the context of the –85 promoter, and all are required to obtain any enhancer activity in the strong –898 promoter.

In summary, we have shown that the core region of the second-intron enhancer of the apoB gene is composed of the binding sites for nine liver nuclear proteins (Fig. 6). The well-characterized transcription factor HNF-1 binds to the very 5' end of the footprinted sequences, on the 5' half of a 20-bp palindrome. Mutations that prevented binding of HNF-1 showed that this factor is essential for the function of both the core enhancer and the 443-bp enhancer fragment. Deletion experiments showed that the HNF-1 binding site functioned synergistically with other protein-binding sites within the core enhancer. The C/EBP site alone was not sufficient to elicit this synergistic effect; sequence elements containing the binding site for protein II were also required.

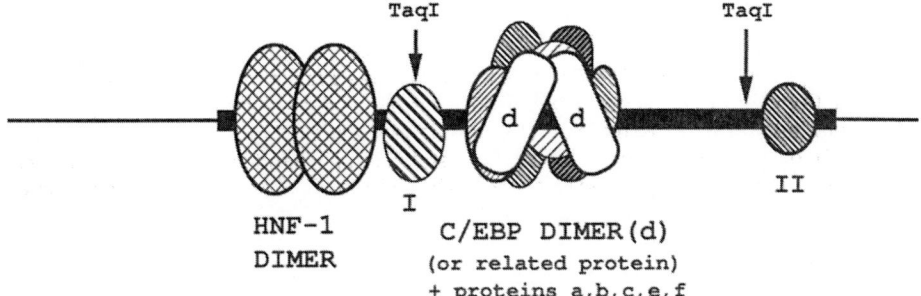

FIG. 6. Proposed arrangement of protein factors binding to the apoB core enhancer. The thick black line represents the 97-bp footprint of the core enhancer, and the location of the cutting sites for TaqI are shown. HNF-1 (cross-hatched ellipses) and C/EBP (d) are shown binding as homodimers. The five other proteins (a, b, c, e, f) that bind to the same or overlapping sites as C/EBP are shown as shaded ellipses. The 3'-most 14 bp of the footprint are bound by protein II.

Cooperativity between trans-acting factors has been well documented by others [7,10,14,21,22,31]. Cooperativity could occur by two different mechanisms: cooperative binding to DNA or cooperative trans-activation, in which two or more factors interact in such a way as to have a synergistic effect on some rate-limiting step in the assembly of the basal transcription complex. There is evidence that both of these mechanisms can operate.

The transcription factor HNF-1 is a divergent member of the homeodomain family of proteins [2,13] and has been implicated in the liver-specific transcription of many genes (for a review, see [25]). Although initially thought to be strictly liver-specific, functional HNF-1 protein has also been detected at comparable levels in rat kidney [35] and in the human intestine-derived cell line CaCo-2 [3]. HNF-1 mRNA is present at high levels in the kidney and intestine of rats and mice and in mouse stomach and rat spleen, as well as in the liver [2,19,35]. In fact, none of the transcription factors that have been implicated in the transcription of liver-specific genes (C/EBP, HNF-1, HNF-3, HNF-4) are expressed in a strictly liver-specific manner [35]. This has led to the suggestion that liver-specific transcription requires the simultaneous expression of all these factors (and perhaps others). Furthermore, many of the genes that are considered to be liver-specific are expressed in other tissues also. In the case of the apoB gene, the fact that HNF-1 is also expressed at high levels in the intestine suggests that it may contribute to apoB expression in that tissue.

Our experiments identified a binding site for C/EBP, another factor implicated in liver-specific expression, within the core enhancer. Mutagenesis of this site showed that it also is important for the activity of the enhancer, and that proteins binding here act synergistically with proteins bound at adjacent sites. In addition, the binding site for C/EBP overlaps at least partially with the binding sites for five other proteins. Three of these are related to C/EBP in that their binding is eliminated by competition with an oligonucleotide containing the binding site for C/EBP and by mutation of the C/EBP binding site. It seems likely that the four related mouse liver proteins that bind to the C/EBP site of the apoB core enhancer are homo- or heterodimers of members of the C/EBP family. Clearly, only a single dimeric protein can bind to this site at any one time. Thus, *in vivo* there may be competition for binding to this site that could modulate the activity of the enhancer. The function of proteins c and f that are clearly distinct from the C/EBP proteins but appear to bind to overlapping sites is unclear at this time.

The results in Figures 2 and 5 indicate that the mechanism of action of the enhancer may be different when it is placed close to the transcription start site of a weak apoB promoter than when it is placed at a distance from a strong apoB promoter. All the protein-binding sites in the core enhancer are required for significant transcriptional activation when the enhancer is 898 bp from the transcription start site of the strong apoB promoter. In contrast, individual protein-binding sites are able to function independently when placed 85 bp from the start site of a weak apoB promoter. Thus, a complex array of proteins bound to the core enhancer may be required to act cooperatively to enhance transcription at a distance.

Acknowledgments

We are indebted to Drs. Dirk Mendel and Gerald Crabtree for providing us with the mouse liver extract enriched for HNF-1, together with the β-28 oligonucleotide, the HNF-1 antiserum, and the HNF-1 expression plasmids. This work was supported by Program Project Grant HL41633 (to B.L.W.) from the National Institutes of Health.

References

1. Akira, S., H. Isshiki, T. Sugita, O. Tanabe, S. Kinoshita, Y. Nishio, T. Nakajima, T. Hirano, and T. Kishimoto. 1990. A nuclear factor for IL-6 expression (NF-IL6) is a member of a C/EBP family. EMBO J. 9: 1897-1906.
2. Baumhueter, S., D. B. Mendel, P. B. Conley, C. J. Kuo, C. Turk, M. K. Graves, C. A. Edwards, G. Courtois, and G. R. Crabtree. 1990. HNF-1 shares three sequence motifs with the POU domain proteins and is identical to LF-B1 and APF. Genes Dev. 4: 372-379.
3. Brooks, A. R., B. D. Blackhart, K. Haubold, and B. Levy-Wilson. 1991. Characterization of tissue-specific enhancer elements in the second intron of the human apolipoprotein B gene. J. Biol. Chem. 266: 7848-7859.
4. Brooks, A. R. and B. Levy-Wilson. 1992. HNF-1 and C/EBP are essential for the activity of the human apolipoprotein B gene second intron enhancer. Mol. Cell. Biol. 12: 1134-1148.
5. Brunzell, J. D., A. D. Sniderman, J. J. Albers, and P. O. Kwiterovich Jr.. 1984. Apoproteins B and A-I and coronary artery disease in humans. Arteriosclerosis 4: 79-83.
6. Cao, Z., R. M. Umek, and S. L. McKnight. 1991. Regulated expression of three C/EBP isoforms during adipose conversion of 3T3-L1 cells. Genes Dev. 5: 1538-1552.
7. Carey, M., Y. S. Lin, M. R. Green, and M. Ptashne. 1990. A mechanism for synergistic activation of a mammalian gene by GAL4 derivatives. Nature 345: 361-364.
8. Chang, C. J., T. T. Chen, H. Y. Lei, D. S. Chen, and S. C. Lee. 1990. Molecular cloning of a transcription factor, AGP/EBP, that belongs to members of the C/EBP family. Mol. Cell. Biol. 10: 6642-6653.
9. Costa, R. H., D. R. Grayson, K. G. Xanthopoulos, and J. E. Darnell Jr.. 1988. A liver-specific DNA-binding protein recognizes multiple nucleotide sites in regulatory regions of transthyretin, α 1 -antitrypsin, albumin, and simian virus 40 genes. Proc. Natl. Acad. Sci. USA 85: 3840-3844.

10. Courey, A. J., D. A. Holtzman, S. P. Jackson, and T. Tjian. 1989. Synergistic activation by the glutamine-rich domains of human transcription factor Sp1. Cell 59: 827-836.
11. Courtois, G., J. G. Morgan, L. A. Campbell, G. Fourel, and G. R. Crabtree. 1987. Interaction of a liver-specific nuclear factor with the fibrinogen and α 1 -antitrypsin promoters. Science 238: 688-692.
12. Descombes, P., M. Chojkier, S. Lichtsteiner, E. Falvey, and U. Schibler. 1990. LAP, a novel member of the C/EBP gene family, encodes a liver-enriched transcriptional activator protein. Genes Dev. 4: 1541-1551.
13. Frain, M., G. Swart, P. Monaci, A. Nicosia, S. Stampfli, R. Frank, and R. Cortese. 1989. The liver-specific transcription factor LF-B1 contains a highly diverged homeobox DNA binding domain. Cell 59: 145-157.
14. Giniger, E. and M. Ptashne. 1988. Cooperative DNA binding of the yeast transcriptional activator GAL4. Proc. Natl. Acad. Sci. USA 85: 382-386.
15. Goldstein, J. L. and M. S. Brown. 1977. The low-density lipoprotein pathway and its relation to atherosclerosis. Annu. Rev. Biochem. 46: 897-930.
16. Gorski, K., M. Carneiro, and U. Schibler. 1986. Tissue-specific in vitro transcription from the mouse albumin promoter. Cell 47: 767-776.
17. Grayson, D. R., R. H. Costa, K. G. Xanthopoulos, and J. E. Darnell. 1988. One factor recognizes the liver-specific enhancers in α 1 -antitrypsin and transthyretin genes. Science 239: 786-788.
18. Johnson, P. F., W. H. Landschulz, B. J. Graves, and S. L. McKnight. 1987. Identification of a rat liver nuclear protein that binds to the enhancer core element of three animal viruses. Genes Dev. 1: 133-146.
19. Kuo, C. J., P. B. Conley, C. L. Hsieh, U. Francke, and G. R. Crabtree. 1990. Molecular cloning, functional expression, and chromosomal localization of mouse hepatocyte nuclear factor 1. Proc. Natl. Acad. Sci. USA 87: 9838-9842.
20. Landschulz, W. H., P. F. Johnson, E. Y. Adashi, B. J. Graves, and S. L. McKnight. 1988. Isolation of a recombinant copy of the gene encoding C/EBP. Genes Dev. 2: 786-800.
21. Lin, Y. S., M. F. Carey, M. Ptashne, and M. R. Green. 1988. GAL4 derivatives function alone and synergistically with mammalian activators in vitro. Cell 54: 659-664.
22. Lin, Y. S., M. Carey, M. Ptashne, and M. R. Green. 1990. How different eukaryotic transcriptional activators can cooperate promiscuously. Nature 345: 359-361.
23. Ludwig, E. H., B. Levy-Wilson, T. Knott, B. D. Blackhart, and B. J. McCarthy. 1991. Comparative analysis of sequences at the 5' end of the human and mouse apolipoprotein B genes. DNA Cell Biol. 10: 329-338.
24. Mendel, D. B., L. P. Hansen, M. K. Graves, P. B. Conley, and G. R. Crabtree. 1991. HNF-1α and HNF-1β (vHNF-1) share dimerization and homeo domains, but not activation domains, and form heterodimers in vitro. Genes Dev. 5: 1042-1056.
25. Mendel, D. B. and G. R. Crabtree. 1991. HNF-1, a member of a novel class of dimerizing homeodomain proteins. J. Biol. Chem. 266: 677-680.
26. Mueller, C. R., P. Maire, and U. Schibler. 1990. DBP, a liver-enriched transcriptional activator, is expressed late in ontogeny and its tissue specificity is determined posttranscriptionally. Cell 61: 279-291.
27. Paulweber, B., M. Onasch, B. P. Nagy, and B. Levy-Wilson. 1991. Similarities and differences in the regulatory elements at the 5' end of the human apolipoprotein B gene between hepatic and intestinal cells. J. Biol. Chem., in press.
28. Paulweber, B. and B. Levy-Wilson. 1991. The mechanisms by which a human apolipoprotein

B gene enhancer and reducer interact with the promoter are different in cells of hepatic and intestinal origin. J. Biol. Chem., in press.

29. Poli, V., F. P. Mancini, and R. Cortese. 1990. IL-6DBP, a nuclear protein involved in interleukin-6 signal transduction, defines a new family of leucine zipper proteins related to C/EBP. Cell 63: 643-653.

30. Sanger, F., S. Nicklen, and A. R. Coulson. 1977. DNA sequencing with chain-terminating inhibitors. Proc. Natl. Acad. Sci. USA 74: 5463-5467.

31. Schule, R., M. Muller, H. Otsuka-Murakami, and R. Renkawitz. 1988. Cooperativity of the glucocorticoid receptor and the CACCC-box binding factor. Nature 332: 87-90.

32. Sniderman, A., S. Shapiro, D. Marpole, B. Skinner, B. Teng, and P. O. Kwiterovich, Jr.. 1980. Association of coronary atherosclerosis with hyperapobetalipoproteinemia [increased protein but normal cholesterol levels in human plasma low density (β) lipoproteins]. Proc. Natl. Acad. Sci. USA 77: 604-608.

33. Steinberg, D., S. M. Grundy, H. Y. L Mok, J. D. Turner, D. B. Weinstein, W. V. Brown, and J. J. Albers. 1979. Metabolic studies in an unusual case of asymptomatic familial hypobetalipoproteinemia with hypoalphalipoproteinemia and fasting chylomicronemia. J. Clin. Invest. 64: 292-301.

34. Williams, S. C., C. A. Cantwell, and P. F. Johnson. 1991. A family of C/EBP-related proteins capable of forming covalently linked leucine zipper dimers *in vitro*. Genes Dev. 5: 1553-1567.

35. Xanthopoulos, K. G., V. R. Prezioso, W. S. Chen, F. M. Sladek, R. Cortese, and J. E. Darnell Jr.. 1991. The different tissue transcription patterns of genes for HNF-1, C/EBP, HNF-3, and HNF-4, protein factors that govern liver-specific transcription. Proc. Natl. Acad. Sci. USA 88: 3807-3811.

36. Young, S. G.. 1990. Recent progress in understanding apolipoprotein B. Circulation 82: 1574-1594.

37. Zhang, H., R. Scholl, J. Browse, and C. Somerville. 1988. Double stranded DNA sequencing as a choice for DNA sequencing. Nucleic Acids Res. 16: 1220.

38. Zhou, D. X. and T. S. B. Yen. 1991. The ubiquitous transcription factor Oct-1 and the liver-specific factor HNF-1 are both required to activate transcription of a hepatitis B virus promoter. Mol. Cell. Biol. 11: 1353-1359.

Abbreviations

The abbreviations used are: apo, apolipoprotein; LDL, low density lipoprotein(s); kb, kilobase(s); CAT, chloramphenicol acetyltransferase; PCR, polymerase chain reaction; BMV, Brome Mosaic virus.

STRUCTURE-FUNCTION RELATIONSHIPS OF APOLIPOPROTEIN B-100

LAWRENCE CHAN

ABSTRACT. Apolipoprotein (apo) B-100 is a huge protein that has been difficult to study by traditional protein chemistry techniques. Other experimental approaches, such as investigations in cultured cells, and in human subjects with specific apoB mutations also have their limitations. A novel approach using transgenic mice has yielded interesting information on the low density lipoprotein-associating function of apoB-100. In future, transgenic animals expressing site-specific mutant apoB molecules will be a valuable tool to study the structure-function relationship of this complex but functionally important protein in lipid metabolism.

Apolipoprotein (apo) B-100 is the major protein in low density lipoproteins (LDL) and a physiological ligand for the LDL receptor. Its primary structure was first reported in 1986 [1-5]. It is only now, seven years later, that we begin to have some understanding of the structure-function relationships of this unique protein.

ApoB-100 serves two major functions: lipid binding and LDL receptor binding. The lipid-binding properties of apoB-100 must also account for the fact that apoB-100 is the only protein in LDL and it does not dissociate from the latter. This is in contrast to the soluble apolipoproteins (apoA-I, A-II, C-I, C-II, C-III and E), which also spontaneously bind to lipid. However, during the metabolic conversion of very low density lipoproteins (VLDL) to LDL, they dissociate from the lipoprotein particles and are absent from LDL. The ligand function of apoB-100 is also dependent on its unique LDL-associating properties. ApoB-100 is a competent ligand for the LDL receptor only when it is present on LDL. For example, apoB-100 is not a competent ligand in large VLDL particles. Instead, apoE, a soluble apolipoprotein, serves this function. Therefore, the two major functions of apoB-100 are closely interrelated.

There are four approaches that have been taken to analyze the lipid- and LDL-binding properties of apoB-100: (i) binding of proteolytic apoB peptides to lipid in vitro, (ii) expression and characterization of different lengths of apoB-100 in hepatoma cells in vitro, (iii) characterization of truncated apoB-100 fragments in patients with familial hypobetalipoproteinemia, and (iv) use of transgenic mice to examine apoB transgene product distribution.

Tryptic apoB-100 fragments were allowed to spontaneously associate with dimyristoylphosphatidylcholine vesicles in vitro, and the vesicle-bound peptides were isolated by ultracentrifugal flotation. Using this procedure, Yang et al. purified 13 apoB-100 lipid-binding peptides [6]. These peptides were characterized by their high hydrophobicity and predicted β-sheet content. They were distributed throughout the

45

A. L. Catapano et al. (eds.), Drugs Affecting Lipid Metabolism, 45–47.
© 1993 Kluwer Academic Publishers and Fondazione Giovanni Lorenzini.

length of apoB-100. Although they contribute to the lipid-binding activity of apoB-100, these peptides cannot account for apoB-100 being the only protein in LDL because lipid-binding peptides can also be isolated by a similar procedure from the soluble apolipoproteins which are absent from LDL.

Yao et al. [7] expressed different lengths of apoB-100 N-terminal fragments in rat hepatoma cell lines using cytomegalovirus promoter driven cDNA constructs. When they characterized the lipoproteins produced by these cells, they found that the apoB fragments were distributed in different particles according to the length of the apoB-100 peptide produced. In cells that express the longest construct (apoB-53, i.e., one that spans the N-terminal 53% of apoB-100), the B-53 peptide was found to be associated with high density lipoproteins (HDL) and VLDL, but not LDL. Their observations suggest that more than 53% of apoB-100 sequence was required for its association with LDL.

The most rigorous assay for human apoB-100 sequence requirement for LDL association must be in the natural host. Individuals with familial hypobetalipoproteinemia produce different lengths of N-terminal apoB-100 sequence [8]. The distribution of the truncated apoB fragments among the different lipoprotein particles has been investigated by different laboratories. It appears that when less than 30% of apoB-100 is predicted to be produced, the truncated protein is not detectable in the patient's plasma, indicating that either it is not produced or it is rapidly turned over. For apoB-100 molecules that fall between 37% and 50% of the full-length protein, the truncated protein is generally present in HDL, VLDL and LDL. Therefore, although there is enough sequence information for the protein to stay associated with LDL, it is also associated, inappropriately, with HDL. These experiments in nature strongly suggest that more than 50% of apoB-100 N-terminal sequence is required for its specific association with VLDL and LDL but not HDL. An alternative explanation is that perhaps the C-terminal 50% of apoB-100 sequence contains important information which allows the protein to specifically associate with LDL.

In order to address the issue of the importance of C-terminal sequences in the lipoprotein distribution of apoB-100, Xiong et al. produced transgenic mice that express the following human apoB sequence: apoB (1-56 / 2878-3925 / 4528-4536) [9]. The DNA construct contains 4.5 kb in the 5' flanking DNA and the first three introns. An apoB mini-mRNA of the predicted size was detected at high level in the liver and small intestine, and at much lower level in muscle. An immunoreactive apoB miniprotein was detected in total plasma and in LDL, but not in HDL or lipoprotein-free plasma. It was also absent from VLDL which might be explained by the very low level of the miniprotein present in this class of lipoproteins.

Taken together, the 4 experimental approaches on apoB expression and its lipoprotein distribution indicate that the longer the apoB peptide, the more likely it is to be exclusively present in VLDL and LDL, its natural host particles. In addition, it appears that apoB sequences in the C-terminal half of the molecule, especially those defined by Xiong et al. (i.e., residues 2878-3925), seem to be more competent than the N-terminal half of the molecule in allowing apoB-100 to be tightly associated with the lipoprotein particles during the metabolic conversion of VLDL to LDL when other apoproteins dissociate from the particles.

Only limited information is available on the potential LDL receptor-binding domain of apoB-100. By sequence comparison, two regions of apoB-100, domain A (residues 3147-3157) and domain B (residues 3359-3367), were found to display homology to the apoE receptor-binding domain. They were postulated to be important for LDL receptor binding in apoB-100. Oligopeptide reconstitution experiments indicate that residues 3345-3381, which encompass domain B, may be a bona fide LDL-receptor-binding region for apoB-100 [3].

ApoB-100 is a highly complex protein of enormous size. It has been difficult to study the structure-function relationships of this highly unique protein. Recently, Xiong et al. (Xiong, W., Zsigmond, E., and Chan, L., unpublished observation) generated transgenic mice that produce full-length human apoB-100. The protein was synthesized at high level in the liver and small intestine, and was present in both plasma VLDL and LDL. It is apparent that the transgenic mice serve as a good in vivo model to study apoB-100 function. In future, the production of site-specific apoB mutants in these animals will allow us to study the role of individual amino acid residues in apoB in LDL receptor binding.

References

1. Chen, S.-H., Yang, C.-Y., Chen, P.-F., Setzer, D., Tanimura, M., Li, W.-H., Gotto, A.M.Jr., and Chan, L. (1986) 'The complete cDNA and amino acid sequence of human apolipoprotein B-100', J. Biol. Chem. 261, 12918-12921.
2. Knott, J., Pease, R.J., Powell, L.M., Wallis, S.C., Rall, S.C. Jr., Innerarity, T.L., Blackhart, B., Taylor, W.H., Marcel, Y.L., Milne, R., Johnson, D., Fuller, M., Lusis, A.J., McCarthy, B.J., Mahley, R.W., Levy-Wilson, B., and Scott, J. (1986) 'Complete protein sequence and identification of structural domains of human apolipoprotein B', Nature 323, 734-738.
3. Yang, C-Y., Chen, S-H., Gianturco, S.H., Bradley, W.A., Sparrow, J.T., Tanimura, M., Li, W-H., Sparrow, D.A., DeLoof, H., Rosseneu, M., Lee, F-S., Gu, Z-W., Gotto, A.M., Jr., and Chan, L. (1986) 'Sequence, structure, receptor-binding domains and internal repeats of human apolipoprotein B100', Nature 323, 738-742.
4. Law, S.W., Grant, S.M., Higuchi, K., Hospattankar, A., Lackner, K., Lee, N., and Brewer, H.B., Jr. (1986) 'Human liver apolipoprotein B100 cDNA: complete nucleic acid and derived amino acid sequence', Proc. Natl. Acad. Sci. USA 83, 8142-8146.
5. Cladaras, C., Hadzopoulou-Cladaras, M., Nolte, R.T., Atkinson, D., and Zannis, V.I. (1986) 'The complete sequence and structural analysis of human apolipoprotein B100: relationship between apoB100 and apo-B48 forms', EMBO J. 5, 3495-3507.
6. Yang, C.-Y., Kim, T.W., Pao, Q., Chan, L., Knapp, R.D., Gotto, A.M., Jr., and Pownall, H.J. (1989) 'Structure and conformational analysis of lipid-associating peptides of apolipoprotein B-100 produced by trypsinolysis'. J. Protein Chem. 8, 689-699.
7. Yao, Z., Blackhart, B.D., Linton, M.F., Taylor, S.M., Young, S.G., and McCarthy, B.J. (1991) 'Expression of carboxyl-terminally truncated forms of human apolipoprotein B in rat hepatoma cells', J. Biol. Chem. 266, 3300-3308.
8. Young, S.G. (1990) 'Recent progress in understanding apolipoprotein B', Circulation 82, 1574-1594.
9. Xiong, W., Zsigmond, E., Gotto, A.M. Jr., Lei, K.Y., and Chan, L. (1991) 'Locating a low density lipoprotein-targeting domain of human apolipoprotein B-100 by expressing a minigene construct in transgenic mice', J. Biol. Chem. 266, 20893-20898.

CONTRIBUTION OF HELIX-HELIX INTERACTIONS TO THE STABILITY OF APOLIPOPROTEIN-LIPID COMPLEXES

B. Vanloo, M. Rosseneu, M. De Pauw, L. Lins
R. Brasseur and J-M. Ruysschaert

ABSTRACT. The sequences of the human apo A-I and A-IV proteins contain respectively seven and eleven helical repeats of 17 residues, which were fully characterized. In discoidal lipid-apoprotein complexes, these helixes are oriented parallel to the phospholipid acyl chains around the edge of the disc, and antiparallel to each other. The residues on the side of the contiguous helixes are in close vicinity and can form salt bridges. Computer modeling of apo A-I- and apo A-IV-DPPC discoidal complexes, by energy minimisation procedures, suggests that electrostatic interactions between charged residues can significantly contribute to the stability of the apoprotein-lipid complexes.

INTRODUCTION.

The sequence of the plasma HDL apolipoproteins is characterized by the occurrence of several amphipathic alpha-helical segments of 17 residues (1). Hydrophobic residues are segregated on one face of such amphipathic helix and the hydrophilic residues on the opposite side (2). These helixes have a high degree of internal homology and Segrest et al. (3) proposed that these helixes might be involved in lipid-apolipoprotein binding.

    In the model proposed for the association of the helical amphipathic segments of the apolipoproteins with phospholipids, the helixes are oriented parallel to the phospholipid acyl chains around the edge of the discoidal complexes (4). In apo A-I and apo A-IV, these 17-residue helixes are interrupted by short non-helical peptides,

A. L. Catapano et al. (eds.), Drugs Affecting Lipid Metabolism, 49–56.
© 1993 Kluwer Academic Publishers and Fondazione Giovanni Lorenzini.

most of which contain a proline residue. These segments
have a strong helix-breaking tendency and can be
responsible for the anti-parallel orientation of the
contiguous helixes. In this configuration, the distances
between amino acid residues located along the sides of
adjacent helixes are small (5-10 Å). Ion pairing and salt
bridge formation are therefore theoretically possible
between these residues.

In this paper we carried out a full characterisation
of the amphipathic helixes of apo A-I and apo A-IV and
investigated ionic interactions between contiguous
helixes. An estimation of the stability of the different
pairs of helixes is derived from the calculation of the
energy of interaction between contiguous helixes at a
water/lipid interface after energy minimisation (5). Our
data suggest that ionic interactions can contribute to
the stabilisation of the protein structure in
reconstituted HDL and to the cooperativity of the helixes
of apo A-I and apo A-IV.

CALCULATION METHODS.

The helical repeats identified in apo A-I and A-IV, using
a hydrophobicity autocorrelation matrix, are in agreement
with previous reports (6).

For each pair of helixes, the lowest energy
structure was calculated as the sum of the London-van der
Waals energy, the Coulomb's electrostatic energy and the
potential energy of rotation of the torsional angles.

We considered repeats of apo A-I and A-IV consisting
of two alpha-helical segments separated by a 3-5 residue
peptide. We obtained the lowest energy conformations for
this entire segment by a systematic calculation of the
torsional angles phi and psi for the residues in the
linker peptide using the stereoalphabet procedure (7).
The conformation with the lowest energy was subsequently
obtained using a simplex minimisation procedure (5).

The molecular hydrophobicity potential (MHP) and the
electrostatic potential were calculated (5) for a 39-
residue peptide, consisting of two helixes separated by a
non-helical segment. They were calculated in a plane
perpendicular to the average orientation of the long axes
of the helixes, which was moved every 2 Å along this
direction (6).

The electrostatic energy was calculated for all
positions of an electron moving around the peptide, by
assuming a value of 16.5 for the dielectric constant and
by taking into account all atomic charges of the
molecule. Isoenergetic contour lines were drawn at
distances corresponding to energy differences of 1
Kcal/mol.

The energy of interaction between a pair of helixes was calculated after energy minimisation at the water/lipid interface. This interaction energy consists of the sum of the van der Waals and of the electrostatic energy of interaction as described above (5). Only atomic interactions between contiguous helixes were considered.

Calculations were performed on an Olivetti CP486 microcomputer equipped with an Intel 80486 arithmetic co-processor, using the PC-PROT+ (Proteins Analysis Programs) and the PC-TAMMO+ (Theoretical Analysis of Molecular Membrane Organization) procedures.

RESULTS.

Seven helical repeats in apo A-I and eleven in human apo A-IV were identified and characterized (6). A two-dimensional representation of the electrostatic potential around helical residues 146-162 and 190-206, representative for the helixes of apo A-I, is illustrated on Fig.1. In Fig.1A, there is a clustering of positive charges around the N-terminal and of negative charges around the C-terminal end of the helix, which is typical for most of the helixes of apo A-I. However, in some helixes the charges are evenly distributed along the axis of the helix as illustrated in Fig. 1B.

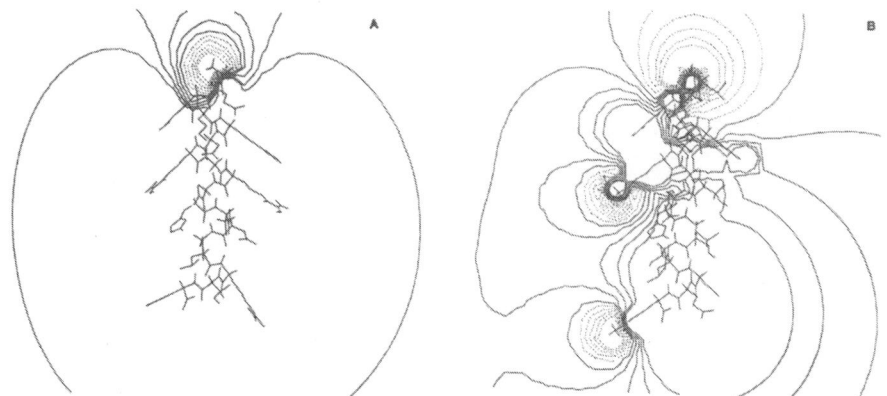

Figure 1. Representation of the electrostatic isopotential lines of 2 helixes of human apo A-I. (—) positive energy and (---) negative energy. A: 146-162; B: 190-206.

In the model previously proposed and supported by experimental data obtained by attenuated total infrared spectroscopy (4, 6), the helical repeats were oriented parallel to the lipid acyl chains. The proline

residues starting the 22-mer repeats created beta-turns,
reversing the orientation of the contiguous helixes (4,
6). The energy minimisation procedure consisted therefore
of the calculation of the most stable structure for two
helixes separated by a three to five residue segment able
to reverse the orientation of the helixes.

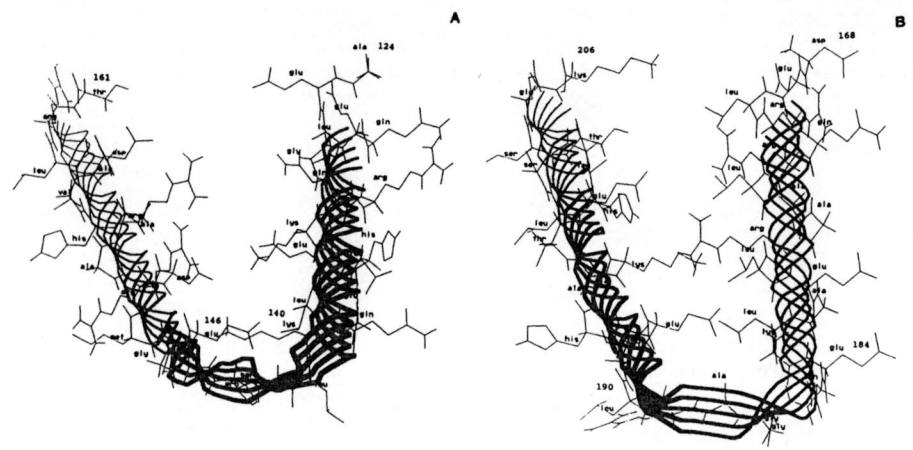

Figure 2. Computer modeling of 2 pairs of helixes
separated by an extended beta-strand in human apo A-I.
The helical residues are A: 124-140; 146-161, B: 168-184;
190-206.The beta-strand residues are A: 141-145, B: 185-
190.

        Such an intervening sequence consisted mostly of a
central proline flanked by one or two residues on each
side.   The   length   of   these   segments   was   varied
systematically   from   three   to   five   residues   and   the
minimal   energy   was   calculated   for   all   structure
combinations.
        The lowest conformational energy was reached when
two   17-residue   helical   segments   were   separated   by   a
stretch   of   five   amino   acids   in   an   extended   beta-strand
conformation. Any other combination of X-Pro-X, X-Pro-X-X
or X-X-Pro-X had a beta-turn configuration and did not
yield any stable structure. This is probably due to the
steric   hindrance   caused   by   the   side   chain   residues
located along the edges of the contiguous helixes such as
arginine,   lysine,   aspartic   and   glutamic   acid.   Five
residues   in   an   extended   beta-strand   conformation   are
therefore a prerequisite to span the distance between the
two helixes. The 17-residue helical repeats of apo A-I
and A-IV and the corresponding beta-strands are listed in
Table   2.   As   previously   described   (6),   these   helixes
have a high degree of homology both within and between

apoprotein sequences. The sequences of the beta-strands are also highly homologous and a consensus sequence of L-X-P-L-L and L-X-P-L-A can be derived for apo A-I and A-IV respectively.

A systematic analysis of the angles phi and psi followed by the Simplex energy minimisation method show that the axes of the helixes of apo A-I and A-IV are almost parallel in the lowest energy structure (Fig.2), with angles varying between 0 and 25°. The residues susceptible to form salt bridges between contiguous helixes in apo A-I and A-IV, are either conserved in the different species or replaced by residues with the same charge (6).

TABLE 1: Sequences of the helical and extended beta-strand segments in apo A-I and apo A-IV.

BETA-STRANDS		HELICAL REPEATS	
APO A-I		**APO A-I**	
64-68	LGPVT	102-118	DDFQKKWQEEMELYRQK
97-101	VQPYL	124-140	AELQEGARQKLHELQEK
119-123	VEPLR	146-162	EEMRDRARAHVDALRTH
141-145	LSPLG	168-184	DELRQRLAARLEALKEN
163-167	LAPYS	190-206	AEYHAKATEHLSTLSEK
185-189	GGARL	223-239	ESFKVSFLSALEEYTKK
207-211	AKPAL		
CONSENSUS	LXPLL		
APO A-IV		**APO A-IV**	
60-64	LVPFA	98-114	NEVSQKIGDNLRELQQR
93-97	LLPHA	120-136	DQLRTQVNTQAEQLRRQ
115-119	LEPYA	142-158	QRMERVLRENADSLQAS
137-141	LDPLA	164-180	DELKAKIDQNVEELKGR
159-163	LRPHA	186-202	DEFKVKIDQTVEELRRS
181-185	LTPYA	208-224	QDTQEKLNHQLEGLTFQ
203-207	LAPYA	230-246	EELKARISASAEELRQR
225-229	KKNA	252-268	EDVRGNLKGNTEGLQKS
247-251	LAPLA	292-308	ENFNKALVQQMEQLRQK
287-291	VEPYG	314-330	GDVEGHLSFLEKDLRDK
309-313	LGPHA		
CONSENSUS	LXPLA		

The interaction energy of a pair of helixes separated by a beta-strand segment at a lipid/water interface is calculated as the sum of van der Waals and electrostatic interactions between respectively induced and permanent dipoles, and of hydrophobic interactions calculated as

TABLE 2. Interaction energies (Kcal/mole peptide) between pairs of helixes of apo A-I linked by an extended beta-strand.

1st	helices Beta-strand	2nd	E_{tot}	$E_{v.d.W.}$	E_{pho}	$E_{electr.}$
102-118	119-123	124-140	0.1	-0.3	0.2	0.2
124-140	141-145	146-162	-9.2	-2.5	0	-6.7
146-162	163-167	168-184	-7.1	-0.8	0.04	-6.4
168-184	185-189	190-206	-9.2	-0.9	0.3	-8.7

the energy of transfer from an aqueous to an apolar phase. These energies listed in Table 2 for the pairs of adjacent helixes in apo A-I, show that the most stable pairs are 124-162 and 168-206. The greater stability of these pairs of helixes was predominantly due to stronger electrostatic interactions.

The electrostatic and hydrophobic potentials around the pair of helixes spanning residues 146-184 of apo A-I are illustrated in Fig.4 and 5. The 3D representation of the electrostatic potential shows that in a phospholipid-peptide complex, most of the negatively charged residues are on the outer face of the helixes facing the aqueous

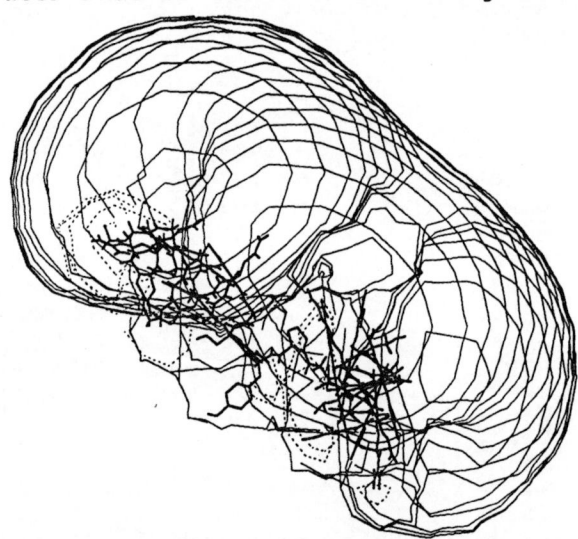

Figure 4. Representation of the electrostatic isopotential lines for the pair of helixes of apo A-I between residues 146-184. (———) positive energy, (---) negative energy.

phase. In contrast most of the positive arginine and
lysine residues occur along the edge of the helixes and
are involved in salt bridge formation with residues of
opposite charge.
Fig.5 illustrates the hydrophobic and hydrophilic
potentials around the same pair of helixes. It clearly
shows that the two hydrophobic faces are directed towards
the lipid core and the hydrophilic sides of the helixes
are directed towards the aqueous phase.

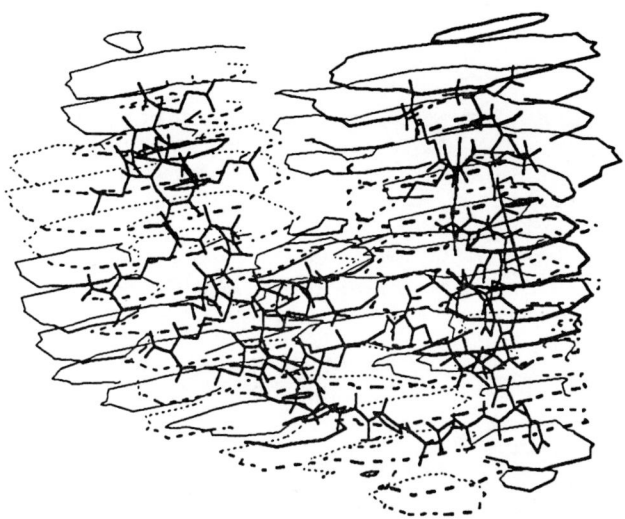

Figure 5. Representation of the hydrophilic (——) and
hydrophobic (---) isopotential lines for the pair of
helixes of apo A-I between residues 146-184.

DISCUSSION.

According to the conformational analysis of the helixes
of apo A-I and A-IV, ionic interactions between residues
of contiguous helical repeats can significantly
contribute to the stabilisation of the apoprotein-
phospholipid discoidal complexes. Such interactions
probably account for the high cooperativity observed in
apoprotein-lipid complex formation.
The importance of the cooperativity between
apolipoprotein helical repeats was further supported by
the results obtained with synthetic peptide analogs.
Segrest et al.(3) showed that the LCAT activation and the
surface properties of dimeric peptides consisting of two
helical repeats separated by a proline, mimicked more
closely the properties of an apoprotein than any
monomeric peptide. The role of the beta-strand segment to
ensure a proper match of the apolar faces of the helixes

seems therefore critical. Moreover, the crystal structure of the N-terminal domain of apo E (8) shows that it consists of four helixes which form a 2 by 2 bundle. Most of the charged residues, including 24 acidic and 24 basic amino acids, participate in intramolecular salt bridges, seven of which between pairs of helixes.
We postulate that the same type of interaction is responsible for the cooperativity of the phospholipid transition in the apo A-I and A-IV complexes and probably in other apoproteins including apo E.

REFERENCES.

1. Boguski, M. S.,Freeman, M., Elshourbagy, N. A.,Taylor, J. M., and Gordon, J. I. (1986) 'On computer-assisted analysis of biological sequences: proline punctuation, consensus sequences, and apolipoprotein repeats', J. Lipid Res. 27, 1011-1034.
2. Segrest, J. P., Jackson, R. L., Morrisett, J. D., and Gotto, A. M. (1974) 'A molecular theory of lipid-protein interactions in the plasma lipoproteins', FEBS Lett. 38, 247-253.
3. Segrest, J. P., De Loof, H., Dohlman, J. G., Brouillette, C. G., and Anantharamaiah, G. M. (1990) 'Amphipathic helix motif: classes and properties', Proteins 8, 103-117.
4. Brasseur, R., De Meutter, J., Vanloo, B., Goormaghtigh, E., Ruysschaert, J. M., and Rosseneu, M. (1990) 'Mode of assembly of amphipathic helical segments in model high density lipoproteins', Biochim. Biophys. Acta. 1043, 245-252.
5. Brasseur, R. (1988) 'Calculation of the three-dimensional structure of saccharomyces cerevisiae cytochrome b inserted in a lipid matrix', J. Biol. Chem. 263, 12571-12575.
6. Brasseur, R., Lins, L.., Vanloo, B., Ruysschaert, J. M., and Rosseneu, M. (1992) 'Molecular modelling of the amphipathic helixes of the plasma apolipoproteins' Proteins: Structure, Function, and Genetics 13, 246-257.
7. De Coen, J. L., and Ralston, E. (1973) 'Conformational energy of peptides: application to the study of the conformation of oxytocin-like peptides' in H. Nesvada (ed), Peptides, North-Holland Publishers, Amsterdam, pp. 335-342.
8. Wilson, C., Wardell, M. R., Weisgraber, K. H., Mahley, R. W., and Agard, D. A. (1991) 'Three-dimensional structure of the LDL receptor binding domain of human apo E', Science 252, 1817-1822.

Oxidatively Modified LDL and Atherosclerosis

DANIEL STEINBERG, M.D., Ph.D.

Abstract

A growing body of evidence indicates that oxidative modification of LDL enhances its potential atherogenicity in a number of different ways. It has also been clearly demonstrated that oxidative modification <u>does</u> occur *in vivo* and that administration of some antioxidant compounds slows the progression of atherosclerosis in LDL receptor-deficient rabbits and in cholesterol-fed rabbits. Whether the antiatherosclerotic effect of these compounds is limited to their ability to directly protect LDL against oxidation or whether they have significant additional biological effects is not clear. Recent studies on the mechanisms that may be involved in cell-catalyzed oxidation of LDL are reviewed and discussed. Finally, the pros and cons of undertaking clinical testing of the oxidative modification hypothesis are presented.

INTRODUCTION

The oxidative modification hypothesis (1) proposes that native low density lipoprotein (LDL) has only a limited atherogenic potential compared to that of oxidatively modified LDL (Ox-LDL). Actually the hypothesis also implies that the difference is large enough such that inhibition of LDL oxidation should slow the progression of atherosclerotic lesions. Several recent reviews have summarized the extensive and growing body of evidence that oxidative modification of LDL does indeed occur *in vivo* and that inhibition of oxidation of LDL can slow the progression of atherosclerotic lesions, at least in experimental animals (2-8). The purpose of the present paper is to highlight some recent advances in our understanding of the mechanisms involved in oxidation of LDL, the many different ways in which it is potentially more atherogenic than native LDL, the evidence that antioxidants work *in vivo* in experimental animals, and the evidence, still quite limited, that the hypothesis may hold for the human disease.

A. L. Catapano et al. (eds.), Drugs Affecting Lipid Metabolism, 57–68.

MECHANISMS OF LDL OXIDATION

The fact that LDL is extremely labile and undergoes spontaneous oxidative damage in the presence of copper or iron has been known for many years. These transition metals catalyze the conversion of lipid hydroperoxides to peroxy radicals, initiating a chain reaction or propagation reaction that dramatically increases the number of lipid hydroperoxides per particle. Esterbauer has proposed (9) that the LDL particles must contain at least one (or a few) lipid hydroperoxides if this mechanism is to operate. The fact that cell-catalyzed oxidation of LDL is blocked by the chelation of metal ions suggests that similar considerations apply to cell-catalyzed LDL oxidation. A central issue then becomes: How is the *first* lipid peroxide introduced? Two general possibilities suggest themselves:

1.   *The cells release reactive forms of oxygen that can generate lipid peroxides in LDL in the surrounding medium.*

Superoxide anion is the most likely participant because it is reasonably stable and can readily cross the plasma membrane. Hydrogen peroxide is another plausible candidate. Hydroxyl radicals are much too short-lived and too highly reactive for this role. Superoxide anion itself is probably incapable of directly oxidizing lipids (10). However, in the presence of transition metals it can give rise to hydroxyl radicals which are highly reactive. This might account for the requirement for metal ions in the medium during oxidative modification of LDL. Recent studies show that LDL has copper ion closely associated with it, although that copper can be mostly removed by treatment with EDTA (11).

The oxidation of LDL by smooth muscle cells, monocytes and fibroblasts (12-14) is strongly inhibited by superoxide dismutase (SOD), implying an important role for superoxide anion in these systems. On the other hand, SOD has very little effect on oxidation of LDL by macrophages (15) and by endothelial cells (16). Obviously different mechanisms can be operative in different cell types. Furthermore, it is perfectly possible that any given cell type may utilize more than one mechanism.

The cell sources of superoxide anion that are important in LDL oxidation have yet to be identified. Xanthine oxidase would be a candidate but studies in our laboratory failed to show any effect of allopurinol on cell-induced oxidation of LDL (S. Parthasarathy, unpublished results). DPNH oxidase is a major source of superoxide anion, especially in activated leukocytes. Resting monocytes, however, release very little and yet they are perfectly capable of oxidizing LDL. Whether or not activation of leukocytes importantly enhances LDL oxidation remains unclear and certainly has yet to be tested *in vivo*. In principle, *any* of the systems that are involved in electron transport could be sources of superoxide anion but there is thus far little work assessing their roles.

2. *The cells first oxidize their own membrane lipids and then transfer lipid hydroperoxides to the LDL in the surrounding medium.*

Cyclooxygenase and lipoxygenase are the two best-studied membrane enzymes that can directly oxidize fatty acids. A role for cyclooxygenase has been ruled out on the basis of studies showing no inhibition by aspirin or indomethacin (15,16). Several lines of evidence have been presented compatible with a significant role for lipoxygenase, at least in the case of macrophages and endothelial cells. These lines of evidence include the following: 1) purified soybean lipoxygenase in a cell-free system can oxidatively modify LDL (17); 2) a number of lipoxygenase inhibitors, including inhibitors that are *not* themselves nonspecific antioxidants, inhibit the oxidative modification of LDL by endothelial cells and macrophages (15, 16); 3) macrophage-rich atherosclerotic lesions strongly express mRNA for 15-lipoxygenase (15-LO) and also stain positively for 15-LO protein (18,19); interestingly, mRNA for 5-LO and 12-LO were not detectable using similar methods; 4) incubation of labeled arachidonic acid with lesioned rabbit aortic tissue generates 15-LO products whereas incubation with normal rabbit artery does not (20).

Recent studies have added further evidence supporting a role for 15-LO. Conrad *et al.* (21) have found that interleukin-4, and only interleukin-4 among the large number of cytokines tested, dramatically increases the expression of 15-LO in monocytes. In collaboration with Dr. Sara M. Rankin and Dr. Sampath Parthasarathy, we have shown that IL-4 treatment of freshly isolated human monocytes almost doubles the rate at which they can oxidatively modify LDL (assessed in terms of the rate at which the Ox-LDL is degraded by macrophages). As shown in Table 1 this increased

TABLE 1. Interleukin-4 stimulates monocyte oxidation of LDL

LDL Treatment	Macrophage Degradation ($\mu g/5h/mg$)
No cell control	1.21 ± 0.46
Incubated with monocytes	2.28 ± 0.53
Incubated with monocytes + IL-4	4.72 ± 1.09
Incubated with monocytes + IL-4 + 20 μM indomethacin	4.25 ± 1.16
Incubated with monocytes + IL-4 + 20 μM ETYA	2.23 ± 0.61

ability to oxidatively modify LDL was not inhibited by indomethacin but was inhibited by ETYA, as would be expected if the increase were attributable to an increase in 15-LO activity. We might note parenthetically that circulating monocytes exhibit almost no detectable 15-LO activity and yet they do oxidatively modify LDL, albeit at a low rate. Thus it is clear that different mechanisms for oxidative modification can be operative in a given cell type. A major source of IL-4 is the T-cell and it is now generally accepted that a significant number of T-cells is present even in very early atherosclerotic lesions (22). Moreover, these are in an activated state (23) and could thus very well be producing significant amounts of lymphokines, including IL-4. Whether or not this kind of T-lymphocyte-monocyte interaction is important in the atherogenic process remains to be established.

Sparrow and Olszewski (24), while confirming that ETYA can inhibit both the 15-LO activity of macrophages and their ability to oxidatively modify LDL, call attention to a striking difference in the concentrations of inhibitor required. They suggest that the difference is so large that 15-LO is unlikely to be involved in macrophage oxidation of LDL. This might be persuasive if one knew that 15-LO activity is *rate-limiting* in LDL oxidation by cells but we do not know that. After the membrane cell lipids have been oxidized, they must be transferred to the LDL particle in the medium. After that, there must be a series of propagation reactions and a host of complex secondary changes that eventually alter the configuration of LDL to one recognized by the scavenger receptor. *Any* of these many steps might in fact be the rate-limiting step. Furthermore, the assay of 15-LO activity utilized a 30-min exposure of cells to labeled linoleic acid whereas the assay for LDL oxidation involved an overnight incubation. Finally, the kinetics may be quite different when the substrate is free linoleic acid and when the substrate is a complex mixture of membrane phospholipids. As reported at these meetings by Ho *et al.* (25), a partially purified rabbit reticulocyte 15-LO showed an IC_{50} for ETYA of 0.03 μM when linoleic acid was the substrate. When LDL was the substrate the IC_{50} was 50-fold greater (15 μM).

MECHANISMS BY WHICH OX-LDL IS POTENTIALLY MORE ATHEROGENIC THAN NATIVE LDL

The oxidative modification hypothesis was put forward initially to account for the generation of foam cells from monocyte/macrophages (26,27), but it very quickly became clear that Ox-LDL might be atherogenic in additional ways. It was found to be chemotactic for monocytes (but not for neutrophils) (28); it was found to inhibit the motility of tissue macrophages (29); and, as shown by Morel, DiCorleto and Chisolm, it was cytotoxic, at least in the absence of serum proteins (30). Over the past several years Ox-LDL has been shown to have a large number of additional biological properties:

TABLE 2. Biological Properties of Oxidized LDL

1.	Recognized by scavenger receptor(s) (26,27).
2.	Chemotactic for monocytes (28).
3.	Inhibits macrophage motility (29).
4.	Cytotoxic (30).
5.	Immunogenic (31).
6.	Stimulates release of MCP-1 from endothelial cells and SMC (32).
7.	Stimulates release of MCSF from endothelial cells (33).
8.	Inhibits EDRF-dependent arterial dilatation (34).
9.	Activates T-cells (35).
10.	Increases adhesion of monocyte to endothelial cells (36-38).
*11.	Inhibits PDGF secretion by macrophages (39).
12.	Increases expression of tissue factor activity on endothelial cells (40,41).
13.	Stimulates endothelin secretion by macrophages (42).
14.	Increases glutathione content of macrophages (43).
15.	Increases secretion of plasminogen activator inhibitor-1 (AI-1) by endothelial cells (44).
16.	Increases release of interleukin-1 from monocyte/macrophages (35,45).

* The only property that might be *anti*atherogenic.

Some of these biological effects can be seen in LDL that has undergone only minimal degrees of oxidative modification. Thus the ability of Ox-LDL to stimulate release of MCP-1 and of MCSF, as studied in Dr. Alan Fogelman's laboratory, can be conferred by minimal oxidation and they have referred to such oxidized LDL as "MM-LDL" (32,33). The extent of oxidation in "MM-LDL" is so slight that it is still a ligand for the LDL receptor (and is *not* a ligand for the acetyl LDL receptor). As discussed in detail elsewhere (2), the oxidation of LDL involves a continuum of changes and it is necessary to specify exactly how a given preparation of "Ox-LDL" was made. Alternatively (or in addition) investigators should utilize one or more criteria for characterizing Ox-LDL preparations operationally (e.g., potency in stimulating release of MCP-1, cytotoxicity, chemotactic activity, etc.).

The fact that Ox-LDL can stimulate the release of IL-1 is especially pertinent to the transition from fatty streak lesion to fibrous plaque. That transition presumably depends upon the stimulation of smooth muscle cell growth and the deposition of connective tissue matrix. Ox-LDL could, as we now understand it, play a role in this key transition.

The inhibition of endothelial-dependent relaxation by Ox-LDL implies the possibility that abnormalities in vascular tone could begin even before there are mechanical factors affecting constriction and dilatation of the artery.

In summary, there are now 15 or more potential links between Ox-LDL and atherosclerosis and its complications. Which of these are pathophysiologically important will only emerge after appropriate *in vivo* studies have been done.

THE EVIDENCE *IN VIVO* THAT OXIDATIVE MODIFICATION OF LDL IS SIGNIFICANT

The evidence that oxidative modification of LDL does indeed occur *in vivo* has been summarized elsewhere (1,2). The most critical evidence comes from animal studies showing that antioxidants slow the progression of experimental atherosclerosis, as summarized in Table 3. The list is confined to those studies in which the design limited the possibility that the effect might be due to a cholesterol-lowering effect of the drug. There are a number of other studies in which antioxidant compounds, including probucol, have been administered and in which an antiatherosclerotic effect has been seen, but because there were significant differences in cholesterol levels the observed effects can't necessarily be ascribed to the antioxidant properties of the drug administered.

TABLE 3. Effects of Antioxidants in Experimental Atherosclerosis

Agent	Reduction in Lesion Area	Authors
1) Probucol in WHHL rabbits	87%	Kita *et al.* (46)
2) Probucol in WHHL rabbits	70%	Carew *et al.* (47)
3) Probucol (and its analogues) in WHHL rabbits	30-42%	Mao *et al.* (48)
4) Probucol in cholesterol-fed rabbits	No effect	Stein *et al.* (49)
5) Probucol in cholesterol-fed rabbits	79%	Daugherty *et al.* (50)
6) Butylated hydroxytoluene in cholesterol-fed rabbits	70%	Björkhem *et al.* (51)
7) N,N'-diphenyl-phenylenediamine in cholesterol fed rabbits	71%	Sparrow *et al.* (52)

Six of the seven studies showed a significant inhibitory effect of the antioxidant. The reason for the absence of an effect in the study by Stein *et al.* (49), even though it was quite similar in design to that of Daugherty *et al.* (50), is not apparent. The recent studies using antioxidants other than probucol (51,52) are especially welcome because probucol has a number of biological effects in addition to its antioxidant effect. The fact that butylated hydroxytoluene and N,N'-diphenyl-phenylenediamine also work suggests that the results obtained with probucol *do* relate to its properties as an antioxidant, at least in part. It is still possible that some of the other biological effects of probucol contribute to its overall effectiveness. Indeed, recent studies in this laboratory suggest that probucol could have important effects *within* the cell.

We had shown previously that endothelial cell or macrophages previously incubated with probucol, washed and then allowed to act on LDL were less able to oxidize it. However, since probucol is highly insoluble, it could not be ruled out that some of the drug remained adsorbed to the cell surface after washing and took up residence in the LDL added in the subsequent incubation, i.e., enough to protect it against oxidative modification. Dr. Parthasarathy devised a probucol analog -- probucol diglutarate -- which is highly water-soluble and which regenerates probucol spontaneously at a slow rate (53). This made it possible to incubate cells with the water-soluble derivative in order to increase the intracellular concentration of the drug and then wash to remove the drug in the medium. As shown in Table 4, these pretreated cells showed a markedly reduced capacity to oxidatively modify fresh LDL added to the medium. The implication is that probucol can act *intracellularly* to inhibit cell-catalyzed oxidation of LDL.

TABLE 4. Evidence that Probucol May Act Intracellularly to Inhibit LDL Oxidation

Mouse peritoneal macrophages were preincubated 3 hr with probucol diglutarate, a highly water-soluble derivative, the medium was changed, and LDL was added for a second incubation (24 hr). Oxidation of LDL was assessed in terms of thiobarbituric-reactive substances (TBARS) and the rate of degradation by macrophages (Mac. Degn.)

	TBARS nmol/mg protein	Mac. Degn. (μg/5 hr/ mg protein)
Unincubated LDL	3.2	1.5
LDL + untreated macrophages	21.8	5.5
LDL + macrophages pretreated with probucol diglutarate (30 μM)	3.3	1.4

In view of these findings, it is important that we not jump to the conclusion that the relative efficacy of antioxidants in relationship to atherogenesis can be inferred by simply measuring the extent to which the circulating LDL is protected against oxidation. If the intracellular site of action is important, different antioxidants could differ widely in their effectiveness against atherosclerosis even though they are similar in terms of how well they protect the isolated LDL particle against oxidation.

RELEVANCE OF OXIDATIVE MODIFICATION TO THE HUMAN DISEASE

There is as yet no large, double blind intervention study to demonstrate that anti-oxidants affect the human disease. The closest we can come is the preliminary report from the Physicians' Health Survey presented at the 1990 meetings of the American Heart Association (54). The Physicians' Health Survey was undertaken to test the hypothesis that aspirin might prevent coronary heart disease and that β-carotene might prevent cancer. In view of the emerging evidence that oxidative modification of LDL might play a role in atherogenesis, a subset of the men who had clinical evidence of coronary artery disease at the beginning of the study (some seven years ago) was examined for the possibility that β-carotene might be having an effect on coronary events. Indeed, it was reported that in this subset the men on β-carotene had a significantly lower number of major cardiovascular events (infarction, bypass surgery, angioplasty or stroke). The results were marginally significant at a little less than $p = 0.05$. The study is continuing with the major cohort of over 20,000 men (who did not have clinical coronary disease at the beginning of the study) and data should become available in about three or four years.

In September of 1991 the National Heart, Lung, and Blood Institute sponsored a workshop on "Antioxidants and Atherosclerosis" which I was privileged to chair (55). About 40 experts on various aspects of the problem spent a day and a half reviewing all of the relevant evidence relating to the oxidative modification hypothesis. Their conclusion was that the case was strong enough to justify clinical intervention trials at this time using natural antioxidants. Used at reasonable doses, the natural antioxidants (β-carotene, alpha-tocopherol, ascorbic acid) are without toxic side effects and their use can be justified to explore this hypothesis in humans. The group felt that it was premature to launch intervention trials using drugs, however. There is intense interest in this problem and some studies are already under way. A definitive answer could be available in a matter of four or five years.

References

1. Steinberg, D., Parthasarathy, S., Carew, T.E., Khoo, J.C. and Witztum, J.L. (1989) 'Beyond cholesterol: modifications of low density lipoprotein that increase its atherogenicity', N. Engl. J. Med. 320, 915-924.
2. Witztum, J.L. and Steinberg, D. (1991) 'Role of oxidized low density lipoproteins in atherogenesis', J. Clin. Invest. 88, 1785-1792.
3. Hoff, H.F. and O'Neil, J.A. (1991) 'Oxidation of LDL: role in athero-genesis', Klinische Wochenschrift 69, 1032-1038.
4. Steinbrecher, U.P. (1991) 'Role of lipoprotein peroxidation in the pathogenesis of atherosclerosis', Clin. Cardiol. 14, 865-867.
5. Chisolm, G.M. III (1991) 'Antioxidants and atherosclerosis: a current assessment', Clin. Cardiol. 14, I25-I30.
6. Luc, G. and Fruchart, J.C (1991) 'Oxidation of lipoproteins and atherosclerosis', Am. J. Clin. Nutr. 53, 206S-209S.

7. Ylä-Herttuala, S. (1991) 'Biochemistry of the arterial wall in developing atherosclerosis', Ann. N.Y. Acad. Sci. 623, 40-59.
8. Parthasarathy, S., Steinberg, D. and Witztum, J.L. (1992) 'The role of oxidized low density lipoproteins in the pathogenesis of atherosclerosis', Ann. Rev. Med. 43, 219-225.
9. Esterbauer, H., Rotheneder, M., Striegl, G., Waeg, G., Ashy, A., Sattler, W. and Jürgens, G. (1989) 'Vitamin E and other lipophilic antioxidants protect LDL against oxidation', Fat Sci. Technol. 91, 316-324.
10. Bedwell, S. and Jessup, W. (1987) 'Effects of oxygen-centered free radicals on low density lipoprotein structure and metabolism', Biochem. Soc. Trans. 15, 259-260.
11. Kuzuya, M., Yamada, K., Hayashi, T., Naito, M., Asai, K. and Kuzuya, F. (1992) 'Role of lipoprotein-copper complex in copper catalyzed peroxidation of low density lipoprotein', Biochim. Biophys. Acta 1123, 334-341.
12. Hiramatsu, K., Rosen, H., Heinecke, J.W., Wolfbauer, G. and Chait, A. (1987) 'Superoxide initiates oxidation of low density lipoprotein by human monocytes', Arteriosclerosis 7, 55-60.
13. Cathcart, M.K., McNally, A.K., Morel, D.W. and Chisolm, G.M. (1989) 'Superoxide anion participation in human monocyte-mediated oxidation of low density lipoprotein and conversion of low density lipoprotein to a cytotoxin', J. Immunol. 142, 196-199.
14. Heinecke, J.W., Baker, L., Rosen, H. and Chait, A. (1986) 'Superoxide-mediated modification of low density lipoprotein by arterial smooth muscle cells', J. Clin. Invest. 77, 757-761.
15. Rankin, S.M., Parthasarathy, S. and Steinberg, D. (1991) 'Evidence for a dominant role of lipoxygenase(s) in the oxidation of LDL by mouse peritoneal macrophages', J. Lipid Res. 32, 449-456.
16. Parthasarathy, S., Wieland, E. and Steinberg, D. (1989) A role for endothelial cell lipoxygenase in the oxidative modification of low density lipoprotein', Proc. Natl. Acad. Sci. USA 86, 1046-1050.
17. Sparrow, C.P., Parthasarathy, S. and Steinberg, D. (1988) 'Enzymatic modification of low density lipoprotein by purified lipoxygenase plus phospholipase A2 mimics cell-mediated oxidative modification', J. Lipid Res. 29, 745-753.
18. Ylä-Herttuala, S., Rosenfeld, M.E., Parthasarathy, S., Glass, C.K., Sigal, E., Witztum, J.L. and Steinberg, D. (1990) 'Colocalization of 15-lipoxygenase mRNA and protein with epitopes of oxidized low density lipoprotein in macrophage-rich areas of atherosclerotic lesions', Proc. Natl. Acad. Sci. USA 87, 6959-6963.
19. Ylä-Herttuala, S., Rosenfeld, M.E., Parthasarathy, S., Sigal, E., Särkioja, T., Witztum, J.L. and Steinberg, D. (1991) 'Gene expression in macrophage-rich human atherosclerotic lesions. 15-lipoxygenase and acetyl low density lipoprotein receptor messenger RNA colocalize with oxidation specific lipid-protein adducts', J. Clin. Invest. 87, 1146-1152.

20. Henriksson, P., Hamberg, M. and Diczfalusy, U. (1985) 'Formation of 15-HETE as a major hydroxyeicosatetraenoic acid in the atherosclerotic vessel wall', Biochim. Biophys. Acta 834, 272-274.

21. Conrad, D.J., Kuhn, H., Mulkins, M., Highland, E. and Sigal, E. (1992) 'Specific inflammatory cytokines regulate the expression of human monocyte 15-lipoxygenase', Proc. Natl. Acad. Sci. USA 89, 217-221.

22. Jonasson, L., Holm, J., Skalli, O., Gabbiani, G., Bondjers, G. and Hansson, G.K. (1986) 'Regional accumulation of T-cells, macrophages and smooth muscle cells in the human atherosclerotic plaque', Arteriosclerosis 6, 131-138.

23. Hansson, G.K., Holm, J. and Jonasson, L. (1989) 'Detection of activated T lymphocytes in the human atherosclerotic plaque', Am. J. Pathol. 135, 169-175.

24. Sparrow, C.P. and Olszewski, J. (1992) 'Cellular oxidative modification of low density lipoprotein does not require lipoxygenases', Proc. Natl. Acad. Sci. USA 89, 128-131.

25. Ho, P.P.K., Towner, R.D. and Lin, C.C. (1992) 'Enzymatic modification of low density lipoprotein by a mammalian 15-lipoxygenase mimics oxidative modification by intact macrophages,' XI International Symposium on Drugs Affecting Lipid Metabolism, p. 98 (abstract); Circulation, in press.

26. Henriksen, T., Mahoney, E.M. and Steinberg, D. (1981) 'Enhanced macrophage degradation of low density lipoprotein previously incubated with cultured endothelial cells: recognition by receptors for acetylated low density lipoproteins', Proc. Natl. Acad. Sci. USA 78, 6499-6503.

27. Steinbrecher, U.P., Parthasarathy, S., Leake, D.S., Witztum, J.L. and Steinberg, D. (1984) 'Modification of low density lipoprotein by endothelial cells involves lipid peroxidation and degradation of low density lipoprotein phospholipids', Proc. Natl. Acad. Sci. USA 81, 3883-3887.

28. Quinn, M.T., Parthasarathy, S. and Steinberg, D. (1985) 'Endothelial cell-derived chemotactic activity for mouse peritoneal macrophages and the effects of modified forms of low density lipoprotein', Proc. Natl. Acad. Sci. USA 82, 5949-5953.

29. Quinn, M.T., Parthasarathy, S., Fong, L.G. and Steinberg, D. (1987) 'Oxidatively modified low density lipoproteins: a potential role in recruitment and retention of monocyte/macrophages during atherogenesis', Proc. Natl. Acad. Sci. USA 84, 2995-2998.

30. Morel, D.W., DiCorleto, P.E. and Chisolm, G.M. (1984) 'Endothelial and smooth muscle cells alter low density lipoprotein in vitro by free radical oxidation', Arteriosclerosis 4, 357-364.

31. Palinski, W., Ylä-Herttuala, S., Rosenfeld, M.E., Butler, S.W., Socher, S.A., Parthasarathy, S., Curtiss, L.K. and Witztum, J.L. (1990) 'Antisera and monoclonal antibodies specific for epitopes generated during oxidative modification of low density lipoprotein', Arteriosclerosis 10, 325-335.

32. Cushing, S.D., Berliner, J.A., Valente, A.J. et al. (1990) 'Minimally

modified low-density lipoprotein induces monocyte chemotactic protein 1 in human endothelial cells and smooth muscle cells', Proc. Natl. Acad. Sci. USA 87, 5134-5138.

33. Rajavashisth, T.B., Andalibi, A., Territo, M.C., *et al.* (1990) 'Induction of endothelial cell expression of granulocyte and macrophage colony-stimulating factors by modified low density lipoproteins', Nature, 344, 254-257.

34. Kugiyama, K., Kerns, S.A., Morrisett, J.D., Roberts, R. and Henry, P.D. (1990) 'Impairment of endothelium-dependent arterial relaxation by lysolecithin in modified low density lipoproteins', Nature 344, 160-162.

35. Frostegard, J., Wu, R., Giscombe, R., Holm, G., Lefvert, A.K. and Nilsson, J. (1992) 'Induction of T-cell activation by oxidized low density lipoprotein', Arterio. Thromb. 12, 461-467.

36. Berliner, J.A., Territo, H.C., Sevanian, A., Ramin, S., Kim, J.A., Banishad, B., Esterson, M. and Fogelman, A.M. (1990) 'Minimally modified low density lipoprotein stimulates monocyte endothelial interactions', J. Clin. Invest. 85, 1260-1266.

37. Frostegard, J., Haegerstrand, A., Gidlund, M. and Nilsson, J. (1991) 'Biologically modified LDL increases the adhesive properties of endothelial cells', Atherosclerosis 90, 119-126.

38. Lehr, H.A., Hubner, C., Nolte, D., Finckh, B., Beisiegel, U., Kohlschutter, A. and Messmer, K. (1991) 'Oxidatively modified human low density lipoprotein stimulates leukocyte adherence to the microvascular endothelium in vivo', Res. Exper. Med. 191, 85-90.

39. Malden, L.T., Chait, A., Raines, E.W. and Ross, R. (1991) 'The influence of oxidatively modified low density lipoproteins on expression of platelet-derived growth factor by human monocyte-derived macrophages', J. Biol. Chem. 266, 13901-13907.

40. Weis, J.R., Pitas, R.E., Wilson, B.D. and Rodgers, G.M. (1991) 'Oxidized low density lipoprotein increases cultured human endothelial cell tissue factor activity and reduces protein C activation', FASEB J. 5, 2459-2465.

41. Drake, T.A., Hannani, K., Fei, H.H., Lavi, S. and Berliner, J.A. (1991) 'Minimally oxidized low density lipoprotein induces tissue factor expression in cultured human endothelial cells', Am. J. Pathol. 138, 601-607.

42. Martin-Nizard, F., Houssani, H.S., Lestavel-Delattre, S., Duriez, P. and Fruchart, J.C. (1991) 'Modified low density lipoproteins activate human macrophages to secrete immunoreactive endothelin', FEBS Letters 293, 127-130.

43. Darley-Usmar, V.M., Severn, A., O'Leary, V.J. and Rogers, M. (1991) 'Treatment of macrophages with oxidized low density lipoprotein increases their intracellular glutathione content', Biochem. J. 278, 429-434.

44. Latron, Y., Chautan, M., Anfosso, F., Alessi, M.C., Nalbone, G., Lafont, H. and Juhan-Vague, I. (1991) 'Stimulating effect of oxidized low density lipoproteins on plasminogen activator inhibitor-1 synthesis by endothelial cells', Arterio. Thromb. 11, 1821-1829.

45.   Ku, G., Doherty, N.S., Wolos, J.A. and Jackson, R.L. (1988) 'Inhibition by probucol of interleukin-1 secretion and its implication in atherosclerosis', Am. J. Cardiol. 62, 77B-81B.

46.   Kita, T., Nagano, Y., Yokode, M., Ishii, K., Kume, N., Ooshima, A., Yoshida, H. and Kawai, C. (1987) 'Probucol prevents the progression of atherosclerosis in Watanabe heritable hyperlipidemic rabbit, an animal model for familial hypercholesterolemia', Proc. Natl. Acad. Sci. USA 84, 5928-5931.

47.   Carew, T.E., Schwenke, D.C. and Steinberg, D. (1987) 'Antiatherogenic effect of probucol unrelated to its hypocholesterolemic effect: Evidence that antioxidants in vivo can selectively inhibit low density lipoprotein degradation in macrophage-rich fatty streaks slowing the progression of atherosclerosis in the WHHL rabbit' Proc. Natl. Acad. Sci. USA 84, 7725-7729.

48.   Mao, S.J.T., Yates, M.T., Rechtin, A.E., Jackson, R.L. and Van Sickle, W.A. (1991) 'Antioxidant activity of probucol and its analogues in hypercholesterolemic Watanabe rabbits', J. Med. Chem. 34, 298-302.

49.   Stein, Y., Stein, O., Delplanque, B., Fesmire, J.D., Lee, D.M. and Alaupovic, P. (1989) 'Lack of effect of probucol on atheroma formation in cholesterol-fed rabbits kept at comparable plasma cholesterol levels', Atherosclerosis 75, 145-155.

50.   Daugherty, A., Zweifel, B.S. and Schonfeld, G. (1989) 'Probucol attenuates the development of aortic atherosclerosis in cholesterol-fed rabbits', Br. J. Pharmacol. 98, 612-618.

51.   Björkhem, I., Henriksson-Freyschuss, A., Breuer, O., Diczfalusy, U., Berglund, L. and Henriksson, P. (1991) 'The antioxidant butylated hydroxytoluene protects against atherosclerosis', Arterio. Thromb. 11, 15-22.

52.   Sparrow, C., Doebber, T., Olszewski, J., Wu, M., Ventre, J., Stevens, K. and Chao, Y.-S. (1992) 'The antioxidant N,N'-diphenyl-phenylenediamine prevents atherosclerosis in cholesterol-fed rabbits', XI International Symposium on Drugs Affecting Lipid Metabolism, p. 121(abstract)

53.   Parthasarathy, S. (1992) 'Evidence for an additional intracellular site of action of probucol in the prevention of oxidative modification of low density lipoprotein: Use of a new water-soluble probucol derivative', J. Clin. Invest. 89, 1618-1621.

54.   Gaziano, J.M., Manson, J.E., Ridker, P.M., Buring, J.E. and Hennekens, C.H. (1990) 'Beta-carotene therapy for chronic stable angina', Circulation 82, III-201 (Abst.).

55.   Steinberg, D. and Workshop Participants (1992) 'Antioxidants in the prevention of human atherosclerosis', Circulation 85, 2337-2344.

POSTPRANDIAL HYPERLIPIDEMIA AND CORONARY ARTERY DISEASE

Josef R. Patsch

Summary

Postprandial hypertriglyceridemia which puts a stressful challenge to triglyceride transport, is likely to increase the risk of cardiovascular disease because it provides the opportunity for cholesteryl esters to be transferred from LDL and HDL into triglyceride-rich particles conferring on them atherogenic potential. Increased shunting of cholesteryl esters into triglyceride-rich lipoproteins appears to be related to impaired triglyceride metabolic capacity which is indicated by the fasting lipoprotein constellation most frequently associated with coronary artery disease: low HDL cholesterol and a preponderance of small-sized HDL and LDL.

Introduction

Discussion on hypertriglyceridemia including postprandial hyperlipidemia have focussed frequently on the search for an atherogenic lipoprotein which might occur in the postprandial state only. This point of view is referred to as the "Zilversmit hypothesis" (1). According to this hypothesis chylomicrons and their remnants, if enriched in dietary cholesterol possess the potential to cause cholesterol deposition in the arterial wall.

A more comprehensive view of hypertriglyceridemia can also be taken whereby triglyceride transport in general is considered potentially atherogenic, with the postprandial state of challenge constituting a particularly critical and revealing phase. This broader view was labeled the "triglyceride intolerance hypothesis" (2). According to this hypothesis, a low triglyceride clearing capacity constitutes a risk of susceptibility for coronary artery disease (CAD). In other words, CAD risk is not linked exclusively or mainly to accumulation and misdirection of chylomicron remnants in the postprandial state, but rather to a general impairment of triglyceride transport, irrespective of whether this impairment affects the metabolism of triglyceride-rich lipoproteins of intestinal or of hepatic origin. Postprandial lipemia is only the most critical phase of triglyceride transport, and measuring the magnitude of lipemia is only a convenient tolerance test for triglyceride metabolic capacity (2).

A. L. Catapano et al. (eds.), Drugs Affecting Lipid Metabolism, 69–74.
© 1993 Kluwer Academic Publishers and Fondazione Giovanni Lorenzini.

Postprandial hyperlipidemia and coronary artery disease

An individual's triglyceride metabolic capacity, defined as the magnitude of lipemia which occurs after a standardized oral fat load (3), is a strong determinant of his or her plasma HDL cholesterol and, in particular, HDL_2 cholesterol level (3,4). Therefore, we have hypothesized that the powerful negative association between HDL cholesterol and CAD in reality is a positive relationship between triglycerides and CAD (3). If this hypothesis is correct, why then is it so difficult to clearly define the triglyceride-CAD connection itself (5,6). The probably correct answer is that: 1) fasting triglyceride measurements show a large intra-individual variability, and 2) information about long-term triglyceride concentrations in plasma is expressed more appropriately in the HDL_2 cholesterol level rather than in a single fasting triglyceride measurement. A way to take these problems into consideration in epidemiological studies may be to use not a single fasting triglyceride measurement but a measure of triglyceride metabolic capacity under challenge: postprandial lipemia. This should largely eliminate the variability inherent in single triglyceride measurements and represent in a better way to characterize average long-term triglyceride levels.

To our knowledge, three case-control studies have employed postprandial lipemia in subjects with angiographically verified presence or absence of CAD (2,7,8). Groot et al. (7) conducted their investigation with 20 matched pairs of normolipidemic cases and controls. Starting from similar postabsorptive levels, triglycerides rose to higher postprandial peak concentrations and remained elevated for a longer period of time in the normolipidemic cases, leading to an overall lerger magnitude of postprandial lipemia. The largest differences in triglyceride levels occurred at the late postprandial hours, i.e. between 6 and 12 h after ingestion of the test meal. The authors interpret their results in terms of the "Zilversmit hypothesis" (1) because of inefficient clearance of chylomicron remnants. Simpson et al. (8) studied 34 cases, 10 of whom displayed considerable hypercholesterolemia, and 18 controls. Again, the mean magnitude of postprandial lipemia was higher in the patients, irrespective of whether or not the hypercholesterolemic subset was included in the analysis; the postprandial triglyceride curves of cases and controls diverged at the late postprandial hours; and the Zilversmit hypothesis was invoked to relate these data to CAD prevalence. Administration of the lipid-lowering drug fenofibrate to eight controls, eight normo-cholesterolemic and eight hypercholesterolemic subjects attenuated the average magnitude of postprandial lipemia significantly and proportionately within each of these groups, but, interestingly, did not abolish the difference between CAD cases and controls (8).

As would be expected from the differences in postprandial lipemia, reduced HDL cholesterol clearly figured as the fasting characteristic distinguishing normocho-lesterolemic CAD patients in both case-control trials (7,8). Unfortunately, no efforts were made in these studies to weigh the risk factor roles of elevated postprandial triglycerides and concomitantly reduced HDL cholesterol against each other, to establish whether postprandial triglycerides and HDL cholesterol are each independent predictors of disease, or to estimate their quantitative share of the overall CAD risk.

The third study used larger samples and employed multivariate statistical techniques. Patsch et al. studied 101 angiographically characerized subjects and performed multivariate analyses (2). In 61 male subjects with severe CAD and 40 control subjects without CAD as verified by angiography, they measured cholesterol; triglycerides; HDL cholesterol; HDL_2 cholesterol; and apolipoproteins A-I, A-II, and B in fasting plasma and triglycerides before and 2, 4, 6 and 8 hours after a standardized test meal. Both the maximal triglyceride increase and the magnitude of postprandial lipemia (area under the triglyceride curve over 8 hours after the meal) were higher in cases than in control subjects. Single postprandial triglyceride levels 6 and 8 hours after the meal were highly discriminatory ($p<0.001$), and by logistic-regression analysis displayed an accuracy of 68 % in predicting the presence or absence of CAD. In this respect, accuracy was higher than that of HDL_2 cholesterol (64 %) and equal to that of apolipoprotein B (68 %), the most discriminatory fasting parameter. Multivariate logistic-regression analysis was performed to reduce selected postprandial but not fasting triglycerides into the most accurate multivariate model, which also contained the accepted risk factors HDL$_2$ cholesterol, apolipoprotein B, and age. This model classified 82 % of subjects correctly. The authors concluded that triglycerides are independent predictors of CAD in multivariate analyses including HDL cholesterol, provided that a challenge test of triglyceride metabolism such as postprandial lipemia is used. The study suggests that the metabolism of triglycerides is a critical determinant of cholesterol metabolic routing. The findings support the concept that the negative association between HDL cholesterol levels and CAD actually originates in part from a positive relation between CAD and plasma triglycerides, as ascertained in the postprandial state.

Hypertriglyceridemia and atherogenic lipoproteins

The two major lipid species transported in plasma lipoproteins, cholesteryl esters (CE) and triglycerides, show two major biological differences: (1) the former are considered atherogenic while the latter are not, and (2) the latter are degraded by lipases while the former are not. Triglycerides are confined largely to triglyceride-rich lipoproteins, while CE are transported mainly by LDL and HDL. However, in many species including man, there exists a mechanism which can disrupt the fairly strict separation of the two lipids: CE transfer protein (CETP) catalyzes the exchange of CE and triglycerides between all plasma lipoproteins. Triglycerides can thus be transferred from triglyceride-rich lipoproteins to LDL and HDL, and CE, in turn, can be withdrawn from LDL and HDL and incorporated into triglyceride-rich lipoproteins.

Up to a triglycerice level of roughly 270 mg/dl the transfer of CE into a triglyceride- rich lipoprotein/unit time is a linear function of its own concentration, but is independent of the concentration of CE-donor particles like LDL and HDL, and CETP activity (9). At higher triglyceride levels, CETP activity becomes rate-limiting, and CE-transfer to triglyceride-rich lipoproteins per unit time reaches a plateau with respect to triglyceride concentration (9). When these data obtained with VLDL *in vitro* are extrapolated to conditions *in vivo*, concentrations and plasma residence times of the triglyceride-rich lipoproteins are the major variables controlling their CE-enrichment in all states of absorption: in most individuals, the critical triglyceride level of 270 mg/dl is exceeded only briefly, if at all, even during the postprandial period (3,4,10). It is thus reasonable to expect that a quantitative relationship exists between triglyceride metabolic capacity, which determines the concentration and plasma residence time of triglyceride-rich lipoproteins, and the degree of enrichment of triglyceride-rich lipoproteins with CE. Because differences in triglyceride metabolic capacity are large even among normolipidemic individuals (2,3,4,10) the associated differences in the amount of CE transferred to triglyceride- rich lipoproteins must be equally large; in fact, they can be calculated to be in the order of gram quantities of CE during a single day (11). Rather undramatic and hidden differences in the metabolism of triglycerides, the lipid widely considered innocent, thus have grave consequences for the metabolic routing of the dangerous lipid, i.e., cholesterol. The reciprocal crossing-over of CE and triglycerides eventually leads to a lipoprotein constellation termed the "atherogenic lipoprotein phenotype" (12,13). The development of this phenotype can be explained as follows: CE transferred to triglyceride-rich lipoproteins are resistant to lipase action and can thus impede the undisturbed passage of their originally triglyceride-rich acceptor lipoproteins through the lipolytic cascade. Multiple CE-enriched intermediates of intestinal and hepatic origin - for instance, chylomicron remnants and IDL - may accumulate and in this way end up in an atheromatous leason (14); hence, the term "atherogenic". Triglycerides transferred to LDL and HDL, on the contrary, are susceptible to hydrolysis by lipases, which reduces the size of these lipoproteins

(15,16). The result is a preponderance of small LDL ("pattern B" (12,13)) and small HDL (HDL$_3$ (16)), the "lipoprotein phenotype" that is "atherogenic". If the above scenario is corrected, any triglyceride-rich lipoproteins regardless of whether of intestinal or of hepatic origin, can become atherogenic. Any triglyceride-rich lipoprotein holds the poteintial of becoming excessively enriched in CE and, thus, be amenable for endocytic uptake by macrophages and smooth muscle cells in the arterial wall.

Factors at the root of triglyceride intolerance

An individual's triglyceride metabolic capacity as ascertained by the fat load test is a highly reproducible parameter (2,3,10) the magnitude of which depends on a number of factors. These factors are now increasingly being identified. A rather trivial factor should be the activity of lipoprotein lipase (LPL), the enzyme responsible for the initial processing of triglyceride-rich lipoproteins in the circulation. LPL activity is inversely related to the magnitude of lipemia in healthy young subjects (4). This is apparently not true for middle-aged CAD patients (7), suggesting that LPL activity is of only minor importance in these individuals. In contrast, young carriers of a defective LPL gene in single dose displayed pronounced lipemia (17), supporting again the role of LPL as a limiting factor. What at first appears straightforward, therefore, turns out to be a quite complex mechanism: LPL activity may restrict triglyceride metabolic capacity when deficient or in the absence of other limitations, such as in healthy young individuals; it may, however, be overridden as a limiting factor by other, as yet unknown factors associated with conditions such as obesity and age.

Receptor-mediated remnant removal may be a second determinant of triglyceride tolerance, with possible variation of either comptetence of the ligand or activity of the receptor. At the ligand level, apolipoprotein (apo)E isoforms affect clearance of both intestinal and hepatic triglyceride-rich lipoproteins. Compared with apoE3 homozygotes, carriers of the apoE2 allele show delayed clearance of retinyl palmitate with the chylomicron remnant fraction (18); remnants of larger VLDL are also removed more slowly from the blood in these individuals (19). In addition, apoC-I and, to a lesser degree, apoC-II inhibit binding of both intestinal and hepatic triglyceride-rich lipoproteins to their respective receptors (20-22). ApoCs appear to either displace apoE from the lipoprotein surface or interact with and thereby inactivate apoE as a ligand. At the receptor level, variable expression of the LDL receptor certainly influences the removal rate of VLDL remnants. The role of receptor activity in the clearance of chylomicron remnants, however, is far less well understood. Experiments in man have shown that variable expression of the LDL receptor does not produce significant differences in the magnitude of lipemia (23), consistent with the hypothesis that chylomicron remnants are mainly cleared via a different type of receptor, for instance, the LDL receptor-related protein (24). Experiments in mice, however, seem to be at variance with this idea: immunological blockage of the LDL receptor substantially shows down the removal of chylomicron remnants from plasma, elevating the role of the LDL receptor in this process (25).

A third source of variation in triglyceride metabolic capacity may be the hormonal fine-tuning achieved when approaching the postprandial state. When insulin resistance renders postprandial insulin levels insufficient for suppression of VLDL secretion by the liver (26), hepatic triglyceride-rich particles superimposed on chylomicrons will augment postprandial lipemial. It is therefore possible that the CAD risk associated with familial dyslipidemic hypertension syndrome (27) is in part caused by impaired triglyceride metabolic capacity due to hepatic insulin resistance and, consequently, uncontrolled production of VLDL in the postprandial state.

Conclusion

A picture is now taking shape in which low triglyceride metabolic capacity imparts CAD risk. There is now one case-control study available (2) indicating that triglyceride intolerance, as ascertained in the postprandial state, is an independent CAD risk factor. This proof of independence was necessary to justify the claim that impaired triglyceride metabolic capacity underlies the common high-risk lipoprotein constellation of low HDL cholesterol and small-sized HDL and LDL. Clearly, prospective studies will be necessary to substantiate this piece of epidemiologic evidence.

References

1. Zilversmit DB. Atherogenesis. A postprandial phenomenon. Circulation 1979;60:473-485.
2. Patsch JR, Miesenbock G, Hopferwieser T et al. Relation of triglyceride metabolism and coronary artery disease. Studies in the postprandial state. Arteriosclerosis Thromb1992;12:1336-1345.
3. Patsch JR, Karlin JB, Scott LW, Smith LC, Gotto AM Jr. Inverse relationship between blood levels of high density lipoprotein subfraction 2 and magnitude of postprandial lipemia. Proc Natl Acad Sci USA 1983;80:1449-1453.
4. Patsch JR, Prasad S, Gotto AM Jr, Patsch W. High density lipoprotein2: relationship of the plasma levels of this lipoprotein species to its composition, to the magnitude of postprandial lipemia, and to the activities of lipoprotein lipase and hepatic lipase. J Clin Invest 1987;80:341-347.
5. Miesenbock G, Patsch JR. Coronary artery disease: synergy of triglyceride-rich lipoproteins and HDL. Cardiovascular Risk Factors 1991;1:293-299.
6. Austin MA. Plasma triglyceride and coronary heart disease. Arteriosclerosis Thromb 1991;11 :2-14.
7. Groot PHE, Van Stiphout WAHJ, Krauss XH et al. Postprandial lipoprotein metabolism in normolipidemic men with and without coronary artery disease. Arteriosclerosis Thromb 1991;11:653-662.
8. Simpson HS, Williamson CM, Olivecrona T et al. Postprandial lipemia, fenofibrate and coronary artery disease. Atherosclerosis 1990;85:193-202.
9. Mann CJ, Yen FT, Grant AM, Bihain BE. Mechanism of plasma cholesterol ester transfer in hypertriglyceridemia. J Clin Invest 1991;88:2059-2066.
10. Patsch JR. Postprandial lipaemia. Clin Endocrinol Metabol 1987;1:551-580.
11. Miesenbock G, Patsch JR. Postprandial hyperlipidemia: the search for the atherogenic lipoprotein. Curr Opin Lipidol 1992;3:196-201.
12. Austin MA, King M-C, Vranizan KM, Krauss RM. Atherogenic lipoprotein phenotype: a proposed genetic marker for coronary heart disease risk. Circulation 1990;82:495-506.
13. Krauss RM. Low-density lipoprotein subclasses and risk of coronary artery disease. Curr Opin Lipidol 1991;2:248-252.
14. Huff MW, Evans AJ, Sawyez CG, Wolfe BM, Nestel PJ. Cholesterol accumulation in J774 macrophages induced by triglyceride-rich lipoproteins. Comparison of very low density lipoproteins from subjects with Type III, IV, and V hyper-lipoproteinemia. Arteriosclerosis Thromb 1991;11:221-232.
15. Deckelbaum RJ, Granot E, Oschry Y, Rose 1, Eisenberg S. Plasma triglyceride determines structure-composition in low and high density lipoproteins. Arteriosclerosis 1984;4:225-231.
16. Patsch JR, Prasad S, Gotto AM Jr, Bengtsson-Olivecrona G. Postprandial lipemia: a key for the conversion of high density lipoproteins into high density lipoproteins by hepatic lipase. J Clin Invest 1984;74:2017-2023.

17. Miesenbock G, Holzl B, Foger B, Brandstatter E, Paulweber B, Sandhofer F, Patsch JR. Heterozygous lipoprotein lipase deficiency due to a missense mutation as the cause of impaired triglyceride tolerance with multiple lipoprotein abnormalities. J Clin Invest 1993; in press.
18. Weintraub MS, Eisenberg S, Breslow JL. Dietary fat clearance in normal subjects is regulated by genetic variation in apolipoprotein E. J Clin Invest 1987 ;80 :1571-1577.
19. Demant T, Bedford D, Packard CJ, Shepherd J. Influence of apolipoprotein E polymorphism on apolipoprotein B-100 metabolism in normolipidemic subjects. J Clin Invest 1991;88:1490-1501.
20. Kowal RC, Herz J, Weisgraber KH, Mahley RW, Brown MS, Goldstein JL. Opposing effects of apolipoprotein E and C on lipoprotein binding to low density lipoprotein receptor-related protein. J Biol Chem 1990;265:10771-10779.
21. Weisgraber KH, Mahley RW, Kowal RC, Herz J, Goldstein JL,Brown MS. Apolipoprotein C-1 modulates interaction of apolipoprotein E with β-migrating very low density lipoprotein (β-VLDL) and inhibits binding of β-VLDL to low density lipoprotein receptor-related protein. J Biol Chem 1990;265:22453- 22459.
22. Sehayek E, Eisenberg S. Mechanisms of inhibition by apolipoprotein C of apolipoprotein E-dependent cellular metabolism of human triglyceride-rich lipoproteins through the low density lipoprotein receptor pathway. J Biol Chem 1991;266:18259-18267.
23. Eriksson M, Angelin B, Henriksson P, Ericsson S, Vitols S, Berglund L. Metabolism of lipoprotein remnants in humans: studies during infusion of fat and cholesterol in subjects with varying expression of the low density lipoprotein receptor. Arteriosclerosis Thromb 1991;11:827-837.
24. Brown MS, Herz J, Kowal RC, Goldstein JL. The low-density lipoprotein receptor-related protein: double agent or decoy? Curr Opin Lipidol 1991;2:65-72.
25. Choi SY, Fong LG, Kirven MJ, Cooper AD. Use of an anti-low density lipoprotein receptor antibody to quantify the role of the LDL receptor in the removal of chylomicron remnants in the mouse in vivo. J Clin Invest 1991;88:1173-1181.
26. Patsch W, Gotto AM Jr, Patsch JR. The effects of insulin on lipoprotein secretion in rat hepatocyte cultures: the role of the insulin receptor. J Biol Chem 1986;261:9603-9606.
27. Gwynne J. Clinical features and pathophysiology of familial dyslipidemic hypertension syndrome. Curr Opin Lipidol 1992;3:215-221.

GENETIC FACTORS AFFECTING LIPOPROTEIN METABOLISM

Kåre Berg

INTRODUCTION

Genetic as well as environmental factors are of importance for the
population variation in lipid and apolipoproteins. Several of these
variables are known or believed to be of importance for susceptibility
or resistance to atherogenesis.

HYPOTHETICAL MECHANISMS UNDERLYING ATHEROSCLEROTIC DISEASE

Hypothetically, several mechanisms could affect lipid metabolism in an
individual, in a way relevant to risk for atherosclerotic disease,
including the following:

1. Diet or life style could be so unhealthy that cardiovascular disease
develops even in the absence of any genetic predisposition.

2. A single gene may have such a major disruptive effect on lipid
metabolism that atherosclerotic disease is likely to develop, even in
people with a diet and life style that should counteract atherogenesis.
The genetic defect in classical familial hypercholesterolemia is the
best example of such a strong genetic determinant of atherosclerosis
risk. Genes with major effects on lipid metabolism are relatively rare
and account for only a small proportion of cases of atherosclerotic
disease.

3. There may be interaction between genetic factors and environmental
factors, where dietary or life style factors preferentially cause
disease in people with a genetic predisposition to atherosclerosis. For
example, an atherogenic diet could raise cholesterol to a level of
significant cardiovascular risk, in people who because of their genetic
constitution tend to have somewhat high lipid levels (Berg (1990a)).
Plausibly, such interactions could be operative in a substantial
fraction of people who contract coronary heart disease (CHD) at a
relatively early age (prior to age 55-60 in men or 60-65 in women).
Accordingly, it is of utmost importance to identify persons with a

A. L. Catapano et al. (eds.), Drugs Affecting Lipid Metabolism, 75–82.
© 1993 Kluwer Academic Publishers and Fondazione Giovanni Lorenzini.

genetic predisposition to atherosclerotic disease, in order to make it
possible for those with the highest risk to make use of the most
efficient preventive measures. Thus, identification of genes that
influence atherosclerosis risk may become very useful for the attempts
to prevent (or delay) the garden variety of CHD. Genes that influence
absolute risk factor level may conveniently be referred to as "level
genes" to distinguish them from certain other genes (see below).

4. Genes most likely contribute to determining the borders within which
dietary factors or life style factors can cause lipid or apolipoprotein
variation. This notion has led to the development of the "variability
gene concept". With respect to disorders of lipid metabolism, this
would imply that it is important to be as aware of the organism's
reaction to lipid intake and life style factors, as it is to observe
absolute risk factor level under certain ("basic") circumstances (such
as the fasting state). Genes that contribute to determining the limits
to the amount of variation that environmental factors can cause may be
referred to as "variability genes" to distinguish them from "level
genes", as defined above. A method to detect variability genes is
discussed below.

5. Interaction between genetic and environmental factors may be limited
to situations where one specific environmental factor, such as smoking,
is either present or absent. Thus, we have observed a significant
association between normal genes at the cholesteryl ester transfer
protein (CETP) locus and level of high density lipoprotein (HDL)
cholesterol as well as apolipoprotein A-I (apoA-I) (Kondo et al.
(1989)). This association was only present in non-smokers. Accordingly,
smokers may have lower levels of HDL and apoA-I than their genetic
constitution permits.
        It is possible that some of the conflicting results of attempts to
uncover associations between genetic markers and risk factors can be
explained by heterogeneity of the study population with respect to
important environmental factors.

6. Gene - gene interaction may contribute to risk factor level. Thus,
the first example of gene - gene interaction influencing the level of a
CHD risk factor was recently observed (Pedersen and Berg (1989)). The
well established cholesterol-increasing effect of the E4 allele in the
apolipoprotein E (apoE) polymorphism was suppressed when a normal gene
at the low density lipoprotein receptor (LDLR) locus detected as
presence of a PvuII restriction site, was present. We have made this
observation in two different series (Pedersen and Berg (1990)). If
independently confirmed, this observation implies that genotypes at the
LDLR locus must be taken into consideration if the effect of apoE genes
on cholesterol level is to be measured in a meaningful way.

7. If the variability gene concept is valid, it would appear that
interaction between level genes and variability genes could determine
an individual's total risk for atherosclerotic disease. Restrictive
variability genes could be advantageous in people whose level genes

tend to give them a low risk factor level, whereas they could be damaging to people whose level genes tend to give them a higher risk factor level. This concept has led to the development of a model where a person's total genetic risk for atherosclerotic disase results from his combination of level genes and variability genes (Berg (1987), Berg (1990b)).

8. Plausibly, some genes may influence lipid metabolism as well as thrombogenesis/thrombolysis. Genes determining a high level of Lp(a) lipoprotein may have those properties. Lp(a) lipoprotein level is under strict genetic control and a high level of Lp(a) lipoprotein is an independent risk factor for atherosclerosis. Apparent intact Lp(a) lipoprotein is present in atherosclerotic lesions of people with a high Lp(a) lipoprotein level, and this lipoprotein particle may therefore be considered as atherogenic. The long polypeptide chain characteristic of Lp(a) lipoprotein (the Lp(a) polypeptide chain or apolipoprotein(a)) turned out to have very extensive homology with plasminogen, a much smaller protein (McLean et al. (1987)). The homology between plasminogen and the Lp(a) polypeptide chain strongly suggested evolutionary relationship between the two components, and absolute genetic linkage has since been found between the plasminogen locus and the LPA locus. The great similarity of the Lp(a) polypeptide chain with plasminogen also suggested that the Lp(a) lipoprotein particle could interfere with thrombolytic/fibrinolytic processes. Several in vitro studies have yielded results compatible with this hypothesis, but as yet there is no in vivo evidence of interference by Lp(a) lipoprotein with thrombolysis/fibrinolysis. Lp(a) lipoprotein may form a bridge between atherogenesis and thrombogenesis, the two main processes underlying myocardial infarction.

9. Finally, there could be interactions that may be very difficult to decipher, between the above mechanisms or between mechanisms that as of today are unknown.

Some of the items above are further discussed below.

CANDIDATE GENES

Present attempts to identify genes of importance for lipid metabolism or risk for atherosclerotic disease, make use of the "candidate gene approach". With respect to lipid metabolism, any gene whose protein product might plausibly interfere with lipid metabolism is a candidate gene, as is any gene whose product may bridge the gap between atherosclerotic and thrombotic processes. With the advent of DNA technology, many candidate genes have become accessible for study. In the following, emphasis will be on genes affecting lipid metabolism in a way that may contribute to the garden variety of atherosclerotic disease, rather than on rare genes causing monogenic hyperlipidemias. These genes (usually detected as variants in restriction fragment length polymorphisms (RFLPs)) are part of the normal fabric of genes that forms the basis for man's biochemical individuality.

The first studies of CHD risk employing the "candidate gene approach" took place several years before the term "candidate gene" was coined. The early studies were conducted at the lipoprotein or apolipoprotein level, rather than at the DNA level. The first successful studies were reported in 1974 (Berg et al. (1974)) when association between Lp(a) lipoprotein and premature CHD was found. This observation has been confirmed in a long series of studies including one by Rhoads et al. (1986) which uncovered a 28% population attributable risk of contracting myocardial infarction before age 60 for men whose Lp(a) lipoprotein level corresponded to the top quartile of the population distribution of Lp(a) lipoprotein concentrations.

A second study employing the "candidate gene approach" was conducted in the 1970s by Berg et al. (1976). It showed that total serum cholesterol level as well as triglyceride level are associated with phenotypes in the allotypic Ag system of LDL. The results are consistent with results obtained much more recently, employing DNA variation at the apolipoprotein B (apoB) locus, and the lipid associations are internally consistent with associations between the Ag variation and DNA polymorphisms (Berg et al. (1986)).

A third successful use of the "candidate gene approach" was made in the 1970s when the importance of normal genes at the apoE locus for total and LDL cholesterol levels was uncovered (Utermann et al. (1979)).

DNA POLYMORPHISMS AT CANDIDATE LOCI AND RISK FACTOR LEVELS

Attempts to uncover association between DNA variation at candidate loci and lipid or apolipoprotein levels have particularly focused on apolipoprotein loci. Already at an early stage an association was detected between an XbaI polymorphism at the apoB locus and lipid levels (Law et al. (1986)). This observation was soon confirmed (Berg (1986)) and today appears to be one of the firmly established associations between DNA variation and lipid levels. This RFLP reflects substitution of a neutral third base of a codon and therefore does not alter the amino acid sequence of apoB. Thus, the RFLP itself is not responsible for the association. Rather, it reflects normal genetic variation in a functionally important domain which is sufficiently close to cause linkage disequilibrium. Doubtless, a similar mechanism underlies other associations between RFLPs and lipids.

Association with lipid level has also been found with a normal RFLP at the LDLR locus (Pedersen and Berg (1989)), confirming early suggestions from our group that normal genes at the LDLR locus contribute to the population variation in cholesterol (Maartmann-Moe et al. (1981)).

We also considered the CETP locus as a candidate locus with respect to disturbance of lipid metabolism and uncovered a significant association between normal genes at this locus and HDL level as well as apoA-I level (Kondo et al. (1989)). As mentioned above, this association was present only in non-smokers. Recently, Freeman et al. confirmed the association and also that it is present only in non-smokers (Freeman et al. (1992)).

RISK FACTOR LEVEL VERSUS VARIABILITY

Until now, most studies of serum lipids in relation to disease have been conducted on blood samples obtained in the fasting state. Since Western man is postprandial most of the hours of the day, the information from such studies may be incomplete. It is known from animal studies that responder or non-responder strains exist, with respect to lipid intake, and such strain differences are almost certainly genetically determined. More recently, Katan and his coworkers (Katan et al. (1986), Katan and Beynen (1987)) have shown not only that there is a great deal of variation with respect to responses in man to altered fat intake, but also that an individual's response pattern remains unchanged, at least over many years. This finding makes it plausible that genes contribute to the response pattern in man as well as in animals. Presumably, the amount of variation in lipids and apolipoproteins may be of importance for a person's CHD risk as suggested by an early study (Groover et al. (1960)).

There was a need for more dynamic studies than trying to correlate genetic markers with absolute risk factor level, in the way it had traditionally been done. Monozygotic (MZ) twins offered a unique possibility to study genetic influences on variability of components such as cholesterol. MZ twins have identical genes and any difference with respect to a quantitative variable between the two members of a pair must be caused by dietary or life style factors. Genes with a restrictive effect on the amount of variation that dietary factors or life style factors can cause should result in a small within-pair variation in the component under study. Accordingly, comparing within-pair differences between MZ pairs of different genotypes at a candidate locus should make it possible to detect genes with an effect on variability, and examples of such effects have been reported (Berg (1984, 1990b), Humphries et al. (1992)).

There is no need to postulate that a variability gene should not also have an effect on absolute risk factor level. In fact, it would be plausible that some genes had effect on level as well as variability. The important point with this concept is that it emphasizes the potential importance of variability in lipid parameters rather than absolute risk factor levels.

Although the validity of the variability gene concept has been substantiated (Berg (1988), Humphries et al. (1992)), it remains to be seen how useful the concept will be in the attempts to decipher the importance of genetics for disease risks.

Lp(a) LIPOPROTEIN: GENETICS AND ATHEROSCLEROSIS RISK

It is clear from a long series of published papers that a high level of Lp(a) lipoprotein is a CHD risk factor in its own right (for review, see Berg (1992)) and two prospective studies have confirmed this (Dahlén (1990), Rosengren et al. (1990)). Recently, there has been two or three claims that association between Lp(a) lipoprotein and CHD has been sought for but not detected in the population under study. One of

these populations was in fact the population where this association was
first detected. It appears to be a common denominator for these studies
that they have been conducted using a commercially available test kit
whose quality has not been well documented. The technique preferred
until now by most research laboratories is quantitative
immunoelectrophoresis with its excellent possibilities to control for
confounding factors. The structure of the Lp(a) polypeptide chain
including the varying number of "kringle IV" units could cause
significant problems with test techniques other than quantitative
immunoelectrophoresis or for the use of monoclonal antibodies rather
than polyvalent antisera. The failure of at least one of the
commercially available test kits to detect important characteristics of
the Lp(a) lipoprotein particle is an added reason to consider results
obtained with some of the commercially available kits, with a great
deal of caution.

The absolute genetic linkage detected between segregating high
levels of Lp(a) lipoprotein and DNA variation at the plasminogen locus
(see Berg (1992)) forms irrefutable evidence of single locus control of
quantitative Lp(a) lipoprotein variation, confirming numerous previous
reports. The lack of recombination between segregating high levels of
Lp(a) lipoprotein and plasminogen argues very strongly against a
significant effect on high Lp(a) lipoprotein levels by any other locus
than the LPA locus on chromosome 6.

In retrospect, it is not easy to understand why some workers had
problems accepting single locus control of quantitative Lp(a)
lipoprotein variation. Clearly, segregation from heterozygotes with one
gene determining high Lp(a) lipoprotein level and the other a low level
will result in an autosomal dominant pattern and the (near) absence of
offspring with a high Lp(a) lipoprotein level from parents who both
have a very low level further strengthens the autosomal dominant
pattern in the families.

Some workers have erroneously believed that a locus (or loci)
other than the LPA locus must participate in determining Lp(a)
lipoprotein level, since only about 40% of the quantitative variation
is reflected in the size variation that depends on varying numbers of
kringle IV in the Lp(a) polypeptide chain. In reality, the absolute
genetic linkage between segregating high levels of Lp(a) lipoprotein
and plasminogen has for some years now been conclusive evidence against
a second locus with a major effect on Lp(a) lipoprotein level. A
plausible conclusion is that the kringle IV variation is not very close
to the domain in or near the LPA gene that determines Lp(a) lipoprotein
level.

ACKNOWLEDGEMENTS

This work was supported by the Norwegian Council on Cardiovascular
Disease, the Norwegian Research Council for Science and the Humanities,
and Anders Jahres Foundation for the Promotion of Science.

REFERENCES

Berg, K. (1984) 'Twin studies of coronary heart disease and its risk factors', Acta Genet. Med. Gemellol. 33, 349-361.

Berg, K. (1986) 'DNA polymorphism at the apolipoprotein B locus is associated with lipoprotein level', Clin. Genet. 30, 515-520.

Berg, K. (1987) 'Genetics of coronary heart disease and its risk factors', in G. Bock and G.M. Collins (eds.), Molecular Approaches to Human Polygenic Disease, Ciba Foundation Symposium 130, John Wiley & Sons, Chichester, pp. 14-33.

Berg, K. (1988) 'Variability gene effect on cholesterol at the Kidd blood group locus', Clin. Genet. 33, 102-107.

Berg, K. (1990a) 'Molecular genetics and nutrition', in G.H. Bourne (ed.), World Review of Nutrition and Dietetics, Karger, Basel, pp. 49-59.

Berg, K. (1990b) 'Level genes and variability genes in the etiology of hyperlipidemia and atherosclerosis', in K. Berg, N. Retterstøl and S. Refsum (eds.), From Phenotype to Gene in Common Disorders, Munksgaard, Copenhagen, pp. 77-91.

Berg, K. (1992) 'Lp(a) lipoprotein: An important genetic risk factor for atherosclerosis', in A.J. Lusis, J. Rotter and R. Sparkes (eds.), Monogr. Hum. Genet., Karger, Basel, in press.

Berg, K., Dahlén, G. and Frick, M.H. (1974) 'Lp(a) lipoprotein and pre-ß1-lipoprotein in patients with coronary heart disease', Clin. Genet. 6, 230-235.

Berg, K., Hames, C., Dahlén, G., Frick, M.H. and Krishan, I. (1976) 'Genetic variation in serum low density lipoproteins and lipid levels in man', Proc. Natl. Acad. Sci. (USA) 73, 937-940.

Berg, K., Powell, L.M., Wallis, S.C., Pease, R., Knott, T.J. and Scott, J. (1986) 'Genetic linkage between the antigenic group (Ag) variation and the apolipoprotein B gene: Assignment of the Ag locus', Proc. Natl. Acad. Sci. USA 83, 7367-7370.

Dahlén, G. (1990) 'Clinical significance of Lp(a) lipoprotein', in K. Berg, N. Retterstøl and S. Refsum (eds.), From Phenotype to Gene in Common Disorders, Munksgaard, Copenhagen, pp. 163-178.

Freeman, D., Lindsay, G., McCusker, L., Gaffney, D., Packard, C. and Shepherd, J. (1992) 'Plasma HDL-2 concentration is associated with polymorphisms of the cholesteryl ester transfer protein gene (CETP) and smoking status', in Abstracts, European Atherosclerosis Society, 59th EAS Congress, 75.

Groover, M.E., Jernigan, J.A. and Martin, C.D. (1960) 'Variations in serum lipid concentration and clinical coronary disease', Am. J. Med. Sci. 239, 53-59.

Humphries, S.E., Green, F.R., Henney, A.M. and Talmud, P.J. (1992) 'DNA polymorhisms: the variability gene concept and the risk of coronary artery disease', in A.G. Bearn (ed.), Genetics of Coronary Heart Disease, Institute of Medical Genetics, University of Oslo, pp. 123-142.

Katan, M.B. and Beynen, A.C. (1987) 'Characteristics of human hypo- and hyperresponders to dietary cholesterol', Amer. J. Epidemiol. 125, 387-399.

Katan, M.B., Beynen, A.C., De Vries J.H.M. and Nobels, A. (1986) 'Existence of consistent hypo- and hyperresponders to dietary cholesterol in man', Amer J Epidemiol. 123, 221-234.

Kondo, I., Berg, K., Drayna, D. and Lawn, R. (1989) 'DNA polymorphism at the locus for human cholesteryl ester transfer protein (CETP) is associated with high density lipoprotein cholesterol and apolipoprotein levels', Clin. Genet. 35, 49-56.

Law, A., Powell, L.M., Brunt, H., Knott, T.J., Altman, D.G., Rajput, J., Wallis, S.C., Pease, R.J., Priestley, L.M., Scott, J., Miller, G.J. and Miller, N.E. (1986) 'Common DNA polymorphism within the coding sequence of the apolipoprotein B gene associated with altered lipid levels', Lancet i, 1301-1303.

McLean, J.W., Tomlinson J.E., Kuang, W.-J., Eaton, D.L., Chen, E.Y., Fless, G.M., Scanu, A.M. and Lawn, R.M. (1987) 'cDNA sequence of human apolipoprotein (a) is homologous to plasminogen', Nature 330, 132-137.

Maartmann-Moe, K., Magnus, P., Golden, W. and Berg, K. (1981) 'Genetics of the low density lipoprotein receptor: III. Evidence for multiple normal alleles at the low density lipoprotein receptor locus', Clin. Genet. 20, 113-129.

Pedersen, J. and Berg, K. (1989) 'Interaction between low density lipoprotein receptor (LDLR) and apolipoprotein E (apoE) alleles contributes to normal variation in lipid level', Clin. Genet. 35, 331-337.

Pedersen, J.C. and Berg, K. (1990) 'Gene - gene interaction between the low density lipoprotein receptor and apolipoprotein E loci affects lipid levels', Clin. Genet. 38, 287-294.

Rhoads, G.G., Dahlén, G., Berg, K., Morton, N.E. and Dannenberg, A.L. (1986) 'Lp(a) lipoprotein as a risk factor for myocardial infarction', JAMA 256, 2540-2544.

Rosengren, A., Wilhelmsen, L., Eriksson, E., Risberg, B. and Wedel, H. (1990) 'Lipoprotein (a) and coronary heart disease: a prospective case-control study in a general population sample of middle aged men', Br. Med. J. 301, 1248-1251.

Utermann, G., Pruin, N. and Steinmetz, A. (1979) 'Polymorphism of apolipoprotein E. III. Effect of single polymorphic gene locus on plasma lipid levels in man', Clin. Genet. 15, 63-72.

Lipoprotein Assembly: A Potential Target for Drugs Affecting Lipid Metabolism*

Roger A. Davis

Abstract

The human recessive disorder abetalipoproteinemia is associated with a complete inability to assemble and secrete apo B-containing lipoproteins by both the liver and intestine. The gene responsible for this disease does not co-segregate with the apo B gene suggesting it is caused by the loss of some gene product. To gain an understanding of the apparently unique process necessary for apo B secretion, plasmids expressing apo B were transfected into Chinese hamster ovary fibroblasts. Expression of a truncated form (apo B15, consisting of 15% of the N-terminus of the full length protein), which is too short to assemble lipoproteins, resulted in the accumulation of apo B in both cells and culture medium. In contrast, cells transfected with a plasmid encoding apo B53 (which is sufficiently large to allow the assembly and secretion of lipoproteins when expressed in hepatoma cells) did not contain apo B nor did they secrete it despite the presence of apo B mRNA. Incubation with calpain inhibitor I (ALLN) led to the accumulation of apo B53 in cells, showing that it is synthesized, but completely degraded in the absence of the inhibitor. Despite the accumulation of apo B53 in ALLN-treated cells, none was secreted. The inability of Chinese hamster ovary cells to secrete apo B53 cannot be explained by insufficient lipid since stimulation of triglyceride synthesis did not induce secretion. Essentially all of the apo B53 which accumulated in the microsomes from ALLN-treated cells was bound to microsomal membranes and susceptible to degradation by exogenous trypsin, while the lumenal enzyme protein disulfide isomerase was fully protected. These data suggest that translocation is the step in the secretory pathway responsible for sorting apo B into either the secretory or degradation (i.e. default) pathways. Moreover, it appears that apo B requires a unique process, not expressed in Chinese hamster ovary cells, for its translocation. This process required for translocation may be lacking in abetalipoproteinemia. Based on the findings that essentially no toxicity is associated with either the abetalipoproteinemic phenotype or the phenotype created using fibroblast cells reported here, we propose that agents that would create the abetalipoproteinemic phenotype would be useful in treating hyperlipidemic conditions associated with increased plasma apo B levels.

Introduction

Triglyceride-rich lipoproteins consist of a monolayer surface of phospholipid, free cholesterol and specific proteins (apolipoproteins) which surround a hydrophobic core of apolar lipids: triglycerides and cholesterol esters. These lipoproteins serve to transport the apolar

A. L. Catapano et al. (eds.), Drugs Affecting Lipid Metabolism, 83–87.
© 1993 Kluwer Academic Publishers and Fondazione Giovanni Lorenzini.

lipids from their site of synthesis (liver) and absorption (intestine) to peripheral tissues where the lipids are metabolized and imported for anabolic and energy purposes. Clearly, because of the parental role that triglyceride-rich lipoproteins play in the derivation of LDL and HDL, derivation of agents that can control VLDL assembly should provide an ideal means with which to treat hyperlipidemia.

Assembly of Triglyceride-rich Lipoproteins

Essentially all the protein and lipid components of VLDL are synthesized on or within the endoplasmic reticulum. This includes the synthesis of proteins on membrane-bound ribosomes, the synthesis of free cholesterol, cholesterol esters, phospholipids and triglycerides. The proximity of these biosynthetic processes in the endoplasmic reticulum provides all components necessary at the intracellular site where VLDL are first assembled (1). One feature that distinguishes the endoplasmic reticulum in liver from that of tissues not involved in VLDL assembly is the presence in the cisternae of VLDL-like particles having a fairly uniform diameter (1).

VLDL Assembly Requires Apolipoprotein B

The assembly of VLDL requires bringing together individual lipid and protein components necessary to form a thermodynamically stable macromolecular aggregate (i.e. lipoprotein particle). Clearly, several independent lines of evidence show that one apolipoprotein (i.e. apo B) is essential for the assembly and secretion of VLDL. In several forms of the human autosomal dominant disease hypobetalipoproteinemia alteration of the apo B gene leads to forms of apo B that are too short to assemble VLDL (2). When these truncated forms of apo B are expressed in hepatoma cells they reproduce the hypobetalipoproteinemic phenotype i.e. they are too short to assemble lipoproteins (3). Thus, apo B having a minimal size is one essential component of the VLDL assembly pathway.

Apo B has Unusual Characteristics That Allow it to Assemble VLDL

A consistent characteristic of the structural, physical, biosynthetic and metabolic properties of apo B is unusual. These properties interact to allow apo B to serve its two major physiological functions: to assemble VLDL and to direct the metabolism and tissue targeting of plasma lipoproteins.

In normal patients there are two major forms of apo B designated by the percentage of the N-terminal coding region of the largest form possible (i.e. apo B100) (as reviewed in reference 4). The full-length form transcribed by a single apo B gene (apo B100) contains 4536 amino acids as a single peptide chain. In humans apo B100 is synthesized almost exclusively by the liver. In contrast, the other major form of apo B (apo B48) is synthesized by the intestine. In rodents the liver synthesizes both apo B48 and apo B100 (4).

While there are no predicted membrane spanning domains, apo B appears to integrate into membrane bilayers and lipoprotein particles. Unlike other mammalian apolipoproteins, apo B does not exchange between lipoprotein particles. The structural motifs responsible for the association of apo B with lipids are likely to involve different secondary structures that allow the formation of amphipathic faces. These structures include β-sheets having hydrophobic and hydrophilic surfaces, short stretches of amphipathic alpha-helices and β-strands that have the potential to form amphipathic domains (5-8). Using a variety of techniques to probe the structure of apo B, at least 13 separate lipid binding domains have been identified throughout the large molecule . These domains are thought to allow apo B to associate with lipids during the assembly of VLDL.

However, the same property that allows apo B to assemble lipoproteins (i.e. membrane integration) may also act to block its ability to translocate across the endoplasmic reticulum. Amino acid sequences usually containing 18 contiguous hydrophobic residues is one criterion that is known to act to block translocation across the endoplasmic reticulum leading to membrane integration (9-13). While no such sequences can be found in apo B, other structural motifs that may allow membrane integration, may also block translocation. Analysis of apo B translocation shows that it is unusually inefficient (14).

The amount of VLDL apo B that is secreted is variable in response to metabolic state through a post-transcriptional mechanism (15-17). The amount of apo B synthesized appears to be constant, while the amount secreted appears to be highly variable (15). Moreover, apo B shows the unusual property that a significant portion of it is degraded intracellularly (18-20). This intracellular degradation of apo B appears to occur in the endoplasmic reticulum and may be metabolically regulatable (14). Variable translocation of apo B could determine how much apo B enters the VLDL assembly pathway and how much is degraded.

Evidence That a Gene Product In Addition to Apo B is Required for VLDL Assembly

The phenotype of the human disorder abetalipoproteinemia supports the proposal that along with apo B, another gene product is also required for VLDL assembly. This disease is inherited recessively and is caused by a mutation in a gene other than the one coding for apo B (21). Livers of patients with abetalipoproteinemia have apo B mRNA of normal size and slightly higher abundance (22). Since specific apo B epitopes recognized by monoclonal antibodies are present, apo B is synthesized (23,24). However, almost no apo B100 (liver) and apo B48 (intestine) is secreted (25-27). Analysis of intestinal cells obtained from abetalipoproteinemics shows the absence of VLDL particles either in the endoplasmic reticulum or the Golgi (23,24). Thus, it appears that the secretory step that is blocked in abetalipoproteinemia lies before the VLDL assembly step. Since the plasma concentrations of proteins other than apo B are not altered in abetalipoproteinemics (26), the secretory defect is selective for apo B.

Our lab recently investigated an experimental model to identify the apparently unique process necessary for apo B secretion (28). To explore this possibility and the potential role such a process may play in regulating lipoprotein assembly, plasmids encoding truncated forms of apolipoprotein B were transfected into Chinese hamster ovary (CHO) fibroblasts. (The one, encoding apo B53, the N-terminal 53% of apo B100, can direct the assembly and secretion of lipoproteins when expressed in hepatoma cells, while the other, encoding the shorter apo B15, does not direct lipoprotein assembly.) Expression of apo B15 in CHO cells resulted in the accumulation of apo B15 protein in both medium and cells. In contrast, apo B was not detectable in medium or within CHO cells transfected with the plasmid encoding apo B53, despite the expression of apo B53 mRNA. Apo B53 did accumulate within transfected cells incubated with the thiol protease inhibitor N-acetyl-leucyl-leucyl-norleucinal (ALLN), suggesting it is synthesized but completely degraded in the absence of the inhibitor. Apo B53 was not secreted despite its presence within ALLN-treated cells. Essentially all the apo B53 that accumulated in microsomes from ALLN-treated cells was associated with the membrane and was susceptible to degradation by exogenous trypsin, indicating exposure on the cytoplasmic face of the membrane. Thus translocation of B53 across the endoplasmic reticulum membrane is blocked. However the apo B53 bound to concanavalin A, suggesting that it is glycosylated and therefore partly exposed to the lumen as well. Apo B requires a unique process, not expressed in CHO fibroblasts, for its complete translocation and entrance into the secretory pathway. This process might account for the inability of abetalipoproteinemic patients to secrete apo B.

Conclusions Regarding the Discovery of New Hypolipidemic Drugs
    The most effective drugs that are useful in correcting hyperlipidemic states are those that act on cholesterol biosynthesis and triglyceride metabolism. Based on our results, we believe that a new class of drugs that can regulate apo B translocation might offer an additional effective means to control plasma lipoprotein levels. Moreover, our studies in CHO cells and those characterizing abetalipoproteinemia suggest that blocking apo B translocation is not associated with any apparent toxicity. This is probably because the apo B that is not translocated is efficiently degraded. Considering the finding that other than neurologic developmental problems that can be corrected with vitamin E therapy, the abetalipoproteinemic phenotype is associated with longevity and hypolipidemia, pharmacologic induction of a less severe abetalipoproteinemia in adulthood may have a profoundly beneficial effect in preventing atherosclerosis and other pathological conditions associated with hyperlipidemia.

References
1.   Alexander, C.A., Hamilton, R.L. and Havel, R.J. (1976) J. Cell Biol. 69:241-263.
2.   Young, S.G. (1990) Circulation 82:1574-1594.
3.   Yao, Z., Blackhart, B.D., Linton, M.F., Taylor, S.M., Young, S.G. and McCarthy, B.J. (1991) J. Biol. Chem. 266, 3300-3308.
4.   Kane, J.P. (1983) Apolipoprotein B: structural and metabolic heterogeneity. Ann. Rev. Physiol. 45, 637-650.
5.   Yang, C.-Y., Chen, S.-H., Gianturco, S.H., Bradley, W.A., Sparrow, J.T., Tanimura, M., Li, W.-H., Sparrow, D.A., DeLoof, H., Rosseneu, M., Lee, F.-S., Gu, Z.-W., Gotto, A.M., Chan, L. (1986) Sequence, structure, receptor-binding domains and internal repeats of human apolipoprotein B-100. Nature 323, 738-742.
6.   Yang, C.-Y., Gu, Z.-W., Weng, S.-a, Kim, T.W., Chen, S.-H., Pownall, H.J., Sharp, P.M., Liu, S.-W., Li, W.-H., Gotto, A.M., Chan, L. (1989) Structure of apolipoprotein B-100 of human low density lipoproteins. Arteriosclerosis 9, 96-108.
7.   Chen, G.C., Hardman, D.A., Hamilton, R.L., Mendel, C.M., Schilling, J.W., Zhu, S., Lau, K., Wong, J.S., Kane, J.P. (1989) Distribution of lipid-binding regions in human apolipoprotein B-100. Biochemistry 28, 2477-2484.
8.   Cladaras, C., Hadzopoulou-Cladaras, M., Nolte, R.T., Atkinson, D., Zannis, V.I. (1986) The complete sequence and structural analysis of human apolipoprotein B-100: relationship between apoB-100 and apoB-48 forms. EMBO Journal 5, 3495-3507.
9.   Blobel, G. (1980) Proc. Natl. Acad. Sci. USA 77:1496-1500.
10.   Gething, M.-J. and Sambrook, J. (1982) Nature 200:598-603.
11.   Boeke, J.D. and Model, P. (1982) Proc. Natl. Acad. Sci. USA 79:5200-5204.
12.   Rose, J.K. and Bergmann, J.E. (1982) Cell 30:753-762.
13.   Yost, C.S., Hedgpeth, J. and Lingappa, V.R. (1983) Cell 34:759-766.
14.   Davis, R.A., Thrift, R.N., Wu, C.C. and Howell, K.E. (1990) J. Biol. Chem. 265, 10005-10011.
15.   Leighton, J.K., Joyner, J., Zamarripa, J., Deines, M. and Davis, R.A. (1990) J. Lipid Res. 31:1663-1668.
16.   Davidson, N.O., Powell, L.M., Wallis, S.C. and Scott, J. (1988) J. Biol. Chem. 203:13482-13485.
17.   Pullinger, C.R., North, J.D., Teng, B.-B., Rificini, V.A., Ronhild de Brito, A.E. and Scott, J. (1989) J. Lipid Res. 30:1065-1077.
18.   Borchardt, R.A. and Davis, R.A. (1987) J. Biol. Chem. 262, 16394-1642.
19.   Davis, R.A., Prewett, A.B., Chan, D.C.F., Thompson, J.J., Borchardt, R.A. and Gallaher, W.R. (1989) J. Lipid Res. 30, 1185-1196.
20.   Sato, R., Imanaka, T., Takatsuki, A. and Takano, T. (1990) J. Biol. Chem. 265, 11880-11884.

21. Talmud, P.J., Lloyd J.K., Muller, D.R., Collins, D.R., Scott, J. and Humphries, S. (1988) *J. Clin. Invest.* **82**, 1803-1806.
22. Lackner, K.J., Monge, J.C., Gregg, R.E., Hoeg, J.M., Triche, T.J., Law, S.W. and Brewer, H.B., Jr. (1986) *J. Clin. Invest.* **78**, 1707-1712.
23. Dullaart, R.P.F., Speelberg, B., Schuurman, H.J., Milne, R.W., Havekes, L. Marcel, Y.L., Genze H.J., Hulshox, M.M. and Erkelens, D.W. (1986) *J. Clin. Invest.* **78**, 1397-1404.
24. Bouma, M.E., Beucler, I., Pessah, M., Heinzmann, C., Lusis, A.J., Naim, H.Y., Ducastelle, T., Leluyer, B., Schmitz, J., Infante, R. and Aggerbeck, L.P. (1990) *J. Lipid Res.* **31**, 1-15.

25. Kayden, H.J. (1972) Ann. Rev. Med. 23:285-296.
26. Herbert, P.N., Assman, G., Gotto, A.M. and Fredrickson, D.S. (1983) in *Metabolic Basis of Inherited Disease, 5th Edition,* eds. Stanbury, J.B., Wyngaarden, J.B., Fredrickson, D.S., Goldstein, J.L., and Brown, M.S., (McGraw-Hill, New York, NY), pp 589-691.
27. Malloy, M.J. and Kane, J.P. (1982) Med. Clin. N. Am. 66:469-488.
28. Thrift, R.N., Drisko, J., Dueland, S., Trawick, J.D. and Davis, R.A. (1992) (In Press).

*Work supported by NIH grant HL 41624

STRUCTURAL FEATURES THAT DETERMINE THE FUNCTIONAL PROPERTIES OF
THE LOOP REGION OF HUMAN LIPOPROTEIN LIPASE

Louis C. Smith, Roger D. Knapp, Fabrizia Faustinella and Lawrence Chan

ABSTRACT - Lipoprotein lipase, hepatic triglyceride lipase, and pancreatic lipase have
high sequence homology. The crystal structure of human pancreatic lipase and site
specific mutagenesis of lipoprotein lipase and hepatic lipase demonstrate an Asp-His-Ser
catalytic triad covered by a peptide loop bounded by a conserved disulfide bridge.
Substitution of the loop of lipoprotein lipase with either six or twenty-two residues of the
hepatic lipase loop gives mutants with complete and partial activity, respectively. Partial
or complete substitution with the pancreatic lipase loop produces an inactive protein.
Comparison of the primary sequences and the predicted secondary structures identify
Glu^{220} and a large hydrophobic moment of the first predicted α-helical region as structural
features of lipoprotein lipase that distinguish it from hepatic and pancreatic lipase and may
account for the much greater hydrolytic activity of lipoprotein lipase on a triolein substrate.

Hydrolysis of triglyceride by lipoprotein lipase (LPL) at the vascular wall is the key process
for utilization of the fatty acids derived from diet as well as endogenously synthesized
lipoproteins [1]. Full activity of LPL requires apolipoprotein C-II (apoC-II), a lipid
associating protein in the macromolecular substrate. Based on primary sequence
homology to pancreatic lipase [2] as well as studies involving site-directed mutagenesis
[3,4], the catalytic domain of LPL consists of Ser^{132}, Asp^{156}, and His^{241}. The functional
domains proposed for LPL, other than the catalytically active site, include apoC-II and
heparin binding sites, a catalytic domain, a site for dimer formation, and a lipid binding
site. The location of these functional domains of LPL remain to be identified.

The crystallographic data show that pancreatic lipase (PL) contains a 23-amino acid
disulfide bridged loop which covers the catalytic domain and prevents access of the
substrate to the catalytic pocket (Figure 1). Because of its location, movement of the
lipase loop is necessary to allow hydrolysis of lipid substrates. This movement of a loop
has been elegantly illustrated by crystallographic studies of an inhibitor covalently bound
to the active site serine of a fungal lipase [5]. The loop that covers the active site is the

A. L. Catapano et al. (eds.), Drugs Affecting Lipid Metabolism, 89–96.
© 1993 Kluwer Academic Publishers and Fondazione Giovanni Lorenzini.

structural feature which accounts for the interfacial activation phenomena originally observed by Sarda and Desnuelle [6]. Conservation of most disulfide bonds between LPL, hepatic lipase (HL), and PL suggests that all enzymes in this family have similar tertiary structures [7].

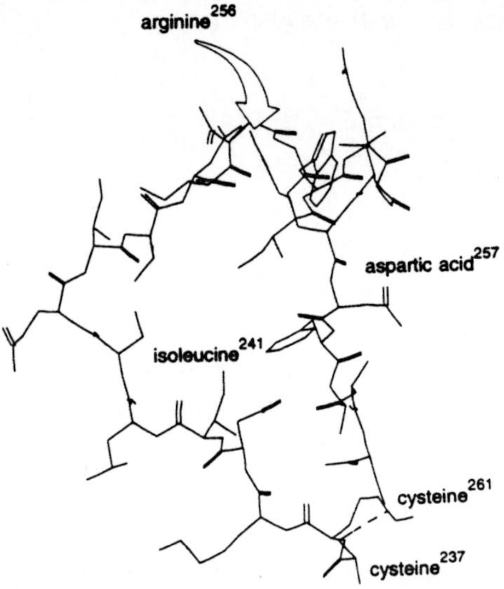

Figure 1. The Peptide Loop that Covers the Active Site of Human Pancreatic Lipase.

The primary sequences of the loop region of the lipase family are presented in **Table I.**

```
        humlpl          FQPGCNIGEAIRVIAERGLGDVD.QLVKC
        bovlpl          FQPGCNIGEALRVIAERGLGDVD.QLVKC
        muslpl          FQPGCNIGEAIRVIAERGLGDVD.QLVKC
        cknlpl          FQPGCNLGEALRLIAEKGFSDVD.QLVKC
        gplpl           FQPGCNIQDALRVISQKGFGDMD.QLVKC

        humhl           FQPGCHSLELYRHIAQHGFNAIT.QTIKC
        rabhl           FQPGCHFLELYKHIAQHGLNALS.QTIKC
        rathl           FQPGCHFLELYKHIAEHGLNAIT.QTIKC

        humpl           EMPGCKKNILSQIVDIDGIWEGTRDFAAC
        pigpl           QMPGCQKNILSQIVDIDGIWEGTRDFVAC
        dogpl           EMPGCKKNALSQIVNLDGIWEGTRDFVAC

   LPL consensus        FQPGCNL-eAlRvI--rGlgDvD.QLVKC
   HL consensus         FQPGCH-LELYkHIA-HGlNAit.QTIKC
   PL consensus         -MPGCkKNiLSQIVdIDGIWEGTRDFAAC

Overall Consensus       --PGCb---o-+-o---Go--ob-b-o-C
```

Table I. Sequence Homolog of the Loop Region of Lipases. Lower case abbreviations of the single letter amino acid code denote the location of conservative substitutions; the site of an Arg insertion in the PL loop by a period; hydrogen bonding residues by b; hydrophobic residues by o; and positively charged residues by +.

Inspection of the sequence data reveals that only the guinea pig loop is variable, with three residues, Gly[219], Ala[226], and Glu[227], that differ from other LPL species. Otherwise, the residues are completely conserved. Whether the three variant residues affect the comparative physical and enzymatic properties of guinea pig LPL is not known. By contrast, the substitution of Ser for Phe in the HL loop is expected to produce substantial effects on lipid binding properties of the loop. Moreover, the tripeptide containing Ala and Thr flanking a hydrophobic residue in HL bears little resemblance to the corresponding LPL tripeptide of two Asp residues on either side of a hydrophobic residue. The sequence similarity of loop region of LPL and HL to that of PL is limited. Easily identified features are (a) Gly at the center of the loops, (b) hydrogen bonding potential at the beginning and end of the loops, (c) five hydrophobic residues at various locations throughout the loop and (d) a positive charge in the center of the first helical region. To evaluate the structure-function relationships in the LPL loop, we expressed mutants of LPL in which the structural characteristics of the loop were altered by interchanging part and all of the loop regions of HL and PL [3].

Lipoprotein lipase (wild-type):	(wt)	NIGEAIRVIAERGLGDVD.QLVK
LPL-hepatic lipase (partial):	(LPL-pH)	HSLELYRHIAERGLGDVD.QLVK
LPL-hepatic lipase (complete):	(LPL-cH)	HSLELYRHIAOHGFNAIT.OTIK
LPL-pancreatic lipase (partial):	(LPL-pP)	KKNALSOIIAERGLWEGTRDFVA
LPL-pancreatic lipase (complete):	(LPL-cP)	KKNALSOIVNLDGIWEGTRDFVA

	LPL activity (munits/dish)		LPL mass (µg/dish)		specific activity (munits/µg)	
	cell	media	cell	media	cell	media
wild-type	530 ± 41.5	1750 ± 130	17 ± 2.1	50 ± 3.5	31	35
LPL-pH	500 ± 40	1700 ± 131	16 ± 1.9	48 ± 3	31	35
LPL-cH	310 ± 38	1050 ± 100	16 ± 2.5	47 ± 2.8	19	22
LPL-pP	0	0	6.5 ± 1.9	21 ± 1.8	0	0
LPL-cP	0	0	7 ± 1.7	20 ± 2	0	0

Table II. Lipoprotein Lipase Activity in Wild-Type LPL and Loop Mutants Produced in COS Cells. The data and experimental conditions are described by Faustinella et al. [3]. The substrate was tri-[1-^{14}C]-oleoylglycerol.

The partial-replacement chimeric LPL containing a partial HL sequence, expressed *in vitro*, was fully active, with a specific activity identical to that of the wild-type enzyme (Table II). The complete-replacement HL chimeric molecule was also active, with a specific activity approximately 60% that of the wild-type enzyme. By contrast, replacement of the LPL loop with the pancreatic lipase loop, either partially (replacing 6 of 22 residues) or completely (replacing the 22 LPL loop residues with a 23-residue pancreatic lipase loop produced inactive proteins). Although immunoreactive protein was synthesized and secreted in both cases. The observed absence of activity in the case of the PL mutants can be attributed to the differences in sequences, illustrated in **Figure 1**. The highly conserved Glu[220] in LPL corresponds to Ile[241] in PL. An absolutely conserved Gln[234] in

LPL corresponds to Asp[257] in PL. The other major sequence difference is the insertion of Arg[256] in the PL loop.

The results of the loop replacement construction can be interpreted from two perspectives: charge distribution and the hydrophobic/hydrophilic balance. The charge of the amino acid residues along the loop of LPL, and the HL mutants is shown in **Figure 2A**. The charge differences between LPL and HL toward the carboxyl terminal portion of the loop apparently are responsible for the reduced rate of triglyceride hydrolysis by the LPL mutant containing the complete HL loop. Additional studies with site-specific mutants of the LPL loop will be necessary to determine whether the principal effect of the ala-ile-thr substitution in lieu of asp-val-asp is exerted on K_m or K_{cat}.

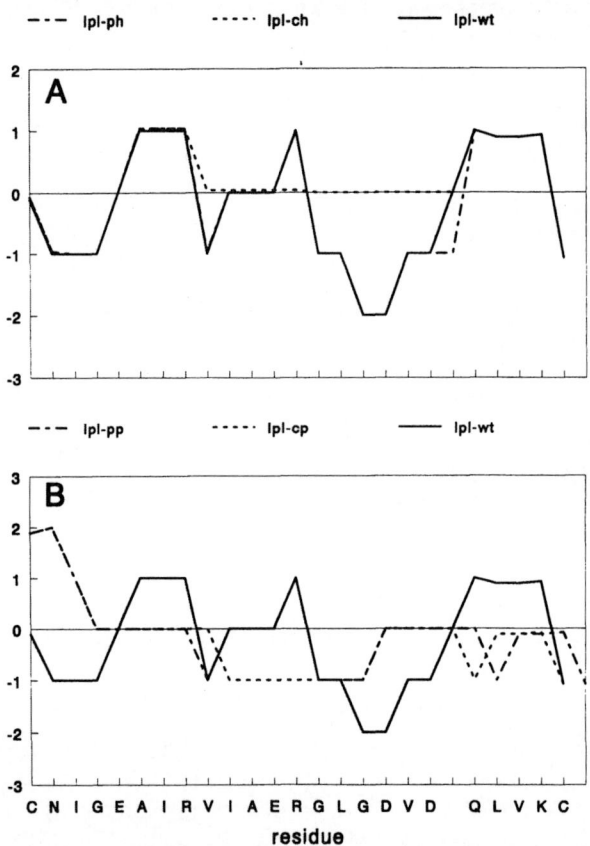

Figure 2. Charge Distribution of the Loop Region of LPL and the Mutant Enzymes.
The sequence of LPL is given as reference. An R is inserted between D and Q in the PL mutants. The upper panel (A) is calculated from LPL and the HL mutant. The lower panel (B) is calculated from LPL and the PL mutants.

The second perspective focuses on the properties of the loop determined by hydrophobic-hydrophilic balance of amino acid side chains. The method described by Pownall et al. [8] uses the free energy of transfer of amino acids from water to hydrocarbon for the hydrophobicity scales and assumes a helical arrangement of the peptide. The helical moment for each residue is represented as a vector directed from the helical axis through its position on the circumference of the helix. The polar hydrophilic vector is converted to a negative free energy contribution by rotation through 180°. The value of the ratio of the hydrophobic and hydrophilic vectors is one measure of the amphipathic character of the sequence region. The resultant from the projection of the hydrophobic and hydrophilic vector takes into account the relative position on the helix as well as the magnitude of the respective moment.

As shown in **Figure 3**, the first region of LPL has an unusually large hydrophobic moment, assuming an α-helical conformation of the loop. This feature is also retained in both HL mutants. The hydrophobic face of LPL is bounded by glutamic acid residues and contains Arg[223], a positively residue conserved among all lipases. In other regions of the loop, the effect of hydrophobic moment on the properties of LPL and either HL or PL mutants is minimal **(Figure 3 & 4)**, possibly due to the lack of an α-helical conformation of the sequence. For all enzymes, there is no appreciable hydrophilic helical moment **(Figure 5)**.

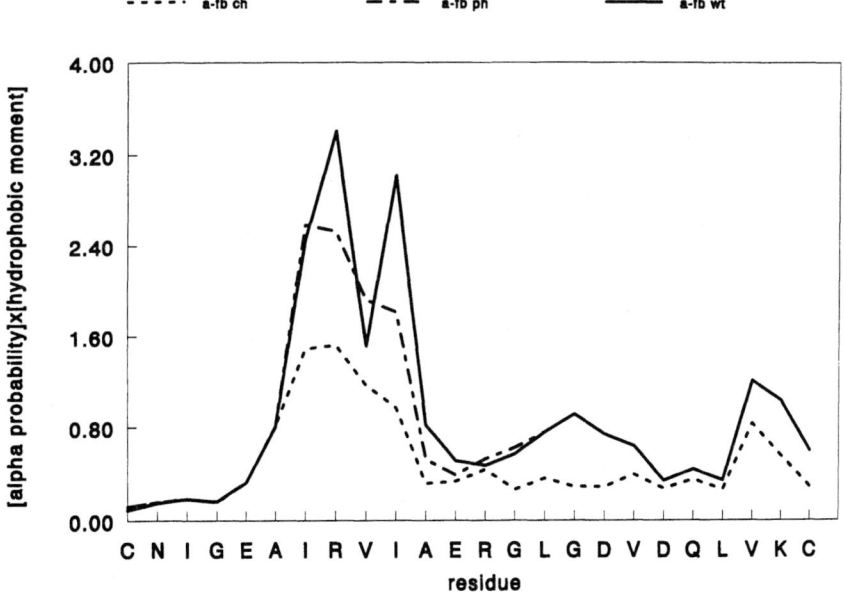

Figure 3. Hydrophobic Helical Moments of LPL and HL mutant enzymes. The sequence of LPL is given as reference. The hydrophilic moment has been calculated as described by Pownall et al. [8].

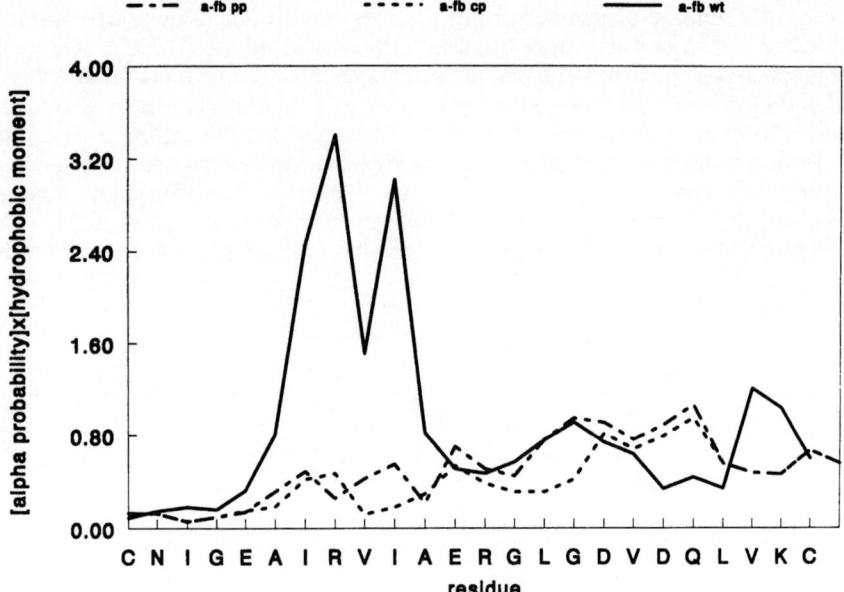

Figure 4. Hydrophobic Helical Moments of LPL and PL Mutant Enzymes.

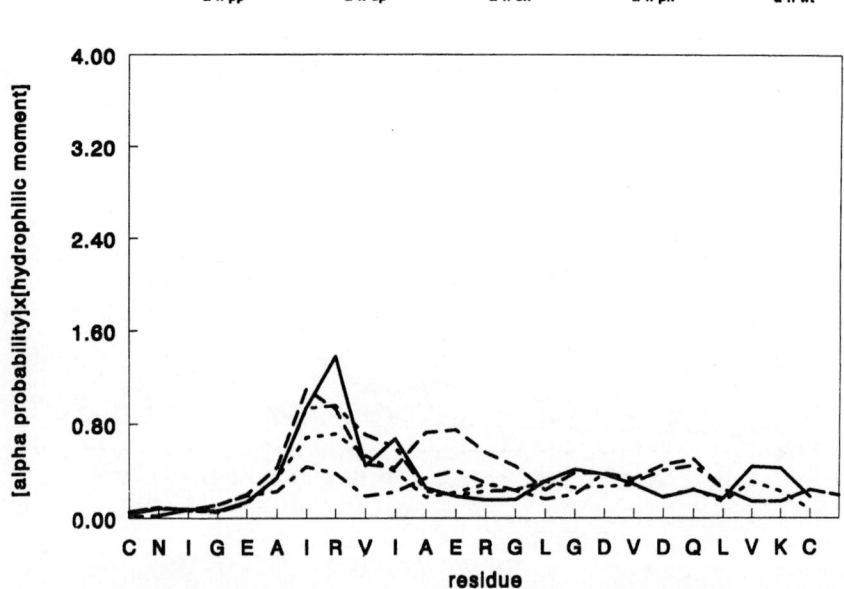

Figure 5. Hydrophilic Helical Moments of LPL and the Mutant Enzymes.

The most striking difference between LPL and the PL mutant enzymes is the angle between the hydrophobic and hydrophilic moments along the sequence of the loop (**Figure 6**). Throughout the PL loop, the resultant of the helical moments is large and highly variable in its orientation. By contrast, the angle between the hydrophobic and hydrophilic moments of the loop of LPL is small, relatively invariant and not significantly different from that of either HL loop mutant.

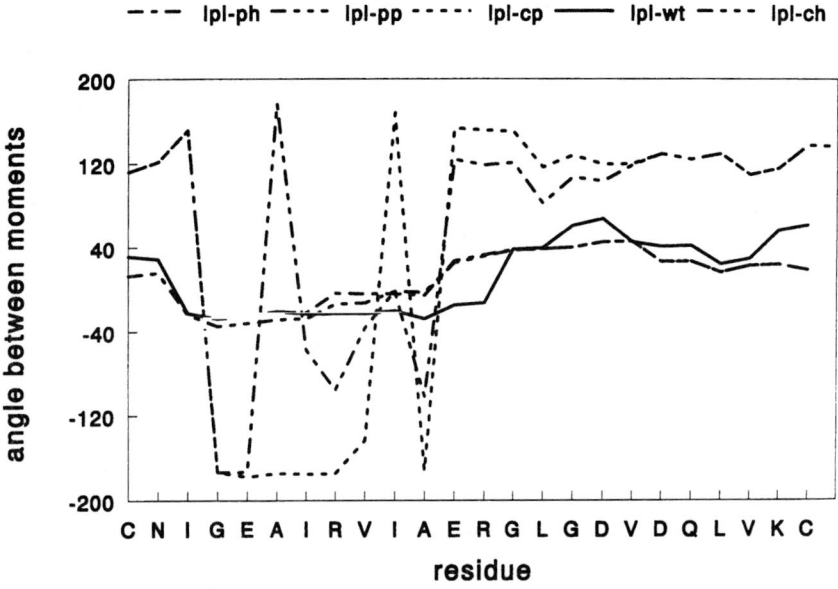

Figure 6. The Resultant of the Hydrophobic and Hydrophilic Moments of LPL and Mutant Enzymes.

As noted previously [3], there are substantial differences in the size and surface properties of the respective physiological substrates for these three enzymes. The loop regions of LPL and hepatic triglyceride lipase should have a high degree of functional similarity and large hydrophobic helical moments in order to interact with and penetrate the interfacial region of the plasma lipoproteins. LPL utilizes as substrates almost exclusively the large triglyceride-rich chylomicrons and very low density lipoproteins. Hepatic triglyceride lipase acts on a much more diverse group of lipoprotein particles, with significant hydrolysis of both phospholipids and triglycerides in very low density, intermediate density, and high density lipoproteins. The surface monolayers of the plasma lipoproteins are complex. They contain primarily phosphatidylcholine, cholesterol, several apolipoproteins, and other relatively soluble lipid components that rapidly equilibrate with the surface. By contrast, the bile salt micellar substrates for pancreatic lipase are dominated by the negatively charged bile acids. For PL, the helical moments and the variation in the orientation of the resultant of the helical moments suggest that formation of the PL-bile salt complex does not require penetration of the loop into the interfacial region of the micelle. Thus, from the perspective of the lipid-water interface of the respective substrates, the properties of the loop region of these lipases and their role in substrate binding would be similar for LPL and hepatic triglyceride lipase on one hand but quite different for pancreatic lipase on the other hand.

An unambiguous understanding of the structure-function relationships of LPL clearly requires a crystal structure [9]. Molecular engineering, however, has provided important evidence for the functional loop domain of LPL involved in hydrophobic substrate binding. The surface loop of LPL that shields the active center of the enzyme does not have an absolute sequence requirement, but has function equivalents with different primary sequences.

This work was supported by HL-27341 (LCS, RDK), HL-16512 (LC) and March of Dimes Birth Defects Foundation (LC). We are indebted to Dr. Fritz Winkler for the x-ray coordinates of the structure of human pancreatic lipase.

References

1.   Smith LC, Pownall HJ. in Lipolytic enzymes (Bergstrom B, Brockman HL eds.) Elsevier, Amsterdam, 1983, pp. 264-305.
2.   Winkler FK, D'Arcy A, Hunziker W. Nature 1990;343:771-774.
3.   Faustinella F, Smith LC, Chan L. Biochemistry 1992;31:7219-7223.
4.   Emmerich J, Beg OU, Peterson J, Previato L, Brunzell JD, Brewer HB Jr., Santamarina-Fojo S. J Biol Chem 1992;267:4161-4165.
5.   Derewenda U, Brzozowski AM, Lawson DM, Derewenda ZS. Biochemistry 1992;31:1532-1541.
6.   Sarda L, Desnuelle P. Biochem Biophys Acta 1958;30:513-521.
7.   Yang C-H, Gu ZW, Yang HX, Rohde MF, Gotto AM, Pownall HP. J Biol Chem 1989;264:16822-16827.
8.   Pownall HP, Knapp RD, Gotto AM, Massey JB. FEBS Lett 1983;159:17-23.
9.   Smith LC, Faustinella F, Chan L. Curr Opin Struct Biol 1992;2:490-496.

Molecular Genetics of Lipoprotein Lipase Deficiency

Michael R. Hayden and Yuanhong Ma

Summary

Prior recognition and selection of patients for analysis was based on the phenotype of chylomicronemia. However, mutations in the LPL gene might also result in a milder clinical phenotype. The clue to detection of these changes in the LPL gene might be to be to investigate patients who present with chylomicronemia when exposed to specific environmental stresseswhile continuing with only moderate hypertriglyceridemia in the resting state.

The first mutations which were described in the LPL gene occurred in a patient with undetectable levels of LPL mass and activity in plasma and constituted a major deletion and a duplication [1]. Since this report in 1989, many different DNA sequence alterations have been identified to cause LPL deficiency [2]. A summary of the sequence alterations which have beenreported from our laboratories is shown in Figure 1. As can be seen, the majority of thesecomprised missense mutations, mostly in exons 4, 5 and 6. In most instances, different mutations segregate in unrelated families and distinct population groups.

Exceptions to this, are the substitution of leucine for proline at amino acid 207 which constitutes approximately 73% of the mutant alleles in patients with LPL deficiency from Quebec, Canada [3]. The prevalence, spatial distribution and genealogy of this mutation in the Quebec population has been determined [4]. Genealogical reconstruction has revealed that thismutation has been traced to 16 founders all of whom migrated to Quebec in the early 17th Century from the northwestern part of France, especially from the regions of Perche.

A. L. Catapano et al. (eds.), Drugs Affecting Lipid Metabolism, 97–100.
© 1993 Kluwer Academic Publishers and Fondazione Giovanni Lorenzini.

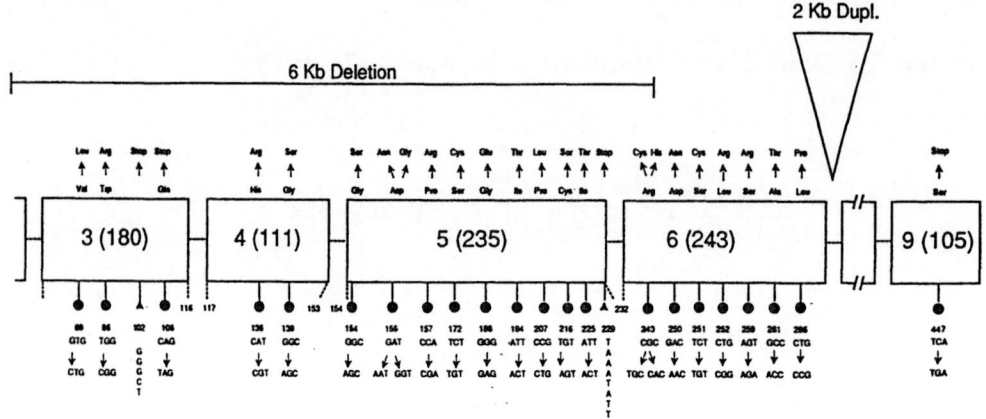

Figure 1 : Summary of mutations in the LPL gene

Another mutation found in higher frequency in different populations is the substitution in exon 5 of glycine for glutamic acid at residue 188. This mutation has been found in unrelated affected persons of different ancestries, including those of French Canadian, British, Polish, Dutch, German and East Indian descent [5-6]. This mutation has also been found in all probands of Indian descent in Cape Town, South Africa [7]. These affected Indian kindreds have been independently traced to immigrants who arrived in South Africa during the first half of this century. No definite genetic relationship between these particular families was established despite the fact that they came from four villages very close to the town of Khed, approximately 150 km from Bombay. A common original ancestral origin for the 188 mutation has been postulated, possibly predating the spread of the Caucasian populations [5].

Most of the mutations shown in Figure 1 represent missense mutations and their functional significance has clearly been demonstrated by in vitro site directed mutagenesis studies [1,3,5,7,8-16]. Other mechanisms for production of a catalytically defective protein includeinsertions resulting in frameshifts. A frameshift mutation resulting from an insertion of 5'-GGGCT-3' at residue 102 results in the formation of a premature stop codon in exon 4 and a truncated protein [13]. This LPL protein is not detectable with the 5D2 monoclonal antibodythat has epitope specificity to residue 400 in the carboxy terminus portion of the LPL protein [17]. Another frameshift mutation at the 3' end of exon 5 is due to an insertion of 5'-TAAATATT-3' after the second nucleotide of codon 229. This mutation also results in a frameshift which is expected to produce a truncated protein of 238 residues, including 9 foreign residues at its C terminal [17,18].

Acknowlegements

Part of the contents of this manuscript have been presented orally to the meeting of the Biochemical Society in London, 1992 and will be included in the proceedings of the meeting. I would like to thank Dr. J.J. Kastelein, Dr. J.D. Brunzell and Dr. H. Funke for collaboration andsupport in providing information concerning mutations in their patients that they have analyzed. This work is supported by grants from the Medical Research Council of Canada, the British Columbia Heart and Stroke Foundation and The Canadian Genetic Disease Network.Dr. Hayden is an established investigator of the British Columbia Children's Hospital and Dr. Yuanhong Ma is a postdoctoral fellow supported by the Medical Research Council of Canada.

References

1. Langlois, S., Deeb, S., Brunzell, J., Kastelein, J.J., Hayden, M.R. (1989) P.N.A.S. 88, 948-952.
2. Hayden, M.R., Ma, Y., Brunzell, J., Henderson, H.E. (1991) Current Opinion in Lipidology 2(2), 104-110.
3. Ma, Y., Henderson, H.E., Ven Murthy, M.R., Roederer, G., Monsalve, M.V., Clarke, L.A., Julien, P., Brunzell, J., Hayden, M.R. (1991) New Engl. J. Med. 324, 1761-1766.
4. Normand, T., Bergeron, J., Fernandez-Margallo, T., Bharucha, A., Ven Murthy, M.R., Julien, P., Gagne, C., Dionne, C., De Braekeleer, M., Hayden, M.R. (1992) Human Genet. 89, 671-675.
5. Monsalve, M.V., Henderson, H.E., Roederer, G., Julien, P., Deeb, S., Kastelein, JJP, Peritz, L., Devlin, J., Bruin, T., Ven Murthy, M.R., Gagne, C., Davignon, J., Lupien, P.J., Brunzell, J.D., Hayden, M.R. (1991) J. Clin. Invest. 86, 728-734.
6. Emi, M., Wilson, D.E., Iverius, P.H., Wu, L., Hata, A., Hegele, R., Williams, R.R., Lalouel, J.M. (1990) J. Biol. Chem. 265, 5910-5916.
7. Henderson, H.E., Hassan, F., Berger, G.M.B., Hayden, M.R. (1992) J. Med. Genet. 29, 119- 122.
8. Ma, Y., Bruin, T., Tuzgol, S., Wilson, B.I., Roederer, G., Liu, M-S., Davignon, J., Kastelein, J.J.P., Brunzell, J.D., Hayden, M.R. (1992) J. Biol. Chem. 267(3),1918-1923.
9. Ma, Y., Wilson, B.I., Bijvoet, S., Henderson, H.E., Cramb, E., Roederer, G., Ven Murthy, M.R., Julien, P., Bakker, H.D., Kastelein,

J.J.P., Brunzell, J.D., Hayden, M.R. (1992) Genomics 13(3), 649-653.
10. Bruin, T., Kastelein, J.J.P., van Diermen, D.E., Ma, Y., Henderson, H.E., Stuyt, P.M.J., Stalenhoef, A.F.H., Sturk, A., Brunzell, J.D., Hayden, M.R. (1992) Eur. J. Biochem. 208(2), 267-272.
11. Ma, Y., Liu, M-S., Ginzinger, D., Frohlich, J., Brunzell, J.D., Hayden, M.R. (1992) J. Clin. Invest., in press.
12. Henderson, H.E., Devlin, R., Peterson, J., Brunzell, J.D., Hayden, M.R. (1990) Mol. Biol. & Med.7,511-517.
13. Devlin, R.H., Deeb, S., Brunzell, J.D., Hayden, M.R. (1990) Am. J. Hum. Genet. 46,112- 119.
14. Henderson, H.E., Ma, M.F., Hassan, F., Monsalve, M.V., Winkler, F., Gubernator, K., Firth, J., Brunzell, J.D., Hayden, M.R. (1991) J. Clin. Invest. 87(6), 2005-2011.
15. Bruin, T., Tuzgol, S., Mulder, W.J., van den Ende, A.E, Hayden, M.R., Kastelein, J.J.P., submitted.16. Ma, Y., Liu, M-S., Chitayat, D., Beisiegel, U., Benliane, P., Forsythe, I., Brunzell, J.D., Hayden, M.R. (1992) submitted.
17. Liu, M-S., Ma, Y., Hayden, M.R., Brunzell, J.D. (1992) Biochim. et Biophys. Acta 1128, 113-115.
18. Faustinella, F., Chang, A., van Biervliet, J.P., Rosseneau, M., Vnaimont, N., Smith, C., Chen, S.H., Chan, L. (1991) J. Biol. Chem. 266,14418-14424.

A NEW CASE OF LIPOPROTEIN LIPASE DEFICIENCY

A. CAPURSO, G. PEPE , G. CHIMIENTI , F. RESTA, M. LOVECCHIO, A.M. COLACICCO

ABSTRACT

We describe a new case of lipoprotein lipase (LPL) deficiency in a 33 year old man with a history of milky serum, severe hypertriglyceridemia with hyperchylomicronemia and recurrent episodes of acute pancreatitis.

Analysis of the complete coding sequence, with intronic boundaries, and the promoter region of the LPL gene of the propositus revealed a G-->C transversion at the 5' donor splice site of intron 1. We suggest that this mutation is not compatible with normal mRNA processing and it is responsible for the defect in our patient.

INTRODUCTION

Lipoprotein lipase (LPL-triacylglycerolprotein acylhydrolase) has a pivotal role in the metabolism of plasma lipoproteins.

Active LPL is a noncovalently linked homodimer of a glycoprotein of 448 amino acids, 54 KD m.w. (1,2). It is synthesized mainly by parenchimal cells of adipose tissue, heart and muscle. It is then transported to the luminal surface of capillary endothelial cells where it presumably binds to heparan sulfate.

To hydrolyze triglycerides to di- and monoglycerides and free fatty acids, LPL requires the binding of a specific co-factor, the apolipoprotein (apo) C-II.

The LPL gene has been mapped on the short arm of human chromosome 8 (3). It extends over 30 kb and consists of 10 exons interrupted by 9 introns (4-6).

Human LPL cDNA has been cloned and its sequence reported. It includes a region of 1425 nucleotides coding for a protein of 475 aminoacids which becomes a mature protein of 448 residues after cleavage of a 27 residue signal peptide (5,6).

LPL deficiency is a rare autosomal recessive disorder occurring with a carrier frequency of 1/500 in most parts of the world, one notable exception being Quebec (2,7). Fasting plasma from these patients reveals type I hyperlipoproteinemia with triglyceride concentration above 2000 mg/dl, normal or slightly elevated cholesterol in total plasma and in very low density

A. L. Catapano et al. (eds.), Drugs Affecting Lipid Metabolism, 101–106.
© 1993 Kluwer Academic Publishers and Fondazione Giovanni Lorenzini.

lipoproteins (VLDL), and markedly reduced cholesterol concentration in low and high density lipoproteins (LDL and HDL). LPL activity in post-heparin plasma is typically absent, in the presence of normal levels of apo C-II. Hepatic lipase (HL) is normal.

The clinical syndrome of LPL deficiency is characterized by severe hypertriglyceridemia with chylomicronemia, abdominal pain, recurrent acute pancreatitis, lipaemia retinalis, eruptive xantomata, hepato-splenomegaly and failure to thrive.

Several LPL gene mutations have been identified (7-23): 10 of them were missense mutations, 4 non sense mutations, 1 frameshift, 2 splice site mutations (intron 2), 1 large deletion (6 kb) and 1 duplication (2 kb).

We describe a new case of LPL deficiency due to a point mutation in the 5' splice site of intron 1.

METHODS

Clinical Data

The proband is a 33 year old male. He presented at the age of 16 with a history of severe recurrent abdominal pain and milky serum. The first serum lipid analysis revealed a typical hyperlipoproteinemia phenotype I, with chylomicronemia and a triglyceride level of 2160 mg/dl. The electrophoresis of post-heparin plasma failed to show the typical increase in pre beta and beta electrophoretic mobility and measurement of post heparin lipolytic activity (PHLA) with radiolabeled triolein showed none or only trace amounts of LPL activity while HL activity was normal. Apo C-II, evaluated in native serum by radial immunodiffusion and in VLDL by isoelectric focusing, was normal.

Subsequently, the patient entered the hospital several times suffering from recurrent pancreatitis. In these circumstances, his serum triglyceride level was above 3000 mg/dl. A low fat diet (20 g/day) and substitution of fats with medium chain triglycerides (MCT) reduced the level of serum triglycerides below 1000 mg/dl.

On physical examination, using ecotomography and C.T.scan, the patient showed a normal physical growth, typical lipaemia retinalis, moderate hepatomegaly but no splenomegaly, Histological examination of liver biopsy showed the presence of steatosis, scattered foci of hepatocyte necrosis and slight fibrosis of portal areas. Cutaneous eruptive xantomata were never observed.

Recent fasting plasma lipoprotein values were: triglycerides 1910; cholesterol 269; LDL-cholesterol 39; HDL-cholesterol 11 (expressed in mg/dl).

Laboratory methods

Blood samples were obtained in the fasting state from the proband, parents and siblings. Post-heparin plasma was obtained from blood taken 10 mins after an intravenous bolus of heparin administred at 60 U/kg body mass. Protease inhibitor aprotinin (trasylol) was added to the samples at 25 IU/ml. Aliquots were either assayed immediately or stored at -80° C.

Lipoprotein fractionation (by preparative ultracentrifugation, delipidization and isoelectric focusing of apolipoproteins), cholesterol and triglyceride evaluation and serum apolipoproteins quantitation with specific antibodies, were all performed as previously reported (24). Plasma lipoprotein (a) level (Lp(a)) was evaluated by enzyme immuno-assay (IMMUNOZYM Lp(a)-Immuno AG A-1220 WIEN).

Quantitation of PHLA was performed as previously reported with (3H)triolein as substrate and inhibition of LPL activity with protamine sulfate (24).

DNA was extracted from peripheral blood cells according to standard procedure. All nine translated exons, with corresponding intron-exon boundaries, and the 5' non transcribed regulatory region of the LPL gene were separately amplified by P.C.R. as previously described (25) with suitable primers. The amplification products were sequenced using the Sanger procedure.

RESULTS

The plasma lipid and apoprotein values of the proband and his family are reported in Table I.

The values of PHLA, evaluated several times in duplicate, were found to be slightlly variable. In particular while hepatic lipase (HL) activity was in the normal range, lipoprotein lipase (LPL) activity was between 0 and 1.5 umol FFA/ml/hr, i. e. absent or 1/10 of the normal values.

To determine the molecular basis of the disease in the propositus, the gross structure of the LPL gene was examined by hybridization of pLPL35 probe to the genomic DNA digested with different restriction enzymes. No obvious rearrangements were found (data not shown). Then the entire LPL gene was analyzed in detail, using P.C.R. followed by DNA sequence analysis. When compared to the normal sequence, only a single base change was found, a G to C transversion at the first nucleotide of intron 1.

Table I. Lipid and apolipoprotein values of proband and kindred.
The values of lipids and apoproteins are expressed in mg/dl. TG = triglycerides. CH = total cholesterol. LDL = LDL-cholesterol. HDL = HDL-cholesterol. A-I = apoprotein A-I (and so forth).

TG	84	140	962	80	50	96	1901	1678
CH	157	227	248	180	200	44	269	177
LDL	101	164	43	105	134	95	39	36
HDL	39	35	16	59	56	63	12	14
A-I	126	111	82	---	---	150	73	72
A-II	33	39	20	---	---	29	25	25
C-II	4.2	3.4	3.2	---	---	4.1	3.2	3.3
C-III	9.6	11.8	6.8	---	---	8.3	7.0	6.9
B	67	87	51	---	---	59	49	50
E	4.3	5.5	3.2	---	---	3.5	3.0	3.1
Lp(a)	41.9	41.0	---	---	---	12.3	2.7	2.5

DISCUSSION

We have presented some preliminary data of a new case of LPL deficiency.

The propositus showed a typical pattern of hyperlipoproteinemia phenotype I (hyperchylomicronemia type I) with recurrent pancreatitis. He never had cutaneous eruptive xantomata or splenomegaly, but did have hepatomegaly. Histological examination of liver biopsy documented a marked steatosis with some focal necrosis of hepatocytes and initial fibrosis of portal areas.

The parents, who were not consanguineous, had never suffered from pancreatitis but interestingly the mother appeared to be rather hypercholesterolemic with a serum cholesterol level ranging between 223 and 302 mg/dl while serum triglycerides were constantly below 180 mg/dl. These data make the inheritance of LPL deficiency quite complex and possibly linked to other gene defects.

Clinical features, particularly the inactivity of lipoprotein lipase enzyme, made the diagnosis of LPL deficiency in our patient possible, The LPL mass of the proband, determined with ELISA method using a monoclonal antibody, was undetectable (kindly performed by M.R. Taskinen). We suggest therefore that the trace amounts of LPL activity found in some determinations are depending on the sensibility of the method.

Molecular studies were performed by analyzing the complete coding sequence, with intronic boundaries, and the promoter region of the LPL gene of our patient. The only mutation found anywhere along the sequenced region was a G->C change which distroys the conserved GT dinucleotide at the 5' donor splice site of intron 1, a mutation as yet not described in the litterature for LPL defects. Although we have not direct evidence that this mutation alters the mRNA processing (the study of the patient's mRNA is still in progress in our Laboratory) it is known that a point mutation at this site can drastically affect correct splicing and hence enzyme production.

In conclusion we suggest that defective mRNA splicing, due to the mutation at the junction site of intron 1, is responsible for the LPL deficiency in our patient.

ACKNOWLEDGEMENTS

We are indebted with Prof. Marja-Riitta Taskinen, Third Dept. of Medicine, University of Helsinki, Finland, for evaluating LPL mass. Prof. A.L. Catapano and Dr. P. Roma, Dept. of Pharmacology University of Milan, have also evaluated PHLA activity of the proband. The skilful assistance of Dr. M. Di Tommaso, M.C. D'Amelio, M.L. Fulgido, M. Attolini and V. Di Perna is also acknowledged.

Supported by M.U.R.S.T. grants, C.N.R. Progetto Finalizzato Invecchiamento-PF 40, and C.N.R. Progetto Finalizzato Dieta Mediterranea.

REFERENCES

1.   Iverius, Per-Henrik., Ostlund-Lindquist, Ann-Margret (1976) 'Lipoprotein Lipase from bovine milk. Isolation procedure, chemical characterization and molecular weight analysis', J. Biol. Chem. 251, 7791-7795.

2.   Brunzel, John D. (1989) 'Familial Lipoprotein Lipase deficiency and other causes of the chylomicronemia syndrome', in C.R. Scriver, A.L. Beaudet, W.S. Sly, D. Valle (eds), The Metabolic Basis of Inherited Disease, McGraw-Hill Co. Publisher, New York, pp. 1165-1180.

3.   Sparks, R.S., Zollner, S., Klisak, I., Kirkgessner, T.G., Komaromy, M.C., Mohandas, T., Schotz. M.C. and Lusis A.J. (1987) 'Human genes involved in lipolysis of plasma lipoproteins: mapping of loci for lipoprotein lipase to 8p22 and hepatic lipase to 15q21', Genomics 1, 138-144.

4.   Deeb, S.S. and Peng, R. ((1989) 'Structure of the human lipoprotein lipase gene', Biochemistry 28, 4131-4135.

5.   Kirchgesser, T.G., Svenson, K.L., Lusis, A.J. and Schotz, M.C. (1987) 'The sequence of cDNA encoding lipoprotein lipase', J. Biol. Chem. 262, 8463-8466.

6.   Wion, K.L., Kirchgessner, T.G., Lusis, A.J., Schotz, M.C., Lawn, R.M. (1987) 'Human lipoprotein lipase complementary DNA sequence', Science 235, 1638-1641.

7.   Monsalve, M.V., Henderson, H., Roederer, G., Julien, P., Deeb,   S., Kastelein, J.J.P., Peritz, L., Devlin, R., Bruin, T., Murthy, M.R.V., Gagne, C., Davignon, J., Lupien, P.J., Brunzell, J.D., and Hayden, M.R. (1990) 'A missense mutation at codon 188 of the human lipoprotein lipase gene is frequent cause of lipoprotein lipase deficiency in persons of different ancestries', J. Clin. Invest. 86, 728-734.

8.   Devlin, R.H., Deeb, S., Brunzell, J. and Hayden, M.R. (1990) 'Partial gene duplication involving exon-Alu interchange results in lipoprotein lipase deficiency', Am. J. Hum. Genet. 46, 112-119.

9.   Langlois, S., Deeb, S., Brunzell, J.D., Kastelein, J.J.P. and Hayden M.R. (1989) 'A major insertion accounts for a significant proportion of mutations underlying human lipoprotein lipase deficiency', Proc. Natl. Acad. Sci. USA 86, 948-952.

10.   Ameis, D., Kobayashi, D.J., Davis, R.C., Ben-Zeev, O., Malloy,   M.J.,   Kane,   J.P., Lee, G., Wong, H., Havel, R.J. and Schotz, M.C. (1991) 'Familial hyperchylomicronemia (Type I hyperlipoproteinemia) due to a single missense mutation in the lipoprotein lipase gene', J. Clin. Invest. 87, 1165-1170.

11.   Beg, O.U., Meng, M.S., Skarlatos, S.I., Previator, L., Brunzell, J.D., Brewer, H.B. Jr., and Fojo, S.S. (1990) 'Lipoprotein lipase (Bethesda): a single amino acid sobstitution (Ala176-Thr) leads to abnormal heparin binding and loss of enzymatic activity', Proc. Natl. acad: Sci. USA 87, 3474-3478.

12.   Emi, M., Wilson, D.E., Iverius, P.H., Wu, L., Hata, A., Hegele, R., Williams, R.R., and Lalouel, J.M. (1990) 'Missense mutation (Gly-Glu188) of humal lipoprotein lipase imparting functional deficiency', J. Biol. Chem. 265, 5910-5916.

13.   Emi, M., Hata, A., Robertson, M., Iverius, P.H., Hegele, R., and Lalouel, J.M. (1990) 'Lipoprotein lipase deficiency resulting from a nonsense mutation in exon 3 of the lipoprotein lipase gene', Am. J. Hum. Genet. 47, 107-111.

14.   Hata, A., Emi, M., Luc, G., Basdevant A., Gambert, P., Iverius, P.H., and Lalouel J.M. (1990) 'Compound Heterozygote for Lipoprotein Lipase Deficiency: Ser-Thr 244 and Transition in 3' Splice Site of Intron 2 (AG-AA) in the Lipoprotein Lipase Gene', Am. J. Hum. Genet. 47, 721-726.

15.   Henderson, H.E., Devlin R., Peterson, J., Brunzell, J.D., and Hayden, M.R. (1990) 'A frameshift mutation in exon 3 of the lipoprotein lipase gene causes a premature stop codon and lipoprotein lipase deficiency', Mol. Biol. Med. 7, 511-517.

16.   Dichek, H.L., Fojo, S.S., Beg, O.U., Skarlatos S.I., Brunzell, J.D., Cutler, G.B.Jr., and Brewer, B.Jr. (1991) 'Identification of Two Separate Allelic Mutations in the Lipoprotein Lipase Gene of a Patient with Familial Hyperchylomicronemia Syndrome', J. Biol. Chem. 266, 473-477.

17.   Gotoda, T., Murase, T., Ishibashi, S., Shimano, H., Harada, K., Yamada, N., (1990) '
Splicing, Nonsense, and Missense Mutations in Familial Lipoprotein Lipase Deficiency',
Arteriosclerosis 10, abs. 833.
18.   Bruin, T., Tuzgol, S., Bijvoet, S.M., Brunzell, J.D., Hayden, M.R., Kastelein, J.J., (1991)
'Lipoprotein Lipase Deficiency in the Netherlands', International Atherosclerosis Society abs. 219.
19.   Henderson, H.E., Ma, Y., Hassan, M.F., Monsalve, M.V., Marais, A.D., Winkler, F.,
Gubernator, K., Peterson, J., Brunzell, J.D., Hayden, M.R., (1991) 'Amino acid substitution (Ile 194-
>Thr) in exon 5 of the lipoprotein lipase gene causes lipoprotein lipase deficiency in three
unrelated probands. Support for a multicentric origin', J. Clin. Invest. 87, 2005-2011.
20.   Funke, H., Wiebush, H., Paulweber,B., Assman, G., (1990) 'Identification of the
Molecular Defect in Patient whith Type I Hyperlipidemia ', Arteriosclerosis 10 abs. 830.
21.   Paulweber, B., Wiebusch, H., Miesenboeck, G., Funke, H., Assmann, G., Hoelzl, B.,
Sippl, M.J., Friedl, W., Patsch, J. R., Sandhofer, F., (1991) 'Molecular basis of lipoprotein lipase
deficiency in two Austrian families with type I hyperlipoproteinemia', Atherosclerosis 86, 239- 250.
22.   Ma, Y., Henderson, H. E., Murthy, M. R., V., Roederer, G., Monsalve, M. V., Clarke, L. A.,
Normand, T., Julien, P., Gagne, C., Lambert, M., Davignon, J., Lupien, P. J., Hayden, M. R. (1991)
'A Mutation in the Human Lipoprotein Lipase Gene as the Most Common Cause of Familial
Chylomicronemia in French Canadians', N. Engl. J. Med. 324, 1761-1766.
23.   Faustinella, F., Chang, A., Van Biervliet, J. P., Rosseneu, M., Vinaimont, N., Smith, L. C.,
Chen, S. H., Chan, L., (1991) 'Catalytic triad residue mutation (Asp 156--> Gly) causing familial
lipoprotein lipase deficiency. Co-inheritance with a nonsense mutation (Ser 447-->Ter) in a Turkish
family', J. Biol. Chem. 266, 1418-1424.
24.   Capurso, A., Mogavero, A.M., Resta, F., Di Tommaso, M., Taverniti, R., Turturro, F., La
Rosa, M., Marcovina, S., and Catapano, A.L. (1988) 'Apolipoprotein C-II deficiency: detection of
immunoreactive apolipoprotein C-II in the intestinal mucosa of two patients', J. Lipid Res. 29, 703-
711.
25.   Crecchio, C., Capurso A., Pepe, G. (1990) 'Identification of the mutation responsible for
a case of plasmatic apolipoprotein CII deficiency (Apo CII-Bari)', Biochem. Biophys. Res.
Commun. 29, 1118-1127.

Modulation of Triglyceride Metabolism by Diet and Drugs

Henry J. Pownall, Patricia Pace, Roger D. Knapp, Antonio M. Gotto, Jr. and Peter H. Jones

ABSTRACT. Lipoprotein lipase is a key enzyme in the mobilization of fat from triglyceride-rich particles in human plasma. The composition of very low density lipoproteins (VLDL) and chylomicrons, which are secreted by the liver and the intestine, respectively, are important determinants of the composition, structure and catabolism of high (HDL) and low density lipoproteins (LDL). HDL and LDL communicate with triglyceride-rich lipoproteins through the action of cholesteryl ester transfer protein (CETP) which exchanges the triglycerides of the latter for the cholesteryl esters of the former . Therefore, the amounts of triglyceride in VLDL and chylomicrons are important determinants of the triglyceride content and the metabolic fates of HDL and LDL. Under fasting conditions the major donor of triglycerides to LDL and HDL are the VLDL. Therefore, factors that affect fasting triglycerides are likely to have an effect on metabolism of all lipoproteins including the chylomicrons.

Fibrates: In hypertriglyceridemia, there is frequently some underlying compromise of the lipolytic capacity of the plasma compartment and the release of non-esterified fatty acids (NEFA) from adipose tissue is poorly controlled. There is an array of lipid abnormalities that frequently characterize hypertriglyceridemia. These are decreased plasma lipoprotein lipase activity, elevated plasma NEFA, low HDL-cholesterol, low or undetectable HDL_2-cholesterol, and small dense LDL. These effects are not independent of each other and may be due only to the elevations in plasma NEFA that are due to increased release by adipose tissue. Beginning with an increase in the release of NEFA by adipose tissue the remainder of the lipid abnormalities can be explained on the basis of known activities in the plasma compartment. The increased plasma NEFA stimulates additional hepatic triglyceride synthesis and secretion of apoB-100 in the VLDL [1-5]. This enlarged pool of VLDL-triglyceride exchanges with the cholesteryl esters of HDL and LDL through the action of CETP. The resulting triglyceride-rich HDL_2 and LDL are transient because they are rapidly converted to HDL_3 and small dense LDL, respectively. This is mediated by the activity of hepatic lipase (HL). The increase in postprandial lipemia that is found in hypertriglyceridemic subjects is likely due to competition of the large numbers of VLDL with the chylomicrons for the limited numbers of sites for binding to the lipoprotein lipase on

A. L. Catapano et al. (eds.), Drugs Affecting Lipid Metabolism, 107–113.
© 1993 Kluwer Academic Publishers and Fondazione Giovanni Lorenzini.

the capillary endothelium.

Many of these clinical symptoms are greatly reduced with fibrate therapy and it is interesting to examine how their reductions may be related to the primary mechanism by which fibrates elicit their therapeutic effects. *In vitro* [3, 7] and *in vivo* *[8]* fibrates inhibit the release of free fatty acids from fat cells. It appears that the major physiologic effects that are found *in vivo* can be explained on the basis of this single activity. All other effects such as lower plasma triglycerides, increased HDL-cholesterol, decreased LDL and VLDL triglycerides, decreased postprandial lipemia and increased lipoprotein lipase follow mechanistically from an inhibition of lipolysis in adipose tissue. With the inhibition of lipoprotein lipase in adipose tissue there is a decrease in the plasma concentration of NEFA. With a reduction in this important precursor, hepatic triglyceride synthesis declines. As a consequence there is a decrease in VLDL and apoB-100 secretion [1]. With a decrease in both the number of VLDL particles and their respective triglyceride contents, the pool of triglycerides that are available for exchange with the LDL and HDL is reduced. In the absence of transport of additional triglycerides to HDL and LDL, there is little or no substrate for HL and the conversion of LDL and HDL to their smaller analogs does not occur.

Omega-3 Fatty Acids: Substitution of a diet of polyunsaturated fats for one containing saturated fats its generally acknowledged to reduce plasma cholesterol. Reductions in plasma triglycerides can also be achieved via dietary interventions. Omega-3 fatty acids are one the most potent hypolipidemic components of diet [9, 10]. The most common of these are eicosapentaenoic acid (EPA) and docosahexaenoic acid (DHA), both of which are major components of the oils that are found in cold water fish. Much of the past work has focused on the effects of omega-3 fatty acids in liver where they can inhibit a number of enzymes involved in hepatic triglyceride synthesis including acylCoA:diacylglycerol acyltransferase [11] and phosphatidate phosphohydrolase [12]. Alternatively, n-3 fatty acids may reduce hepatic fatty acids by increasing β-oxidation [13] or inhibiting VLDL assembly through the reductions in PC synthesis [14] which have been shown to be obligatory for the assembly of secretion-competent VLDL [15]. More recent studies suggest that omega-3 fatty acids may alter the flux of NEFA between plasma and adipose tissue. As a consequence, plasma NEFA are dramatically reduced and there is less fatty acid available for hepatic triglyceride synthesis [16-19]. This may explain the reduction in both fasting and postprandial lipemia that occur after consuming a diet that is rich in omega-3 fatty acids. However, the role of increased lipolytic susceptibility of the chylomicrons that are secreted when a saturated fat load is replaced by one of polyunsaturated fat load cannot be discounted [20, 21].

Ethanol: In contrast, to fibrates and n-3 fatty acids, excessive ethanol (ETOH) consumption increases HTG [22]. Moreover, dietary challenges of fat and ETOH appear to unmask lipid abnormalities that might be ignored if only fasting plasma lipid levels were measured [23-25]. It has been proposed that ETOH inhibits lipolytic activity in adipose tissue leading to a decrease in plasma NEFA [26] and that this effect is mediated by acetate that is derived from the oxidation of ETOH [27, 28]. With the decreased NEFA one would expect less hepatic triglyceride synthesis and, in the absence of other effects, lower plasma VLDL-TG. Instead plasma VLDL-TG increases in response to an acute dose of ETOH. Moreover, recent studies have shown that an acute ETOH load has little effect on several parameters of lipid metabolism in adipose tissue including plasma insulin, NEFA, and catecholamines [29]. Herein, we summarize some recent findings on the mechanisms by which n-3 fatty acids, fibrates and ETOH affect plasma TG concentrations.

Results and Discussion

Effects of Lopid: Six Type IIA subjects were placed on an American Heart Association Step 1 diet for three months. At the end of this interval two tests were conducted. First, the lipoproteins were isolated from a unit of plasma after an overnight fast after which the lipid composition of each lipoprotein class was determined. Second, each subject was give an oral fat tolerance test according to Patsch [30]. The subjects continued the Step 1 diet for another three months during which they were given the hypotriglyceridemic drug, gemfibrozil (1.5 g bid). At the end of this test interval the lipoprotein compositions and postprandial lipemia were again determined. Two notable differences between the control and test intervals were seen in response to the reduced plasma triglyceride levels. First, the triglyceride content of all lipoprotein classes was reduced (Table 1). Second, the magnitude

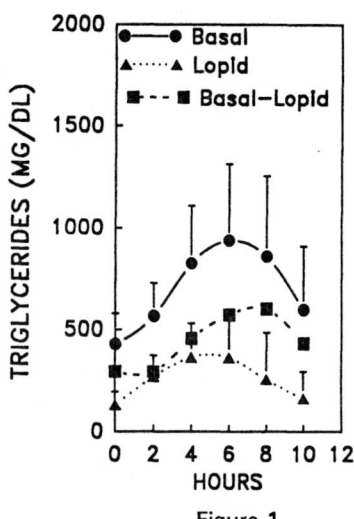

Figure 1

and the duration of postprandial lipemia was much lower after fibrate treatment (Figure 1). Lopid was particularly effective in reducing the lipemia in the late postprandial phase; this finding is significant because delayed clearance is highly correlated with the incidence of coronary artery disease [31].

Table 1

Composition of Lipoproteins After Lopid Therapy

	HDL		LDL		VLDL	
	Basal	+ Lopid	Basal	+ Lopid	Basal	+ Lopid
Protein	50.	50	17.6	16.9	5.8	9.1
Phospholipid	20.5	19.5	17.2	16.9	14.4	20.6
Triglyceride	3.5	2.0*	5.1	2.3*	55.	54.7
Free Cholesterol	1.0	1.3	5.7	6.1	4.0	6.1
Cholesteryl Ester	25.	27.2	54.4	57.8	20.8	9.5

*Different from basal value, $p < 0.005$.

These data support the model described above in the following way. The lower triglyceride to protein ratio found in the VLDL after drug treatment is likely due to a reduction in the amount of fatty acid that is available for glycero-lipid synthesis. With lower plasma levels of endogenously synthesized lipoproteins, a greater fraction of plasma lipoprotein lipase can be committed to the hydrolysis of chylomicrons, resulting in their more rapid disappearance with drug treatment. With reduced concentrations of plasma triglycerides in both VLDL and chylomicrons, there is a smaller pool of triglyceride to exchange with the LDL and HDL and their respective triglyceride contents are also reduced [32, 33].

Omega-3 Fatty Acids   We have compared the effects of rat chow with and without corn oil or menhaden oil on the plasma NEFA, triglyceride and lipoprotein levels in male Sprague-Dawley rats (180-225 g). Animals were fed either a control chow diet or the chow diets plus either 10% corn oil or 10 % menhaden oil, which is rich in omega-3 fatty acids. Animals were maintained on these diets for 3, 7, and 14 days, after which at least four animals in each group were sacrificed. At each of the time intervals, some or all of the following measurements were made as follows: 1] liver and plasma triglyceride by an enzymatic assay (Boerhinger-Manheim), 2] NEFA (Boehringer- Mannheim), 3] fatty acid composition of the plasma and liver triglycerides and plasma NEFA by gas chromatography of the methyl esters produced by transesterification, 4] plasma insulin levels by radioimmunoassay and the plasma cholesterol levels of the HDL and apolipoprotein B-containing proteins.

After nineteen days, there was the expected reduction in the plasma triglyceride levels of animals on the menhaden oil that was associated with a decrease in the plasma cholesterol in the apoB-containing lipoproteins but no changes in HDL-cholesterol (Table 2). Plasma insulin levels were highest in the animals on the menhaden oil but the differences among the three diets never reached statistical significance.

Table 2
Plasma Lipid Levels

Analyte	Plasma/Tissue Concentration		
	Chow	Corn Oil	Menhaden Oil
HDL-Cholesterol, mg/dl	29.3 ± 9	30.7 ± 3	30.6 ± 1
(LDL + VLDL)-cholesterol, mg/dl	11.8 + 1	8.2 ± 1	3.7 ± 1
Liver-triglyceride, mg/g	2.6 ± .5	4.9 ± 1	8.4 ± 1
Plasma Triglyceride	66. ± 15	58. ± 11	35. ± 7
Plasma NEFA	398. ± 146	489. ± 173	257. ± 35

Interestingly, there was a positive correlation between plasma NEFA and plasma triglycerides (data not shown). This correlation was observed in spite of rather large differences within groups of animals. These data support the model described above in which the plasma NEFA levels may determine, in part, the amount of VLDL-triglyceride that is secreted by the liver.

Ethanol: Following an over night fast, six subjects were given several different fat tolerance tests (50 g/m^2 body area). These were composed of saturated fat. These tests were repeated with the addition of 40 ml ethanol in the form of dry white wine. Following each fat load, plasma levels of triglyceride and NEFA were determined as a function of time The fatty acid data are summarized in Table 3. These data show that there was little change in the plasma levels of arachidonate acid, which was not a component of the fat load. This was observed even if ethanol was added to the fat load. In contrast, oleate and palmitate, which compose a major fraction of the fat load, increased between t = 0 to t = 4 h after the standard fat load. Addition of ethanol to the fat load was associated with significant reduction in the plasma levels observed at four hours. This effect was assigned to an inhibition of lipoprotein lipase.

Table 3

Postprandial NEFA (μmol/ml) after a Saturated Fat Load with and without Ethanol Fatty Acid

	Sat Fat		Sat Fat + ethanol	
	0 h.	4 h.	0 h.	4 h.
$C_{14:0}$	0.026	0.14	0.018	0.053*
$C_{16:0}$	0.40	0.68	0.32	0.38*
$C_{16:1}$	0.046	0.08	0.030	0.03*
$C_{18:0}$	0.11	0.21	0.11	0.16
$C_{18:1}$	0.42	0.68	0.33	0.26**
$C_{18:2}$	0.44	0.51	0.36	0.30*
$C_{20:4}$	0.067	0.08	0.051	0.05**
$C_{20:5}$				
$C_{22:6}$				
Total	1.51	2.38	1.22	1.23*

Fat vs fat + ethanol; *p < 0.05, **p < 0.01.

Summary: These data show various ways that diets and drugs can effect changes in plasma triglycerides and NEFA and that these two parameters of lipid metabolism are mechanistically connected. Some of the effects have been observed before but interpreted differently or in a slightly different light. Different tissue sites are loci for the three different drug and diet effects. Adipose tissue is the likely site of action of both n-3 fatty acids and fibrates although other more complex activities may be involved, especially in the former case. Our most notable finding was the connection between oral ethanol and lipolysis. We have compelling evidence that ethanol inhibits lipoprotein lipase activity but the mechanism remains unknown. Although other investigators assigned the lipemic effects of ethanol to the liver, our evidence clearly points to an effect that is in the plasma compartment. This is important because it makes investigation of the mechanism simpler than if a tissue site was involved.

At this point it is difficult to make dietary recommendations except in subject where hyperlipidemic subjects are prone to bouts of pancreatitis. For these persons prudent use of ethanol in combination with saturated fat would be advised. The literature contains arguements both for and against the reduction of plasma triglycerides to reduce the risk of coronary artery disease [34]. On one hand high HDL-cholesterol is induced by ethanol while at the same time producing a transient increase in plasma triglycerides and reduced risk of coronary artery disease. Additional mechanistic and clinical studies will be needed to clarify this important health question.

Literature Cited

1.   Dixon JL, Furukawa S, and Ginsberg HN. J Biol Chem 1991; 266:5080.
2.   Erickson SK, and Fielding PE. J Lipid Res 1986; 27:875.
3.   Stirling C, McAleer M, Reckless HPD, Campbell RR, Mundy D, Betteridge DJ, and   Foster K. Chemical Science 1985; 68:83.
4.   Goh EH and Heimberg M. Biochem. Bilphys. Res. Commun. 1973; 55:382-388.
5.   Soler-Argilaga C, Wilcox HG and Heimberg M. J Lipid Res 1976; 17:139.
6.   Elkeles RS, Ashwell M, Priest R, and Dkurrant M. Proc Roy Soc Med 1976; 69(Supplement 2):98.
7.   Carlson LA. Proc Roy Soc Med 1976; 69 (Supplement 2):101.
8   Rifkind B. Metabolism 1966; 15:673.
9.   Harris WS. J Lipid Res 1989; 30:785.
10.   Nestel PJ. Annu Rev Nutr 1990; 10:149.
11.   Rustan AC, Nossen JO, Christiansen EN, and Drevon CA. J Lipid Res 1988; 29:1417.
12.   Wong SH and Marsh JB. Metabolism 37:1177.
13.   Yamazaki RK, Shen T, and Schade GB. Biochim Biophys Acta 1987; 920:62.
14.   Homan R, Grossman JE, and Pownall HJ. J Lipid Res 1991; 32:231-241.
15.   Yao, ZM, and Vance DE. J Biol Chem 1987; 263:2998.
16.   Stacpoole PW, Alig J, Kilgore LL, Ayala CM, Herbert PN, Zech LA, and Fisher WR. 1988. Metabolism 37:944-951.
17.   Tsai CE, Wooten JT, and Otto DA. Nutr Res 1989; 9:673.
18.   Baltzell JK, Wooten JT, and Otto DA. Lipids 1991; 26:289.
19.   Bick D, Pao Q, and Pownall HJ (abstract) FASEB Journal 1992; 6:A370.
20.   Hulsmann WC, Oerdemanus MC, and Jansen H. Biochim Biophys Acta 1980; 618:364-9.
21.   Weintraub MS, Zechner R, Brown A, Eisenberg S, and Breslow JL. J Clin Invest 1988; 82:1884-93.
22.   Lieber, CS, and Pignon, J.-P. In: J Shepherd and JC Fruchart, eds. Human plasma lipoproteins: Chemistry, Physiology and Pathology. 1989:245-80.
23.   Weintraub MS, Eisenberg S, and Breslow JL. J Clin Invest 1987; 79:1110.

24. Wilson, DE, Schreibman PH, Brewster AC, and Arky RA. J Lab Clin Med. 1970; 75:264-74.
25. Chait A, Mancini M, February AW, and Lewis B. Lancet 1972; 2:62-4.
26. Jones DP, Perman ES, and Lieber CS. J Lab Clin Med 1965; 66:804-13.
27. Crouse JR, Gerson CD, DeCarli LM, and Lieber CS. J Lipid Res 1968; 9:509-12.
28. Abramson, EA, and Arky, RA. J Lab Clin Med 1968; 72:105-17.
29. Frayn KN Coppack SW, Walsh PE, Butterworth HC, Humphreys SM, and Pedrosa HC. Metabolism 1990; 39:958
30. Patsch JR, Karlin JV, Scott LW, Gotto AM Jr. Proc Natl Acad Sci *USA* 1983; 80:1449
31. Patsch JR, Hopferwieser Th, Muhlberger V, Knapp E, Braunsteiner H, Gotto AM, Dunn K, and Patsch W. Postprandial lipemia in patients with coronary artery disease. Arteriosclerosis 1990; 10:766a
32. Deckelbaum RJ, Granot E, Oschry Y, Rose L, and Eisenberg S. Arteriosclerosis 1984; 4:225.
33. Mann CJ, Yen FT, Grant AkMk, and Bihain BE. J Clin Invest 1991; 88:2059.
34. Austin MA. Arteriosclerosis and Thrombosis. 1991; 11:2-14.
35. Assman G, Gotto AM, and Paoletti R., eds. Report of an international committee for the Evaluation of hypertriglyceridemia as a vascular risk factor. Amer J Cardiol 1991; 681A

DRUGS AFFECTING REVERSE CHOLESTEROL TRANSPORT

G. FRANCESCHINI, G. CHIESA, L. CALABRESI, C.R. SIRTORI

ABSTRACT. Reverse cholesterol transport identifies a series of metabolic events resulting in the transport of excess cholesterol from peripheral tissues to the liver. High density lipoproteins (HDL) are the vehicle of cholesterol in this reverse transport, a function believed to explain the inverse correlation between plasma HDL levels and atherosclerosis. An attempt to stimulate, by the use of drugs, this transport process may hold promise in the prevention and treatment of arterial disease. Among the agents affecting lipoprotein metabolism, only probucol exerts significant effects on reverse cholesterol transport, by stimulating the activity of the cholesteryl ester transfer protein and consequently altering HDL subfraction composition/distribution. Another approach to the stimulation of reverse cholesterol transport consists in raising plasma HDL levels; studies in animals, either by exogenous supplementation or by endogenous overexpression, have shown a consistent benefit in terms of atherosclerosis regression and/or non progression. It is thus time for thinking at different future treatments of atherosclerosis, combining the classical lipid-lowering treatments with innovative methods to promote cholesterol removal from the arterial wall.

1. The reverse cholesterol transport

The reverse cholesterol transport was originally defined by Glomset in 1968 [1], as the complex mechanism by which the excess cholesterol in peripheral cells is transported to the liver, the only organ in the human body responsible for cholesterol elimination. This process appears to be dependent on high density lipoproteins (HDL) [2], thus explaining the well established negative correlation between plasma HDL levels and atherosclerosis [3].

The whole process of reverse cholesterol transport can be subdivided into three major steps (Figure 1), occurring at the peripheral cell, plasma and liver levels. Initially, cholesterol, in the unesterified form, is taken up by HDL; small, pre-β-migrating particles, containing only apolipoprotein A-I as protein component, seem to be the most efficient in the process [4]. However, other apolipoproteins, either in lipoprotein particles [5] or in lipid-free form [6], have the

A. L. Catapano et al. (eds.), Drugs Affecting Lipid Metabolism, 115–120.
© 1993 Kluwer Academic Publishers and Fondazione Giovanni Lorenzini.

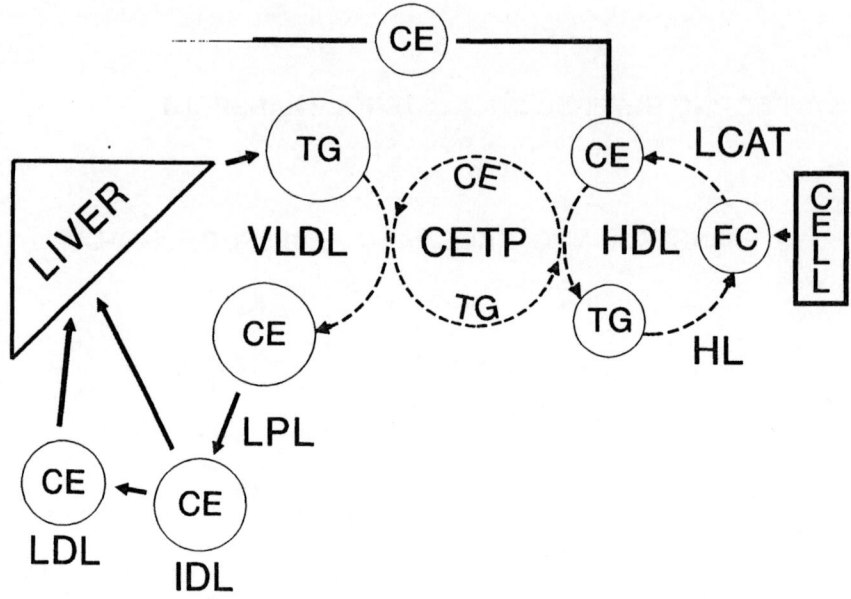

Figure 1. Physiology of reverse cholesterol transport

capacity of promoting cholesterol efflux from a variety of cells. Cholesterol de-
sorbs from the plasma membrane into the extracellular fluids by a diffusion-
limited process, being then incorporated into acceptor particles. Apolipoproteins can also interact with a specific cell surface receptor, promoting the translocation of excess cholesterol from intracellular to membrane pools [2].

The second step in reverse cholesterol transport occurs in plasma and involves the interaction of HDL with other lipoproteins, enzymes and transfer proteins, resulting in a continuous remodeling of HDL particles with changes in
size, lipid and apolipoprotein composition [2]. The cellular unesterified cholesterol incorporated into small HDL is esterified by the lecithin:cholesterol acyltransferase (LCAT) enzyme [1] and the newly synthesized cholesteryl esters
are exchanged for very low density lipoprotein (VLDL) triglycerides [7], by the
"cholesteryl ester transfer protein" (CETP or LTP-I) [8]. Once the triglyceride
content in the new large HDL reaches a threshold value, triglycerides and
phospholipids are hydrolyzed by hepatic lipase (HL), converting the large, triglyceride-rich HDL_2 back into small, triglyceride- and cholesteryl ester-poor
HDL_3 [2]. Other factors, i.e. lipoprotein lipase and phospholipid transfer protein (LTP-2), may be involved in the HDL conversion process; their physiological role in the reverse cholesterol transport is at present unclear, although LPL
and LTP-2 may supply phospholipids to HDL, as substrates for the LCAT reaction [2].

The third and final step in reverse cholesterol transport consists in the delivery of the cholesteryl esters synthesized in plasma to the liver. This last process
can occur through different mechanisms, possibly species-specific [9]. In man,

the major pathway for cholesterol delivery to the liver is dependent on low density lipoproteins (LDL) [10], which interact with specific receptors recognizing apo B [11]. The CETP-mediated transfer of cholesteryl esters from HDL to VLDL-LDL is thus essential for the transport of cholesterol from periphery to liver. In CETP-deficient animals, i.e. rat, dog and pig [12], or even in humans homozygous for a genetic CETP deficiency [13], HDL directly transport cell-derived cholesterol to the liver were cholesteryl esters are taken up either as a whole HDL particle or by a process independent from particle uptake [9].

2. Effects of drugs on the reverse cholesterol transport

Numerous pharmacological substances can modify plasma HDL levels in man; among these, several lipid-lowering drugs, antihypertensive agents, hormones and microsomal enzyme inducers [14]. Drug-induced elevations of HDL-cholesterol (HDL-C) levels have been associated with a reduction of cardiovascular risk [15, 16], possibly secondary to an improved reverse cholesterol transport, but only few studies have examined the effect of drugs on this process.

Treatments with lipid-lowering agents affect HDL subfraction distribution in both normo- and hyperlipidemic subjects (Figure 2), but the exact mechanisms responsible for these modifications are generally poorly understood. Pure cholesterol-lowering agents, i.e. anion exchange resins and HMG-CoA reductase inhibitors, generally minimally affect plasma HDL levels and subfraction distribution [14, 17], although prolonged treatments may result in enhanced plasma HDL_2-C levels [18, 19], possibly secondary to an increased cholesterol esterification [19] and/or decreased CETP activity [20]. Fibric acid derivatives

	HDL-SUB	LCAT	CETP
RESINS	=	=/↑	↓
STATINS	=	↑	=/↓
FIBRATES	↑HDL_3	=/↓	=
NIC. ACID	↑HDL_2↑HDL_3	=	=
PROBUCOL	↓↓HDL_2↓HDL_3	=	↑↑
FISH-OIL	↑HDL_2↓HDL_3	↓	↓

Figure 2. Effects of drugs on reverse cholesterol transport

increase plasma HDL$_3$-C [17], either through an increased flux of surface material derived from the stimulated VLDL lipolysis or by increasing hepatic lipase activity [2]. Minor changes were observed in patients treated with acipimox, while the parent compound, nicotinic acid, reportedly increases both HDL$_2$ and HDL$_3$ levels [2], probably by inhibiting hepatic lipase. Probucol, the most powerful agent in promoting the regression of peripheral cholesterol deposits [21], dramatically lowers plasma HDL, and particularly HDL$_2$ levels, mainly through a direct stimulation of CETP activity [22] (Figure 2). By this mechanism, and by a stimulation of the uptake of cell cholesterol by HDL [23], probucol may exert the antiatherogenic effect observed in humans [21] and experimental animals [24].

3. Future developments

Reverse cholesterol transport is the result of a complex mechanism, with several, different metabolic steps. There is, at present, little information on the relative importance of the single steps on the efficiency of the whole process *in vivo*, especially in man. Furthermore, *in vivo* studies are necessary to definitely prove that a promotion of reverse cholesterol transport reverts the atherogenic process in man. However, it seems to us that this field provides promising targets for the treatment of atherosclerotic disease.

A great effort is needed in order to identify treatments that specifically act on reverse cholesterol transport; probucol is the prototype of drugs promoting reverse cholesterol transport, preventing atherosclerosis development and inducing a regression of tissue lipid deposits. In addition to chemical agents, recombinant proteins seem to be the great promise for the future. HDL infusions in cholesterol fed rabbits prevent atherosclerosis development [25] and even promote regression [26]. Furthermore, apo A-I overexpression, doubling the plasma levels in transgenic mice, converts atherosclerosis-susceptible into resistant animals [27].

Based on these findings, it is time to look at different approaches to the treatment of atherosclerotic vascular disease, not only based on prevention, but also on an attempt to cure the disease, by treatments causing a rapid regression of the lesions. In this scenario, a great advantage will come from the development of more sophisticated non-invasive techniques allowing a direct visualization of the arterial wall [28] and thus the identification of the patients with clinically significant arterial lesions. These patients will be then placed into a "regression program", with the objective of a rapid, monitored regression of the lesions. At the moment, the best "regression program" seems to be a combination of LDL-apheresis [29], to remove atherogenic lipoproteins, simultaneous infusion of HDL analogues, and probucol.

4. References

1. Glomset, J.A. (1968) 'The plasma lecithin:cholesterol acyltransferase reaction', J. Lipid Res. 9, 155-167.

2. Franceschini, G., Maderna, P. and Sirtori, C.R. (1991) 'Reverse cholesterol transport: physiology and pharmacology', Atherosclerosis 88, 99-107.
3. Miller, G.J. and Miller, N.E. (1975) 'Plasma high-density lipoprotein concentration and development of ischaemic heart disease', Lancet i, 16-19.
4. Castro, G.R. and Fielding, C.J. (1988) 'Early incorporation of cell-derived cholesterol into pre-beta-migrating high density lipoprotein', Biochemistry 27, 25-29.
5. Steinmetz, A., Barbaras, R., Ghalim, N., Clavey, V., Fruchart, J.C. and Ailhaud, G. (1990) 'Human apolipoprotein A-IV binds to apolipoprotein A-I/A-II receptor sites and promotes cholesterol efflux from adipose cells', J. Biol. Chem. 265, 7859-7863.
6. Hara, H. and Yokoyama, S. (1991) 'Interaction of free apolipoproteins with macrophages. Formation of high density lipoprotein-like lipoproteins and reduction of cellular cholesterol', J. Biol. Chem. 266, 3080-3086.
7. Nichols, A.V. and Smith, L. (1965) 'Effect of very low-density lipoproteins on lipid transfer in incubated serum', J. Lipid Res. 6, 206-210.
8. Chajek, T. and Fielding, C.J. (1978) 'Isolation and characterization of a human serum cholesteryl ester transfer protein', Proc. Natl. Acad. Sci. USA 75, 3445-3449.
9. Reichl, D. and Miller, N.E. (1989) 'Pathophysiology of reverse cholesterol transport: insights from inherited disorders of lipoprotein metabolism', Arteriosclerosis 9, 785-797.
10. Sniderman, A., Marpole, D. and Teng, B. (1978) 'Low density lipoprotein: a metabolic pathway for return of cholesterol to the splanchnic bed', J. Clin. Invest. 61, 867-874.
11. Goldstein, J.L. and Brown, M.S. (1977) 'The low-density lipoprotein receptor pathway and its relation to atherosclerosis', Annu. Rev. Biochem. 46, 897-930.
12. Ha, Y.C. and Barter, P.J. (1982) 'Differences in plasma cholesteryl ester-transfer activity in sixteen vertebrate species', Comp. Biochem. Physiol. 71, 265-269.
13. Yamashita, S., Sprecher, D.L., Sakai, N., Matsuzawa, Y., Tarui, S. and Hui, D.Y. (1990) 'Accumulation of apolipoprotein E-rich high density lipoproteins in hyperalphalipoproteinemic human subjects with plasma cholesteryl ester transfer protein deficiency', J. Clin. Invest. 86, 688-695.
14. Sirtori, C.R. and Franceschini, G. (1990) 'Pharmacological modifications of high density lipoproteins', in L.A. Carlson (ed.), Disorders of HDL, Smith-Gordon Co, London, pp. 197-202.
15. Levy, R.I., Brensike, J.F., Epstein, et al. (1984) 'The influence of changes in lipid values induced by cholestyramine and diet on progression of coronary artery disease: results of the NHLBI Type II Coronary Intervention Study', Circulation 69, 325-337.
16. Manninen, V., Elo, O., Frick, H., et al. (1988) 'Lipid alterations and decline in the incidence of coronary heart disease in the Helsinki Heart Study', J. Amer. Med. Ass. 260, 641-651.
17. Franceschini, G., Sirtori, M., Vaccarino, V., Gianfranceschi, G., Chiesa, G. and Sirtori, C.R. (1989) 'Plasma lipoprotein changes after treatment with pravastatin and gemfibrozil in patients with familial hypercholesterolemia', J. Lab. Clin. Med. 114, 250-259.
18. Neuman, M.P., Neuman, H.R., and Neuman J. (1991) 'Significant increase

of high-density lipoprotein$_2$-cholesterol under prolonged simvastatin treatment', Atherosclerosis 91, S11-S19.

19. Desager, J.P., Horsmans, Y, and Harvengt, C. (1991) 'Lecithin:cholesterol acyltransferase activity in familial hypercholesterolemia treated with simvastatin and simvastatin plus low-dose colestipol', J. Clin. Pharmacol. 31, 537-542.

20. Savolainen, M.J., Kervinen, K., Hannuksela, M., Seppanen, S. and Kesaniemi A. (1991) 'Lovastatin and colestipol decrease plasma cholesteryl ester transfer protein activity', 9th International Symposium on Atherosclerosis, Abs p. 36.

21. Yamamoto, A., Matsuzawa, Y., Yokoyama, S., Funahashi, T., Yamamura, T. and Kishino, B. (1986) 'Effects of probucol on xanthomata regression in familial hypercholesterolemia', Am. J. Cardiol. 57, 29H-35H.

22. Franceschini G, Chiesa G. and Sirtori C.R. (1991) 'Probucol increases cholesteryl ester transfer protein activity in hypercholesterolemic patients', Eur. J. Clin. Invest. 21, 384-388.

23. Goldberg, R.B. and Mendez, A. (1988) 'Probucol enhances cholesterol efflux from cultured human skin fibroblasts', Am. J. Cardiol. 62, 57B-59B.

24. Kita, T., Nagano, Y., Yokode, M., Ishii, K., Kume, N., Ohshima, A., Yoshida, H. and Kawai, C. (1987) 'Probucol prevents the progression of atherosclerosis in WHHL rabbit, an animal model of familial hypercholesterolemia', Proc. Natl. Acad. Sci. USA 84, 5928-5931.

25. Badimon, J.J., Badimon, L., Galvez, A., Dische, R. and Fuster, V. (1989) 'High density lipoprotein plasma fractions inhibit aortic fatty streaks in cholesterol-fed rabbits', Lab. Invest. 60, 455-462.

26. Badimon, J.J., Badimon, L. and Fuster, V. (1990) Regression of atherosclerotic lesions by high density lipoprotein plasma fraction in the cholesterol-fed rabbit, J. Clin. Invest. 85, 1234-1241.

27. Rubin, E.M., Krauss, R.M., Spangler, E.A., Verstuyft, J.G. and Clift, S.M. (1991) 'Inhibition of early atherogenesis in transgenic mice by human apolipoprotein AI', Nature 353, 265-267.

28. Sheikh, K.H., Davidson, C.J., Kisslo, K.B., et al. (1991) 'Comparison of intravascular ultrasound, external ultrasound and digital angiography for evaluation of peripheral artery dimensions and morphology', Am. J. Cardiol. 67, 817-822.

29. Franceschini, G., Busnach, G., Vaccarino, V., Calabresi, L., Gianfranceschi, G. and Sirtori, C.R. (1988) 'Apheretic treatment of severe familial hypercholesterolemia: comparison of dextran sulfate cellulose and double membrane filtration methods for low density lipoprotein removal', Atherosclerosis 73, 197-202.

HIGH DENSITY LIPOPROTEINS: FUNCTION IN REVERSE CHOLESTEROL TRANSPORT AND MAINTENANCE OF CELLULAR INTEGRITY.

G. SCHMITZ, K.J. LACKNER

ABSTRACT. High density lipoproteins (HDL) have long been known to play an important role in reverse cholesterol transport. This has served as an explanation for the epidemiologic observation that HDL-cholesterol and apolipoprotein (apo) A-I are inversely correlated with the risk for coronary artery disease. More recent data indicate that HDL is involved in several other mechnisms such as coagulation, immunomodulation, cell proliferation, and detoxification. It appears that specific subclasses of HDL may serve different fuctions. One potentially important discovery is the presence of clusterin in a specific HDL-fraction. Clusterin, which is also known as complement lysis inhibitor or apoJ, has been shown to be associated with slow migrating HDL in isotachophoresis. Since it has a high affinity to damaged cell membranes, it may play an important role in targeting of HDL to sites of tissue damage and repair. Studies regarding the function of clusterin containing HDL particles are likely to permit new insights into the antiatherogenic mechanisms related to HDL. Of particular importance will be the interaction of these particles with the cells of the vessel wall. To this end more refined methods to isolate functional HDL subclasses are necessary.

1. Introduction

HDL has been shown to have antiatherogenic functions in several epidemiologic studies [1-5]. In animal models it has been possible to retard the development of atherosclerosis by infusion of HDL or by the overexpression of apoA-I in transgenic mice [6-8] The exact mechanisms of this protective effect have not been elucidated in detail. The currently favored hypothesis is that removal of excess cholesterol from peripheral cells is the most important protective function of HDL [9,10]. However, there is evidence that only specific HDL subclasses may be important for the protection from atherosclerosis. It may be possible that minor components of serum HDL are in fact more important than was anticipated until now. Thus, it is important to analyze HDL subclasses and their composition using more refined methods. This may permit the identification of components of specific HDL subclasses that exert vasoprotective effects. Analytical and preparative isotachophoresis (ITP) is one such method among others like gradient gel electrophoresis, gradient ultracentrifugation or immunoaffinity methods. Using ITP it is possible to separate serum HDL into six fractions, which have been shown to interact specifically with human monocyte/macrophages [11].

A. L. Catapano et al. (eds.), Drugs Affecting Lipid Metabolism, 121–129.
© 1993 Kluwer Academic Publishers and Fondazione Giovanni Lorenzini.

2. HDL associated Proteins (see also Table 1)

2.1.   ApoA-I

The major protein in HDL is apolipoprotein (apo) A-I, which is a 28 kD protein. ApoA-I has been shown to be involved in the specific binding of HDL to cell surface receptors [12-14]. It is probably the major cofactor for the LCAT reaction in plasma [15]. These two properties of apoA-I make it a crucial constituent of reverse cholesterol transport. ApoA-I undergoes several co- and post-translational modifications such as acylation and phosphorylation/dephosphorylation [16,17]. And finally, apoA-I has been shown to be identical to a so called serum prostacyclin stabilizing factor [18]. Absence of apoA-I due to genetic defects has been described and appears to be accompanied by premature vascular disease [19-23].

2.2.   ApoA-II

The other major protein of HDL is apoA-II. ApoA-II is an 8.7 kD protein that is found as a disulfide linked dimer in plasma. The function of this protein has still to be elucidated. It has been implicated in the regulation of the activity of hepatic lipase [24]. A complete lack of apoA-II due to a splice junction mutation has been described. However, the absence of apoA-II does not lead to HDL deficiency or premature atherosclerosis [25].

2.3.   ApoA-IV

ApoA-IV is a minor constituent of HDL. It is primarily synthesized in the intestine and secreted with chylomicrons. The chylomicron pool of apoA-IV seems to be a precursor of HDL apoA-IV. On ITP, it has been found in slow migrating HDL particles. The majority of apoA-IV is not lipoprotein associated. The function of this "free" apoA-IV has still to be elucidated. There is evidence that apoA-IV may be involved in receptor mediated uptake of HDL particles in the liver [26]. Recently it has been suggested that apoA-IV modulates the activity of lipoprotein lipase [27].

2.4.   Lecithin:cholesteryl acyltransferase (LCAT)

Lecithin:cholesterol acyltransferase (LCAT) catalyzes the transfer of acyl groups from phosphatidylcholine to cholesterol, forming cholesteryl ester and lysolecithin. LCAT contributes to the maintenance of a concentration gradient for free cholesterol between cell membranes and HDL [28]. Thus, LCAT is an important component of reverse cholesterol transport. The action of LCAT is mandatory for the maturation of HDL particles [29]. In LCAT deficiency there are mostly disc shaped HDL particles with a very low cholesterol ester content [30,31].

2.5.   Cholesteryl ester transfer protein (CETP)

Cholesteryl ester transfer protein (CETP) is involved in the transfer of cholesteryl esters from HDL to apoB containing lipoproteins. Interestingly, complete lack of CETP is associated with high levels of HDL cholesterol and apoA-I and perhaps longevity [32]. Another potentially interesting function of CETP is related to its structural similarity to lipopolysaccharide (LPS) binding protein [33]. HDL is known to bind LPS and modulate its biologic activity [34]. However, so far no data on physiologic functions of CETP in modulating lipopolysaccharide effects are available.

Table 1: HDL associated proteins

Protein	MW (kDa)	Site of Synthesis	Functions and Properties
ApoA-I	28.4	Intestine, liver	Structural protein of HDL; ligand for specific binding to cells; promotes cellular cholesterol-efflux; cofactor for LCAT; stabilizes prostacyclin; inhibits aCEH in vitro:
ApoA-II	8.7	Liver, (?) intestine	Structural protein of HDL; modulates activity of LCAT and HTGL; activates LPL
ApoA-IV	46	Intestine, liver	Lipid transport; activates LCAT; modulates LPL-activity and HDL-interconversion
ApoC-I	6.6	Liver	Activates LCAT und LPL; inhibits phospholipase-A2; inhibits binding of β-VLDL to LRP
ApoC-II	8.9	Liver	Obligatory cofactor for LPL; activates LCAT
ApoC-III	8.8	Liver	Inhibits uptake of triglyceride rich particles in the liver; modulates LCAT activity
ApoD	19	Liver, intestine, brain, placenta, adrenal, pancreas, spleen	Bilirubin-binding; possibly radical scavenger; involved in wound healing processes
ApoE	34	Ubiquitous; except intestine	Ligand for LDL- and apoE-receptor (LRP?); reverse cholesterol transport; lipid transport in tissues; perhaps immuno- and growth regulatory functions
ApoF	26-32	?	Unknown
ApoH	54	Liver, (? other tissues)	Involved in phospholipid autoantibody reactions; stimulates LPL; binds to platelets
LCAT	63	Liver	Esterifies free cholesterol in lipoproteins (and cell membranes); phospholipase A2-activity; involved in the interconversion of lipoprotein particles and reverse cholesterol transport
CETP	66-74	Liver (non-parenchymal cells?), spleen, intestine, adipose tissue, muscle, adrenal	Lipid transfer between lipoprotein particles; involved in the interconversion of lipoprotein particles and reverse cholesterol transport
Clusterin	35-39	Brain, testes, ovary, liver, heart, lung, spleen	Inhibits cytolysis by C5b-9 complement-complex; binds to heparin;
SAA	11-24	Liver	acute phase protein; function not known, (?) wound healing; modulates LCAT-activity
Paraoxonase	42-45	Liver, kidney	Detoxifies organophosphorous compounds; inhibits lipid peroxidation in lipoproteins
LACI	40-46	Liver	Inhibits factor VII(a)-tissue-factor complex and factor X(a); protects from intravascular coagulation after exposure to endotoxin
LPB-protein	60	Liver, macrophages	Binds lipopolysaccharide; mediates LPS-binding to LPS receptor; regulation of neutrophils in acute inflammation
Elastase	28-31	Leucocytes	Posttranslational modification of apolipoproteins; degradation of apoA-I in preβ-HDL

2.6. ApoC

The C-apolipoproteins apoC-I, apoC-II and apoC-III are minor constituents of HDL. They are primarily involved in the metabolism of triglyceride rich particles. During lipolysis of chylomicrons and VLDL they rapidly exchange to HDL. ApoC-II is the major cofactor of LPL [35]. ApoC-III interferes with the uptake of apoE-containing particles [36]. All three apolipoproteins modify the action of LCAT in vitro. It is not known, whether this property is relevant in vivo.

2.7. ApoD

ApoD is supposedly involved in reverse cholesterol transport. This hypothesis is based on the fact that it copurifies with LCAT and CETP, and that apoD particles bind cholesterol. ApoD belongs to the α2-microglobulin family. Members of this family have a number of functions in the acute phase response and the complement cascade. They are able to bind small hydrophobic ligands such as retinol. It has been speculated that one of the major physiologic functions of apoD may be the binding of heme-related compounds. ApoD has been found to accumulate in tissues under certain stress conditions. It may function in the removal of heme products from these tissues [37,38].

2.8. ApoE

The major function of apoE is in the metabolism of chylomicron and VLDL remnants. The protein is synthesized in several tissues, indicating that it may serve additional functions in cell biology [39]. However, complete absence of apoE leads to severe type III hyperlipoproteinemia with remnant accumulation. There are no additional major metabolic derangements discernible [40]. There is usually some apoE in HDL which may contribute to reverse cholesterol transport by targeting HDL to hepatic receptors for apoE. CETP deficiency leads to a substantial increase in apoE containing HDL particles. This may compensate for the decreased exchange of cholesterol esters to apoB containing particles and restore reverse cholesterol transport via uptake of HDL by apoE receptors [41].

2.9. ApoH

ApoH which is also known as β2-glycoprotein I is mostly associated with HDL but also with other lipoprotein particles [42]. Its function is still not well characterized. It behaves as a "negative" acute phase protein, i.e. that its plasma level decreases during the acute phase response. One interesting aspect of apoH is that it is required as cofactor for the binding of phospholipid or cardiolipin antibodies to their antigen. Thus, free phospholid or cardiolipin is not bound by these antibodies. Only the addition of apoH will restore binding [43]. Whether this property of apoH has physiologic significance is still an unanswered question [44].

2.10. Clusterin

Clusterin is another important addition to the list of minor HDL components with potentially important functions in vasoprotection [45]. It is a 427 amino acid polypeptide that is cleaved posttranslationally. Similar to apoE, it contains potential heparin binding domains. The major function of clusterin is the inhibition of the C5b-9 terminal complement complex. Thus, clusterin inhibits complement mediated cell damage. Since there are several lines of evidence implicating complement mediated events in early atherogenesis, clusterin containing HDL particles may exert distinct antiatherogenic effects, which are not related to reverse cholesterol transport [46].

2.11. Paraoxonase

Paraoxonase is a minor component of HDL. This enzyme is responsible for the hydrolysis of organophosphorous compounds. It has also been shown that it may function as an antioxidant. Thus, it has been speculated that paraoxonase may protect HDL from oxidative modification and preserve the integrity of HDL particles. Patients with HDL deficiency syndromes have low paraoxonase activity [47].

2.12. Serum amyloid A (SAA)

Serum amyloid A (SAA) is an acute phase protein that is found in HDL. Its concentration is related to the amount of unesterified cholesterol. SAA is capable of displacing apoA-I stoichiometrically from HDL particles. The function of SAA in lipoprotein metabolism during the acute phase response remains to be elucidated [48].

2.13. Lipoprotein associated coagulation inhibitor (LACI)

LACI is a potent inhibitor of coagulation. It is associated mainly with HDL but also with other lipoprotein particles. It has been shown that LACI prevents activation of the coagulation system in experimental animals by low doses of tissues factor, which may occur during subthreshold bacteraemia [49,50]. This function of HDL would represent a second mechanism besides LPS binding, by which HDL particles protect the organism from the effects of minor bacteraemia.

3. Cellular Interaction of HDL Subclasses.

Several methods have been developed to isolate HDL subclasses with specific functions. Thses include ultracentrifugation, gradient gel electrophoresis, immunoaffinity chromatography, and isotachophoresis (ITP).

Immunoaffinity chromatography has yielded metabolically distinct HDL subclasses containing only apoA-I without apoA-II (LpAI) or containig apoA-I and apoA-II (LpAI,AII). Both particles contain apoD, apoE, and apoA-IV [51]. Cholesterol efflux from cultured adipose cells is mediated specifically by LpAI but not by LpAI,AII [52].

By gradient gel electrophoresis it has been possible to identify HDL subclasses with preβ-mobility that lack apoA-II. These subclasses - preβ-HDL1,2,3 - are involved in the removal of cellular cholesterol and are remodelled into α-migrating HDL by the action of LCAT [53].

We have used preparative ITP to identify HDL subclasses. This method permits the separation of lipoprotein particles in a matrix free system according to their net charge. Preparative ITP separates three major HDL-fractions, which have been called fast, intermediate and slow migrating HDL. Fast migrating HDL are enriched in apoA-I and promote cholesterol efflux from cells via interaction with specific cellular receptors. During this process they are internalized and resecreted. The slow migrating HDL are rich in apoA-I, apoA-IV and LCAT. They interact with cell membranes and mobilize cholesterol without binding to specific receptors. The driving force of cholesterol removal is a concentration gradient between membrane and HDL particle. This gradient is preserved by the action of LCAT. The intermediate migrating HDL are poor acceptors of cellular cholesterol. They are enriched in apoA-II, apoC-II, apoC-III, and apoE.

In figure 1 the interaction of cells with the different HDL subclasses separated by isotachophoresis is depicted (for explanation see figure legend).

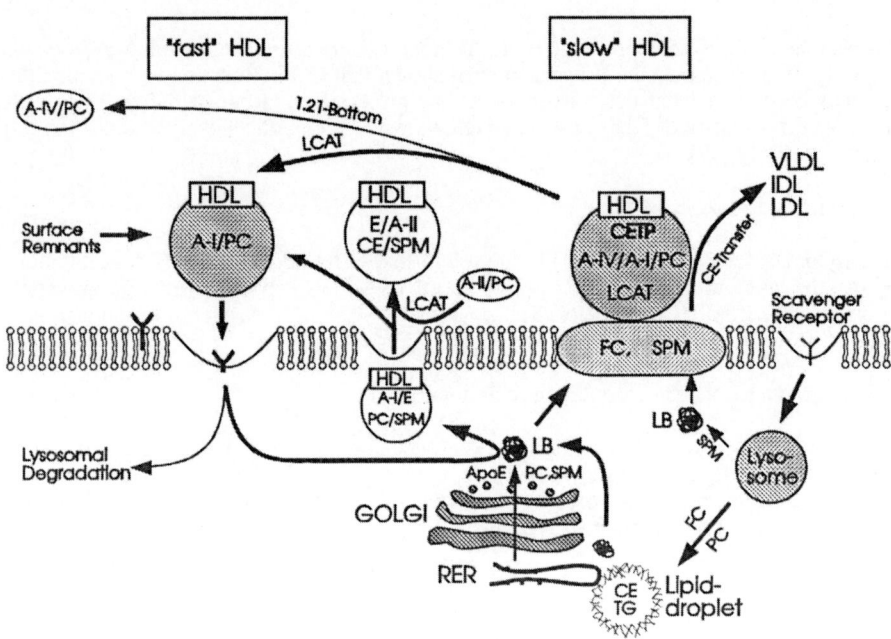

Figure 1:

Interaction of HDL subclasses with macrophages. In addition to physicochemical exchange, there are two major routes by which macrophages can release excess cholesterol. (1) Upon cholesterol loading macrophages form "lamellar bodies" (LB) which originate from lysosomes. These LBs move towards the cell periphery, fuse with the cell membrane and release their lipid components into the extracellular space. Some of the lipids may also associate with the cell membrane. This pathway of lipid and cholesterol release is promoted by apoA-I/A-IV/LCAT-rich slow-migrating HDL. (2) Cholesterol efflux may also be sitimulated by a specific HDL-receptor mediated mechanism in which apoA-I rich fast migrating HDL particles bind to a cell membrane receptor with subsequent internalization. The majority of these HDL particles are not directed to lysosomes but take up cholesterol and are retroendocytosed. The resecreted particles may represent the precursors for apoE/apoA-II rich HDL with intermediate mobility.
PC - phosphatidylcholine; FC - free cholesterol; CE - cholesterol ester; SPM - sphingomyelin;

5. References

1.   Miller GJ, Miller NE. Plasma high-density lipoprotein concentration and development of ischaemic heart disease. Lancet 1975; i:16-8
2.   Maciejko JJ, Holmes DR, Kottke BA, Zinsmeister AR, Dinh DM, Mao SJT. Apolipoprotein A-I as a marker of angiographically assessed coronary-artery disease. N Engl J Med 1983; 309:385-9

3. Castelli WP, Garrison RJ, Wilson PWF, Abbott RD, Kalousdian S, Kannel WB. Incidence of coronary heart disease and lipoprotein cholesterol levels. The Framingham Study. JAMA 1986; 256:2835-8
4. Gordon D, Rifkind BM. High density lipoproteins - the clinical implications of recent studies. N Engl J Med 1989; 321:1311-5
5. Buring JE, O'Connor GT, Goldhaber SZ, Rosner B, Herbert PN, Blum CB, Breslow JL, Hennekens CH. Decreased HDL2 and HDL3 cholesterol, apo A-I and apo A-II, and increased risk of myocardial infarction. Circulation 1992; 85:22-9
6. Badimon JJ, Badimon L, Fuster V. Regression of atherosclerotic lesions by high density lipoprotein plasma fraction in the cholesterol-fed rabbit. J Clin Invest 1990; 85:1234-41
7. Badimon JJ, Badimon L, Galvez A, Dische R, Fuster V. High density lipoprotein plasma fractions inhibit aortic fatty streaks in cholesterol-fed rabbits. Lab Invest 1989; 60:455-61
8. Rubin EM, Krauss RM, Spangler EA, Verstuyft JG, Clift SM. Inhibition of early atherogenesis in transgenic mice by human apolipoprotein AI. Nature 1991; 353:265-7
9. Tall AR. Plasma high density lipoproteins. Metabolism and relationship to atherogenesis. J Clin Invest 1990; 86:379-84
10. Kovanen PT. Atheroma formation: defective control in the intimal round-trip of cholesterol. Eur Heart J 1990; 11 Suppl E: 238-46
11. Nowicka G, Brüning T, Böttcher A, Kahl G, Schmitz G. Macrophage interaction of HDL subclasses separated by free flow isotachophoresis. J Lipid Res 1990; 31:1947-63
12. Schmitz G, Robenek H, Lohmann U, Assmann G. Interaction of high density lipoproteins with cholesteryl ester-laden macrophages: biochemical and morphological characterization of cell surface receptor binding, endocytosis and resecretion of high density lipoproteins by macrophages. EMBO J 1985; 4:613-22
13. Oram JF, Johnson CJ, Aulinskas-Brown T. Interaction of high denisity lipoprotein with its receptor on cultured fibroblasts and macrophages. J Biol Chem 1987; 262:2405-10
14. Monaco L, Bond HM, Howell KE, Cortese R. A recombinant apoA-1-protein A hybrid reproduces the binding parameters of HDL to its receptor. EMBO J 1987; 6:3253-60
15. Fielding CJ, Shore VG, Fielding PE. A protein cofactor of lecithin:cholesterol acyltransferase. Biochem Biophys Res Commun 1972; 46:1493-8
16. Hoeg JM, Meng MS, Ronan R, Fairwell T, Brewer HB Jr. Human apolipoprotein A-I. Post-translational modification by fatty acid acylation. J Biol Chem 1986; 261:3911-4
17. Beg ZH, Stonik JA, Hoeg JM, Demosky SJ, Fairwell T, Brewer HB Jr. Human apolipoprotein A-I. Post-translational modification by covalent phosphorylation. J Biol Chem 1989; 264:6913-21
18. Yui Y, Aoyama T, Morishita H, Takahashi M, Takatsu Y, Kawai C. Serum prostacyclin stabilizing factor is identical to apolipoprotein A-I (apo A-I). A novel function of apo A-I. J Clin Invest 1988; 82:803-7
19. Breslow JL. Familial disorders of high denisty lipoprotein Metabolism. In: The metabolic basis of inherited disease. Scriver CR, Beaudet AL, Sly WS, Valle D (Eds). 8th ed, McGraw-Hill, New York, 1989; Chapt 49:1251-1266
20. Karathanasis SK, Ferris E, Haddad IA. DNA inversion within the apolipoproteins AI/CIII/AIV-encoding gene cluster of certain patients with premature atherosclerosis. Proc Natl Acad Sci USA 1987;84:7198-202
21. Lackner KJ, Schmitz G. Familial high density lipoproteindeficiency with xanthomas is caused by a point mutation in the apolipoprotein A-I gene. Int Atherosclerosis Congress 1989; Abstr 177
22. Ordovas JM, Cassidy DK, Civeira F, Bisgaier CL, Schaefer EJ. Familial apolipoprotein A-I, C-III, and A-IV deficiency and premature atherosclerosis due to deletion of a gene complex on chromosome 11. J Biol Chem 1989; 264:16339-42
23. Matsunaga T, Hiasa Y, Yanagi H, Maeda T, Hattori N, Yamakawa K, Yamanouchi Y, Tanaka I, Obara T, Hamaguchi H. Apolipoprotein A-I deficiency due to a codon 84

nonsense mutation of the apolipoprotein A-I gene. Proc Natl Acad Sci USA 1991; 88:2793-7

24. Jahn CE, Osborne JC jr, Schaefer EJ, Brewer HB jr. In vitro activation of the enzymic activity of hepatic lipase by apoA-II. FEBS Lett 1981; 131:366-8

25. Deeb SS, Takata K, Peng RL, Kajiyama G, Albers JJ. A splice-unction mutation responsible for familial apolipoprotein A-II deficiency. Am J Hum Genet 1990; 46:822-7

26. Steinmetz A, Barbaras R, Ghalim N, Clavey V, Fruchart JC, Ailhaud G. Human apolipoprotein A-IV binds to apolipoprotein A-I/A-II receptor sites and promotes cholesterol efflux from adipose cells. J Biol Chem 1990; 265:7859-63

27. Goldberg IJ, Scheraldi CA, Yacoub LK, Saxena U, Bisgaier CL. Lipoprotein apoC-II activation of lipoprotein lipase. Modulation by apolipoprotein A-IV. J Biol Chem 1990; 265:4266-72

28. McCall MR, Nichols AV, Blanche PJ, Shore VG, Forte TM. Lecithin:cholesterol acytransferase-iduced transformation of HepG2 lipoproteins. J Lipid Res 1989; 30:1579-89

29. Francone OL, Gurakar A, Fielding C. Distribution and functions of lecithin:cholesteryl ester transfer protein in plasma lipoproteins. J Biol Chem 1989; 264:7066-72

30. Carlson LA, Holmquist L. Evidence for deficiency of high density lipoprotein lecithin:cholesterol acyltransferase activity (a-LCAT) in fish eye disease. Acta Med Scand 1985; 218:189-96

31. Norum RA, Gjone E, Glomset JA. Familial Lecithin:cholesterol acytransferase deficiency, including fish eye disease. In: The metabolic basis of inherited disease. Scriver CR, Beaudet AL, Sly WS, Valle D (Eds). 8th ed, McGraw-Hill, New York, 1989; Chapt 46:1181-94

32. Brown ML, Inazu A, Hesler CB, Agellon LB, Mann C, Whitlock ME, Marcel YL, Milne RW, Koizumi J, Mabuchi H, Takeda R, Tall AR. Molecular basis of lipid transfer protein deficiency in a family with increased high-density lipoproteins Nature 1989; 342:448-451

33. Vosbeck K, Tobias P, Müller H, Allen RA, Arfors KE, Ulevitch RJ, Sklar LA. Priming of polymorphonuclear granulocytes by lipopolysaccharides and its complexes with lipopolysaccharide binding protein and high density lipoprotein. J Leukoc biol 1990; 47:97-104

34. Baumberger C, Ulevitch RJ, Dayer JM. Modulation of endotoxic activity of lipopolysaccharide by high-density lipoprotein. Pathobiology 1991; 59:378-83

35. Jackson RL, Tajima S, Yamamura T, Yokoyama S, Yamamoto A. Comparison of apolipoprotein C-II deficient triacylglycerol-rich lipoproteins and trioleylglycero/phophatidylcholine-stabilized particles as substrates for lipoprotein lipase. biochim Biophys Acta 1986; 857:211-7

36. Ito Y, Arzolan N, O'Connell A, Walsh A, Breslow JL. Hypertriglyceridemia as a result of human apo CIII gene expression in transgenic mice. Science 1990; 249-790-3

37. Boyles JK, Notterpek LM, Anderson LJ. Accumulation of apolipoproteins in the regenerating and remyelinating mammalian peripheral nerve. Identification of apolipoprotein D, apolipoprotein A-IV, apolipoprotein E, and apolipoprotein A-I. J Biol Chem 1990; 265:17805-15

38. Peitsch MC, Boguski MS. Is apolipoprotein D a mammalian bilin-binding protein? The New Biologist 1990; 2:197-206

39. Mahley RW. Apolipoprotein E: Cholesterol transport protein with expanding role in cell biology. Science 1988; 240:622-630

40. Ghiselli G, Schaefer EJ, Gascon P, Brewer HB Jr. Type III hyperlipoproteinemia associated with apolipoprotein E deficiency. Science 1981; 214:1239-41

41. Yamashita S, Sprecher DL, Sakai N, Matsuzawa Y, Tarui S, Hui-DY. Accumulation of apolipoprotein E-rich high density lipoproteins in hyperalphalipoproteinemic human

subjects with plasma cholesteryl ester transfer protein deficiency. J Clin Invest 1990; 86:688-95

42. Polz E, Kostner GM. The binding of β2-glycoprotein-I to human serum lipoproteins. Distribution among density fractions. FEBS Lett 1979; 102:183-6

43. McNeil HP, Simpson RJ, Chesterman CN, Krilis SA. Anti-phospholipid antibodies are directed against a complex antigen that includes a lipid-binding inhibitor of coagulation: β2-glycoprotein I (apolipoprotein H). Proc Natl Acad Sci USA 1990; 87:4120-4

44. Jordan-Starck TC, Witte DP, Aronow BJ, Harmony JAK. Apolipoprotein J: a membrane policeman? Curr Opin Lipidol 1992; 3:75-85

45. Jenne DE, Lowin B, Peitsch MC, Böttcher A, Schmitz G, Tschopp J. Clusterin (complement lysis inhibitor) forms a high density lipoprotein complex with apolipoprotein A-I in human plasma. J Biol Chem 1991; 266:11030-6

46. Seifert PS, Hugo F, Hansson GK, Bhakdi S. Prelesional complement activation in experimental atherosclerosis. Terminal c5b-9 complement deposition conincides with cholesterol accumulation in the aortic intima of hypercholesterolemic rabbits. Lab Invest 1989; 60:747-54

47. Mackness MI, Arrol S, Durrington PN. Paraoxonase prevents accumulation of lipoperoxides in low-density lipoprotein. FEBS Lett 1991; 286:152-4

48. Kisilevsky R. Serum amyloid A (SAA), a protein without a function: some suggestions with reference to cholesterol metabolism. Med Hypotheses 1991; 35:337-41

49. Wun T-C, Kretzmer KK, Girard TJ, Miletich JP, Broze GJ Jr. Cloning and characterization of a cDNA coding for the lipoprotein-associated coagulation inhibitor shows that it consists of three tandem Kunitz-type inhibitory domains. J Biol Chem 1988; 263:6001-4

50. Rapaport SI. The extrinsic pathway inhibitor: a regulator of tissue factor-dependent blood coagulation. Thromb Hemost 1991; 66:6-15

51. Cheung MC, Wolf AC, Lum KD, Tollefson JH, Albers JJ. Distribution and localization of lethicin:cholesterol acyltransferase and cholesteryl ester transfer activity in A-I-containing lipoproteins. J Lipid Res 1986; 27:1135-44

52. Fruchart JC, Theret N, Barabas R, Puchois P, Ailhaud G. ApoA-containing lipoprotein particles. Physiological role, quantification and clinical significance. In: Disorders of HDL. Carlson LA (ed). London, Smith-Gordon 1990; pp 71-75

53. Francone OL, Gurakar A, Fielding C. Distribution and functions of lecithin:cholesterol acyltransferase and cholesteryl ester transfer protein in plasma lipoproteins. Evidence for a functional unit containing these activities together with apolipoprotein A-I and D that catalyzes the esterification and transfer of cell-derived cholesterol. J Biol Chem 1989; 264:7066-72

THE EXPRESSION AND REGULATION OF CHOLESTEROL 7α-HYDROXYLASE

J.Y.L. Chiang, W.G. Karam, T.P. Yang and D.P. Wang

ABSTRACT: To study the molecular mechanism of regulation of cholesterol 7α-hydroxylase, the rate-limiting enzyme in bile acid synthesis, we have purified a rat liver cholesterol 7α-hydroxylase, obtained a specific antibody, cloned the cDNA and expressed an active enzyme in E. Coli. Using these reagents, we studied the regulation of 7α-hydroxylase by cholesterol, oxysterols, bile acids, hormones and other drugs. All results indicate that 7α-hydroxylase is regulated at the gene transcriptional level. The human cholesterol 7α-hydroxylase cDNA was cloned and polymorphisms were identified in a human liver. The rat 7α-hydroxylase gene was cloned and several liver specific and ubiquitous regulatory elements were found in the 5'-upstream sequence of the rat gene. Possible mechanisms of regulation of 7α-hydroxylase are proposed.

INTRODUCTION

Cholesterol 7α-hydroxylase (7α-hydroxylase) has long been recognized as the rate-limiting enzyme in bile acid synthesis from cholesterol in the liver. This enzyme activity is thought to be regulated by bile acid feedback, hormones, diurnal rhythm, diet and other factors (1). The mechanisms of regulation of this enzyme, however, remain unknown. To study the molecular mechanism of regulation, purified enzyme, specific antibody, and cDNA clone are required. Only until recently, a highly purified 7α-hydroxylase become available. Reconstitution of an active 7α-hydroxylase using purified enzyme confirmed that this enzyme activity is catalyzed by a cytochrome P450-dependent monooxygenase (2,3). A monospecific antibody against the purified rat enzyme was obtained and used to screen an expression library for 7α-hydroxylase cDNA (2,4). A full-length cDNA contains 3561 bp nucleotides which encode a polypeptide of 503 amino acid residues. The sequence revealed that this P450 enzyme is a product of an unique P450 gene, CYP7, which belongs to the P450 supergene family (4). The rat CYP7 gene was then cloned by screening a genomic library using cDNA as a hybridization probe. The knowledge gained from study cholesterol 7α-hydroxylase in the rat model can now be expanded to study this enzyme in human liver. Polymorphisms of cholesterol 7α-hydroxylase was discovered in the human liver. In this paper, we summarize the regulation of 7α-hydroxylase by bile acids, cholesterol, hormones and

A. L. Catapano et al. (eds.), Drugs Affecting Lipid Metabolism, 131–138.
© 1993 Kluwer Academic Publishers and Fondazione Giovanni Lorenzini. ₁

drugs, the expression of an active 7α-hydroxylase in E. Coli, the effects of oxysterols on 7α-hydroxylase, the cloning and polymorphisms of human 7α-hydroxylase, and the cloning of the rat 7α-hydroxylase gene. We also propose possible mechanisms regulating cholesterol 7α-hydroxylase gene transcription by bile acids.

REGULATION OF CHOLESTEROL 7α-HYDROXYLASE

Western immunoblot and Northern blot hybridization were applied to measure 7α-hydroxylase protein and mRNA levels, respectively, in rat liver. We have demonstrated that 7α-hydroxylase activity varies in parallel with cholesterol 7α-hydroxylase enzyme protein and mRNA levels in rat liver (2,4). Table I summarizes changes in cholesterol 7α-hydroxylase mRNA levels in response to treatment with bile salts, cholesterol, drugs and hormones, in comparison with changes in HMG-CoA reductase mRNA levels in rat liver.

Table I.   A comparison of effects of bile acid, cholesterol, hormones and drugs on cholesterol 7α-hydroxylase and HMG-CoA reductase mRNA levels in rat liver

Treatments	Cholesterol 7α-hydroxylase	HMG-CoA reductase
Bile salts	↓	↓
Cholesterol	↑	→
Mevalonate	↑	→
Cholestyramine	↑	↑
Mevinolin	↓	↑
Thyroid hormone	↑	↑
Dexamethasone	↑	↓

Hydrophobic bile salts, such as chenodeoxycholate and taurocholate reduced 7α-hydroxylase activity and mRNA level in intact rats and bile fistula rats (5,6). Bile salts also strongly inhibited HMG-CoA reductase activity and mRNA levels (7). Cholesterol feeding increased 7α-hydroxylase activity, protein and mRNA levels by two folds in rat liver (4-6). In contrast, cholesterol feeding drastically decreased HMG-CoA reductase activity without much effect on the mRNA level (8). Mevalonate, the product of HMG-CoA reductase increased 7α-hydroxylase mRNA level but had no effect on HMG-CoA reductase mRNA level in rat liver, according to a recent study (8). Cholestyramine, a bile acid sequestrant, increased 7α-hydroxylase activity, protein and mRNA levels and also stimulated HMG-CoA reductase activity and mRNA levels (2,4,9). Mevinolin, a competitive inhibitor of HMG-CoA reductase significantly reduced 7α-hydroxylase mRNA, but increased HMG-CoA reductase mRNA level (10). Therefore, cholesterol or its precursors may directly regulate 7α-hydroxylase gene transcription and bile acid repress the gene transcription. Thyroid hormone rapidly increases both 7α-hydroxylase and HMG-CoA reductase mRNA levels in hypophysectomized rats (11). Dexamethasone increases cholesterol 7α-hydroxylase activity and mRNA levels, but decreases HMG-CoA reductase mRNA level at physiological dosage (12-14). At a higher dosage, dexamethasone drastically reduced 7α-hydroxylase activity, protein and mRNA levels (2,4). Thus, in many instances, activities and mRNA levels of these two rate-limiting enzymes are not regulated in parallel as previously thought.

POSSIBLE MECHANISMS OF REGULATION

Several mechanisms have been suggested to regulate cholesterol 7α-hydroxylase in the liver. It has been proposed that the availability of cholesterol substrate could regulate this enzyme in vivo and that newly synthesized cholesterol is the preferred substrate (1). Therefore, there may be a cross-regulation between de novo synthesis of cholesterol and bile acid synthesis. Second, bile salts are strong detergents which may directly inhibit this enzyme activity in hepatocytes. Third, recent experiments using antibody and cDNA clone revealed that 7α-hydroxylase activity varies in parallel with enzyme protein and mRNA levels. Furthermore, nuclear run-on transcription assay revealed that this enzyme is regulated at the gene transcriptional level by bile salts and cholesterol (5,6). Fourth, post-translational modification, such as activation by phosphorylation and inactivation by dephosphorylation, may also play a role in the short term regulation of activity (15). It is also possible that the stability of enzyme and/or mRNA may play a role in the regulation of enzyme activity in the liver, since 7α-hydroxylase has a very short half-life and its mRNA contains many destabilizing sequences (4,16). While all these are possible, the major mechanism of regulation of 7α-hydroxylase activity appears to be at the gene transcriptional level.

EXPRESSION OF CHOLESTEROL 7α-HYDROXYLASE IN E. Coli

The low enzyme level and difficulty in isolation of cholesterol 7α-hydroxylase from liver microsomes hindered a detailed study of the structure and function relationship of this enzyme. An active 7α-hydroxylase which lacks the N-terminus membrane binding domain has been expressed in E. Coli

(17). This shortened form of enzyme is largely located in the cytosol of E. Coli and could be purified in large quantity. The bacterial enzyme has the same K_m but lower V_{max} than the full-length form isolated from rat liver microsomes (17). These data indicate that the N-terminus hydrophobic segment is not required for enzyme activity and the shortened form is rather soluble. This bacterial expression system provides an unique system to study structure and function relationship by site-directed mutagenesis, to screen activators or inhibitors for drug design and to study active site structure by x-ray crystallography.

EFFECTS OF OXYSTEROLS ON CHOLESTEROL 7α-HYDROXYLASE

The binding of cholesterol substrate and the effects of oxysterols on substrate binding were studied by measuring the Type I cholesterol binding spectra of the purified, expressed 7α-hydroxylase in the presence and absence of oxysterols. Table II shows the effects of 7α-hydroxy-, 7ß-hydroxy- or 7-keto-cholesterol on the spectral dissociation constant (K_s) of cholesterol binding to 7α-hydroxylase. 7-ketocholesterol is a strong competitive inhibitor of 7α-hydroxylase. At the same concentration, 7α-hydroxycholesterol also inhibits this enzyme competitively, but to a lesser extent. On the other hand, 7ß-hydroxycholesterol is not an inhibitor.

Table II. Effects of oxysterols on cholesterol binding to cholesterol 7α-hydroxylase

Oxysterols	K_s
No oxysterol	30
7-ketocholesterol	200
7α-hydroxycholesterol	100
7ß-hydroxycholesterol	30

3 to 12 μM cholesterol were added to titrate the type I spectra of 0.43 μM P450c7 in the presence or absence of 0.5 μM oxysterol. K_s was calculated by a double reciprocal plot of absorbance differences vs. cholesterol concentrations.

The infusion of 7-ketocholesterol (2 mg/ml) in 10 % Intralipid increased 7α-hydroxylase activity, protein and mRNA levels by two to three-fold in the rat (18). Therefore, 7-ketocholesterol inhibited 7α-hydroxylase activity and reduced bile acid synthesis in the rat. Reduced bile acid feedback stimulated transcription of the 7α-hydroxylase gene. Similarly, a high cholesterol diet could cause the malabsorption of bile acids and produces a high level of oxysterols. Both effects will stimulate bile acid synthesis by increasing 7α-hydroxylase gene transcription. Oxysterols are known inhibitors of cholesterol synthesis.

POLYMORPHISMS OF HUMAN CHOLESTEROL 7α-HYDROXYLASE

Human 7α-hydroxylase cDNAs were isolated from a human liver cDNA library. A full-length cDNA contains 2901 nucleotides and encodes a polypeptide of 504 amino acid residues. A comparison of sequences between rat and human 7α-hydroxylase revealed that there is an overall sequence identity of 85 %, which is much higher than the identity between orthologues of other P450 gene families. The putative steroid binding site, aromatic amino acid region and heme binding site are completely conserved in the rat and human sequences. We found two different codons for amino acid residue 100 in these cDNA clones, which are TTT (Phe) and TCT (Ser), (19). In addition, codons 347 and 385 are GAT (Asp) and GAC (Asp), respectively, in all cDNA clones, which are different from the corresponding sequences reported previously (20). Since there is only one 7α-hydroxylase gene in the human genome, it is likely that polymorphisms arise from the presence of two different alleles in this human liver. The significance of 7α-hydroxylase polymorphisms in bile acid synthesis in humans is not known at present.

CHOLESTEROL 7α-HYDROXYLASE GENE STRUCTURE

Rat 7α-hydroxylase gene has been cloned recently (21,22). There are six exons and five introns spanning about 10 kb of the gene. This gene has a 600 bp 5'-flanking region (21,22). To obtain a gene containing a longer 5'-upstream sequence, we used a 5' cDNA probe to screen a genomic library and isolated a 15 kb genomic clone which contains an 8 kb upstream sequence. About 2 kb of the 5'- upstream region has been sequenced. Many liver specific regulatory elements (HNF/LF-B1, TGT3), ubiquitous regulatory elements (NF1, OTF1), steroid responsive elements (TRE, GRE, half sites), and phorbol ester and cAMP responsive elements (AP1 and AP2) were found in this region of gene. However, no oxysterol regulatory element was found in this region. A stretch of 23 "CA" repeats were located near these putative regulatory elements. This pyrimidine-purine repeats may form a Z-DNA structure and play a role in the regulation of gene transcriptions. Functional analysis of these putative regulatory elements in this upstream promotor region is currently being studied.

THE PROPOSED MECHANISMS OF CHOLESTEROL 7α–HYDROXYLASE GENE REGULATION

It seems clear now that hydrophobic bile salts are the physiological regulators of 7α-hydroxylase.   Bile acids returning to the hepatocytes may bind to and stimulate a bile acid binding protein or receptor and repress 7α-hydroxylase gene transcription.   Figure 1 illustrates several possible mechanisms which may regulate the 7α-hydroxylase gene. In mechanism A, bile acid binding protein (BP) may bind to a normal activator (A) and prevent its activation of the gene. The normal activator(s) could be hormones, cholesterol, or other factors. This normal activator may interact with other liver specific factors and exert its regulatory function in the 7α-hydroxylase promotor.   In mechanism B, a bile salt binding protein may bind to a bile salt responsive element (BRE) and neutralize the action of a normal activator. In mechanism C, bile acids exert a direct inhibitory effect on the general transcriptional complexes which bind to the TATA box of the gene.   Many bile acid binding proteins have been identified in cytosol of hepatocytes, but none of these factors have been demonstrated to play a role in the regulation of cholesterol 7α-hydroxylase gene. Experiments are being carried out to examine these mechanisms.

Mechanism A:

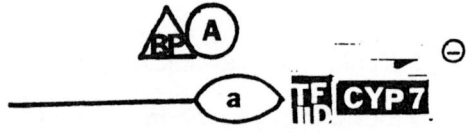

Mechanism B:

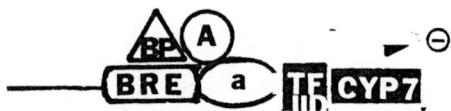

Mechanism C:

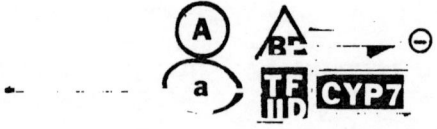

Figure 1: The proposed molecular mechanisms of regulation of the CYP7 gene by bile salts

ACKNOWLEDGMENTS

This research is supported by a NIH grant GM 31584 and a grant-in-aid from American Heart Association Ohio Affiliates (A91-01).

REFERENCES

1. Myant, N.B. and Mitropoulos,K.A. (1979) "Cholesterol 7α-hydroxylase." J. Lipid Res. 18, 135-153.
2. Chiang, J.Y.L., Miller, W.F. and Lin,G.-M. (1990) "Regulation of cholesterol 7α-hydroxylase:Purification of cholesterol 7α-hydroxylase and the immunochemical evidence for the induction of cholesterol 7α-hydroxylase by cholestyramine and circadian rhythm." J. Biol. Chem. 265, 3889-3897.
3. Ogishima, T., Deguchi, S. and Okuda, K. (1987) "Purification and characterization of cholesterol 7α-hydroxylase from rat liver microsomes." J. Biol. Chem. 262, 7646-7650.
4. Li, Y.C., Wang, D.P. and Chiang, J.Y.L. (1990) "Regulation of cholesterol 7α-hydroxylase in the liver: cDNA cloning, sequencing and regulation of cholesterol 7α-hydroxylase mRNA." J. Biol. Chem. 265, 12012-12019.
5. Jelinek, D. F., Andersson, S., Slaughter, C.A. and Russell, D. W. (1990) "Cloning and regulation of cholesterol 7α-hydroxylase, the rate-limiting enzyme in bile acid biosynthesis." J. Biol. Chem. 265, 8190-8197.
6. Pandak, W. M., Li, Y.C., Chiang, J.Y.L., Studer,E.J., Gurley,E.C., Heuman,D.M., Vlahcevic, Z.R. and Hylemon, P.B. (1991) "Regulation of cholesterol 7α-hydroxylase mRNA and transcriptional activity by taurocholate and cholesterol in the chronic biliary diverted rat." J. Biol. Chem. 266, 3416-3421.
7. Duckworth, P.F., Vlahcevic, Z.R., Studer, E.J., Gurley, E.C., Heuman, D.M., Beg, Z.H. and Hylemon, P.B. (1991) "Effect of hydrophobic bile acids on HMG-CoA reductase activity and mRNA levels in the rat." J. Biol. Chem. 266, 9413-9418.
8. Ness, G.C.,Keller, R.K., and Pendleton, L.C. (1991) "Feedback regulation of hepatic HMG-CoA reductase activity by dietary cholesterol is not due to altered mRNA levels." J. Biol. Chem. 266, 14854-14857.
9. Clark, C.F., Fogelman, A.M. and Edwards, P.A. (1985) "Transcriptional regulation of the HMG-CoA reductase gene in rat liver" J. Biol. Chem. 260, 14363-14367.
10. Clark, C.F., Edwards, P.A., Lan, S.F., Tanaka, R.D. and Fogelman, A.M. (1983) "Regulation of HMG-CoA reductase

mRNA levels in rat liver." J. Biol. Chem. Proc. Natl. Acad. Sci. 80, 3305-3308.

11. Ness, G.C., Pendleton, L.C., Li, Y.C. and Chiang, J.Y.L. (1991) "Effect of thyroid hormone on hepatic cholesterol 7α-hydroxylase, LDL receptor, HMG-CoA reductase, farnesyl pyrophosphate synthetase and apolipoprotein A-1 mRNA levels in hypophysectomized rats." Biochem. biophys. Res. Commun. 172, 1150-1156.

12. Leighton, J.K., Dueland, S., Straka, M.S., Trawick, J. and Davis, R.A. (1991) "Activation of the silent endogenous cholesterol 7α-hydroxylase gene in rat hepatoma cells: a new complementation group having resistance to 25-hydroxycholesterol." Mol. Cell. Biol. 11, 2049-2056.

13. Princen, H.M.G., Meijer,P., and Hoffee, B. (1989) "Dexamethasone regulates bile acid synthesis in monolayer cultures of rat hepatocytes by induction of cholesterol 7α-hydroxylase." Biochem. J. 262, 341-348.

14. Simonet, W.S. and Ness, G.C. (1989) "Post-transcriptional regulation of HMG-CoA reductase mRNA in rat liver." J. Biol. Chem. 264, 569-573.

15. Tang, P.M., Finkelstein, J.A.,and Chiang, J.Y.L. (1988) "Expression of hepatic microsomal cholesterol 7α-hydroxylase activity in lean and obese Zucker rats." Biochem. Biophys. Res. Commun. 150, 853-858.

16. Noshiro, M., Nishimoto, M. and Okuda, K. (1990) "Rat liver cholesterol 7α-hydroxylase. Pretranslational regulation for circadian rhythm." J. Biol. Chem. 265, 10036-10041.

17. Li, Y.C. and Chiang, J.Y.L. (1992) "The expression of a catalytically active cholesterol 7α-hydroxylase cytochrome P450 in E. coli." J. Biol. Chem. 266, 19186-19191.

18. Breuer, O., Sudjana-Sugiaman, E., Eggertsen, G., Chiang, J.Y.L. and Bjorkhem, I. (1992) "Cholesterol 7α-hydroxylase is upregulated by the competitive inhibitor 7-oxocholesterol in rat liver." Submitted.

19. Karam, W.G. and Chiang, J.Y.L. (1992) "Polymorphisms of human cholesterol 7α-hydroxylase (CYP7)." Biochem. Biophys. Res. Commun. In press.

20. Noshiro, M. and Okuda, K. (1990) "Molecular cloning and sequence analysis of cDNA encoding human cholesterol 7α-hydroxylase." FEBS Lett. 268, 137-140.

21. Jelinek, D.F. and Russell, D.W. (1990) "Structure of the rat gene encoding cholesterol 7α-hydroxylase." Biochem. 29, 7781-7785.

22. Nishimoto, M., Gotoh,O., Okuda, K. and Noshiro, M. (1991) "Structural analysis of the gene encoding rat cholesterol 7α-hydroxylase, the key enzyme for bile acid biosynthesis." J. Biol. Chem. 266, 6467-6471.

CHOLESTEROL METABOLISM IN NORMO AND GENETICALLY HYPERLIPIDEMIC RATS IN AGING

G. GALLI, M. CANCELLIERI, S. BARATTE', E. DE FABIANI AND E. BOSISIO

ABSTRACT. The changes of cholesterol metabolism in aging was studied in normolipidemic (Brown Norway strain) and in spontaneously hyperlipidemic rats (Yoshida strain). Plasma and hepatic lipid levels and the activity of HMGCoA reductase, cholesterol 7α-hydroxylase were measured at the age of 2, 6 and 18 months. The effect of cholestyramine and simvastatin was also considered. Plasma cholesterol and triglyceride levels were higher in Yoshida and increased with aging. The raise of plasma lipid levels with increasing age was not evident in Brown Norway rats. HMGCoA reductase was higher in Yoshida as compared to Brown Norway, and decreased with aging in both groups. Cholesterol 7α-hydroxylase was higher in Yoshida with respect to Brown Norway and no variation of the activity was observed in aging. Cholestyramine induced HMGCoA reductase and cholesterol 7α-hydroxylase activity in both groups, the stimulation of the enzymes being more pronounced in Brown Norway rats. Treatment with simvastatin reduced HMGCoA reductase activity to the same extent (50%) in both groups at the different ages.

INTRODUCTION

Atherosclerosis is known to progress with age and has a strong genetic component. It is known that serum cholesterol levels increase in older age and other parameters of cholesterol metabolism such as cholesterol synthesis, turnover, absorption and excretion are reported to decrease in aging (1).

Epidemiological studies indicated that high levels of cholesterol contribute to the development of atherosclerosis and therefore augment the risk of coronary heart disease. The control of cholesterolemia by therapy with lipid lowering drugs is therefore recommended to mantain low levels of cholesterol in serum. This type of treatment is life-long and mainly applied to middle-age or elderly patients.

Therefore it seemed of interest to evaluate the changes of cholesterol metabolism with age and the effect of cholesterol lowering drugs on cholesterol metabolism either in adult and aged rats. As experimental models were used a strain of normolipidemic rat (Brown Norway, BN) and a strain of spontaneous hyperlipidemic rat (Yoshida,YOS). This study describes the changes of plasma and hepatic lipid levels and of the cholesterol metabolizing enzymes in the liver of BN and YOS rats at different ages. Cholestyramine and simvastatin were used as drugs.

A. L. Catapano et al. (eds.), Drugs Affecting Lipid Metabolism, 139–143.
© 1993 *Kluwer Academic Publishers and Fondazione Giovanni Lorenzini.*

MATERIALS AND METHODS

Animals

Male Brown Norway rats and Yoshida rats of 2, 6 and 18 months of age were obtained from Charles River. Animals were fed a chow diet costituted by : proteins 16%, lipids 2.5%, carbohydrates 55%, fibers 7.5% and ash 6.5%. They were housed at 21 °C with a light cycle of 14 hrs and had free access to food before sacrifice.

Rats were sacrificed at 9 a.m. and plasma samples were obtained by venipuncture using 1% Na-EDTA as anticoagulant. Plasma cholesterol and triglycerides were determined by enzymatic kits (Boehringer, Mannheim, Germany).

Cholestyramine was given as 4% in the diet for 10 days. Simvastatin was administered by gavage at the dose of 10 mg/kg suspended in 0.5% tragacantha gum and the last dosage was given 2 hrs before the sacrifice. Treatment lasted 10 days. Control animals were given the vehicle only.

Determination of liver lipid levels

Aliquots of the liver were homogenized in chloroform methanol, 2:1; the organic phase was used for the measurement of cholesterol and triglycerides by enzymatic kits.

Determination of liver enzyme activities

Liver microsomes for the determination of HMGCoA reductase activity were prepared following homogenization in 0.3M sucrose, 10mM mercaptoethanol and 50mM NaF and centrifugation of the 10.000 x g supernatant at 105.000 x g for 1 hr at 4 °C. Microsomes for the determination of cholesterol 7α-hydroxylase activity were prepared from livers homogenized in 0.25M sucrose containing 1mM EDTA. Microsomes were washed and suspended in the appropriate buffer as described for each enzyme determination. Protein concentration was determined according to Bradford (2), using bovine serum albumin as standard. HMGCoA reductase activity was assayed with microsomes suspended in 300mM KCl, 1mM EDTA, 5mM dithiothreitol, 50mM phosphate buffer, pH 7.2, under the conditions already described for the evaluation of the active and total form of the enzyme (3). For cholesterol 7α-hydroxylase activity determinations, the microsomal fraction was suspended in 0.1M phosphate buffer, pH 7.4, and the enzyme activity was determined according to (3). In all experiments, zero time control samples were prepared with solvent-inactivated microsomes.

Statistical analysis

Results are expressed as the mean $\pm$ s.d. and statistical analysis was performed according to Duncan, considering the significance limit for $p < 0.05$.

RESULTS AND DISCUSSION

As compared to BN rats , the YOS were slightly hyperphagic and the habit did not change with age. As a consequence, body weight of YOS rats was higher as compared to BN. The liver weight as % of the total body weight was higher in YOS and decreased chronologically in both groups. YOS rats showed higher cholesterol and TG plasma levels. The increase of plasma lipid levels with age was evident only in the YOS strain thus indicating a genetic effect (fig.1).

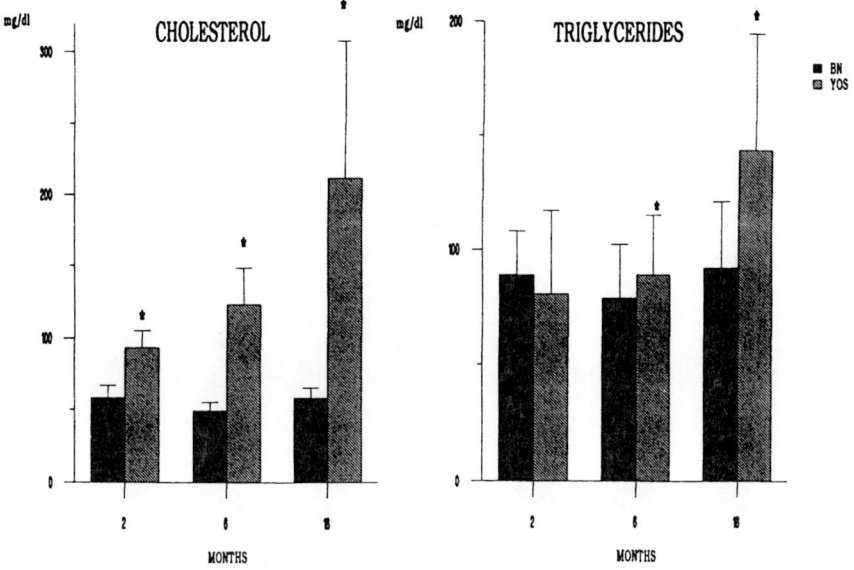

Figure 1. Plasma cholesterol and triglyceride levels in BN and YOS rats. Results are the mean ± s.d.; * significant vs BN.

Cholesterol accumulation was not observed in the liver during aging. The amount of cholesterol (expressed as mg/g liver weight) was similar in the two strain, but considering the total liver mass the hepatic cholesterol pool is higher in YOS with respect to BN rats. TG levels were also higher in YOS as compared to BN group. A slight increase of TG levels was observed in the liver of BN rats during aging. In parallel with the results on liver cholesterol levels, the microsomal free cholesterol was similar in both groups and remained constant during aging.

The total activity of HMGCoA reductase decrased with age in both strains and YOS rats were characterized by a higher activity as compared to BN (fig 2). As regards the expressed fraction of HMGCoA reductase activity, the levels were not statistically different in the two strains. This could mean that the level of cholesterol synthesis is similar in YOS and BN rats, but since the amount of microsomal proteins were higher in YOS, then cholesterol synthesis is elevated in this group with compared to BN.

Cholesterol 7α-hydroxylase activity did not change in aging. The comparison between the two groups indicates for a higher enzyme activity in YOS with respect to BN, either at 2 and 18 months (fig 2). The question remains if the higher levels of enzyme activity are related to a higher *de novo* synthesis of the protein or to a greater availability of the substrate. It is possible that the increased *de novo* synthesis of cholesterol caused the related elevation of 7α-hydroxylase activity. The former hypothesis (increased rate of protein neo-synthesis) is under current investigation by measuring 7α-hydroxylase mRNA levels.

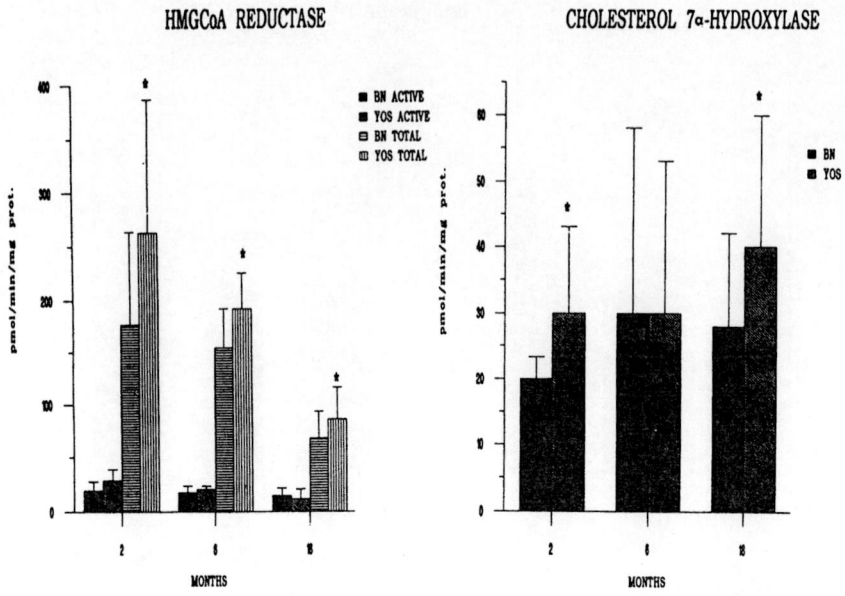

Figure 2. HMGCoA Reductase and cholesterol 7α hydroxylase in BN and YOS rats. Results are the mean ± s.d.; * significant vs BN.

TABLE 1. Cholestyramine effect on HMGCoA Reductase and cholesterol 7α-hydroxylase. Results are expressed as n-fold increase with respect to the basal levels of the enzyme activity.

Age	HMGCoA Rcd		7α-hydroxylase	
	BN	YOS	BN	YOS
2	7.7	2.6	6.8	3.2
18	17	5.2	4.2	1.9

Cholestyramine did not reduce plasma cholesterol in both groups at any age, but its major effect was on cholesterol 7α-hydroxylase and HMGCoA reductase (Table 1). As regards the effect on cholesterol 7α-hydroxylase, the stimulation of the enzyme in BN was twice as high as compared to YOS rats. Similarly HMGCoA reductase in YOS was induced by cholestyramine to a lesser extent than in BN. Therefore the YOS rat seems to be less responsive to the resin induction.

Simvastatin treatment did not exert any effect on plasma lipid levels, at each age. At this respect, BN and YOS rats respond to HMGCoA reductase inhibitors as other rat strain (4). As regards HMGCoA reductase activity, treatment with simvastatin caused a reduction of the enzyme activity of the order of 50% in both strains and the inhibition seems to be similar at 2 and 6 months.

REFERENCES

1.   Uchida, K., Nomura, Y., Kadowaki, M., Takase, H., Takano, K. and Takeuchi, N. (1978) 'Age-related changes in cholesterol and bile acid metabolism in rats', J. Lipid Res. 19, 544-552.
2.   Bradford, M.A. (1976) 'A rapid and sensitive method for quantitation of microgram quantities of protein utilizing the principle of protein dye binding' Anal. Biochem. 72, 248-254
3.   Fantappie', S., Catapano, A.L., Cancellieri, M., Fasoli, L., De Fabiani, E., Bertolini, M. and Bosisio E. (1992) 'Plasma lipoproteins and cholesterol metabolism in Yoshida rats: an animal model of spontaneous hyperlipemia' Life.Sci. 50, 1913-1924
4.   Endo, A. (1981) 'Biological and pharmacological activity of inhibitors of 3-hydroxy-3-methylglutarylcoenzyme A reductase' TIBS,6, 10-12

IN VITRO EFFECT OF THIOL- AND CYSTEINE-CONTAINING COMPOUNDS ON THE IMMUNOLOGICAL REACTIVITY OF HUMAN AND RHESUS MONKEY LIPOPROTEIN(a)

Angelo M. Scanu, Ditta Pfaffinger, Gunther M. Fless and Kazuhiko Makino

Abstract

We have examined samples of human and rhesus monkey plasma both with a single and double-band apo(a) isoforms after incubation in vitro at pH 7.7 with various concentrations (1-20 mM) of N-acetylcysteine (NAC), homocysteine (Hcys), 2- mercaptoethanol (2ME) and dithiothreitol (DTT) for 1 hr at 37°C under a nitrogen atmosphere. Incubated samples when fractionated by SDS-polyacrylamide gel electrophoresis followed by immunoblot analyses reacted less intensively than untreated controls as a function of reductant concentration. These data were corroborated by ELISA using as a capture antibody anti apo(a) and as a developing antibody either anti apoB or anti apo(a). Contrary to apo(a) there were no significant changes in the immunoreactivity of apoB100.

Changes in thiol-induced immunoreactivity were also observed in pure preparations of Lp(a) although, at equivalent stoichiometries, the changes were more marked than those observed with Lp(a) in whole plasma. As assessed by Western blotting the changes in immunoreactivity preceded the dissociation of apo(a) from Lp(a). The dissociation was complete at a 5 mM DTT and 100 mM 2ME.

These results show that thiols and cysteine-containing compounds affect the immunoreactivity of Lp(a) likely the consequence of the cleavage of the intra-kringle disulfides. Should these changes in immunological reactivity also occur in vivo they may introduce a confounding factor when measuring plasma Lp(a) levels by immunologically-based techniques.

Supplementary Key Words:

Lipoprotein(a), apolipoprotein (a), kringles of apolipoprotein(a); thiol compounds and lipoprotein(a); N-acetylcysteine and Lp(a); homocysteine and Lp(a).

A. L. Catapano et al. (eds.), Drugs Affecting Lipid Metabolism, 145–150.

Introduction

It is now known that apo(a) is made of multiple kringle 4 (K4) repeats, each containing three intra-chain disulfide bridges. There is an unpaired cysteine in $K4_{36}$ (1) believed to be disulfide linked to another unpaired cysteine residue located in the carboxyl terminal domain of apoB100 (2, 3). It is also known that treating Lp(a) with relatively high concentrations of dithiothreitol (DTT) or 2-mercaptoethanol (2ME) causes the dissociation of the interchain disulfide bond and the release of apo(a) from apoB100 (2, 3). However, the effect of these and other reducing agents on the intrachain disulfides of the kringles of apo(a) and on the structure of Lp(a) has not been examined in detail. To shed light on the subject we here describe the results of in vitro studies showing that the incubation of either whole plasma or isolated Lp(a) with the cysteine-containing compounds N-acetylcysteine (NAC) and homocysteine (Hcys), and with the thiol reagents 2ME and DTT impacts significantly on the apo(a) immunoreactivity. A report a on the human aspect of this work has appeared (4).

Materials and methods

The studies were carried on healthy male volunteers or rhesus monkeys with plasma Lp(a) protein levels in the range of 5-15 mg/dl with a single band or two band apo(a) isoforms. In a typical experiment 1 ml aliquots of plasma were incubated for 1 h at 37°C at pH 7.7 with 1,2,5,10 and 20 mM concentrations of one of the following reagents: DTT, 2ME, NAC and Hcys. Each tube was purged with nitrogen gas before capping and aliquots of the incubated samples were separated on 2-16% polyacrylamide gradient gels (Pharmacia Fine Chemicals) by electrophoresis in the presence of 0.2% SDS, followed by immunoblotting using a specific polyclonal antibody raised against either human or rhesus monkey Lp(a) in the rabbit (5).

Studies were also carried out on Lp(a) preparations isolated from either human or rhesus plasma essentially according to Fless et al (5) and incubated with 1 to 20 mM of DTT, 2ME, NAC and Hcys followed by a 1 hr incubation at 37°C under nitrogen gas. At the end of the incubation, samples were immediately taken for analyses by ELISA or Western blotting as previously described (6).

Results

A.   STUDIES ON WHOLE PLASMA

Effect of NAC and Hcys. Human plasma samples incubated with either NAC or Hcys exhibited changes in neither total cholesterol or triglycerides but a progressive decrease in Lp(a) immunoreactivity in the presence of increasing concentrations of these reductants as measured by ELISA using either anti apoB100 or anti apo(a) as the developing antibody (Table 1). Contrary to the changes noted with Lp(a), there were no significant modifications in the antigenicity of plasma apoB as assessed by ELISA using anti apoB as both the capture and detecting antibody. Similar results were obtained with rhesus plasma although the ELISA studies were limited to an ELISA system where anti apo(a) was the capture antibody and apo B the developing antibody.

Table 1

Attenuation of Lp(a) immunoreactivity in plasma measured by ELISA as a function of various concentrations of cysteine-containing compounds

Agent	Molarity of agent mM	Capture Antibody Anti apoB / Detecting Antibody Anti apoB	Capture Antibody Anti apo(a) / Detecting Antibody Anti apoB	Anti apo(a) / Anti apo(a)
		% of Control		
NAC	1	96.7	86.9	100.0
	2	95.0	75.1	88.9
	5	88.3	53.8	64.3
	10	98.3	45.0	61.8
	20	83.3	30.1	52.1
D-L Hcys	1	96.7	100.7	100.3
	2	106.7	101.9	92.2
	5	93.3	84.9	88.0
	10	98.3	65.4	76.7
	20	96.7	32.3	54.2

Plasma was incubated with the thiol compounds at 37° C for 1 hr at pH 7.7 under nitrogen gas. All samples remained clear after incubation.

Reproduced by permission from ref. 4.

By Western blotting analyses using a polyclonal anti apo(a) as the detecting antibody, the plasma samples incubated with either NAC or Hcys exhibited a decrease of the immunoreactivity of the band corresponding to the apoB100-apo(a) complex; this decrease started from 10mM concentration of each reagent. The dissociation of apo(a) from Lp(a) was seen at 20mM concentrations; however, the dissociated band was poorly visualized due to the attenuation in immunoreactivity. Overall, the results obtained by ELISA or Western blotting with NAC were comparable to those with Hcys.

Effect of DTT and 2ME. As assessed by ELISA the decrease in immunoreactivity caused by DTT was more severe than that caused by ME at equivalent molar concentrations in keeping with the greater effectiveness of DTT as a reducing agent. Plasma incubated with either 10 or 20 mM DTT formed an irreversible gel which was not observed when either 2ME, NAC or Hcys were used at similar concentrations.

At high concentrations of the reductants, Western blotting of the plasma samples reduced with DTT showed a marked drop in the intensity of the apoB-apo(a) band and a dissociation of apo(a) from Lp(a). In the case of 2ME, the effect on the immunoreactivity was comparatively less marked. A complete dissociation between apoB100 and apo(a) was only seen at high concentrations of the reagent, i.e. 100 mM. The results with rhesus monkey plasma were comparable to those observed with human plasma.

B.   STUDIES ON PURE PREPARATIONS OF LP(A)

ELISA of pure preparations of human Lp(a), incubated with any of the reducing agents employed in this study, exhibited a decrease in immunoreactivity which was significantly higher than that observed in the experiments with whole plasma using either anti apoB100 or anti apo(a) as the detecting antibody. As noted before, loss of immunoreactivity was less severe when measurements were carried out using anti apo(a) as the detecting antibody. Western blotting using anti apo(a) showed an attenuation in immunoreactivity particularly marked in the case of the DTT-treated samples in keeping with the results obtained by ELISA. Complete dissociation of apo(a) from Lp(a) was observed at 5mM DTT and 100mM 2ME and this was accompanied by a marked decrease of immunoreactivity of the dissociated apo(a) band. Immunoblots of the same samples developed in the presence of anti apoB showed that the apoB100 band did not vary in intensity with changing concentrations of thiol in agreement with the results obtained with the ELISA for apoB. Overall, rhesus monkey Lp(a) exhibited a behavior comparabel to that of human Lp(a).

Discussion

The present results show that the cysteine-containing compounds NAC and Hcys and the thiol-containing reagents 2ME and DTT can cause changes in the immunoreactivity of apo(a) likely as a consequence of the destabilization of the disulfide bonds. The concentration dependent effect of the reactants suggests that the cleavage of the intrachain disulfide bonds of the apo(a) kringles occurred well before this glycoprotein was dissociated from apoB100. It is of interest that the loss of apo(a) immunoreactivity was not observed with apoB100, in keeping with the findings of Gries et al. (7) also showing that apoB100 undergoes no significant detectable conformational changes upon reduction. We also observed that purified preparations human and rhesus of Lp(a) were more sensitive to the action of the reductants than in whole plasma at equivalent stoichiometries, suggesting that the plasma may have a quenching action on the reductants. This an explanation is supported by the formation of a gel in the plasma samples that were incubated with high concentrations of DTT. The similarity in results between human and rhesus Lp(a) further underscores the structural similarity between the two species shown in previous studies (8).

Overall, these results point at the critical role played by the disulfide bonds in kringle stability and immunogenicity and the potential problems attending the measurement of plasma Lp(a) levels in the presence of either thiols or cysteine containing compounds. Gavish and Breslow (9) have reported a decrease of the plasma levels of Lp(a) in two patients after a short-term oral intake of NAC in a dosage of 2 or 4 g/day. They interpreted their results to suggest that NAC acted at the hepatocyte level either preventing formation or causing the cleavage of the disulfide linkage between apo(a) and apoB100. While this interpretation is plausible it must be considered tentative until corroborated by measurements of concentrations of tissue NAC. Consideration must be also be given to the fact that apo(a) reduced by NAC may represent an unfavorable compound from the cardiovascular standpoint.

The current studies have also practical implications. Currently the techniques for measuring plasma Lp(a) levels lack standardization, partially due to the variety of antibodies and the varying experimental conditions used in the various laboratories (see for review ref 3). It is now apparent that the examining the plasma of subjects taking drugs with reducing potential on kringle structures may pose an additional level of diffculty. This may also be true for plasminogen(10). Finally, when assessing apo(a) polymorphism by gel electrophoretic techniques, thiols or cysteine containing reagents used for dissociating apo(a) from apoB100 may limit the immunodetection of the isoforms particularly in subjects with low plasma levels of Lp(a).

Acknowledgements

The original work by the authors cited in this manuscript was carried out by USPHS-NHLBI grants #18577. Ms. Jill Voss provided valuable help in preparing this manuscript.

References

1. McLean, J.W., Tomlinson, J.E., Kuang, W-J, Eaton, D.J., Chen, E.Y., Fless, G.M., Scanu, A.M., Lawn, R.M. (1987). 'cDNA sequence of human apolipoprotein(a) is homologous to plasminogen', Nature, 330:132-137.
2. Utermann, G., (1989) 'The mysteries of lipoprotein(a)', Science, 246:904-910.
3. Scanu, A.M. and Fless, G.M. (1990) 'Lipoprotein(a): Heterogeneity and biological relevance', J Clin Invest. 85:1709-1715.
4. Scanu, A.M., Pfaffinger, D., Fless, G.M., Makino, K., Eisenbart, J. and Hinman, J. (1992) 'Attenuation of immunological reactivity of lipoprotein(a) by thiols and cysteine-containing compounds: Structural implications', Arteriosclerosis and Thrombosis 12:424-429.
5. Fless, G.M., ZumMallen, M.E. and Scanu, A.M. (1985) 'Isolation of apolipoprotein(a) from lipoprotein(a)', J. Lipid Res, 26:1224-1229.
6. Fless, G.M., Snyder, M.L., Scanu, A.M. (1989) 'Enzyme-linked immunoassay for Lp(a)', J Lipid Res, 30:651-662.
7. Gries, A., Fievet, C., Marcovina, S., Nimpf, J., Wurm, H., Mezdour, H., Fruchart, J.C., Kostner, G.M. (1988) 'Interaction of LDL, Lp(a) and reduced Lp(a) with monoclonal antibodies against apoB', J Lipid Res, 29:1-8.
8. Makino, K. and Scanu, A.M. (1991) 'Lipoprotein(a): Nonhuman primate models' Lipids 26:679-683.
9. Gavish, D. and Breslow, J.L. (1991) 'Lipoprotein(a) reduction by N-acetyl cysteine', Lancet, 337:203-204.
10. Chalaprawat, M., Scanu, A.M. (1991) 'Effect of N-acetyl cysteine and homocysteine on the immunoreactivity and activity of plasminogen', Arteriosclerosis 11:1568a.

THE INTERACTION OF Lp(a) WITH LIVER CELLS: IMPLICATIONS FOR LIPID
LOWERING THERAPY

G.M.KOSTNER

ABSTRACT.   There is now general agreement that Lp(a) is one of the
most atherogenic lipoproteins. Concerning its pathophysiology, there
are currently two theories discussed: i) Lp(a) interferes with
fibrinolysis in many ways, notably by inhibiting the t-PA mediated
activation of plasminogen. ii) Lp(a) or chemically modified Lp(a) is
taken up by the scavenger pathway, leading to foam cell formation and
cholesterol accumulation in the vessel wall. Little is known today
about the nascent form of Lp(a) and its assembly. From in vivo turnover
studies it appears that Lp(a) is secreted directly from the liver. The
site of Lp(a) catabolism is completely in the dark. In vitro studies
suggest that Lp(a) binds to the LDL-receptor; whether or not this is
also true in vivo is subject of intensive investigations. In order to
shed some light into this question, the interaction of Lp(a) with
cultivated hepatoma cells has been investigated. Other than with
fibroblasts, there seems to be only low affinity, non-saturable binding
of Lp(a) to Hep-G2 and Hep-3B cells. Preincubation of hepatoma cells
with HMG-CoA reductase inhibitors increases Lp(a) binding only
slightly. Preincubation of hepatoma cells with Lp(a) however increases
markedly high affinity LDL-binding. The Lp(a) triggerd LDL-binding
however is not followed by an increase in LDL internalization
degradation, or a decrease of cholesterol biosynthesis.
    Thus lipid lowering drugs acting primarily at the catabolic site of
LDL by stimulating LDL-receptor activity cannot be expected to have
great impacts on plasma Lp(a) levels.

1. INTRODUCTION

1.1. Structure of Lp(a)

Structurally, Lp(a) is best characterized as an LDL particle with one
apo-a protein attached to it by a disulfide bridge. Apo-a is a
glycoprotein, rich in sialic acid. There are approx. 20 genetic
isoforms of apo-a described varying in their molecular weight between
350 - 800 kDa [1]. The Lp(a) plasma concentration was found to
correlate negatively with the molecular weight . The basis of the
genetic size polymorphism has been clarified by molecular biological

151

A. L. Catapano et al. (eds.), Drugs Affecting Lipid Metabolism, 151–159.
© 1993 Kluwer Academic Publishers and Fondazione Giovanni Lorenzini

studies [2]. Apo-a was found to be very homologous to plasminogen
(Plg): The Plg structure is characterized by the presence of 5 so
called "kringles". In the different isoforms of apo-a the kringle-4 of
Plg is repeated between 10 - 40 times. These kringle-4 repeats are 98 -
100 % homologous. Apo-a in addition contains one kringle-5 and the
protease domaine with great homology to the Plg conterparts. Amino acid
560, Arg in Plg is substituted by Ser in apo-a. Thus the Plg activators
t-PA and UK are unable to activate apo-a, exposing proteolytic active
domaines. Yet Lp(a) interferes with Plg binding to its receptor and to
fibrin.

1.2. Metabolism of Lp(a)

We have shown previously that Lp(a) plasma concentrations are
determined mainly by the rate of synthesis. The fractional catabolic
rate of Lp(a) had only a minor influence [3]. By injecting
simultaneously 125-I Lp(a) and 131-I LDL into hypercholesterolemics on
the other hand we found a significant correlation between Lp(a) and LDL
fractional catabolic rates (FCR). As the FCR of LDL is to a major
extent determined by the LDL-receptor activity we speculated that LDL-R
play also a role for the in vivo catabolism of Lp(a).

   Previous publications suggest that Lp(a) does bind to cultured human
skin fibroblasts , but with a reduced affinity as compared to LDL
[4,5]. Martmann-Moe and Berg [6] on the other hand denied specific high
affinity binding . The removal of the apo-a glycoprotein moiety from
Lp(a) yielded a particle which was indistinguishable from LDL with
respect to the affinity to the LDL-R [7,8].

   Since the liver is the main organ for LDL-R mediated catabolism of
apo-B containing lipoproteins, major emphasis has to be given to this
organ in studying the in vivo situation. By infusion of Lp(a) into
transgenic mice with an overexpression of LDL-R in the liver, a
significantly faster catabolism was found as compared to normal mice
[9].

1.3. Factors Interfering with Plasma Lp(a) Levels.

Plasma Lp(a) levels are determined by genetic factors by approx. 50%.
There are however also non-genetic factors known which have some impact
as well. On the other hand, lipid lowering drugs such as cholestyramin
or lovastatin, which increase the LDL-R number in the liver, do not
lower Lp(a) [10].

There are certainly additional studies needed to get deeper insight
into the mode of action of all these factors listed in Tab.1. The
present work was conducted to study the role of the liver in Lp(a)
catabolism.

2. Lp(a) BINDING TO HEPATOMA CELLS

2.1. Material and Methods

Hep-G2 or Hep-3B cells were seeded in multitray petri-dishes in DMEM
containing 20 % FCS and allowed to grow for 2 - 4 days followed by
replacement of the medium by DMEM containing 10 % LPDS and incubation
for 48 h. These cells were studied for LDL and Lp(a) binding by

TABLE 1: Non-Genetic Factors Influencing Lp(a) Levels.

FACTOR/AGENT	LOWERING EFFECT	INCREASING EFFECT
Drugs	See Tab. 2	
ω-3 Fatty acids	+	
Smoking	+	
Pregnancy		+++
Kidney diseases		+++
Acute Phase Reactions		+(+)
Diabetes Mellitus		+

+: low effect;   ++: medium effect;   +++: high effect.

conventional techniques [4]. In another set of experiments, various concentrations of different substances were added to the LPDS medium and cells were further incubated for various periods of time. In most experiments this incubation persisted for 72 h. Cells were now washed, and classical binding studies at 4°C of 125-I labelled LDL in the presence and absence of 50-fold excess of cold LDL were performed. As LDL internalization and degradation is negligible at 4°C, we determined the total radioactivity associated with cells by counting the carefully washed and NaOH solubilized cells in a γ-counter. LDL (d 1.025 - 1.055) was isolated by sequential ultracentrifugation and used within 8-10 days. LDL-free Lp(a) was purified by affinity chromatography using immune specific adsorbers as described earlier [8].

2.2. Results

Fig.1 displays specific binding of LDL (A) or Lp(a) (B) to Hep-G2 cells incubated in LPDS +/- mevinolin (MEV). LDL exhibited high affinity saturable binding with a Kd of approx. 5 nmol/l and a capacity of 150 ng/mg cell protein. In contrast the binding of Lp(a) was non-saturable and of low affinity. Preincubation of Hep-G2 cells with 10^-6 mol/l of mevinolin for 48 hrs increased the capacity of LDL binding by some 45% yet had little influence on Lp(a) binding. Comparable results were obtained with Hep-3B cells, which had a lower capacity for LDL binding (data not shown) .

In order to pursue this topic further, the down regulation of the LDL-R activity by different lipoproteins was studied. As it is known that HDL upregulates LDL-R activity by depleting cells from cholesterol, this lipoprotein was used as a control. The results are shown in Fig. 2: As expected, LDL caused a decrease and HDL caused an increase of LDL-binding in comparison to LPDS. To our surprise, preincubation with Lp(a) - which we expected to behave similarly to LDL, caused a significant increase of LDL association. 50 ug/ml of Lp(a) cholesterol was even more effective as 30 ug/ml of HDL. Scatchard transformation of the binding curves resulted in Kd and Bmax values of Lp(a) or HDL preincubated cells, which were almost identical.

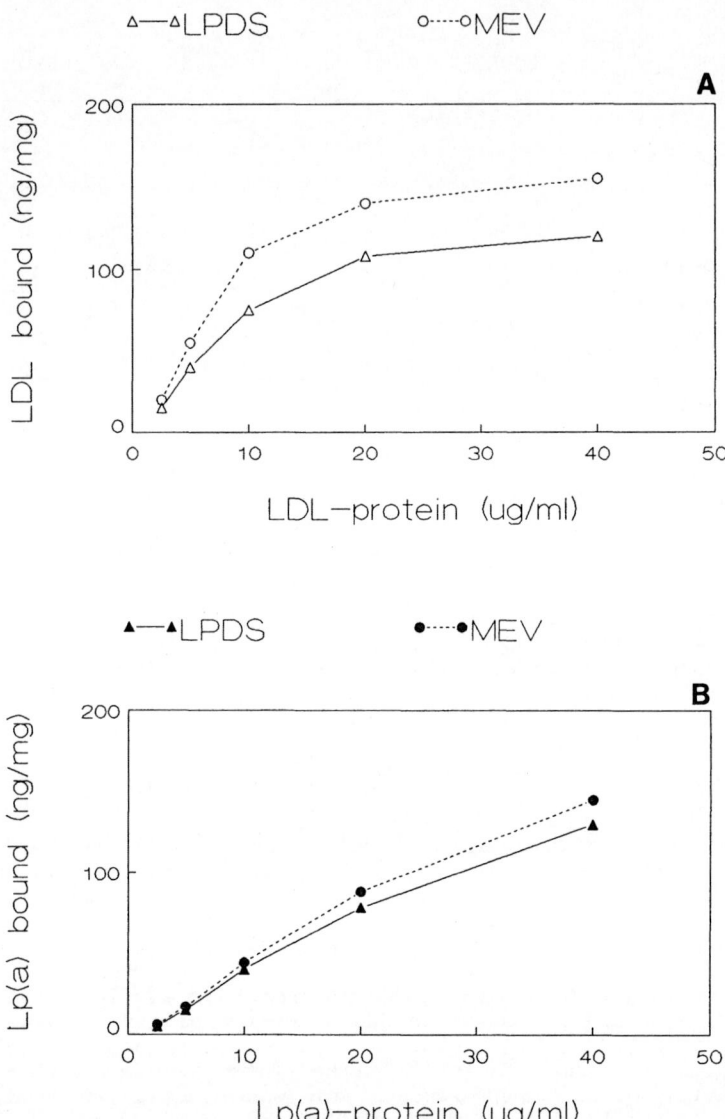

Figure 1. Specific binding of LDL (A) and of Lp(a) (B) to Hep-G2 cells.
Cells were pretreated for 48h with LPDS or with LPDS supplemented with
10^-6 mol/l of mevinolin (MEV). The curves represent total binding
minus unspecific binding.

In order to study the possibility that LDL-receptors were responsible
for the Lp(a) induced LDL binding, monoclonal antibodies against the
LDL-receptor (C-7 clone) were added to Hep-G2 cells before measuring

the LDL binding. In LPDS or HDL pretreated cells, the C-7 antibody completely abolished LDL binding. In the incubates of Hep-G2 cells with Lp(a), the monoclonal LDL-receptor antibody reduced LDL binding by approx. 40 % and even an excess of antibody had no further effect. From these data we concluded that Lp(a) stimulated LDL association to Hep-G2 cells, which is caused by mechanisms distinct from the Brown and Goldstein pathway.

It was also of interest to know, whether preincubation of Hep-G2 cells with Lp(a) would have any effect on endogenous cholesterol biosynthesis. Hep-3B cells were therefore preincubated for 72 h with LPDS supplemented with LDL, Lp(a), apo-a or 10^-6 mol/l of mevinolin, and the incorporation of 14-C labelled octanoate into the non-saponifyable sterol fraction was measured. As shown in Fig. 3 Mevinolin as well as LDL reduced the incorporation of octanoate into the neutral sterol fractions of Hep-3B cells. Lp(a) had a significantly lower effect, whereas apo-a or Plg had no effect whatsoever. Further experiments carried out at 37°C revealed that LDL internalization or degradation into Hep-3B cells is only insignificantly influeneced by Lp(a) or by apo-a.

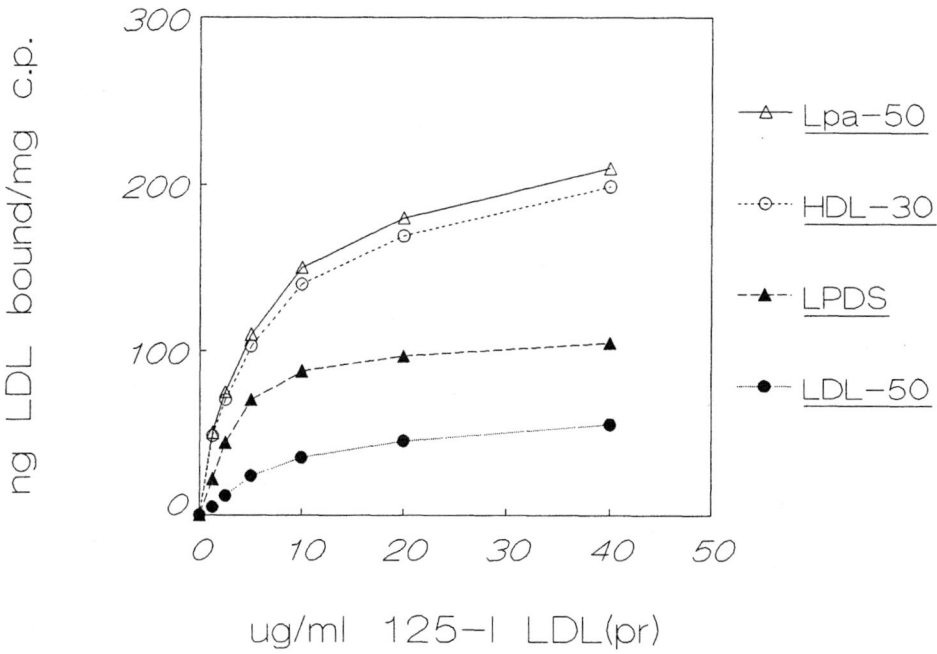

Figure 2. Association of LDL to Hep-2B cells. Cells were preincubated for 72h with LPDS, or with LPDS supplemented with 30 μg/ml HDL, 50 μg/ml LDL or 50 μg/ml Lp(a) and bindig of 125-I LDL was measured at 4°C.

3. CONCLUSION

There are numerous studies published which demonstrate that purified LDL-receptors or LDL-R from peripheral cells bind specifically Lp(a). This binding is mediated by the B-100 component of Lp(a) [4,5,7,8,9].

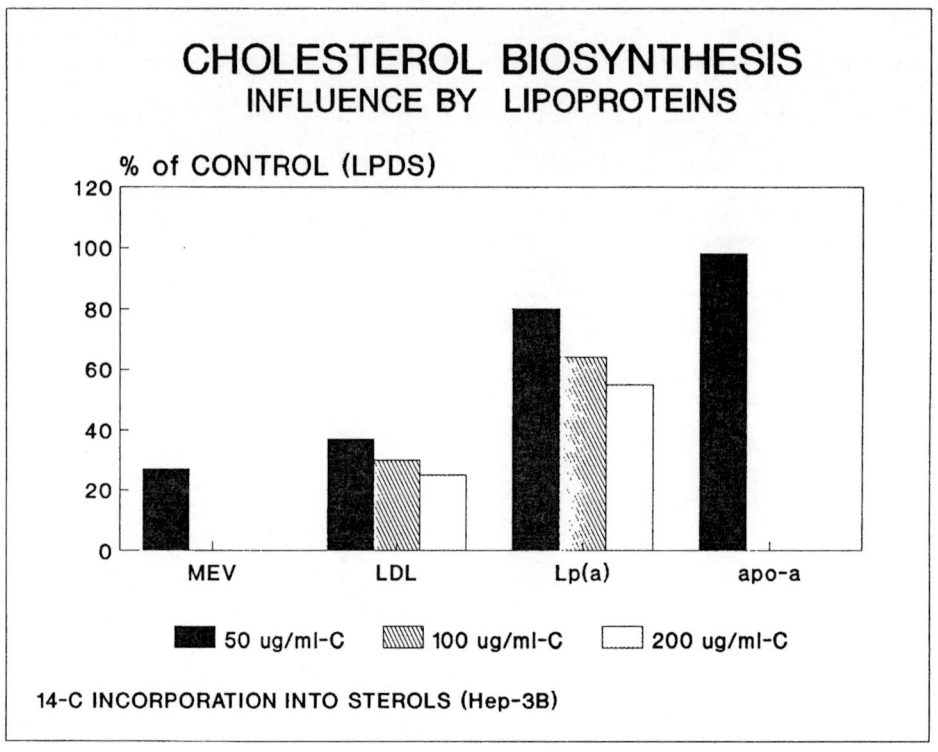

Figure 3. Influenece of cholesterol biosynthesis in Hep-3B cells by LDL and Lp(a). Cells were preincubated for 48h with the indicated agent and the incorporation of 14-C cholesterol into nonsaponifyable sterols was measured.

In the liver, the most important organ for the catabolism of apo-B containing lipoproteins, the situation seems somewhat different. The present studies with Hep-G2 and Hep-3B cells suggest that these cells show a relatively low interaction with Lp(a) via the LDL-receptors as compared to peripheral cells. In vivo, in the presence of large quantities of LDL, this interaction is probably to low to contribute to a major degree to Lp(a) catabolism.

Hepatoma cells on the other hand bind with a high capacity Lp(a) in an LDL-R independent manner. This binding might be mediated by fibronectin, connective tissue proteins or glycosamino glycans and prevents Lp(a) from beeing internalized and degraded. In turn Lp(a) accumulating at the surface of these cells bind LDL with an affinity which is comparable with the binding of LDL to its specific receptor. This portion of LDL is also not internalized or degraded and may be just in equilibrium with the bulk of LDL in the plasma or in the medium in case of our experiments.

Our results are in line with the observations that lipid lowering drugs such as HMG-CoA reductase inhibitors [10] or bile acid sequestrants [11] which increase significantly the LDL-R number on liver cells, have no Lp(a) lowering effects. They do however not explain the well known fact that patients suffering from hypercholesterolemia caused by LDL-R dysfunction [12], or caused by familial defective hyper-apobetalipoproteinemia 13] exhibit significantly increased Lp(a) levels. This open question is currently under investigation in our laboratory.

Coming back to the question of how increased Lp(a) levels may be reduced by drugs it seems clear that at present time the point of approach cannot be a drug which increases Lp(a) catabolism, as we have little information on that mechanism. It certainly seems better to aim at interfering with Lp(a) biosynthesis . There are currently only few agents known which may be useful (Tab.2), many of them however may not be recommendable for long term treatment at high doses.

Table 2. Agents Interfering with Increased Lp(a) Levels.

AGENT	MAXIMAL EFFECT OF REDUCTION	REF.
Stanazolol	60 - 70%	14
Danazolol	60 - 90%	15
Niacin + Neomycin	50 - 60%	16
α-Tocopherol-nicotinate	25 - 30%	17
N-Acetylcysteine*)	50 - 70%	18
LDL-Apheresis	30 - 45 %	19

*) Only at very high doses (4-8 g/d).

There is certainly an urgent need to pursue this important area of research further by investigating open questions of Lp(a) metabolism on one hand and by looking at the physiological function of this peculiar lipoprotein.

ACKNOWLEDGEMENTS

This work was supported by grants from the Austrian Science Fondation, grant Nr. S-4602

4. REFERENCES

4.1. Gaubatz J.W., Ghanem, K.I., Guevara, G.J., Nava, M.L.., Patsch, W. and Morrisett J.D. (1990) 'Polymorphic forms of human apolipoprotein(a): inheritance and relationship of their molecular weights to plasma levels of lipoprotein(a)', J.Lipid Res. 31, 603-613.

4.2. McLean, J.W., Tomlinson, J.E., Kuang, W.J., et al. (1987) 'cDNA sequence of human apolipoprotein-a is homologous to plasminogen', Nature 300, 132 - 137.

4.3. Krempler,F., Kostner, G.M., Bolzano,K., Sandhofer,F. (1980) 'Turnover of Lp(a) in man', J.Clin. Invest. 65, 1483-1490.

4.4. Krempler F, Kostner GM, Roscher A, Haslauer F, Bolzano K, Sandhofer F. (1983) 'Studies on the role of specific cell surface receptors in the removal of lipoprotein(a) in man', J. Clin. Invest. 71, 1431-1441.

4.5. Havekes L, Vermeer BJ, Brugman T, Emeis J. (1981) 'Binding of Lp(a) to the low density liporotein receptor of human fibroblasts', FEBS Lett. 132, 169-173.

4.6. Maartmann-Moe K. and Berg K. (1981) 'Lp(a) lipoprotein enters cultured fibroblasts independently of the plasma membrane low density lipoprotein receptor', Clin. Genet. 20, 352-362.

4.7. Armstrong VW, Walli AK and Seidel D. (1985)'Isolation, characterization and uptake in human fibroblasts of an apo(a)-free lipoprotein obtained on reduction of lipoprotein(a)', J. Lipid Res. 26, 1314-1423.

4.8. Steyrer E, Kostner GM. (1990) 'Interaction of Lp(a) with the B/E-receptor: a study using isolated bovine adrenal cortex and human fibroblast receptors' J.Lipid Res. 31, 1247-1253.

4.9. Hofman, S.L., Eaton, D.L., Brown, M.S., McConnathy W.J., Goldsteim, J.L. and Hammer,R.E. (1990) 'Overexpression of human low density lipoprotein receptors leads to accelerated catabolism of Lp(a) lipoprotein in transgenic mice', J.Clin. Invest. 85, 1542-1547.

4.10.Kostner GM, Gavish D, Leopold B, Bolzano K, Weintraub MS Breslow JL. (1989) 'HMG-CoA reductase inhibitors lower LDL but increase Lp(a) levels: a study of 24 individuals treated with simvastatin or lovastatin' Circulation 80, 1313-1319.

4.11. Vessby B, Kostner GM, Lithell H, Thomis J. (1982) 'Divergent effects of cholestyramin on apolipoprotein Lp(a): A dose response study of the effects of cholestyramin in hypercholesterolemia' Atherosclerosis 44, 61-71.

4.12. Seed M, Hoppichler F, Reaveley D. et al. (1990) 'Relation of serum Lp(a) concentrations and Lp(a) phenotype to coronary heart disease in patients with familial hypercholesterolemia' New Engl. J. Med. 322, 1494-1499.

4.13. Perombelon, Y.F.N. Gallagher,J.J., Myant, N.B., Soutar, A.K., night, B.L. (1992) 'Lpa(a) in subjects with familial defective apolipoprotein B-100', Atherosclerosis 92, 203-212.

4.14. Albers, J.J., Taggart,M.M., Appelbaum-Bowden,D., Haffner,S., Chesnut,C.H. and Hazzard W.R. (1984) 'Reduction of LCAT, apolipoprotein D and the Lp(a) lipoprotein with the anabolic steroid stanazolol'. Biochim.Biophys. Acta 795, 293-298.

4.15. Crook, D., Sidhu,M., Seed,M., O'Donnell and Stevenson J.V. (1992) 'Lp(a) levels are reduced by danazolol, an anabolic steroid', Atherosclerosis 902, 41-47.

4.16. Gurakar,A., Hoeg,J.M., Kostner,G.M., Papadopoulos,N. and Brewer, H.B. (1985) 'Levels of potentially atherogenous lipoprotein Lp(a) decline with neomycin and niacin treatment', Atherosclerosis 57, 293-301.

4.17. Noma,A., Maeda, S., Okuno,M., Abe,A., Muto,Y. (1990) 'Reduction of serum Lp(a) levels in hyperlipidemic patients with α-tocopherol nicotinate', Atheroscleroisis 84, 213-217.

4.18. Gavish,D. and Breslow, J.L. (1991) 'Lp(a) reduction by N-acetylsysteine', Lancet 337, 203-204.

4.19. Ritter,M.M., Sühler,K., Richter, W.and Schwandt,P. (1990) 'Short- and long-term effects of LDL-apheresis on Lp(a) serum levels', Clin.Chim. Acta 195, 9-16.

METABOLISM OF Apo(a) AND ApoB-100 IN HUMAN LIPOPROTEIN(a)

Joel D. Morrisett, John W. Gaubatz, Mauro N. Nava, John R. Guyton, Alan S. Hoffman, Antone R. Opekun, and David L. Hachey.

ABSTRACT. Lipoprotein(a) (Lp(a)) is a plasma lipoprotein highly correlated with cardiovascular and cerebrovascular disease. It contains two major proteins: apoB-100 similar to that present in LDL, and apo(a) which exists in different polymorphic forms with apparent molecular weight (M_r) from 418 to 838 kD. The polymorph M_r is inversely correlated with plasma Lp(a) level, suggesting that the rate of apo(a) synthesis is related to the polymorph size. This possibility has been evaluated by using stable isotope methodology to measure the rates of synthesis of apo(a) in Lp(a) and of apoB-100 in Lp(a), LDL, IDL, and VLDL. The level of isotope enrichment in vivo was used to compute fractional synthesis rates (FSR, d^{-1}) using a non-compartmental model. Five normolipidemic subjects each displaying a unique apo(a) polymorph phenotype were studied. Their mean FSR $\pm$ SD values were: Apo(a) in Lp(a) = 0.162 $\pm$ 0.084; ApoB in Lp(a) = 0.139 $\pm$ 0.073; ApoB in LDL = 0.569 $\pm$ 0.157. From a reduced compartmental model the FSR for ApoB in Lp(a) = 0.130 $\pm$ 0.063; LDL = 0.680 $\pm$ 0.204; IDL = 12.11 $\pm$ 15.72; VLDL = 9.10 $\pm$ 6.58. Although the negative correlation of apo(a) M_r with Lp(a) level was high (r = -0.872), the correlation of apo(a) FSR with apo(a) M_r was low (r = 0.341). The rate of apo(a) synthesis in Lp(a) was quite similar to that of apoB in Lp(a), but the latter was only ~25% of the FSR for apoB in LDL. The FSR for apo(a) was not correlated with plasma cholesterol levels (r = 0.153) but was negatively correlated with plasma triglyceride levels (r = -0.914).

INTRODUCTION

Thus far there have appeared very few reports describing the in vivo metabolism of Lp(a) [1,2,3]. These studies have involved the use of ^{125}I-Lp(a) to monitor the catabolism of this lipoprotein. Several technical problems have limited the value of these studies and their usefulness for understanding the individual metabolic properties of the apo(a) and apoB proteins within Lp(a). An alternative approach for monitoring the metabolic behavior of these individual apoproteins might involve the isolation of pure Lp(a) and the temporary separation of its apo(a) protein by reductive cleavage and ultracentrifugation [4,5]. The isolated apo(a) might then be radiolabeled with ^{125}I and the residual Lp[a-] particle (containing only apoB) labeled with ^{131}I. These two differently labeled species could then be rejoined by mild air oxidation in an attempt to reform the original inter-connecting disulfide bond(s). While there is some precedent in the biochemical literature for believing that Lp(a) could be reconstituted by this method, one would be hard-pressed to demonstrate

A. L. Catapano et al. (eds.), Drugs Affecting Lipid Metabolism, 161–167.
© 1993 Kluwer Academic Publishers and Fondazione Giovanni Lorenzini. ,

unequivocally that the same disulfide bonds present before reduction were also present after re-oxidation. An additional difficulty with this approach would be that individuals who normally have high molecular weight apo(a) polymorphs and low levels of Lp(a) might not be able to provide sufficient amounts of Lp(a) required for the above described biochemical manipulations. Most likely, one would be forced to use heterologous Lp(a) from a donor with a high Lp(a) level but with an apo(a) polymorph that differed from that of the recipient. We have circumvented most of these experimental problems by using an approach involving in vivo labeling of Lp(a) with stable isotopes [6].

METHODS

Criteria for entry into the study included a cholesterol level <240 mg/dl, plasma triglycerides <250 mg/dl, and Lp(a)-protein >3 mg/dl (total-Lp(a) >9 mg/dl) (Table 1).

TABLE 1.   PLASMA CONCENTRATIONS (mg/dl) OF APOLIPOPROTEINS AND LIPIDS FROM STUDY SUBJECTS

SUBJECT	Apo(a) PHENOTYPE	RACE	GENDER	Lp(a) PROTEIN	ApoB	TOTAL CHOL	HDL CHOL	TG
SL	a1, 419 kD	White	M	15	--	148	49	99
SE	a7, 705 kD	Black	M	12	117	178	44	135
GJ	a8, 742 kD	White	M	6	58	139	40	70
BR	a9, 760 kD	White	F	7	105	236	57	76
FW	A10, 796 Kd	White	M	4	104	220	39	125

Study subjects also had plasma glucose, electrolytes and liver enzymes within normal limits and were homozygous for a single apo(a) polymorph. Subjects were admitted to the General Clinical Research Center at The Methodist Hospital and were fasted for 12 h before the study began. The study was initiated by the infusion of a single intravenous bolus of [^{2}H$_4$]-lysine (1.0 mg/kg) followed by constant infusion (0.35 mg/kg) over the next 16 h. Nutrients were provided in the form of a liquid diet (Sustical or Ensure); the subject received 30 kcal/kg/body weight. This diet contained 22% calories from fat and provided 0.88 g/kcal body weight of protein.

The diet was consumed in equal hourly aliquots over the 16 h study period. A 20 ml blood sample was collected into a Vacutainer tube containing EDTA as anti-coagulant at the beginning of the study and at 2 h intervals thereafter. After sedimentation of cells by centrifugation, the plasma was separated into three aliquots for i) measurement of free, unincorporated [^{2}H$_4$]-lysine, ii) isolation of the labeled plasma lipoproteins, and iii) lipid and lipoprotein measurements. One of the three plasma aliquots (2.5 ml) was subjected to sequential ultracentrifugation or immuno precipitation to separate VLDL, IDL, LDL and Lp(a) classes.   Each lipoprotein class was fully delipidated by treatment with cold chloroform:methanol (2:1).   The resulting mixture of apolipoproteins was subjected to SDS/PAGE on 2.75% gels stained with Coomassie Blue.   The bands corresponding to apo(a) and apoB were excised, the protein hydrolyzed, and the resulting amino acids derivatized for analysis by gas chromatography-mass spectrometry [6].

RESULTS

The incorporation of [^{2}H$_4$]-lysine into apoB of Lp(a) and LDL for subject BR is shown in Figure 1.   Incorporation into apoB of Lp(a) was approximately linear, reaching a tracer/tracee molar ratio of ~0.001 by the 16th h.   Isotope incorporation into apoB of LDL exhibited a brief induction period of ~2-3 h after which incorporation increased rapidly, with the tracer/tracee ratio reaching ~0.0025 by the 16th h.   The rather large difference in the rate of isotope incorporation into apoB of Lp(a) and LDL was observed in four additional subjects.   The mean values for the tracer/tracee ratio during the study period are shown in Figure 2.   At 16 h, isotope incorporation is ~3.6 times greater for apoB in LDL than for apoB in Lp(a).   This plot also shows the time-dependent incorporation of [^{2}H$_4$]-lysine into apo(a).   At almost every sampled time-point, incorporation into apo(a) was about the same magnitude as incorporation into apoB from Lp(a).   From individual kinetic curves, fractional synthetic rates (FSR) were calculated for apo(a) and apoB in Lp(a), and apoB in LDL (Table 2).

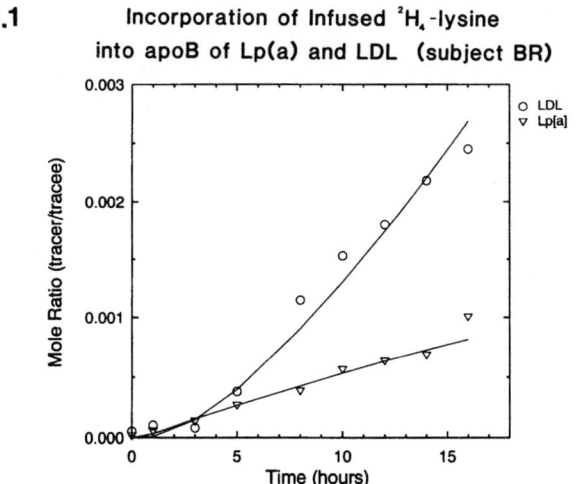

Fig.1   Incorporation of Infused ^{2}H$_4$-lysine
into apoB of Lp(a) and LDL   (subject BR)

Fig. 2   Incorporation of Infused ²H₄-lysine into apo(a) of Lp(a)
and apoB of Lp(a) and LDL (mean of 5 subjects)

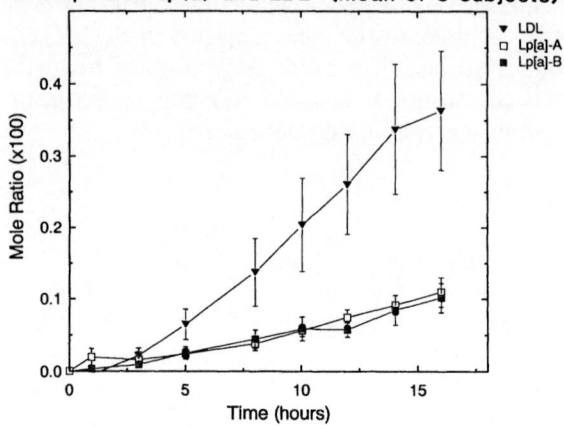

TABLE 2.

Measurement of Apo[a] and ApoB Synthesis in Human Subjects: Fractional Synthesis Rates						
Subject	Apo[a] in Lp[a]		ApoB in Lp[a]		ApoB in LDL	
	FSR	±SD	FRS	±SD	FSR	±SD
SL-1	0.114	±0.028	0.125	±0.017	0.532	±0.085
SE-7	0.085	±0.014	0.086	±0.019	0.600	±0.107
GJ-8	0.239	±0.051	0.129	±0.027	0.425	±0.042
BR-9	0.267	±0.035	0.266	±0.029	0.824	±0.053
FB-10	0.107	±0.018	0.090	±0.036	0.465	±0.030
MEAN	0.162	±0.084	0.139	±0.073	0.569	±0.157

For individuals homozygous for different apo(a) polymorphs spanning almost the full range of molecular weights, the mean FSR for apo(a) was 0.162 day⁻¹, not significantly different from the value of 0.139 obtained for apoB in Lp(a). In contrast, the mean FSR for apoB in LDL was 0.569 day⁻¹, about 3.5-fold greater than that for apoB in Lp(a) (Table 2).

DISCUSSION

Our laboratory [7] has observed that the plasma levels of apoLp(a) are inversely correlated with apo(a) polymorph molecular weight (M_r) (r = -0.461, ρ = 0.0001, n = 686). This type of correlation has also been observed by Utermann et al. [8,9,10] and Rainwater et al. [11]. This effect may be due to i) higher rates of synthesis and/or ii) lower rates of catabolism for individuals with the lower M_r polymorphs. The present study was designed to evaluate the first possibility by measuring the rates of apo(a) synthesis in human subjects displaying different single band polymorphs. For this small group of five subjects, the apo(a) M_r was strongly negatively correlated with the plasma apo(a) concentration (r = -0.872) (Table 3).

However, apo(a) M_r was only weakly correlated with the FSR for apo(a) in Lp(a) (r = 0.341). Nevertheless, the synthesis rate for apo(a) was moderately negatively correlated with the plasma apo(a) concentration (r = -0.448). Hence, it appears that the synthesis rate of apo(a) is only partly responsible for the plasma concentration of this apoprotein. Since the [$^2H_4$]-lysine incorporation into apo(a) and apoB of Lp(a) follow very similar kinetic curves, it is not surprising that the FSR for these two apoproteins in Lp(a) are highly correlated (r = 0.810). One of the more interesting

TABLE 3.   CORRELATIONS   WITH   APOPROTEIN   FRACTIONAL   SYNTHETIC RATES

1.	M_r of apo(a)	with	FSR plasma/apo(a):	r = -0.872
2.	M_r of apo(a)	with	FSR apo(a)/Lp(a):	r = 0.341
3.	Plasma apo(a)	with	FSR for apo(a)/Lp(a):	r = -0.448
4.	FSR for apo(a)/Lp(a)	with	FSR apoB/Lp(a):	r = 0.810
5.	FSR for apoB/Lp(a)	with	FSR apoB/LDL:	r = 0.817
6.	FSR for apoB/Lp(a)	with	Plasma apoB:	r = 0.003
7.	FSR for apoB/LDL	with	Plasma apoB:	r = 0.540
8.	FSR for apo(a)/Lp(a)	with	Plasma TG:	r = -0.914
9.	FSR for apo(a)/Lp(a)	with	Plasma Chol:	r = 0.153

correlations suggested by this study is the inverse relationship between apo(a) synthesis rate and plasma triglyceride level (r = -0.914). This correlation would not have been predicted on the basis of other studies we have conducted in which plasma Lp(a) and triglyceride levels decreased synchronously in Type II diabetic subjects under aggressive treatment [12], and in Type II hyperlipoproteinemics treated with Gemfibrozil [13]. In contrast to triglyceride, plasma cholesterol has almost no correlation to the FSR for apo(a) (r = 0.153).

Admittedly, the size of the study group is small, but there is sufficient consistency in the data at this point to indicate that apo(a) is synthesized at a very low rate, in fact, very near the level of sensitivity of the stable isotope methodology. Unfortunately, this limitation will preclude using the prime-constant infusion protocol to obtain catabolic rate information on this slowly synthesized apoprotein. Counter-balancing this limitation is the advantage that both apo(a) and apoB in Lp(a) can be studied simultaneously and in their native form, without disrupting apoprotein or lipoprotein structure.

ACKNOWLEDGEMENTS: The authors are indebted to Ms. Rosetta Ray for editorial assistance and Ms. Susan Kelly for help with graphics. This project has been supported in part by USPHS grant HL-27341. TBTGA.

REFERENCES

1.   Krempler, F., Kostner, G. M., Bolzano, K. and Sandhofer, F. (1980) J. Clin. Invest. 65, 1483-1490.
2.   Rader, D., Cain, W., Zech, L., Kindt, M., Usher, D. and Brewer, H. B. (1991) Arteriosclerosis 11, 1424a.
3.   Knight, B. L., Wade, D., Seed, M. and Soutar, A. K. (1990) 55th Annual Meeting, European Atherosclerosis Society, Brugge (Abs. 155).
4.   Armstrong, V. W., Walli, A. K. and Seidel, D. (1985) J. Lipid Res. 26, 1314-1323.
5.   Fless, G. M., ZumMallen, M. E. and Scanu, A. M. (1985) J. Lipid Res. 26, 1224-1229.
6.   Lichtenstein, A. H., Cohn, J. S., Hachey, D. L., Millar, J. S., Ordovas, J. M. and Schaefer, E. J. (1990) J. Lipid Res. 31, 1693-1701.
7.   Gaubatz, J. W., Ghanem, K. I., Guevara, G., Jr., Nava, M. L., Patsch, W. and Morrisett, J. D. (1990) J. Lipid Res. 31, 603-613.
8.   Utermann, G., Kraft, H. G., Menzel, H. J., Hopferwieser, T. and Seitz, C. (1988) Hum. Genet. 78, 41-46.

9.   Boerwinkle, E., Menzel, H. J., Kraft, H. G. and Utermann, G. (1989) Hum. Genet. 82, 73-78.

10.   Utermann, G., Menzel, H. J., Kraft, H. G., Duba, H. C., Kemmler, H. G. and Seitz, C. (1987) J. Clin. Invest. 80, 458-465.

11.   Rainwater, D. L., Manis, G. S. and VandeBerg, J. L. (1989) J. Lipid Res. 30, 549-558.

12.   Garber, A. J., Jones, P. H., Ghanem, K. K. and Morrisett, J. D. (1991) 9th International Atherosclerosis Symposium, Chicago, IL, USA, p. 12.

13.   Jones, P. H., Gotto, A. M., Jr., Pownall, H. J., Patsch, W., Herd, J. A., Farmer, J. A., Payton-Ross, C., Cocanougher, B., Ghanem, K. K. and Morrisett, J. D. (1991) Circulation Suppl. II 84, No. 4, Abs.# 1925.

VITAMIN E--ABSORPTION, TRANSPORT IN LIPOPROTEINS, DELIVERY TO TISSUES AND ANTIOXIDANT ACTIVITY

HERBERT J. KAYDEN and MARET G. TRABER

ABSTRACT. Vitamin E, a chain-breaking antioxidant, is the major lipid soluble antioxidant in the plasma. Studies in humans of the absorption and incorporation of vitamin E into lipoproteins have been carried out using *RRR*- and *SRR*- α-tocopherols and *RRR*-γ-tocopherol labeled with different amounts of deuterium. We have investigated normal subjects and patients with abetalipoproteinemia, lipoprotein lipase deficiency, abnormal apolipoprotein B-100 synthesis, and familial isolated vitamin E deficiency. We found that all three labeled tocopherols are absorbed equally and are secreted in chylomicrons. In the liver *RRR*-α-tocopherol is preferentially incorporated into nascent very low density lipoprotein (VLDL), presumably by a hepatic tocopherol binding protein. Therefore, γ- and *SRR*-α-tocopherols do not re-appear in the plasma to the same extent as *RRR*-α-tocopherol. Thus, chylomicrons function to transport various dietary tocopherols from the intestine, while VLDL preferentially transport *RRR*-α-tocopherol into the plasma, where mechanisms of lipoprotein metabolism result in the transfer of α-tocopherol to the other lipoproteins.

1. Introduction

Vitamin E occurs in nature in 8 different forms: α–, β–, γ–, δ–tocopherols, which have a phytyl tail and differ in the number and position of methyl groups on the chromanol ring, and α–, β–, γ–, δ–tocotrienols, which have unsaturated tails. Synthetic α-tocopherol, sold as vitamin E supplements, contains equal amounts of 8 different stereoisomers arising from the three chiral centers in the phytyl tail. All of these various forms of vitamin E differ in their degree of biological activity and antioxidant activity, but these activities are not directly correlated.

Tocopherols and tocotrienols are a lipid soluble, sterically hindered phenols, which react more rapidly with peroxyl radicals than do polyunsaturated fatty acids [1]. Thus, vitamin E is a chain breaking antioxidant, and α-tocopherol is the major lipid soluble antioxidant in the plasma [2, 3].

We have been studying the lipoprotein transport of vitamin E for several years because there are no other plasma tocopherol transport proteins. Using deuterated *RRR*-α-tocopherol we demonstrated that α-tocopherol is transported form the intestine in chylomicrons, then it is secreted in VLDL (very low density lipoproteins) and the label ultimately resides in LDL and HDL (low and high density lipoproteins, respectively) [4]. Tocopherols can be transferred to tissues by

A. L. Catapano et al. (eds.), Drugs Affecting Lipid Metabolism, 169–174.
© 1993 *Kluwer Academic Publishers and Fondazione Giovanni Lorenzini.*

lipoprotein lipase during the hydrolysis of triglyceride in chylomicrons and VLDL [5], and by the uptake of LDL vita the LDL receptor mechanism [6].

Investigations of the discrimination between forms of vitamin E, have suggested that the liver is the source of this discrimination [7-10]. This was demonstrated directly by examining the deuterated tocopherol contents of lipoproteins secreted from perfused livers of monkeys fed a combination of tocopherols labeled with differing amounts of deuterium 24 h prior to sacrifice [11]. These studies demonstrated that the liver preferentially secretes RRR-α-tocopherol in nascent VLDL.

2. Discrimination between forms of vitamin E in humans

2.1 STUDIES IN PATIENTS WITH GENETIC ABNORMALITIES OF LIPOPROTEIN METABOLISM

We have studied the absorption and transport of d_6-RRR-α-tocopherol, d_3-SRR-α-tocopherol and d_2-γ-tocopherol in normal subjects and patients with genetic abnormalities of lipoprotein metabolism [10]. These studies demonstrate that when the plasma contains chylomicrons, it also contains tocopherols in similar proportions to those administered (**FIGURE 1**). This is true in normal subjects up to 9 h post-dosing, or for more prolonged periods in patients who lack lipoprotein lipase, or in patients who have an impaired secretion of lipoproteins containing (apolipoprotein B-100 (not shown).

FIGURE 1. Subjects (4) were given an oral dose containing 50 mg each of d_6-RRR-α-tocopheryl acetate, d_3-SRR-α-tocopheryl acetate, and d_2-RRR-γ-tocopherol, then blood samples were obtained at the indicated intervals. The mean ± SEM of the deuterated tocopherol concentrations (nmol/mL) are shown at each time point in plasma, RBC, chylomicrons, VLDL (d<1.006 g/ml), LDL (1.006<d<1.063) and HDL (d>1.063). ©J. Lipid Res.[10].

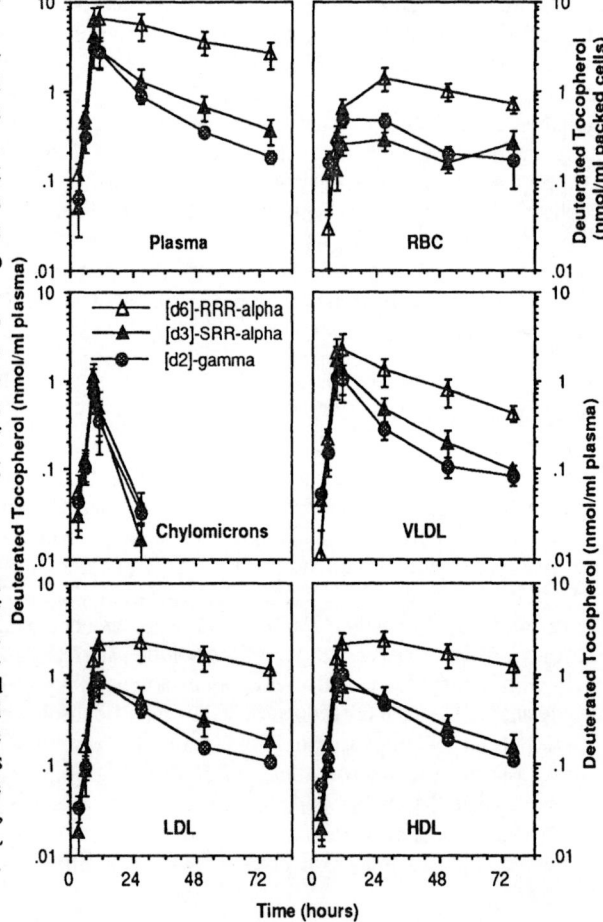

By 24 h the plasma is preferentially enriched in *RRR*-α-tocopherol in normal subjects resulting from the preferential secretion of *RRR*-α-tocopherol in nascent VLDL. (FIGURE 1) and in patients who secrete VLDL albeit with abnormal apolipoprotein B-100 (data not shown).

2.2 TOCOPHEROL BINDING PROTEIN

The studies on discrimination between forms of vitamin E suggest that there is a mechanism in the liver for the preferential enrichment of nascent VLDL with *RRR*-α-tocopherol. A putative mechanism involves an hepatic tocopherol binding protein, which could transfer α -tocopherol from lysosomes to the endoplasmic reticulum where nascent VLDL is assembled.

A tocopherol binding protein has been purified from rat liver [12, 13]. This protein discriminates between tocopherols, preferring to transfer *RRR*-α-tocopherol from liposomes to microsomes in vitro [12]. Extensive investigation of the tissue distribution of this protein has demonstrated that the protein is only found in the hepatocytes of rat liver; it has not been detected using a monoclonal antibody in any other tissues [13]. Furthermore, the protein does not appear to metabolize tocopherol [13], only to transfer it [12].

2.3 PATIENTS WITH FAMILIAL ISOLATED VITAMIN E DEFICIENCY

There is a human genetic abnormality which appears to result from a defect or absence of the tocopherol binding protein. Familial isolated vitamin E deficiency (FIVE deficiency) has been described in 11 patients world-wide [14-24]. Characteristically the patients have nearly undetectable plasma vitamin E levels when consuming a normal diet. They do not have lipid malabsorption syndromes; their gastrointestinal function and lipoprotein metabolism are normal. When given vitamin E supplements (400-1200 IU/day) the patients have normal plasma α-tocopherol concentrations, but upon cessation of the supplements the plasma concentrations decrease dramatically within days to deficient levels (<2 nmol/ml).

The patients do have neurologic abnormalities characteristic of vitamin E deficiency. That is, a peripheral neuropathy caused by the dying back of large calibre axons. All have decreased vibration sense; in some the abnormalities have progressed to the point of areflexia and ataxia. Supplemental vitamin E does halt the progression of the neurologic disorder and in some patients amelioration of symptoms have been reported.

This disorder is not the result of impaired absorption of vitamin E, as shown using large oral doses (100 mg/kg) of unlabeled *all rac*- α-tocopheryl acetate [22], or using small doses (15 mg) of deuterium labeled *RRR*-α-tocopheryl acetate [24]. In this latter study, we observed that incorporation of *RRR*-α-tocopherol into VLDL by the patients was impaired. Further, this impaired secretion in VLDL led to a more rapid disappearance of *RRR*-α-tocopherol from the plasma. It is, thus, likely that the patients lack or have a defective form of the tocopherol binding protein.

Because we have suggested that this protein is necessary for the discrimination between tocopherols, we are in the process of testing FIVE patients to determine whether they can discriminate between tocopherols. Our preliminary observations suggest that there are patients who can and those who cannot discriminate between the natural *RRR* and the synthetic *SRR*-forms of α-tocopherol [25]. d_3-*SRR*-α-tocopherol is not handled differently by patients and controls; in both the *SRR*- α-tocopherol decreases rapidly. Thus, the defect in the patients appears to be an impairment in their abilities to enhance secretion of *RRR*-α-tocopherol into nascent VLDL. Thus, patients who cannot discriminate are likely lacking a functional tocopherol binding protein.

3. Regulation of plasma α-tocopherol

The tocopherol binding protein appears to be critical for the regulation of plasma α-tocopherol. The studies in the FIVE patients suggest that in the apparent absence of the binding protein plasma α-tocopherol concentrations fall rapidly. Thus, the protein is necessary to maintain minimal levels of plasma α-tocopherol. During oral supplementation with large amounts of vitamin E in normal subjects, it has been observed that plasma α-tocopherol concentration increases only 2-3 fold [26-28]. Thus, excess α-tocopherol beyond what the protein can incorporate into VLDL does not increase plasma α-tocopherol. In a preliminary experiment we observed that oral supplementation with α-tocopherol and γ-tocopherol (300 mg of each) to a patient with an indwelling t-tube following gall bladder surgery resulted in an increase in the excretion of both in bile with a simultaneous increase in α-tocopherol in the plasma [8].

Taken together our studies on the absorption, transport and discrimination between forms of vitamin E all lend support to the following concepts: 1) that plasma α-tocopherol levels are regulated, 2) that this regulation is dependent upon the preferential incorporation of *RRR*-α-tocopherol in nascent VLDL by hepatocytes (**FIGURE 2**), 3) that the hepatic tocopherol binding protein is necessary and sufficient to carry out this intrahepatic transfer function, 4) that the lack of this protein results in vitamin E deficiency due to the rapid excretion of vitamin E in bile, and 5) that supplemental vitamin E does not markedly increase plasma α-tocopherol levels beyond 2 to 3 fold because of the limitation of incorporation of α-tocopherol into VLDL by the tocopherol binding protein. Verification of these hypotheses awaits the purification and characterization of the human tocopherol binding protein and the characterization of the precise genetic defects in the FIVE patients.

Regulation of Hepatocyte Vitamin E

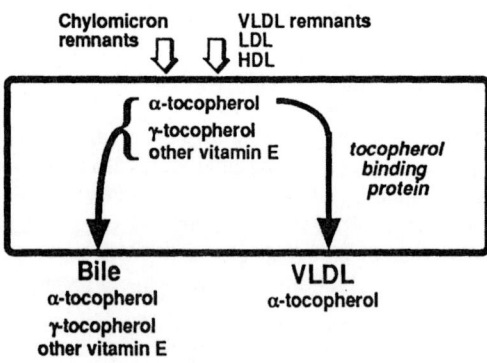

FIGURE 2. Hypothetical mechanism for the regulation of plasma vitamin E by the hepatic tocopherol binding protein. Dietary vitamin E enters hepatocytes in chylomicron remnants. Here the tocopherol binding protein preferentially transfers *RRR*-α-tocopherol to nascent VLDL, perhaps transferring it from lysosomes to the endoplasmic reticulum. Excess α-tocopherol and other forms of vitamin E are excreted in the bile. The nascent VLDL are secreted into the plasma where they are catabolized--a process that results in the preferential enrichment of LDL and HDL with α-tocopherol. Vitamin E is returned to the liver during the course of lipoprotein metabolism. Thus, plasma concentrations of α-tocopherol are regulated by the secretion of α-tocopherol in VLDL, which is regulated by the hepatic tocopherol binding protein.

4. References

1. Burton, G.W. and Ingold, K.U., (1986) 'Vitamin E: applications of the principles of physical organic chemistry to the exploration of its structure and function', Accounts Chem. Res. 19, 194-201.
2. Ingold, K.U., Webb, A.C., Witter, D., et al. (1987) 'Vitamin E remains the major lipid-soluble, chain-breaking antioxidant in human plasma even in individuals suffering severe vitamin E deficiency', Arch. Biochem. Biophys. 259, 224-225.
3. Burton, G.W., Hughes, L. and Ingold, K.U. (1983) 'Antioxidant activity of phenols related to vitamin E. Are there chain-breaking antioxidants better than α-tocopherol?', J. Amer. Chem. Soc. 105, 5950-5951.
4. Traber, M.G., Ingold, K.U., Burton, G.W. and Kayden, H.J. (1988) 'Absorption and transport of deuterium-substituted $2R,4'R,8'R$- α-tocopherol in human lipoproteins', Lipids 23, 791-797.
5. Traber, M.G., Olivecrona, T. and Kayden, H.J. (1985) 'Bovine milk lipoprotein lipase transfers tocopherol to human fibroblasts during triglyceride hydrolysis in vitro', J. Clin. Invest. 75, 1729-1734.
6. Traber, M.G. and Kayden, H.J. (1984) 'Vitamin E is delivered to cells via the high affinity receptor for low density lipoprotein', Am. J. Clin. Nutr. 40, 747-751.
7. Ingold, K.U., Burton, G.W., Foster, D.O., et al. (1987) 'Biokinetics of and discrimination between dietary *RRR*- and *SRR*-α-tocopherols in the male rat', Lipids 22, 163-172.
8. Traber, M.G. and Kayden, H.J. (1989) 'Preferential incorporation of α-tocopherol vs γ-tocopherol in human lipoproteins', Am. J. Clin. Nutr. 49, 517-526.
9. Traber, M.G., Burton, G.W., Ingold, K.U. and Kayden, H.J. (1990) '*RRR*- and *SRR*-α-tocopherols are secreted without discrimination in human chylomicrons, but *RRR*-α-tocopherol is preferentially secreted in very low density lipoproteins', J. Lipid Res. 31, 675-685.
10. Traber, M.G., Burton, G.W., Hughes, L., et al. (1992 In Press) 'Discrimination between forms of vitamin E by humans with and without genetic abnormalities of lipoprotein metabolism', J. Lipid Res.
11. Traber, M.G., Rudel, L.L., Burton, G.W., et al. (1990) 'Nascent VLDL from liver perfusions of cynomolgus monkeys are preferentially enriched in *RRR*- compared with *SRR*-α tocopherol. Studies using deuterated tocopherols', J. Lipid Res. 31, 687-694.
12. Sato, Y., Hagiwara, K., Arai, H. and Inoue, K. (1991) 'Purification and characterization of the α-tocopherol transfer protein from rat liver', FEBS Letters 288, 41-45.
13. Yoshida, H., Yusin, M., Ren, I., et al. (1992) 'Identification, purification and immunochemical characterization of a tocopherol-binding protein in rat liver cytosol', J. Lipid Res. 33, 343-350.
14. Burck, U., Goebel, H.H., Kuhlendahl, H.D., et al. (1981) 'Neuromyopathy and vitamin E deficiency in man', Neuropediatrics 12, 267-278.
15. Laplante, P., Vanasse, M., Michaud, J., et al. (1984) 'A progressive neurological syndrome associated with an isolated vitamin E deficiency', Can. J. Neurol. Sci. 11, 561-564.
16. Harding, A.E., Matthews, S., Jones, S., et al. (1985) 'Spinocerebellar degeneration associated with a selective defect of vitamin E absorption', N. Engl. J. Med. 313, 32-35.
17. Krendel, D.A., Gilchrest, J.M., Johnson, A.O. and Bossen, E.H. (1987) 'Isolated deficiency of vitamin E with progressive neurologic deterioration', Neurology 37, 538-540.

18. Stumpf, D.A., Sokol, R., Bettis, D., et al. (1987) 'Freidreich's disease: V. Variant form with vitamin E deficiency and normal fat absorption', Neurology 37, 68-74.
19. Yokota, T., Wada, Y., Furukawa, T., et al. (1987) 'Adult-onset spinocerebellar syndrome with idiopathic vitamin E deficiency', Ann. Neurol 22, 84-87.
20. Traber, M.G., Sokol, R.J., Ringel, S.P., et al. (1987) 'Lack of tocopherol in peripheral nerves of vitamin E-deficient patients with peripheral neuropathy', N. Engl. J. Med. 317, 262-265.
21. Kohlschütter, A., Hubner, C., Jansen, W. and Lindner, S.G. (1988) 'A treatable familial neuromyopathy with vitamin E deficiency, normal absorption, and evidence of increased consumption of vitamin E', J. Inher. Metab. Dis. 11, 149-152.
22. Sokol, R.J., Kayden, H.J., Bettis, D.B., et al. (1988) 'Isolated vitamin E deficiency in the absence of fat malabsorption - familial and sporadic cases: Characterization and investigation of causes', J. Lab. Clin. Med. 111, 548-559.
23. Trabert, W., Stober, T., Mielke, V., et al. (1989) 'Isolierter Vitamin-E-Mangel', Fortschr. Neurol. Psychiat. 57, 495-501.
24. Traber, M.G., Sokol, R.J., Burton, G.W., et al. (1990) 'Impaired ability of patients with familial isolated vitamin E deficiency to incorporate α-tocopherol into lipoproteins secreted by the liver', J. Clin. Invest. 85, 397-407.
25. Traber, M.G., Sokol, R.J., Burton, G.W., et al. (1991) 'Further evidence for the impaired function of a hepatic α-tocopherol binding protein in patients with familial isolated vitamin E deficiency', Arterio. Thromb. 11, 1610a.
26. Dieber-Rotheneder, M., Ruhl, H., Waig, G., et al. (1991) 'Effect of oral supplementation with d-α-tocopherol on the vitamin E content of human low density lipoproteins and resistance to oxidation', J. Lipid Res. 32, 1325-1332.
27. Dimitrov, M.V., Meyer, C., Gilliland, D., et al. (1991) 'Plasma tocopherol concentrations in response to supplemental vitamin E', Am J Clin Nutr 53, 723-729.
28. Farrell, P. and Bieri, J.G. (1975) 'Megavitamin E supplementation in man', Am J. Clin. Nutr. 28, 1381-1386.

ROLE OF THE MACROPHAGE SCAVENGER RECEPTOR IN THE 9-HYDROXY-OCTADECADIENOIC ACID MEDIATED EXPRESSION OF INTERLEUKIN 1β

G. KU, C.E. THOMAS AND R.L. JACKSON

ABSTRACT. Interleukin 1β (IL-1β) is a macrophage-derived cytokine that has been implicated as playing a central role in the pathogenesis of atherosclerosis. In this report, we show that macrophage-oxidized LDL (M-LDL), minimally-modified LDL (MM-LDL) and Cu^{2+}-oxidized LDL (Cu^{2+}-LDL) induced IL-1β in human peripheral blood monocyte-derived macrophages. One agent present in these oxidized LDL that mediates this induction is 9-hydroxyoctadecadienoic acid (9-HODE), an oxidation product of linoleic acid. 2,4-Decadienal and 2-octenal which are derived from linoleate and are found in extensively oxidized LDL also induced IL-1β. Acetylated LDL (ALDL) did not induce IL-1β. However, in the presence of 9-HODE, ALDL significantly enhanced 9-HODE-induced IL-1β release. A role for the scavenger receptor in the presentation of 9-HODE to macrophages is consistent with the finding that minimally-modified ALDL (MM-ALDL) were more potent than MM-LDL in inducing IL-1β. However, the scavenger receptor may be involved in the down-regulation of the IL-1β response since pretreatment of macrophages with ALDL inhibited the subsequent 9-HODE effect. Lipid-loaded macrophages became refractory to the IL-1β inductive effect of 9-HODE, implying that foam cell formation may be a protective mechanism whereby the release of the growth promoting cytokine IL-1β by 9-HODE is down-regulated. This putative negative regulatory mechanism for oxidized LDL-mediated IL-1β induction is ineffective against lipopolysaccharide (LPS)-induced IL-1β release. In this regard, ALDL pretreatment enhanced LPS-induced IL-1β release, consistent with the ex vivo finding that LPS-stimulated aortae from cholesterol-fed rabbits had higher cellular content of IL-1 than aortae from control rabbits.

A. L. Catapano et al. (eds.), Drugs Affecting Lipid Metabolism, 175–181.
© 1993 Kluwer Academic Publishers and Fondazione Giovanni Lorenzini.

1. Introduction

Many hypotheses have been proposed to explain the pathogenesis of atherosclerosis. Some of these include the "response-to-injury hypothesis" [1], the "lipid peroxidation hypothesis" [2,3], the "LDL oxidative modification hypothesis" [4], the "antioxidant hypothesis" [5] and recently [6-8] we have proposed a "cytokine hypothesis" that attempts to unify the other hypotheses into a single one and places IL-1β at the center of the atherosclerotic process. As IL-1β has been shown to induce smooth muscle cell proliferation [9-11] and its mRNA levels are increased in atherosclerotic tissue [12,13], we reasoned that lipid oxidation products present in oxidized LDL may stimulate the expression and/or the secretion of IL-1β. In this regard, we recently demonstrated that 9-HODE stimulates IL-1β release from human macrophages [14]. In the present report, we have extended these studies and have shown that pretreatment of macrophages in vitro with ALDL inhibits the 9-HODE induced release of IL-1β, suggesting a protective mechanism whereby foam cell formation down-regulates the induction of the growth promoting cytokine, IL-1β.

2. Materials and Methods

Human peripheral blood mononuclear cells were isolated with Leucoprep tubes (Becton Dickinson). Monocyte-derived macrophages were enriched by plastic adherence (3×10^6 mononuclear cells per well of 24-well plate for 1 h at 37°C), after which fresh medium RPMI-1640 was added to adherent cells. To prepare acetylated LDL (ALDL), human plasma-derived LDL (d=1.019-1.063 g/ml) were treated with sodium acetate and anhydrous acetic acid according to the method of Fraenkel-Conrat [15], dialyzed, and detoxified through a pre-packed endotoxin affinity column (Pierce). The detoxified ALDL tested negative for the induction of IL-1β and tumor necrosis factor alpha release (ELISAs from Cistron). Cu^{2+}-LDL and M-LDL were prepared as described previously [14]. MM-LDL and MM-ALDL were prepared by incubating LDL or ALDL with 6 μM $CuSO_4$ for 13 min. Oxidation was stopped by the addition of 18 μM EDTA. 9- and 13-HODE were obtained from Cayman Chemical, 1-octanal, 2-octenal and 2,4-decadienal from Aldrich and 2-hexenal and 1-decanal from Sigma. LPS was from Salmonella typhimurium Re mutant (Ribi Immunochem.).

To test the effect of cholesterol diet on rabbit IL-1α induction, female New Zealand albino rabbits (1 kg weight) were individually caged and fed with 100 g standard chow (Purina) or supplemented with 1% cholesterol per day for 10 wk, after which the thoracic aortae were aseptically removed and cultured in 35 mm tissue culture dishes with medium RPMI-1640 or 200 ng/ml LPS for 24 h. Secreted (from culture supernatants) and cell-associated (from homogenized aortae) IL-1α were measured with a RIA (Cytokine Sci.).

3.   Results

3.1. EFFECTS OF MODIFIED LDL AND OXIDIZED LIPIDS ON IL-1β EXPRESSION

The data shown in Table 1 demonstrate that LDL modified by either Cu^{2+} oxidation or incubation with human macrophages markedly induced the release of IL-1β from human monocyte derived macrophages, whereas native LDL and ALDL were without effect.

TABLE 1.   Induction of IL-1β release from human macrophages by modified LDL and linoleic acid oxidation products

Addition	Concentration	pg IL-1β/10^6 cells
None	–	14 ± 1
LDL	300 µg/ml	22 ± 2
Cu^{2+}-LDL	300 µg/ml	140 ± 3
M-LDL	300 µg/ml	110 ± 2
ALDL	300 µg/ml	14 ± 1
MM-LDL	300 µg/ml	34 ± 5
MM-ALDL	300 µg/ml	115 ± 16
9-HODE	33 µM	60 ± 1
13-HODE	33 µM	19 ± 4
9-HODE	10 µM	10 ± 1
9-HODE + ALDL	10 µM + 100 µg/ml	108 ± 10
2,4-decadienal	100 µM	160 ± 5
1-decanal	100 µM	4 ± 3
2-octenal	100 µM	53 ± 3
1-octanal	100 µM	2 ± 1
2-hexenal	100 µM	9 ± 5

While ALDL was ineffective, MM-ALDL caused an 8-fold increase in IL-1β release. Consistent with our previous report [14], 33 µM 9-HODE induced a IL-1β release; whereas, 13-HODE, a 15-lipoxygenase mediated product of linoleic acid, was 3 times less active. Hydroperoxy fatty acids can be cleaved to yield a variety of other products, including α,β-unsaturated aldehydes. Table 1 shows that 2,4-decadienal and, to a lesser extent, 2-octenal, induced IL-1β release. The results shown for these aldehydes were obtained after incubation of macrophages for only 5 min. The reason for the short incubation time is that α,β-unsaturated aldehydes are extremely reactive in promoting Michael addition and, therefore, prolonged exposure of macropages to these aldehydes could lead to permanent protein adducts and cytoxicity.

3.2. ROLE OF THE MACROPHAGE SCAVENGER RECEPTOR IN IL-1β INDUCTION

In the next experiment, macrophages were first pre-incubated with ALDL
for 6 h, the lipoprotein removed and then 9-HODE added. With these
experimental conditions, the cells were clearly loaded with lipid as
evidenced by phase microscopy. Subsequent addition of 9-HODE was
associated with a 30% diminished release of IL-1β relative to the
untreated cells (Figure 1).

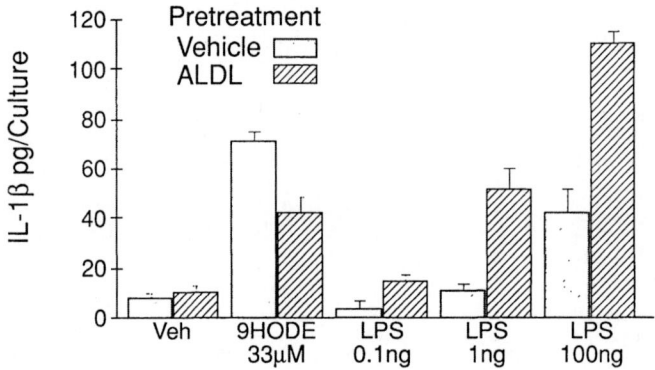

Figure 1. ALDL-pretreatment suppresses 9-HODE- but enhances LPS-
induced IL-1β release. Cultures of human peripheral blood monocyte-
derived macrophages (3x10⁶) in 24-multiwell plates were incubated with
medium RPMI-1640 (vehicle, open bar) or 200 μg/ml ALDL (filled bar)
for 6 h, washed and then 9-HODE (33 μM) or 0.1, 1 and 100 ng/ml LPS
were added for another 24 h. Secreted IL-1β was measured with an
IL-1β ELISA. Data are mean ± SEM of quadruplicate cultures.

LPS is a potent stimulant for the induction of IL-1β. As is shown in Figure 1, pretreatment of macrophages with ALDL further enhanced the LPS effect some 2-4 fold.

3.3. EFFECTS OF CHOLESTEROL-FEEDING ON RABBIT AORTIC IL-1α LEVELS

Since foam cell formation is the hallmark of atherosclerosis in cholesterol-fed rabbits, we next quantitated aortic IL-1α levels ex vivo in the presence and absence of LPS. In this experiment, rabbits were fed normal chow or chow supplemented with 1% cholesterol for 10 wk. Then, the animals were sacrificed and the thoracic aortae were removed; >60% of the aortae was covered with lipid filled lesions.

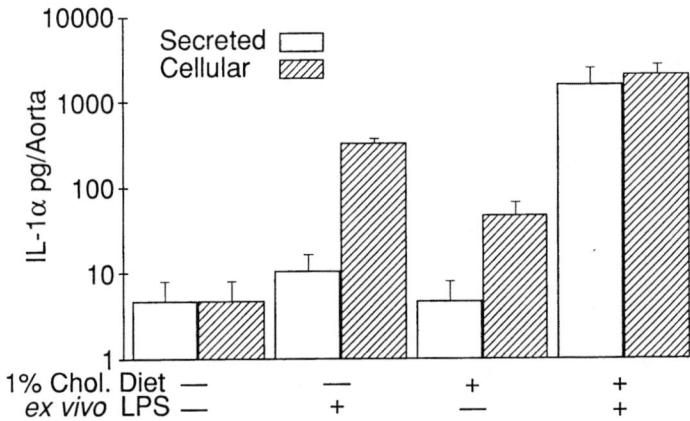

Figure 2. Enhancement of cholesterol diet-induced rabbit aortic IL-1α production by LPS. Thoracic aortae were aseptically removed and cultured in medium RPMI-1640 in the presence or absence of 200 ng/ml LPS for 24 h. Secreted and cell-associated (from homogenized aortae) IL-1α were measured with an IL-1α RIA. Data are mean ± SEM of groups of 4 rabbits.

The aortae were divided lengthwise into equal segments and were incubated in the presence and absence of LPS. The data in Figure 2 show that cholesterol feeding caused an 8-fold increase in cellular IL-1α levels (8 vs 70 pg IL-1α per aorta). However, the secreted levels of IL-1α were not affected by cholesterol feeding. Consistent with recent reports by Libby and coworkers [16], LPS addition to aortae from vehicle-treated rabbits was associated with an approximately 100-fold increase in cellular IL-1α, but again no significant increase in the secreted form of the cytokine. Finally, when LPS was added to the aortae obtained from the cholesterol-fed rabbits, IL-1α levels were increased both in the cell and the medium (Figure 2).

4. Discussion

While there is much interest on the role of oxidatively modified lipoproteins in the pathogenesis of atherosclerosis, few reports have appeared as to the components in oxidized LDL that mediate the cellular changes associated with the disease. For reasons that have been reviewed elsewhere [6-8], we have postulated that the cytokine IL-1β plays an important role in atherosclerosis by enhancing the expression of cell adhesion receptors, monocyte chemotactic proteins and growth factors.

The present results indicate that oxidation products of linoleic acid markedly influence the synthesis and release of IL-1β from activated macrophages. While it is well known that racemic mixtures of 9-HODE and 13-HODE are present in atherosclerotic tissue [17], it is not known if these lipid oxidation products are responsible for IL-1β synthesis in vivo. It is of considerable interest that lipid loading of macrophages decreases the levels of IL-1β, a finding that suggests that the scavenger receptor mediated uptake of modified LDL plays a protective role.

Finally, LPS is one of the most potent stimulators of IL-1β. The data shown in Figure 2 suggest that LPS is even more potent when the macrophage are lipid loaded. This finding may have physiological consequences when a patient with atherosclerotic disease develops a bacterial infection.

5. References

1. Ross, R. (1986) 'The pathogenesis of atherosclerosis - an update', N. Engl. J. Med. 314, 488-500.
2. Yagi, K. (1984) 'Increased serum lipid peroxides initiate atherogenesis', BioEssays 1, 58-60.
3. Hennig, B. and Chow, C.K. (1988) 'Lipid peroxidation and endothelial cell injury: Implication in atherosclerosis', Free Rad. Biol. Med. 4, 99-106.

4. Steinberg, D., Parthasarathy, S., Carew, T.E., Khoo, J.C., and Witztum, J.L. (1989) 'Beyond cholesterol. Modification of low density lipoprotein that increases its atherogenicity', N. Engl. J. Med. 320, 915-924.

5. Gey, K.F., Puska, P., Jordan, P., and Moser, U.K. (1991) 'Inverse correlation between plasma vitamin E and mortality for ischemic heart disease in cross-cultural epidemiology', Am. J. Clin. Nutr. 53, 326S-334S.

6. Jackson, R.L., Ku, G., and Thomas, C.E. (1992) 'Antioxidants: A biological defense mechanism for the prevention of atherosclerosis', Medicinal Research Rev., In press.

7. Ku, G., Akeson, A.L., Mano, M., Thomas, C.E., and Jackson, R.L. (1991) 'Products of oxidized linoleate mediate the release of interleukin-1β from human macrophages', Trans. Assoc. Am. Physci. 104, 107-112.

8. Ku, G. and Jackson, R.L. (1992) 'The pathogenesis of atherosclerosis: A cytokine hypothesis', In 'Xenobiotic Induced Inflammation: Roles of Cytokines and Growth Factors', Academic Press.

9. Libby, P., Warner, S.J.C., Friedman, G.B. (1988) 'Interleukin 1: A mitogen for human vascular smooth muscle cells that induces the release of growth inhibitory prostanoids', J. Clin. Invest. 81, 487-498.

10. Ku, G., Doherty, N.S. Wolos, J. A., and Jackson, R.L. (1988) 'Inhibition by probucol of interleukin-1 secretion and its implication in atherosclerosis', Am. J. Cardiol. 62, 77B-81B.

11. Libby, P., Ordovas, J.M., Bitinyl, L.K., Auger, K.R., and Dinarello, C.A. (1986) 'Inducible interleukin-1 gene expression in human vascular smooth muscle cell', J. Clin. Invest. 78, 1432-1438.

12. Ross, R., Masuda, J., Raines, E.W., Gown, A.M., Katsuda, S., Sasahara, M., Malden, L.T., Masuko, H., and Sato, H. (1990) 'Localization of PDGF-B protein in macrophages in all phases of atherogenesis', Science 248, 1009-1012.

13. Wang, A.M., Doyle, M.V., and Mark, D.F. (1989) 'Quantitation of mRNA by the polymerase chain reaction', Proc. Natl. Acad. Sci. USA 86, 9717-9721.

14. Ku, G., Thomas, C.E., Akeson, A.L., and Jackson, R.L. (1992) 'Induction of interleukin 1 beta expression from human peripheral blood monocyte-derived macrophages by 9-hydroxyoctadecadienoic acid', J. Biol. Chem. In press.

15. Fraenkel-Conrat, H. (1957) 'Methods for investigating the essential groups for enzyme activity', Methods in Enzymol. 4, 247-269.

16. Clinton, S.K., Fleet, J.C., Loppnow, H., Solomon, R.N., Clark, B.D., Cannon, J.G., Shaw, A.R., Dinarello, C.A., and Libby, P. (1991) 'Interleukin-1 gene expression in rabbit vascular tissue in vivo', Am. J. Pathol. 138, 1005-1014.

17. Brooks, C.J.W., Harland, W.A., Steel, G. and Gilbert, J.D. (1970) 'Lipids of human atheroma: Isolation of hydroxyoctadecadienoic acids from advanced aortal lesions', Biochim. Biophys. Acta 202, 563-566.

OXIDATIVE DAMAGE TO CIRCULATING LDL

P. AVOGARO, G. CAZZOLATO, D.M. KRAMSCH, A. SEVANIAN, H.
HODIS   and G. BITTOLO BON

ABSTRACT. A minor, more electronegatively charged, sub-fraction (LDL⁻) was
isolated from plasma LDL by ion exchange HPLC and characterized as a mildly oxidized
LDL. In samples obtained from normal donors HPLC analysis of OPA derivatized
amino-acids, reverse phase HPLC of phospho-lipids and GC analysis of oxysterols was
performed in both normally charged LDL (nLDL) and LDL⁻. In LDL⁻ a significant
decrease of aspartic acid, histidine, threonine, isoleucine, leucine and lysine was found,
whereas serine, glycine and alanine increased. Among phospholipid classes there was a
decrease in phosphatidylcholine and an increase in lysophosphatidylcholine in LDL⁻ as
compared to nLDL; also the percentage content of phosphoinositol, phosphatidtlserine
and phosphatidylhetanolamine was increased in LDL⁻. Furthermore, a specific increase in
cholestan-3,5-diene-7-one and 7-β-hydroxycholesterol, along with an increase in total
oxysterols were found in LDL⁻. Some of the observed characteristics (reduction of
histidine and lysine residues, increase of lyso-phosphatidylcholine and presence of
oxysterols) have been previously reported in LDL oxidized by metal ions or by
endothelial cells cultures. These data support the hypothesis that the LDL⁻ subfraction
may originate from native LDL, through a mild oxidative process occurring "in vivo".

INTRODUCTION

Several lines of evidence suggest that oxidative modification of LDL may play an
important role in atherogenesis [1]. LDL can be oxidized in vitro by a variety of cultured
cells (endothelial cells, monocyte-macrophages, smooth muscle cells) [2-4] or following
incubation with transition metal ions such as Cu^{++} [5]. Recent studies have shown that
oxidative modifications of LDL also occur in vivo [6, 7]. It was assumed that this
modification occurs primarily in the intima, in microdomains sequestered from the many
plasma antioxidants [1]. There are, however, several indications that a modest degree of
oxidative modification of LDL occurs in the circulation [8-10], so that plasma LDL
might be "primed" for more rapid cell-mediated oxidative modifications [11]. By the use

A. L. Catapano et al. (eds.), Drugs Affecting Lipid Metabolism, 183–190.
© 1993 Kluwer Academic Publishers and Fondazione Giovanni Lorenzini.

of ion exchange chromatography, a more electronegative LDL subfraction (LDL⁻) has been isolated in human plasma, which displays many of the characteristics of an vivo oxidized LDL [12-14]. The present study was undertaken to determine whether LDL- has a different amino acid and phospholipid composition and an increased oxysterol content.

MATERIAL AND METHODS

Venous blood, drawn after a 14-hr fast from 8 normal donors, was collected in test tubes containing ethylendiamine tetraacetic acid (EDTA; 1 mg/ml). The blood was immediately centrifuged at 1500 x g. LDL (d = 1.020-1.063 g/ml) were separated through preparative ultracentrifugation from freshly drawn plasma, according to Havel et al. [15]. After separation, LDL were dialyzed 24 hr under N_2 stream at 4° C in the dark against a TRIS-HCl 0.01M, pH 7.2, containing EDTA (10 mM). LDL subfractions were separated by analytic IE-HRLC using a 700B Bio-Rad (Milano - Italy) liquid chromatographyc system equipped with a 7.8 x 50 mm MA-7Q column, according to Cazzolato et al. [13]. The effluent was monitored at 280 nm, and the areas of the obtained peaks were integrated by IBM based workstation. The method allows the separation of two LDL subfractions: the major one shows the usual chemico-physical and biological characteristics of a normal LDL (nLDL), the minor corresponds to the more electronegative LDL- subfraction [13,14]. For amino acid analysis, aliquots of delipidated LDL subfraction proteins were hydrolyzed at 110° C in HCL for 24 hr in evacuated sealed tubes. The hydrolysates were evaporated, washed in distilled water, evaporated again to dryness, derivatized with fluoroaldehyde reagent (OPA) and then analyzed by HPLC[16] utilizing a 700B Bio-Rad system equipped with a 4 x 150 Bio-Sil ODS.5S column. The effluent was monitored utilizing a Perkin-Elmer LS-5 fluorometer (ex 360, em 455 nm). The amino acid standards were obtained from Sigma (St. Louis, MO) and Pierce (Rockford, IL). For cholesterol oxides and phospholipid analysis lipids were extracted from normal LDL and LDL-, by CHCL3:MEOH (2:1) containing 0.01% BHT. The chloroform extract was applied onto "diol" solid-phase extraction columns. The cholesterol and cholesterol oxide fractions were eluted with toluene ethylacetate (3:2) and subjected to cold alkaline saponification. Following methylation of lipids with diazomethane, the residue upon evaporation was derivatized with N,O,- bis(trimethysilyl)trifluoroacetamide (BSTFA) to form the corresponding othotrimethysilyl (O-TMS) ethers, and analyzed by capillary gas chromatography [17]. All procedures were performed under nitrogen in subdued light in the presence of 0.01% BHT and 50 µM EDTA.

The fraction containing phospholipid was analyzed by reversed-phase HPLC, monitoring the effluent with a Beckman Diode Array detector.

	nLDL	LDL⁻	P
Asp	10.23 + .37	8.73 + .46	< .05
Glu	12.13 + .32	11.32 + .91	n.s.
Ser	8.20 + .24	12.01 + .78	< .005
His	2.66 + .26	1.30 + .25	< .01
Gly	6.02 + .58	13.50 + .98	< .001
Thr	6.34 + .16	4.13 + .45	< .005
Arg	4.34 + .16	4.30 + .25	n.s.
Ala	6.50 + .24	8.69 + .69	< .05
Tyr	3.35 + .21	2.90 + .21	n.s.
Met	1.59 + .14	1.41 + .11	n.s.
Val	6.19 + .13	5.71 + .29	n.s.
Phe	6.92 + .40	7.43 + .63	n.s.
Ile	6.72 + .15	4.23 + .26	< .001
Leu	11.71 + .36	8.37 + .32	< .001
Lys	7.23 + .28	4.08 + .49	< .001

Tab. 1: mean ($\pm$ SEM) amino acid composition of apoB from normally charged LDL (nLDL) and LDL⁻. All values are expressed as nmol of amino acid/100 nmol of total amino acids.

RESULTS

The amino acid composition of the delipidated protein from normally charged LDL (nLDL) and from LDL- are reported in tab. 1. The composition of nLDL apoB-100 is similar to that reported by Kane et al. [18]. LDL⁻ shows an increased content of serine, glycine and alanine, while the amount of aspartic acid, histidine, threonine, isoleucine, leucine and lysine are significantly reduced. In general, polar uncharged amino acids are increased and non polar aminoacids are decreased in LDL-. The main variations observed concern the increase in serine (+ 46%) and glycine (+ 126%) and the decrease of histidine (-51%) and lysine (- 43%). The reduction of histidine and lysine has been observed also in LDL oxidized by copper [19].

In both nLDL and LDL⁻ the oxysterol content is low. In LDL-, however, almost all the examined cholesterol oxides are increased, with more marked increase of 3,5-diene, 7-α- and 7-β-hydroxy-cholesterol and cholestane triol (Tab. 2).

	nLDL	LDL⁻
7-α-hydroxy	0.05	0.51
3,5-diene	0.26	1.39
7-β-hydroxi	0.02	0.41
5-β-epoxide	0.16	0.28
α-epoxide	0.38	0.50
cholestane triol	0.03	0.24
7-keto	0.15	0.15
25-hydroxy	0.04	0.19
total	1.09	3.67

Tab. 2: individual cholesterol oxides as a percent of the cholesterol content in human nLDL and LDL- (arithmetic mean of 3 duplicate samples).

The proportion of phosphatidylcholine (PC) in LDL⁻ is half that found in nLDL (82.9 ± 2.0 vs 44.3 ± 10.4 % of total phospholipids), whereas the lysophosphatidylcholine (LPC) content is significantly higher in LDL⁻ (7.3 ± 1.7 vs 12.1 ± 2.4 % of total phospholipida. The LPC/PC ratio is increased by 2.4 fold in LDL⁻. The values of the 234/202 wavelength ratios measured in individual phospholipids are significantly higher in PC and LPC of LDL⁻, thus indicating a greather conjugated diene content in these two phospholipids.

DISCUSSION

Oxidized LDLs display a number of effects which are not shared by native LDL. Some of these effects are noxious altering the expression of some growth factors and cytokines by endothelial cells and macrophages, together with inhibition of EDRF-NO, of prostacyclin synthesis and evoking the production of a monocyte-chemotactic protein [20-22]. It is unclear which are the primary determinants of these newly acquired properties of LDL; whether this is a function of damage to the protein component (apoB-100) through a derangement of its amino acidic composition or protein structure, an alteration of the phospholipid composition, or to an increased level in the content of oxysterols. Variations in phospholipids content during in vitro oxidation, by metal ions or cells, provokes an extensive conversion of lecithin to lisolecithin catalyzed by a phospholipase A2 activity reported by present in LDL apoB-100 [23]. Recently the damaging effect of lyso-lecithin been attributed to yet another mechanism: it was found that EC-modified LDL, but not native LDL, makes a precontracted artery refractory to the relaxing effect of acetilcholine [22]. Albumin treatment reduces the elevated content of lysolecithin and at the same time attenuates its inhibitory effect on endothelium-dependent relaxation [22]. Our observations with LDL⁻ demonstrate a marked dectrease of lecithin, coupled with an increase in lysolecithin. LDL oxidation produces numerous oxysterols, many of which are cytotoxic [24-27]. The cell uptake of oxysterols is greater when serum is present; moreover toxicity is greater for growing than for relatively quiescent cell [26-27]. Among oxysterols, cholestane-triol was the most toxic while the potencies of the epoxides and other oxysterols was less, buth nevertheless remarkable [25]. It should noted that oxysterols content in LDL⁻ is low, probably due to the limited degree of oxidation; the content of oxysterols in human LDL⁻ is, however, higher than in nLDL.

These data confirm of our previous experimental observations obtained with cynomolgus monkeys fed an atherogenic diet [28]. In cholesterol feed monkeys a increase in LDL⁻ was obtained versus controls, and most of the LDL-associated oxisterols was recorded in LDL⁻. Despite the derangement of apoB-100 and its fragmentation and/or aggregation, scanty information exists about its amino acid composition [19]. Only few amino acids undergo significant variations following oxidation by copper; in particular a reduced content of histidine (-52%) lysine (-15%) proline (-10%) methionine (-6%) has been shown, while aspartic acid is increased (+6%). Our analysis has confirmed previous data, in particular the reduction in relative content of lysine and histidine. The differences bethween our data and the data obtained in vitro are probably due to the difference of the modification process occurring in vivo. The observed significant variations could be determined to the presence of apoB aggregates in LDL⁻, or by different proteins wich are assimilated by LDL during its circulatory lifetime. In vitro experiments have shown in LDL modified by endothelial cells the presence of a protein probably: produced by endothelial cells itself [29]. The amino acid changes reflect damage induced by oxidation of apoB, with formation of new epitopes or alterations in epitopes involved in binding to the LDL-receptor. The structural modifications recorded in LDL⁻ are similar to most of modifications described in "in vitro" oxidized LDL. It is, therefore, probable that despite its small mass the circulating LDL⁻ may display some toxic and biological effects on endothelial cells a/or other cells of the arterial wall.

REFERENCES

1. Steinberg, D., Parthasarathy, S., Carew, T.E., Khoo, J.C., and Witztum, J.L. (1989) 'Beyond cholesterol: modifications of low density lipoprotein that increase its atherogenicity', N. Engl. J. Med. 320, 915-924.
2. Henriksen, T., Mahoney, E.M., and Steinberg, D. (1981) 'Enhanced macrophage degradation of low density lipoprotein previously incubated with cultured endothelial cells: recognition by receptors for acetylated low density lipoproteins', Proc. Natl. Acad. Sci. USA 78, 6499-6503.
3. Heinecke, J.W., Baker, L., Rosen, H., and Chait,A. (1986) 'Superoxide-mediated modification of low density lipoprotein by arterial smooth muscle cells', J. Clin. Invest. 77, 757-763.
4. Parthasarathy, S., Printz, D.J., Boyd, D., Joy, L., and Steinberg, D. (1986) 'Macrophage oxidation of low density lipoprotein generates a form recognized by the scavenger receptor', Arteriosclerosis 6, 505-510.

5. Heinecke, J.W., Rosen, H., and Chait, A. (1987) 'Iron and copper promote modification of low-density lipoprotein by human arterial smooth muscle cells in culture', J. Clin. Invest. 74, 1890-1984.

6. Palinsky, W., Rosenfeld, M.E., Yla-Herttula, S., Gurtner, G.C., Socher, S.S., Butler, S.W., Parthasarathy, S., Carew, T.E., Steinberg, D., and Witztum, J.L. (1989) 'Low-density lipoprotein undergoes oxidative modification in vivo', Proc. Natl. Acad. Sci. USA 86, 1372-1376.

7. Haberland, M., Fong, D., and Cheng, L. (1988), ' Malondialdehyde-altered proteins occurs in atheroma of Watanabe heritable hyperlipidemic rabbits', Science 241, 215-218.

8. Yagi, K. (1987) 'Lipid peroxides and human diseases' Chem. Phys. Lipids 45, 337-351.

9. Morel, D.W., and Chisolm, G.M. (1989) 'Antioxidant treatment of diabetic rats inhibits lipoprotein oxidation and cytotoxicity', J. Lipid Res. 30, 1827-1834.

10. Harats, D., Ben-Naim, M., Dabach, Y., Hollander, G., Havivi, E., Stein, O., and Stein, Y. (1990) 'Effect of vitamin C and E supplementation on susceptibility of plasma lipoproteins to peroxidation induced by acute smoking', Atherosclerosis 85, 47-54.

11. Witztum, J.L., and Steinberg, D., (1991) 'Role of oxidized low density lipoproteins in atherogenesis', J. Clin. Invest. 88, 1185-1192.

12. Avogaro, P., Bittolo-Bon, G., and Cazzolato, G., (1988) 'Presence of a modified low density lipoprotein in humans', Arteriosclerosis 8, 79-81.

13. Cazzolato, G., Avogaro, P., and Bittolo-Bon, G., (1991) ' Characterization of a more electronegatively charged LDL subfraction by ion exchange HPLC', Free Radical Biol. Med. 11, 247-253.

14. Avogaro, P., Cazzolato, G., and Bittolo-Bon, G., (1991) 'Some questions concerning a small, more electronegative LDL circulating in human plasma', Atherosclerosis 91, 163-171.

15. Havel R.J., Eder H.A., and Bragdon J.H., (1955) 'The distribution and chemical composition of ultracentrifugally separated lipoproteins in human serum', J. Clin. Invest. 34,1345-1351.

16. Jones B.N., and Gillifan J.P., (1983) 'O-Phtalaldialdehyde precolumn derivatization and reversed-phase HPLC of polypeptide hydrolysates and physiological fluids', J. Chromatography 266, 471-482.

17. Hodis H.N., Crawford D.W., ans Sevanian A., (1991) 'Cholesterol feeding increses plasma and aortic tissue cholesterol oxide levels in parallel: further evidence for the role of cholesterol oxidation in atherosclerosis', Atherosclerosis 89, 117-126.

18. Kane J.P., Hardman D.A., and Paulus H.P., (1980) 'Heterogeneneity of apolipoprotein B: isolation of a new species from human chylomicrons', Proc. Natl. Acad. Sci. USA 77, 2465-2469.

19. Fong L.G., Parthasarathy S., Witztum J.L., and Steinberg D., (1987) 'Nonenzymatic oxidative cleavage of peptide bonds in apoprotein B-100', J. Lipid Res. 28, 1466-1477.

20. Quinn M.T., Parthasarathy S., Fong L.G., and Steinberg D., (1987) 'Oxidatively modified low density lipoproteins: a potential role in recruitment and retention of monocyte/macrophages during atherogenesis', Proc. Natl. Acad. Sci. USA 84, 2995-2998.

21. Berliner J.A., Territo M.C., Sevanian A., Ramin S., Kim J.A., Esterson M., and Fogelman A.M., (1990) 'Minimally modified LDL stimulates monocyte endothelial interactions', J. Clin. Invest. 85, 1260-1266.

22. Kugiyama K. Kerns S.A., Morrisett J.D., Roberts R., and Henry P.D., (1990) 'Impairment of endothelium-dependent arterial relaxation by lisolecithin in modified low density lipoproteins', Nature 344, 160-162.

23. Parthasarathy S., and Barnett J., (1990) 'Phospholipase A2 activity of low density lipoprotein: evidence for an intrinsic phospholipase A2 activity of apolipoprotein B-100', Proc. Natl. Acad. Sci. Usa 87, 9741-9745.

24. Zhang H., Harkamal J.K.B., and Steinbrecher U.P. ,(1990) Effect of oxidatively modified LDL on cholesterol esterification in cultured macrophages', J. Lipid Res. 31, 1361-1369.

25. Peng S.K., Hu B., and Morin R.J., (1991) 'Angiotoxicity and atherogenicity of cholesterol oxides', J. Clin. Lab. Ana. 5, 144-152.

26. Sevanian A., Berliner J., and Patterson H., (1991) 'Uptake, metabolism and cytotoxicity of isolmeric cholesterol-5,6-epoxides in rabbit aortic endothelial cells', J Lipid Res. 32, 147-155.

27. Chisolm G.M., Kimberly C., and Penn M.S., (1992) 'Lipoprotein oxidation and lipoprotein-induced cell injury in diabetes', Diabetes 41 (Suppl. 2), 61-66.

28. Hodis H.N., Kramsh D.M., Sevanian A., Avogaro P., Bittolo-Bon G., Cazzolato G., Hwang G., and Peterson H. 'Biochemical and cytotoxic characteristics of an in vivo circulating oxidized low density lipoprotein (LDL-)', in the press.

29. Van Hinsberg V.H.M., Sheffer M., Haveks L., Kempen H.J.R. (1986) 'Role of endothelial cells in the modification of low density lipoproteins', Biochim. Biophys. Acta 878, 49-64.

DIETARY ADVICE FOR THE PREVENTION OF ARTERIAL THROMBOSIS

Mario Mancini, Angela Rivellese and Giovanni Di Minno

ABSTRACT. Epidemiological, clinical and experimental studies support the concept that a high dietary intake of saturated fatty acids and cholesterol is associated with a high occurrence of thrombotic complications of atherosclerosis. On the other hand, when unsaturated fatty acids, expecially N-3 fats from marine sources, are substituted for saturated fats in the diet, the occurrence of thrombosis is greatly reduced. The mechanisms through which these unsaturated fats lower the occurrence of thrombotic episodes are still unclear. However, several clinical reports show that, in addition to a lowering effect on plasma lipids, these fats also affect major functions of hemostatically active cells such as platelets, monocytes and endothelial cells. The data available do not allow to estabilish the dose and/or the type of fish oil(s) that exert maximal antithrombotic effects. However the evidence available speaks in favor of the fact that a low intake of saturated fats and cholesterol, a higher intake of marine oils should be recommended to lower the occurrence of the thrombotic complications of atherosclerosis.

KEY WORDS: Diet, N-3, fatty acids, thrombosis prevention.

SATURATED FATS, ATHEROSCLEROSIS AND THROMBOSIS

In 1916, deLangen first reported a direct association between dietary intake of cholesterol and fats and incidence of atherosclerosis in humans.[1] In the following years, a series of clinical and epidemiological studies[2-5] confirmed the impact of dietary factors on blood lipids, and established a significant correlation between a prolonged intake of saturated fats and cholesterol and vascular mortality for thrombotic complications of atherosclerosis.[6-8] On the other hand, two major intervention studies[9-11] suggested that a decrease in serum cholesterol by long-term reduction of saturated fats and cholesterol in the diet was associated with a reduced cardiovascular mortality. Further support for the association between saturated dietary fats and thrombotic complications of atherosclerosis emerged from some studies in humans [12,13] showing a correlation between dietary fats and activation of the major thrombogenic mechanisms of platelets. This was also

191

A. L. Catapano et al. (eds.), Drugs Affecting Lipid Metabolism, 191–197.

confirmed by a series of experimental observations.[14-17] The combined
data were taken to suggest an association between a high intake of sa
turated fatty acids and cholesterol and arterial thrombosis.

UNSATURATED FATS, ATHEROSCLEROSIS AND THROMBOSIS

In the Seven Countries Study, cardiovascular mortality was negatively
related to the % consumption of monounsaturated fats such as olive
oil.[8]   Studies in Greenland Eskimos show that these subjects, whose
diet is particularly rich in N-3 fatty acids from marine sources, have
a lower than anticipated rate of myocardial infarction   (i.e. 3-5%,
that is 1/10-1/4 of that reported for Danes).[18,19] This was confirmed
in a Japanese population,[20] and suggested that unsaturated fatty acids
of the N-3 series might be beneficial. Such a concept also emerges
from the Zuptphen Study.[21] This is a retrospective study in which a
large group of men were followed for 20 yrs. It was concluded that a
daily intake of 30 g of fish produced almost a 50% reduction in overall mortality. This conclusion was further supported by the Western
Electric Study (Table I).[22]

TABLE 1. FISH CONSUMPTION AND 25-YEAR CHD MORTALITY.
         THE WESTERN ELECTRIC STUDY

FISH CONSUMPTION (g/day)	MEN AT RISK (n)	CAUSES OF DEATH (%)				
		CHD	OTHER CVD	MALIGNANT TUMORS	OTHER CAUSES	TOTAL DEATHS
0	205	20	7	6	7	40
1-17	686	19	6	10	4	39
18-34	779	16	4	10	5	35
>35	261	13	6	10	5	35
Total	1931	16	5	10	5	36
p value		<.0008	NS	NS	NS	<.05

(SHEKELLE et al. N.Engl.J.Med. 313, 820,1985)

Recently, a prospective clinical trial (DART) has been conducted in
the United Kingdom on 2,000 survivors of myocardial infarction. The
subjects enrolled were advised to increase the amount of fatty fish in
their diet or to consume 1g/d supplementations of N-3 fats.[23]   In the
2 yrs that followed the admission to the study, these subjects showed
a 29% decrease in overall mortality.
Platelets are thought to be a major target of N-3 fatty acids, and
these cells are likely to mediate vascular reocclusion following percutaneous coronary angioplasty.[24,25] Therefore, several studies were
carried out (Table II) to evaluate the effectiveness of this type of
unsaturated fats in the prevention of this reocclusion. Altogether,

the data[26-29] are inconclusive with respect to the question.

TABLE 2. N-3 AND PREVENTION OF VASCULAR OCCLUSION
AFTER CORONARY ANGIOPLASTY

AUTHOR	DOSE	RESTENOSIS RATE	ANGINA
SLACK 1987	1.8-2.7g	not determined	↓
DEHMER 1988	5.4g	16 vs 36% (p<0.02)	↓
GRIGG 1989	3.0g	29 vs 31% (NS)	↓
REIS 1989	6.0g	34 vs 23% (NS)	↓
MILNER 1989	4.5g	22 vs 35% (p<0.04)	↓

In addition to polyunsaturated fats, hemostatically active drugs
(e.g. aspirin) were employed in all cases. In all studies, a small
number of patients (<200) was enrolled. On the other hand, in some of
the studies[26,29] a suitable control (olive or corn oil) was omitted;
the dose and type of fish oil employed in each case was different; and
therapy was started 1 week prior to operation in one study and less
than 1 day in advance in others. Finally, in two cases, evaluation of
the restenosis rate was based on exercise tests rather than on angiography (see [31] and [32] for a review of this area).

UNSATURATED FATS: POTENTIAL ANTITHROMBOTIC MECHANISMS.
In vitro and in vivo studies suggest different mechanisms through
which N-3 fatty acids may produce their antithrombotic effect. A major
suggestion derives from the evidence that these substances affect pro-
staglandin and thromboxane synthesis as well as plasma levels of cholesterol and triglycerides. However, in the following years, it has
been documented that, in addition to a lowering effect on prostaglandins, LDL and VLDL-cholesterol, these fats also affect major functions
of hemostatically active cells such as platelets, monocytes and endothelial cells.

TABLE 3. N-3 FATTY ACIDS AND CVD: POSSIBLE INFLUENCES

PLASMA TRIGLYCERIDES	↓	Sanders, 1985
VLDL-CHOLESTEROL	↓	Nestel, 1984
LDL-CHOLESTEROL	↓	Subbaiah, 1989
HDL-CHOLESTEROL	↑	Sanders, 1986
PG AND TX SYNTHESIS (plts)	↓	Goodnight, 1990
VASCULAR PGI_2	↑	De Caterina, 1990
LTB_4 (neutr)	↓	Lee, 1984
LTB_4 (mono)	↓	Lokesh, 1988
EDRF RELEASE (arteries)	↑	Shimokawa, 1989
MEMBRANE FLUIDITY	↑	Terano, 1983
MONOCYTE ADHESION (EC)	↓	Kim, 1990
IL-1 AND TNF_α (mono)	↓	Enders, 1989
PDGF (EC)	↓	Fox, 1989
FGF (plts)	↓	Smith, 1989
PLASMA FIBRINOGEN	↓	Schmidt, 1990

These concepts, reviewed in [30-35] and summarized in Table III, are now under intensive investigation in several labs, and are likely to represent important directions to be followed to understand the antithrombotic potential of N-3 fatty acids.

CONCLUSIONS AND PERSPECTIVES

A high intake of saturated fatty acids is associated with a high occurrence of thrombotic complications of atherosclerosis. It is also clear that, at least in some clinical settings, when unsaturated fats - expecially N-3 fats from marine sources - are substituted for saturated fats in the diet, the occurrence of thrombotic events is reduced. The data presently available do not allow to estabilish the dose and/or the type of fish oil(s) that exert maximal antithrombotic effects. Likewise, although suggestive, there is only limited experience on the effectiveness of such an approach in some clinical conditions at high risk for thrombotic complications of atherosclerosis (Table IV). The evidence available, however, justifies that a low intake of saturated fats and cholesterol, a higher intake of marine oils may be recommended to lower the occurrence of thrombotic complications of atherosclerosis.

TABLE 4.   RECOMMENDATIONS

	SFA	MUFA	PUFA N-3	N-6
HYPERLIPIDEMIA	↓	↑	↑	↑
DIABETES	↓	↑	?	-
HYPERTENSION	↓	-	?	?
THROMBOSIS	↓	↑	↑	↑

REFERENCES

1. De Langen, C.D. (1916) 'Cholesterol exchange and pathology of race'. Presse Med. 24: 332-333.

2. Enholm, C., Huttunen, J.K., Pietinen, P., et Al. (1982) 'Effect of diet on serum lipoproteins in a population with a high risk of coronary heart disease'. N. Engl. J. Med. 307: 850-855.

3. Ferro-Luzzi, A., Strazzullo, P., Scaccini, C., et Al. (1984) 'Changing the Mediterranean diet: effects on blood lipids'. Am. J. Clin. Nutr. 40: 1027-1037.

4. Dougherty, R.M., Galli, C., Ferro-Luzzi, A. and Iacono, JM. (1987) 'Lipid and phospholipid fatty acid composition of plasma, red blood cells and platelets, and how they are affected by dietary lipids: a study of normal subjects from Italy, Finland and the USA'. Am. J. Clin. Nutr. 45: 443-455.

5. Olsson, A.G., Holmquist, L., Walldius, G. et al. (1988) 'Serum lipoproteins and fatty acids in relation to ischaemic heart disease in northen and southen european males'. Acta Med. Scand. 223: 3-13.

6. Keys, A. (1965) 'Dietary survey methods in studies on cardiovascular epidemiology'. Voeding 26: 464-482.

7. Kannel, W.B. and Castelli, W.A. (1979) 'Cholesterol in the prediction of atherosclerotic disease. New perspectives from the Framingham study'. Ann. Int. Med. 90: 85-92.

8. Keys, A., Menotti, A., Karvonen, M.J. et Al. (1986) 'The diet and 15-year mortality in the seven countries study'. Am. J. Epidemiol. 124: 903-915.

9. Hjermann, I., Byre, K.V., Holme, I. and Leren P. (1981) 'Effect of diet and smoking intervention on the incidence of coronary heart disease. Report From the Oslo Study Group of a randomized trial in healthy men'. Lancet 2: 1303-1310.

10. Multiple Risk Factor Intervention Trial Research Group. (1981) 'Multiple Risk Factor Intervention Trial'. JAMA 248: 1465-1477.

11. Hjermann, I., Holme, I. and Leren, P. (1986) 'Oslo Study Diet and anti-smoking Trial. Results after 102 months'. Am. J. Med. 80 (suppl 2A): 7-11.

12. Tremoli, E., Petroni, A., Socini, A. et Al. (1986) 'Dietary intervention in North Karelia, Finland, and South Italy. Modification of thromboxane B_2 formation in platelets of male subjects only'. Atherosclerosis 59: 101-111.

13. Renaud, S., Morazain, N., Godsey, F., et Al. (1986) 'Nutrients, platelet function and composition in nine groups of French and British farmers'. Atherosclerosis 60: 37-48.

14. MacIntyre, D.E., Hoover, R.L., Smith, M. et Al. (1984) 'Inhibition of platelet function by cis-unsaturated fatty acids'. Blood 63: 848-857.

15. Buchanan, M.R., Crozier, G.L., Haas T.A. (1988) 'Fatty acid metabolism and the vascular endothelial cell'. Haemostasis 18: 360-375

16. Ulbricht, T.L. and Southgate, D.A.T. (1991) 'Coronary heart disease: seven dietary factors'. Lancet 338: 985-992.

17. Nordoy, A. and Goodnight, S.H. Dietary lipids and thrombosis. (1990) 'Relationship to atherosclerosis'. Arteriosclerosis 10:149-163.

18. Djeberg, J., Bang, H.O., Stoffersen, H.O., Moncada, S. and Vane, J. (1978) 'Eicosapentaenoic acid and prevention of thrombosis and atherosclerosis'. Lancet 2: 117-119.

19. Djeberg, J. and Bang, H.O. (1979) 'Hemostatic function and platelet polyunsaturated fatty acids in Eskimos'. Lancet 2: 1128-1130.

20. Hirai, A., Terano, T., Saito, H., Tamura, Y. and Toshida, S. (1987) 'Clinical and epidemiological studies of eicosapentaenoic acid in Japan'. In: Proc AOCS short course on polyunsaturated fatty acids and eicosanoids. American Oil Chemists Society, Lands WEM Ed. 9-24.

21. Kromhout, D., Bosscheiter, E.D. and DeLezzenne Coulander, C. (1985) 'The inverse relation between fish consumption and 20 year mortality from coronary heart disease'. N Engl J Med 312:1205-9.

22. Shekelle, R.B., MacMillan Shryoc, A. et al. (1981) 'Diet, serum cholesterol and death from coronary heart disease (the Western Electric Study)'. N Engl J Med 304:65-70.

23. Burr, M.L., Fehiky, A.M., Gilbert, J.F., et al. (1989) 'Effects of changes in fat, fish and fibre intakes on death and myocardial infarction: diet and reinfarction trial (DART)'. Lancet II:757-61.

24. King, J.F., Manley, J.C. and al-Wathiqui, M.H. (1989) 'Restenosis after angioplasty: mechanisms and clinical experience'. Cardiol Clin 7:853-64.

25. Liu, M.W., Roubin, G.S. and King, S.B. (1989) 'Restenosis after angioplasty: potential biologic determinants and role of intimal hyperplasia'. Circulation 79:1374-87.

26. Dehemer, G.J., Pompa, J.J., van der Bergh. E.K., Eichorn, E.J., Prewitt, J.B., Campbell, W.B., Jennings, L., Willerson, J.T. and Schmitz, J.M. (1988) 'Reduction in the rate of early restenosis after coronary angioplasty by a diet supplemented with N-3 fatty acids'. N Engl J Med 319:733-740

27. Grigg, L.E., Kay, T.W.H., Valentine, P.A., et al. (1989) 'Determinants of restenosis and lack of effect of dietary supplementation with eicosapentanoic acid on the incidence of coronary artery restenosis after angioplasty'. J Am Coll Cardiol 13: 665-72.

28. Reis, G.J., Boucher, T.M., Sipperly, M.E., Silverman, D.J. et al. (1989) 'Randomized trial of fish oil for prevention of restenosis after coronary angioplasty'. Lancet II:177-81.

29. Milner, M.R., Gallino, R.A., Leffinwell, A., Descalzi Pichard, A., Brooks-Robinson, S., Rosenberg, J., Little, T. and Lindsay, J. (1989) 'Usefulness of fish oil supplements in preventing clinical evidence of restenosis after percutaneous transluminal coronary angioplasty'. Am J Cardiol 64:294-9.

30. Kinsella, J.E., Loresh, B. and Stone, R.A. (1990) 'Dietary N-3 polynsaturated fatty acids and amelioration of cardiovascular disease: possible mechanisms'. Am J Clin Nutr 52:1-28.

31. Goodnight SH. 1991 'Fish oil and vascular disease'. Trend Cardiovasc Med 1: 112-116.

32. Slack, J.D., Pinkerton, C.A., VanTassel, J., Orr, C.M., Scott, M., Allen, B. and Nasser, W.K. (1989) 'Can oral fish oil supplement minimize restenosis after percutaneous transluminal coronary angioplasty?' J Am Coll Cardiol 9:64A.

33. Dehemer, G.J. (1990) 'Another piece of the fish oil puzzle'. Circulation 82:624-8.

34. Leaf, A. (1990) 'Cardiovascular effects of the fish oils. Beyond the platelet'. Circulation 82:624-8.

35. Di Minno, G. and Mancini, M. (1992) 'Drugs affecting plasma fibrinogen levels'. Cardiovas. Drug Ther. 6: 25-27,

Drugs Affecting High-Density Lipoprotein and Triglyceride Metabolism

A. M. GOTTO, JR.

Both observational and interventional epidemiological data have established plasma level of high-density lipoprotein cholesterol (HDL-C) as a strong independent, inverse predictor of the development of coronary heart disease (CHD) [1,2]. The first major clinical trial to demonstrate a significant correlation between raising HDL-C level and lowering the incidence of CHD events was the 5-year, randomized, double-blind Helsinki Heart Study, which used diet plus gemfibrozil versus diet plus placebo in symptom-free dyslipidemic men [3]. It is also the Helsinki data set that has recently provided evidence that highest risk for CHD entails elevation of plasma triglyceride: reanalysis showed the highest risk (and greatest treatment benefit) among patients who had a low-density lipoprotein cholesterol (LDL-C) to HDL-C ratio of more than 5 and a triglyceride level of more than 200 mg/dl (2.3 mmol/L) [4]. Highest risk by a like stratification (total to HDL cholesterol ratio > 5, HDL-C < 35 mg/dl [0.91 mmol/L], triglyceride ≥ 200 mg/dl) was found in 4-year data from the observational Prospective Cardiovascular Münster (PROCAM) study [5]. However, the relation between plasma triglyceride level and CHD remains unclear; whether hypertriglyceridemia may be a causative factor or merely a marker for CHD is debated on both metabolic and epidemiological grounds [6].

The panel of the U.S. National Institutes of Health (NIH) Consensus Development Conference on Triglyceride, High Density Lipoprotein, and Coronary Heart Disease (February 1992) concluded that preclinical and clinical data support a causal role for low HDL-C levels in the development of CHD but do not allow the conclusion of comparable causality for triglyceride elevation in this disease [7]. The clinical assessment and treatment recommendations of the consensus panel define low HDL-C as values less than 35 mg/dl and borderline and distinct hypertriglyceridemia as values between 250 and 500 mg/dl (2.82–5.65 mmol/L) and greater than 500 mg/dl, respectively, as determined by repeat fasting samples [7].

Other bodies have recommended lower cutoff values for elevated triglyceride—e.g., the 200 mg/dl used by the International Committee for the Evaluation of Hypertriglyceridemia as a Vascular Risk Factor [8] and by the European Atherosclerosis Society [9]. The 1992 NIH consensus panel emphasizes that the first line and mainstay of therapy for low HDL-C and/or elevated triglyceride is hygienic measures—in chief, diet and weight control, exercise, and smoking cessation. The panel found no consensus for the use of drugs in isolated moderate triglyceride elevation or low HDL-C. It is the panel's recommendation that when HDL-C is low and triglyceride is between 250 and 500 mg/dl in the setting of a desirable LDL-C, drug therapy

A. L. Catapano et al. (eds.), Drugs Affecting Lipid Metabolism, 199–213.
© 1993 *Kluwer Academic Publishers and Fondazione Giovanni Lorenzini.*

may be considered when hygienic measures fail and CHD or a strong risk profile is present. When the plasma triglyceride level exceeds 500 mg/dl, drug therapy may be warranted to reduce the risk of pancreatitis if hygienic measures fail. Drug therapy may be considered as initial treatment in addition to hygienic intervention if triglyceride exceeds 500 mg/dl and a history of pancreatitis is present.

It should be noted that treatment recommendations by a consensus panel do not serve as official guidelines in the United States; treatment guidelines for dyslipidemia are issued by the National Cholesterol Education Program (NCEP), a program of the National Heart, Lung, and Blood Institute of the NIH. However, the adult guidelines last issued—in 1987 [10]—antedate many of the important new findings on HDL and triglyceride and are based chiefly on LDL-C level; thus, the 1992 consensus panel's recommendations represent an effort to extend the NCEP algorithm. Revised NCEP adult guidelines are scheduled for release in 1993.

None of the large-scale clinical trials reported to date was specifically designed to test either a hypothesis of raising HDL-C level or a hypothesis of lowering triglyceride level to decrease CHD risk, although a number of these trials have assessed these lipid levels throughout their study period. The correlations thus demonstrated—in particular, the strong correlation with HDL-C level—and the general success of lipid intervention in CHD risk provide rationale for treatment of low HDL-C and elevated triglyceride. The rationale for treating triglyceride elevation includes the view that some triglyceride-rich lipoproteins are atherogenic, notably very-low-density lipoprotein (VLDL) remnant and postprandial remnant lipoproteins, and the association of triglyceride elevation with a number of conditions predisposing to early atherosclerosis (e.g., the presence of small, dense LDL particles, extended postprandial lipemia).

Of the five classes of drugs approved in the United States for the treatment of hyperlipidemia, two are highly effective in reducing plasma triglyceride levels: nicotinic acid and the fibric-acid derivatives. Nicotinic acid and gemfibrozil also raise HDL-C levels substantially. The 3-hydroxy-3-methylglutaryl coenzyme A (HMG-CoA) reductase inhibitors have a modest effect on lowering triglyceride and raising HDL-C. The bile-acid sequestrants are neutral in effect on or may even increase triglyceride levels; they raise HDL-C levels by only about 2% to 3%. Probucol is reported to be neutral in effect on plasma triglyceride and lowers HDL-C by about 30%.

Nicotinic Acid

Nicotinic acid has favorable effects on all the major lipid fractions, typically reducing (at a dosage of 3–4 g/day) plasma triglyceride by about 30% to 40%, total cholesterol by 10% to 20%, and LDL-C by 20% or more, and increasing HDL-C by 15% to 30%. In the severe hypertriglyceridemia of type V hyperlipidemia, treatment with nicotinic acid has been reported to increase LDL-C and HDL-C, with a concomitant fall in VLDL-C. This effect occurred when the baseline LDL-C level was low. When its baseline level was high, the LDL-C concentration decreased even in the face of hypertriglyceridemia [11]. Increases in HDL-C may be especially marked in normotriglyceridemic individuals. The presumed cardiovascular benefit of the aggregate improvement in lipid profile and the drug's good safety record, low cost, and single-agent association in a major clinical trial with decreased all-cause mortality have made nicotinic acid a first-choice agent in the treatment of dyslipidemia. Unfortunately, the side effects of nicotinic acid are frequent; flushing is the most common adverse effect, but may be blunted with prophylactic aspirin. The use of the drug is limited in patients with diabetes mellitus, gout, or peptic ulcer disease because of its potential for exacerbating these conditions.

Reduction in all-cause mortality was seen in long-term follow-up of the Coronary Drug Project, which gave nicotinic acid, estrogen, dextrothyroxine, clofibrate, or placebo to men who had experienced at least one myocardial infarction. Mean time on trial for the nicotinic acid, clofibrate, and placebo groups was 6.2 years, at which time there was a significant decrease in nonfatal myocardial infarctions with nicotinic acid but no benefit with clofibrate [12]. (Estrogen and dextrothyroxine had been discontinued early because of increased side effects or mortality.) Mean decreases among the nicotinic acid recipients in total cholesterol and triglyceride were 10% and 26% for 5 years on trial. Mortality follow-up 9 years later showed a significant 11% lower all-cause mortality (versus placebo) for nicotinic acid recipients [13].

Diminished overall mortality was also reported from the nonblinded, 5-year Stockholm Ischemic Heart Disease Secondary Prevention Study, which used nicotinic acid not as a single agent but in combination with clofibrate to treat male and female myocardial infarction survivors. The drug regimen lowered triglyceride a mean 19%, and benefit was related to triglyceride concentration in two ways: it occurred only in patients with a triglyceride concentration above 130 mg/dl (1.5 mmol/L), and it was most pronounced among patients in whom triglyceride was lowered 30% or more [14]. CHD mortality in the latter subgroup was reduced 60%, and in the entire treatment group, cardiac and overall mortality rates were reduced 36% and 26%, all significant reductions.

In addition, nicotinic acid in combination regimens has been associated with coronary atherosclerotic lesion nonprogression or regression in several angiographically monitored trials. In the Cholesterol Lowering Atherosclerosis Study (CLAS) [15,16] and the Familial Atherosclerosis Treatment Study (FATS) [17], both conducted among men, it was given with colestipol, and in the University of California, San Francisco, Arteriosclerosis Specialized Center of Research (UCSF-SCOR) Intervention Trial, conducted among men and women with heterozygous familial hypercholesterolemia, it was given in various combinations with colestipol and/or lovastatin [18]. In CLAS, investigators in a 6-week prerandomization trial confirmed that each participant could tolerate the 30 g of colestipol and 3 to 12 g of nicotinic acid [15]. Also in CLAS, the best predictor of improved coronary artery status in the drug-treated group was apolipoprotein (apo) C-III content in HDL; the CLAS drug treatment made no major changes in total apo C-III levels but changed the lipoprotein fractions in which apo C-III was transported, increasing the fraction in HDL and decreasing the fraction in VLDL and LDL [19]. In FATS, LDL-C was reduced to a greater extent in the group receiving lovastatin plus colestipol than in the group receiving nicotinic acid plus colestipol (46% versus 32%, versus 11% for control), but HDL-C was markedly increased among nicotinic acid recipients in comparison with the other two study groups (43%, 15%, and 5%). A higher percentage of nicotinic acid recipients had regression as the only angiographic change (39% versus 32% for lovastatin and 11% for control), and increased HDL-C level was one of three factors that on multivariate analysis correlated independently with regression (the others being decreased apo B level and reduced systolic blood pressure) [17].

Despite more than 30 years' experience with nicotinic acid, its complete mechanism of action is not known [20–22]. One of its major actions is in adipose tissue, where it has an insulin-like antilipolytic effect, so that there is decreased triglyceride breakdown into unesterified fatty acids. The reduced flux of free fatty acids into the liver leads to reduced synthesis and secretion of VLDL. This sequence reduces plasma triglyceride level. One animal study [23] showed nicotinic acid to increase tissue lipoprotein lipase activity, which would also decrease plasma triglyceride.

The reduction in VLDL likely also accounts for the reduction in LDL, although some reports have indicated a direct suppression of cholesterol biosynthesis in the liver, where nicotinic acid may have other direct effects as well. The increase in HDL-C may derive from reduced catabolism of HDL [24]; results of a human study using the nicotinic acid derivative acipimox have suggested a mechanism of interference with hepatic lipase activity [25]. Interference with hepatic lipase would point to an increase in HDL_2, the major substrate of the enzyme. Indeed, Johansson and Carlson in a study of the effect of nicotinic acid on HDL subfractions in hyperlipidemic patients found significantly increased HDL_2, especially in the largest HDL_{2b}, and significantly decreased HDL_3 [26]. Wahlberg et al. found generation of HDL_2 during nicotinic acid treatment to correlate positively with amount of HDL_3 available at the beginning of therapy, regardless of type of hyperlipidemia [27]. However, other studies, such as one by Franceschini et al. using acipimox [28], have failed to show an increase in HDL_2. Consonant with an increased HDL_2 to HDL_3 ratio is the description of nicotinic acid as increasing apo A-I plasma concentration and decreasing apo A-II concentration through alteration of the turnover rate of the major apolipoproteins in HDL [24].

Nicotinic acid appears to be more clinically active than its derivatives. However, some of the derivatives, notably acipimox, have improved tolerability.

Fibric-Acid Derivatives

Like nicotinic acid, the fibric-acid derivatives substantially reduce plasma levels of triglyceride (by about 30–40%), increase those of HDL-C (by about 10–20%), and affect LDL-C depending on the type of hyperlipidemia being treated. In cases of pure and combined hypercholesterolemia, LDL-C is generally decreased by 5% to 20% (more in the pure form than the combined); in type IV hyperlipidemia, however, LDL levels are unchanged or even slightly raised by fibric-acid derivatives. Data from the Helsinki Heart Study suggest that both elevated risk of CHD and the treatment effect of gemfibrozil depend more on the level of HDL-C than on the level of LDL-C in men with elevated LDL-C and no evidence of CHD [4]. Fibric-acid derivatives are also indicated in type III hyperlipidemia. Fibrates reduce the proportion of triglyceride in LDL and HDL, increase that of cholesterol in these lipoproteins, and increase the cholesterol to apo B ratio in LDL [29]. Bezafibrate in hyperlipidemic and normolipidemic rats has been shown to reduce serum total cholesterol and triglyceride levels, and it increases the ratio of HDL to non-HDL cholesterol in hypercholesterolemic rats (reviewed in Monk and Todd [30]). The same pattern holds for normolipidemic nonhuman primates, in which most of the reduction in total cholesterol has been shown to come from lower LDL-C [30]. Gemfibrozil and clofibrate, the two fibric-acid derivatives approved for use in the United States, are respectively recommended at 1,200 and 2,000 mg daily in divided doses; bezafibrate and fenofibrate, which are commonly used in Europe, are administered at 600 and 300 mg daily, respectively, in divided doses.

The fibrates have caused hepatomegaly and sometimes hepatic tumors in rats when given at very high doses, but no such effects have been observed in primates. In fact, the fibric-acid derivatives only rarely confer even dose-limiting side effects. However, clofibrate use is rare in the United States because of the finding of increased all-cause mortality in a World Health Organization cooperative trial [31]. One major side effect of clofibrate in the WHO trial was gallstone formation [32]. It appears that all the commonly used fibric-acid derivatives have lithogenic potential, although this effect seems most severe in the case of clofibrate. The WHO data also indicated that some muscle fatigue resulted from clofibrate therapy, but this effect was not evaluated and similar muscular effects have not been reported for the other fibrates. Sirtori et al. speculate that because myalgia and muscle pain may arise from clofibrate side-chain interaction with the chloride-channel receptor, compounds with longer side chains (e.g., gemfibrozil) and those with additional rings (e.g., bezafibrate and fenofibrate) may have different or no actions there [32].

The fibrates derive from p-chlorophenoxyisobutyric acid (see Figure). The configuration of gemfibrozil has been proved vital to its effect on plasma triglyceride and HDL-C. Data obtained from Dr. Roger Newton of Parke-Davis Pharmaceutical Research Division show the structure–activity relationships of the methyl groups on the ring and side chain on HDL-C and triglyceride in rats. 3,4-Dimethyl substitution of the ring obliterated antitriglyceride activity; activity was also markedly reduced by 2,4-dimethyl substitution. However, gemfibrozil with dimethyl substitutions at the 2,3 and 3,5 positions reduced plasma triglyceride levels by about the same amount as the parent compound. (These data are also presented in Creger et al. [33].) Studies of effects of chain spacing on plasma lipid fractions in rats showed low specificity in effects on triglyceride but high specificity in effects on HDL-C. Antitriglyceride activity was abolished when one or zero carbon spacers were present, but plasma triglyceride was reduced by 38% when two were present and was reduced maximally (74–84%) when three to seven were present [33]. HDL-C in cholesterol-fed rats was increased, however, only when three carbon spacers were in place [34].

One of the fibric-acid derivatives' actions is thought to be through the activation of postheparin plasma lipoprotein lipase, which effects triglyceride hydrolysis and the formation of intermediate-density lipoprotein (IDL) and LDL particles [35]. This activity also may be the means by which HDL levels are increased. Fenofibrate at 300 mg/day given for 8 weeks to patients with severe CHD, some normocholesterolemic and some hypercholesterolemic, reduced postprandial lipemia by stimulating lipoprotein lipase activity 37% and consequently increasing chylomicron triglyceride lipolysis [36]. Through the reduction of chylomicron triglyceride levels, the cholesteryl ester transfer protein (CETP)–mediated exchange of HDL cholesteryl ester for chylomicron triglyceride may have been reduced. In addition, increased chylomicron lipolysis may have enhanced transfer of surface free cholesterol to HDL. In any case, plasma HDL-C was increased 10% with fenofibrate administration in this study [36]. Bezafibrate [37] and gemfibrozil [38] likewise activate lipoprotein lipase.

Fibric-acid derivatives affect lipoprotein structure and composition as well. In hypertriglyceridemia, the fraction of small, dense LDL is abnormally high. Eisenberg et al.

Gemfibrozil

Fenofibrate

Clofibrate

Bezafibrate

found that bezafibrate reversed the LDL size and density abnormalities associated with hypertriglyceridemia [39]; others have noted similar results with gemfibrozil [40,41] and fenofibrate [37]. Gavish et al. found the same effect of bezafibrate in type IIa hyperlipidemia [42]. Also in hypercholesterolemic patients, fenofibrate enhanced the fractional catabolic pathway of LDL by both receptor- and non-receptor-mediated pathways [37].

It is believed that fibrates confer clinical benefit, like nicotinic acid, by inhibiting the release of free fatty acids from adipose tissue, thus reducing the production of VLDL in the liver [29]. The benefits of reducing VLDL may be in part due to the consequent effect on apo E. A review and analysis by Grundy and Vega cited studies whose results suggest that the presence of apo E on triglyceride-rich lipoproteins may facilitate their binding to lipoprotein receptors on macrophages, promoting the formation of foam cells. These reviewers also theorized that apo E–rich VLDL in hypertriglyceridemia may be as atherogenic as LDL in hypercholesterolemia because the apo E has enhanced affinity for lipoprotein receptors on arterial walls [43].

It has also been reported that fibrates stimulate VLDL apo B catabolism in hypertriglyceridemia [35]. Shepherd et al., for example, found that bezafibrate reduced the mean residence time of VLDL apo B in plasma from 3.4 hours to 1.0 hour and increased the VLDL remnant apo B (S_f 12–100) plasma concentration by 30% in hypertriglyceridemic patients (type IV and type V hyperlipidemia) after 4 weeks of therapy [44]. Bezafibrate-induced decreases in plasma apo B in patients with types IIa and IIb hyperlipidemia were likewise significant [42]. Vega and Grundy found that, overall, gemfibrozil therapy did not significantly increase LDL apo B levels in their hypertriglyceridemic patients, but the apo B to cholesterol ratio in LDL and the fractional clearance of LDL apo B were significantly reduced [45]. An analysis by Shepherd et al. found that in hypertriglyceridemic patients fenofibrate and bezafibrate each decreased the triglyceride to apo B ratio in VLDL 73% and increased the LDL-C to LDL apo B ratio 22% [37].

HDL composition abnormalities in hypertriglyceridemia are much like those of the LDL particles: the particles are cholesteryl ester poor, have a low cholesteryl ester to protein ratio, and are smaller and denser than normal. Grundy and Vega have theorized that hypertriglyceridemia may accelerate the clearance of apo A-I from HDL, thus lowering HDL-C concentrations [43]. Although bezafibrate increases plasma apo A-I levels, it increases HDL-C by an even greater proportion (5.1% versus 33.7% in Eisenberg et al. [39]); these values may indicate a normalization of lipoprotein parameters, much as the paradoxical fibrate-induced increase in LDL does. Gemfibrozil [38] but not bezafibrate [44] increases apo A-I concentration and turnover in hypertriglyceridemic subjects.

As noted above, gemfibrozil was evaluated as a single agent in the Helsinki Heart Study. At the end of 5 years of treatment, total cholesterol, LDL-C, and triglyceride decreased 10%, 11%, and 35%, respectively, and HDL-C increased 11% versus placebo [3]. These changes were associated with a 34% decrease in CHD death. In the initial analyses, the greatest effect of gemfibrozil treatment was seen in patients with type IIb hyperlipidemia [3]; recent reanalysis showed particular benefit in patients with a high LDL-C to HDL-C ratio and triglyceride elevation. Clofibrate plus nicotinic acid reduced all-cause and CHD mortality rates in the above-described Stockholm trial [14], but clofibrate as a single agent was without benefit in the Coronary Drug Project [12] (see "Nicotinic Acid"). Fenofibrate was shown in angiographic examination of minor narrowings (diameter reduction 43 ± 14%) in 44 patients to generally be associated with cessation of progression or even regression of plaques [46]. Angiographically evident benefit correlated with total and LDL cholesterol levels, which were lowest in those patients experiencing regression.

Reductase Inhibitors

The chief effect of the HMG-CoA reductase inhibitors is to lower total and LDL cholesterol and apo B levels. Total cholesterol is reduced by about 15% to 30%, LDL-C is reduced by about 20% to 40%, and the fall in apo B corresponds to reductions in LDL-C and VLDL-C. These drugs also yield modest changes in HDL-C and plasma triglyceride levels: HDL-C rises by about 5% to 10%, and triglyceride falls by about 10% to 20%, with these changes somewhat greater in patients who have low HDL-C and high triglyceride. The three reductase inhibitors approved by the U.S. Food and Drug Administration (FDA)—lovastatin, pravastatin, and simvastatin—are quantitatively comparable in lipid effects when administered at equivalent dosages [47]. The reductase inhibitors have proved extremely safe. Myositis and alteration of liver enzymes are the major potential side effects. Myositis with single-agent use has been rare; frequency is increased when reductase inhibitors are used in combination with other agents in a synergistic manner (fibrates, nicotinic acid, cyclosporine, erythromycin).

The reductase inhibitors increase LDL-receptor activity, which promotes direct removal of both LDL and VLDL particles [48]. Clearance of VLDL remnants by the LDL receptor may contribute to decreases in triglyceride levels. However, the reductase inhibitors' chief mechanism is interference with the rate-limiting step of cholesterol biosynthesis, namely, the conversion of HMG-CoA to mevalonic acid. Hunninghake recently reviewed [47] the evidence that other mechanisms are operant as well, and that the lipid-lowering mechanisms of these agents may vary according to the type of hyperlipidemia. Possible compositional changes in apo B–containing lipoproteins could affect uptake by the LDL receptor and residence time in plasma, regulation of cellular cholesterol biosynthesis, or lipoprotein atherogenic potential. Hunninghake notes Miettinen's recent report that reductase inhibitors can reduce cholesterol absorption in the intestine [49], and the preclinical studies that show direct beneficial effects on the arterial wall [50] and decreased growth of malignant and nonmalignant cells [51].

As noted above, a reductase inhibitor in combination drug therapy was associated with coronary atherosclerotic lesion nonprogression or regression in the FATS and UCSF-SCOR trials [17,18]. At the American College of Cardiology 41st Annual Scientific Session (16 April 1992, Dallas, Texas), David Blankenhorn preliminarily described like results (unpublished) at 2 years in the placebo-controlled Mevinolin Atherosclerosis Regression Study (MARS), which used diet plus high-dose lovastatin as a single agent.

Bile-Acid Sequestrants

The effectiveness of the bile-acid sequestrants as single agents or in combined drug therapy for reducing CHD is evident from the results of the 7-year Lipid Research Clinics Coronary Primary Prevention Trial (LRC-CPPT) [52,53], in which diet plus cholestyramine yielded significantly decreased myocardial infarction and deaths from CHD, and from the findings of the above-cited CLAS [15,16], FATS [17], and UCSF-SCOR [18] trials, in which colestipol was given with diet and another hypolipidemic agent or agents.

The bile-acid sequestrants work through interruption of the enterohepatic recirculation of bile acids, resulting in a compensatory increase in hepatic synthesis of cholesterol and in hepatic expression of LDL receptors. The latter effect leads to lowering of plasma LDL-C levels, by as much as 20% to 25%. This decrease is often accompanied by increased plasma levels of VLDL and triglyceride. How the triglyceride increase may occur has recently been discussed in detail by Ericsson and Angelin [54].

Enterohepatic circulation of bile acids may be of regulatory importance to hepatic biosynthesis of triglyceride, perhaps through a link of phosphatidic acid phosphatase activity [54]. Angelin et al. in patients with familial hypercholesterolemia found cholestyramine at 16 g/day increased VLDL triglyceride levels by 50% at 5 to 7 weeks (secondary to 85%-enhanced VLDL production), the effect counteracted by an approximately 40%-enhanced fractional catabolic rate of VLDL triglyceride [55]. In addition, VLDL particle size was transiently increased. Witztum et al. found similar changes in their series of normotriglyceridemic subjects treated with colestipol [56].

Ericsson and Angelin in their review speculate that with increased cholesterol production, cholesterol is channeled not only for synthesis of bile acids but also to VLDL formation. The demonstration that administration of reductase inhibitors during cholestyramine therapy reduces plasma triglyceride levels [57] supports this hypothesis. The authors note as well the possibility that the increased uptake of VLDL remnant particles upon the up-regulation of LDL-receptor activity may stimulate VLDL synthesis, through the enrichment of hepatocytes with fatty acids. An increase in lipoprotein lipase activity may also be present. The findings of transient changes in VLDL size point to an adaptive mechanism. It is of interest, as Ericsson and Angelin note, that bile-acid overproduction can be an antecedent to hypertriglyceridemia [58] and that expression of LDL receptors has been described as enhanced in hypertriglyceridemic subjects [59]. These findings suggest that in some forms of hypertriglyceridemia, enhanced VLDL production secondary to bile-acid malabsorption is often compensated for by increased catabolism, until age or obesity leads to an overload of elimination capacity [54].

VLDL and triglyceride levels also rose in patients who underwent partial ileal bypass surgery for cholesterol lowering in the Program on the Surgical Control of the Hyperlipidemias (POSCH) [60]. At 10 years, VLDL levels were 35% higher and triglyceride levels were 34% higher than corresponding values in the control group. Ileal bypass works somewhat like bile-acid resins in interrupting bile-acid enterohepatic circulation. The 38% lowering of LDL-C in the POSCH surgical group probably represents the maximum of LDL lowering achievable with interruption of recirculation of bile acids. The POSCH surgical group also had diminished rates of myocardial infarction, CHD death, and CHD lesion progression.

Probucol

Whether the decrease in HDL-C with probucol administration represents a clinical problem is controversial since this apparently unfavorable lipoprotein change stands in contrast to associated antiatherosclerotic activity. A number of animal studies have shown an association of probucol administration with decreased progression of atherosclerosis despite minimal LDL-C lowering [61]. The effects may be related to probucol's demonstrated antioxidant activity [62,63]. It is also possible that probucol enhances reverse cholesterol transport, as in the apparently increased removal of cholesteryl esters from tendinous xanthomas, which have been found to regress during such therapy [64].

Franceschini et al. reported that probucol given in hypercholesterolemic patients led to the net mass transfer of cholesteryl esters from HDL to lower-density lipoproteins, through increased CETP activity [65]. With probucol administration, the HDL_2 subfraction was markedly affected (disappearing almost completely in some patients) but HDL_3 was not significantly affected; HDL-

C dropped 30%, apo A-I decreased 23% (apo A-I has been proposed as the critical protein for the synthesis and remodeling of HDL), and cholesteryl ester transfer activity increased 30%. Ying et al. in rabbits found that probucol's effect on HDL apo A-I was only prominent in hypercholesterolemia; they ascribed the decrease in HDL-C or apo A-I with probucol administration to decreased synthesis and increased fractional catabolism of HDL apo A-I [66]. Recently, McPherson et al. reported that probucol treatment of hypercholesterolemic patients significantly increased mean CETP and apo E concentrations and significantly lowered mean HDL_2 and apo A-I concentrations [67]. The changes in CETP, apo E, and HDL_2 are consistent with current models of reverse cholesterol transport in which CETP delivers cholesteryl esters from HDL to lower-density lipoproteins, with apo E facilitating hepatic uptake. Other results have contradicted the Franceschini and McPherson findings: for example, Bagdade et al. suggested that probucol reverses the accelerated cholesteryl ester transfer found in hypercholesterolemia [68], and Cortese at al. found a greater effect on HDL_3 than HDL_2 [69]. Further complicating understanding of the role of CETP activity in atherogenesis is the finding by Inazu et al. of no premature atherosclerosis in Japanese families who had CETP deficiency (due to a gene mutation) and elevated HDL-C; the authors concluded that this lipoprotein profile was potentially antiatherogenic [70].

Clarification of whether an antiatherosclerotic effect of probucol derives from antioxidant effects and/or lipoprotein changes may come from a clinical trial under way in Sweden to test the hypothesis that probucol administration will lead to angiographic regression of obstructive femoral vascular disease [71].

Exogenous Hormones

Progestins and estrogens may be considered agents affecting HDL and triglyceride metabolism. In general, progesterone and estrogen have opposite effects on lipid metabolism [72].

Progesterone reduces the secretion of VLDL and may reduce remnant particle clearance and down-regulate LDL receptors. It has been reported that progesterone receptor activity is enhanced by estrogen, and estrogen may be necessary to elicit a progesterone effect [73]. Progesterone appears to increase hepatic lipase activity. Hence, effects of progesterone, exerted through its androgenic activity, are to increase LDL-C levels and to decrease triglyceride and HDL-C (especially HDL_2) levels.

Estrogen has been reported to decrease hepatic lipase activity and may slightly reduce the activity of adipose tissue lipoprotein lipase. Estrogen is also believed to enhance LDL receptor–mediated lipoprotein uptake, and it appears to promote synthesis and/or secretion of apo A-I in the liver. Thus, estrogen therapy in postmenopausal women increases plasma triglyceride and HDL-C and decreases LDL-C levels [72,73]. It is believed that estrogen enhances the production of larger, less dense, and presumably less atherogenic LDL particles. The effects appear to vary with type of compound, dosage, and route of administration [72]. The increase in HDL-C and decrease in LDL-C may be induced by orally but not transdermally administered estrogens [74,75].

Extensive epidemiological data have shown decreased relative risk of CHD among postmenopausal women taking estrogen-replacement therapy [76,77]. In the 10-year follow-up of the Nurses' Health Study, estrogen use was associated with reductions in both CHD incidence and mortality, with a relative risk for major coronary disease of 0.56 for estrogen users and 0.40 for the subgroup taking unopposed oral conjugated estrogen [76]. At least part of such benefit may relate to changes in plasma lipid levels. Some angiographic evidence is also available: in a series by Hong et al., 22% of postmenopausal women taking estrogen had 25% or greater luminal diameter narrowing in a major coronary artery, compared with 68% of postmenopausal women not using estrogen [78]. The estrogen users had a higher mean HDL-C level, and the women not taking estrogen had a higher mean total to HDL cholesterol ratio; otherwise, lipid values were comparable between the groups. Postmenopausal hormone replacement for the prevention of CHD has not been approved by the FDA. However, it could well turn out upon further research that hormone-replacement therapy would be one preferred form of treatment of dyslipidemia in postmenopausal women.

The increase in plasma triglyceride level with estrogen treatment would be of concern only in patients with substantially elevated triglyceride, that is, higher than 250 or 300 mg/dl (2.82 or 3.39 mmol/L). The effect on plasma triglyceride level can be minimized by using a fairly low dose of estrogen. When estrogen is given in women with an intact uterus, the concomitant use of progesterone is recommended to reduce the risk of endometrial cancer. As noted above, progesterones with androgenic effects (e.g., those of the 21-nortestosterone class) will tend to oppose the effects of estrogen on lipids. Agents such as desogestrel have little or no androgenic effect.

Combinations of Agents

Drug combinations may be considered to maximize the reduction of LDL-C, or to achieve optimal effects on lipid levels in mixed hyperlipidemia. Combined therapy is sometimes required in severe hypertriglyceridemia to prevent abdominal pain and pancreatitis.

Combinations of a reductase inhibitor and a fibrate or nicotinic acid have proved efficacious in mixed hyperlipidemia in which there is modest hypertriglyceridemia and high total cholesterol, in familial combined hyperlipidemia, and in diabetic dyslipidemia [43]. However, because severe myopathy has been reported with such combinations, close monitoring is required, and routine use is not recommended.

When severe hypertriglyceridemia is present in mixed dyslipidemia, gemfibrozil may be combined with nicotinic acid, or one of these two drugs may be combined with a bile-acid sequestrant. As noted, progestins can significantly reduce plasma triglyceride levels, although this is not an approved FDA indication; they might be used in combination with gemfibrozil or nicotinic acid but do not have an FDA indication for triglyceride lowering.

Summary

Like elevations of LDL-C, low levels of HDL-C are now recognized as being causal in the development of CHD. The evidence is not as strong for triglyceride, although triglyceride levels are generally higher in patients with CHD and a great deal of evidence supports the atherogenicity of remnant lipoproteins from chylomicrons or VLDL. Triglyceride levels of 250 mg/dl (2.82 mmol/L) and higher and HDL-C levels under 35 mg/dl (0.91 mmol/L) are considered abnormal. Treatment consists primarily of hygienic measures, except in patients who have marked elevations of triglyceride and thus are at risk for pancreatitis. Efficacy of drug treatment to raise HDL-C or reduce triglyceride levels for the prevention or treatment of CHD has not been established. Drugs should be considered only after nonpharmacologic measures have been unsuccessful and in patients at high risk for coronary events, such as diabetics and patients with existing peripheral atherosclerotic disease, concomitant elevations of LDL-C, chronic renal disease, a strong risk factor profile, or familial combined hyperlipidemia or other familial dyslipidemias in which there is a strong family history of CHD. The most effective drugs for decreasing plasma triglyceride and raising HDL-C are nicotinic acid and the fibric-acid derivatives. Reductase inhibitors have modest effects on reducing triglyceride and raising HDL.

References

1. Grundy SM, Goodman DEW, Rifkind BM, et al. The place of HDL in cholesterol management: A perspective from the National Cholesterol Education Program. Arch Intern Med 1989;149:505–510.
2. Gordon DJ, Probstfield JL, Garrison RJ, et al. High-density lipoprotein cholesterol and cardiovascular disease: Four prospective American studies. Circulation 1989;79:8–15.
3. Manninen V, Elo MO, Frick MH, et al. Lipid alterations and decline in the incidence of coronary heart disease in the Helsinki Heart Study. JAMA 1988;260:641–651.
4. Manninen V, Tenkanen L, Koskinen P, et al. Joint effects of serum triglyceride and LDL cholesterol concentrations on coronary heart disease risk in the Helsinki Heart Study: Implications for treatment. Circulation 1992;85:37–45.
5. Assmann G, Schulte H. Triglycerides and atherosclerosis: Results from the Prospective Cardiovascular Münster Study. Atheroscler Rev 1991;22:51–63.
6. Austin MA. Plasma triglyceride and coronary heart disease (review). Arterioscler Thromb 1991;11:2–14.
7. National Institutes of Health. Consensus Development Conference Statement: Triglyceride, High Density Lipoprotein, and Coronary Heart Disease, February 26–28, 1992. Bethesda, MD: NIH (in press). Available from: Office of Medical Applications and Research, National Institutes of Health, Federal Building Room 618, Bethesda, MD 20892, U.S.A.
8. The International Committee for the Evaluation of Hypertriglyceridemia as a Vascular Risk Factor. The hypertriglyceridemias: Risk and management. Am J Cardiol 1991;68:1A–42A.
9. European Atherosclerosis Society Study Group. The recognition and management of hyperlipidemia in adults: A policy statement of the European Atherosclerosis Society. Eur Heart J 1988;9:571–600.
10. The Expert Panel. Report of the National Cholesterol Education Program Expert Panel on detection, evaluation, and treatment of high blood cholesterol in adults. Arch Intern Med 1988;148:36–69.
11. Carlson LA, Olsson AG, Ballantyne D. On the rise in LDL and HDL in response to the treatment of hypertriglyceridemia in Type IV and Type V hyperlipoproteinemias. Atherosclerosis 1977;26:603–609.
12. The Coronary Drug Project Research Group. Clofibrate and niacin in coronary heart disease. JAMA 1975;231:360–381.
13. Canner PL, Berge KG, Wenger NK, et al. Fifteen year mortality in Coronary Drug Project patients: Long-term benefit with niacin. J Am Coll Cardiol 1986;8:1245–1255.
14. Carlson LA, Rosenhamer G. Reduction of mortality in the Stockholm Ischaemic Heart Disease Secondary Prevention Study by combined treatment with clofibrate and nicotinic acid. Acta Med Scand 1988;223:405–418.
15. Blankenhorn DH, Nessim SA, Johnson RL, et al. Beneficial effects of combined colestipol–niacin therapy on coronary atherosclerosis and coronary venous bypass grafts. JAMA 1987;257:3233–3240. Erratum JAMA 1988;259:2698.

16. Cashin-Hemphill L, Mack WJ, Pogoda JM, et al. Beneficial effects of colestipol–niacin on coronary atherosclerosis. A 4-year follow-up. JAMA 1990;264:3013–3017.

17. Brown G, Albers JJ, Fisher LD, et al. Regression of coronary artery disease as a result of intensive lipid-lowering therapy in men with high levels of apolipoprotein B. N Engl J Med 1990;323:1289–1298.

18. Kane JP, Malloy MJ, Ports TA, et al. Regression of coronary atherosclerosis during treatment of familial hypercholesterolemia with combined drug regimens. JAMA 1990;264:3007–3012.

19. Blankenhorn DH, Alaupovic P, Wickham E, et al. Prediction of angiographic change in native human coronary arteries and aortocoronary bypass grafts. Lipid and nonlipid factors. Circulation 1990;81:470–476.

20. Shepherd J. The action of nicotinic acid and its analogues on lipoprotein metabolism. Atheroscler Rev 1991;22:207–212.

21. Fattore PC, Sirtori CR. Nicotinic acid and derivatives. Curr Opin Lipidol 1991;2:43–47.

22. Walldius G. Probucol and nicotinic acid: Old drugs, new findings and new derivatives. Curr Opin Lipidol 1992;3:34–39.

23. Nikkila EA, Pykalisto O. Induction of adipose tissue lipoprotein lipase by nicotinic acid. Biochim Biophys Acta 1968;152:421–423.

24. Shepherd J, Packard CJ, Patsch JR, et al. Effects of nicotinic acid therapy on plasma high density lipoprotein subfraction distribution and composition and on apolipoprotein A metabolism. J Clin Invest 1979;63:858–867.

25. Taskinen MR, Nikkila EA. Effects of acipimox on serum lipids, lipoproteins and lipolytic enzymes in hypertriglyceridemia. Atherosclerosis 1988;69:249–255.

26. Johansson J, Carlson LA. High density lipoprotein particle size subclass alterations by treatment with nicotinic acid. In: Carlson LA, ed. Disorders of HDL. London: Smith-Gordon and Company, 1990, pp. 203–208.

27. Wahlberg G, Walldius G, Olsson AG, et al. Effects of nicotinic acid on serum cholesterol concentrations of high density lipoprotein subfractions HDL_2 and HDL_3 in hyperlipoproteinaemia. J Intern Med 1990;228:151–157.

28. Franceschini G, Bernini F, Michelagnoli S, et al. Lipoprotein changes and increased affinity of LDL for their receptors after acipimox treatment in hypertriglyceridemia. Atherosclerosis 1990;81:41–49.

29. Tikkanen MJ. Fibric acid derivatives. Curr Opin Lipidol 1992;3:29–33.

30. Monk JP, Todd PA. Bezafibrate: A review of its pharmacodynamic and pharmacokinetic properties, and therapeutic use in hyperlipidemia. Drugs 1987;33:539–576.

31. WHO cooperative trial on primary prevention of ischaemic heart disease using clofibrate to lower serum cholesterol: Mortality follow-up. Report of the Committee of Principal Investigators. Lancet 1980;2(8191):379–385.

32. Sirtori CR, Calabresi L, Werba JP, et al. Tolerability of fibric acids. Comparative data and biochemical bases. Pharmacol Res 1992;26:243–260.

33. Creger PL, Moersch GW, Neuklis WA. Structure/activity relationship of gemfibrozil (CI-719) and related compounds. Proc R Soc Med 1976;69(suppl 2):3–10.

34. Roth BD, Newton RS. Phenoxyacetic acids and lipid-lipoprotein metabolism. In: Witiak DT, Newman HAI, Feller DR, eds. Antilipidemic Drugs: Medicinal, Chemical and Biochemical Aspects, vol.17. Amsterdam: Elsevier, 1991, pp. 225–255.

35. Schwandt P. Fibrates and triglyceride metabolism. Eur J Clin Pharmacol 1991;40(suppl 1):S41–S43.

36. Simpson HS, Williamson CM, Olivecrona T, et al. Postprandial lipemia, fenofibrate and coronary artery disease. Atherosclerosis 1990;85:193–202.
37. Shepherd J, Griffen B, Caslake M, et al. The influence of fibrates on lipoprotein metabolism. Atheroscler Rev 1991;22:163–169.
38. Saku K, Hynd BA, Gartside PS, et al. Mechanism of action of gemfibrozil in increasing HDL and lowering triglycerides. J Clin Invest 1985;75:1702–1712.
39. Eisenberg S, Gavish D, Oschry Y, et al. Abnormalities in very low, low, and high density lipoproteins in hypertriglyceridemia: Reversal toward normal with bezafibrate treatment. J Clin Invest 1984;74:470–482.
40. Tilly-Kiesi M, Tikkanen MJ. Low density lipoprotein density and composition in hypercholesterolaemic men treated with HMG CoA reductase inhibitors and gemfibrozil. J Intern Med 1991;229:427–434.
41. Huttunen JK, Manninen V, Manttari M, et al. The Helsinki Heart Study: Central findings and clinical implications. Ann Med 1991;23:155–159.
42. Gavish D, Oschry Y, Fainaru M, et al. Change in very low-, low-, and high-density lipoproteins during lipid lowering (bezafibrate) therapy: Studies in type IIa and type IIb hyperlipoproteinemia. Eur J Clin Invest 1986;16:61–68.
43. Grundy SM, Vega GL. Two different views of the relationship of hypertriglyceridemia to coronary heart disease. Implications for treatment. Arch Intern Med 1992;152:28–34.
44. Shepherd J, Packard CJ, Stewart JM, et al. Apolipoprotein A and B (S$_f$ 100–400) metabolism during bezafibrate therapy in hypertriglyceridemic subjects. J Clin Invest 1984;74:2164–2177.
45. Vega GL, Grundy SM. Gemfibrozil therapy in primary hypertriglyceridemia associated with coronary heart disease: Effects on metabolism of low-density lipoproteins. JAMA 1985;253:2398–2403.
46. Hahmann HW, Bunte T, Hellwig N, et al. Progression and regression of minor coronary arterial narrowings by quantitative angiography after fenofibrate therapy. Am J Cardiol 1991;67:957–961.
47. Hunninghake DB. HMG CoA reductase inhibitors. Curr Opin Lipidol 1992;3:22–28.
48. Grundy SM. HMG-CoA reductase inhibitors for treatment of hypercholesterolemia. N Engl J Med 1988;319:24–33.
49. Miettinen TA. Inhibition of cholesterol absorption by HMG-CoA reductase inhibitors. Eur J Clin Pharmacol 1991;40(suppl 1):S19–S21.
50. Senaratue MP, Thomson AB, Kappagoda CJ. Lovastatin prevents the impairment of endothelium dependent relaxation and inhibits the accumulation of cholesterol in the aorta in experimental atherosclerosis in rabbits. Cardiovasc Res 1991;25:568–578.
51. Sebti SM, Tkalcevio GI, Jani JP. Lovastatin, a cholesterol biosynthesis inhibitor, inhibits the growth of H-*ras* oncogene transformed cells in nude mice. Cancer Commun 1991;3:141–147.
52. Lipid Research Clinics Program. The Lipid Research Clinics Coronary Primary Prevention Trial results. I. Reduction in incidence of coronary heart disease. JAMA 1984;251:351–364.
53. Lipid Research Clinics Program. The Lipid Research Clinics Coronary Primary Prevention Trial results. II. The relationship of reduction in incidence of coronary heart disease to cholesterol lowering. JAMA 1984;251:365–374.
54. Ericsson S, Angelin B. Effect of bile acid sequestrants on triglyceride metabolism. Atheroscler Rev 1991;22:149–153.

55. Angelin B, Leijd B, Hultcrantz R, et al. Increased turnover of very low density lipoprotein triglyceride during treatment with cholestyramine in familial hypercholesterolaemia. J Intern Med 1990;227:201–206.
56. Witztum JL, Schonfeld G, Weidman SW. The effects of colestipol on the metabolism of very low density lipoproteins in man. J Lab Clin Med 1976;88:1008–1018.
57. Illingworth DR, Bacon SP, Larsen KK. Long-term experience with HMG-CoA reductase inhibitors in the therapy of hypercholesterolemia. Atheroscler Rev 1988;18:161–187.
58. Angelin B, Hershon KC, Brunzell JD. Bile acid metabolism in hereditary forms of hypertriglyceridemia: Evidence for an increased synthesis rate in monogenic familial hypertriglyceridemia. Proc Natl Acad Sci U S A 1987;44:5434–5438.
59. Vega GL, Grundy SM. Studies on mechanisms for enhanced clearance of low density lipoproteins in patients with primary hypertriglyceridemia. J Intern Med 1989;226:5–15.
60. Buchwald H, Varco RL, Matts JP, et al. Effect of partial ileal bypass surgery on mortality and morbidity from coronary heart disease in patients with hypercholesterolemia: Report of the Program on the Surgical Control of the Hyperlipidemias (POSCH). N Engl J Med 1990;323:946–955.
61. Kita T, Nagano Y, Yokode M, et al. Probucol prevents the progression of atherosclerosis in Watanabe heritable hyperlipidemic rabbit, an animal model for familial hypercholesterolemia. Proc Natl Acad Sci U S A 1987;84:5928–5931.
62. Parthasarathy S, Young SG, Witztum JL, et al. Probucol inhibits oxidative modification of low density lipoprotein. J Clin Invest 1986;77:641–644.
63. Kita T. Oxidized lipoproteins and probucol. Curr Opin Lipidol 1991;2:36–38.
64. Yamamoto A, Matsuzawa Y, Yokoyama S, et al. Effects of probucol on xanthomata regression in familial hypercholesterolemia. Am J Cardiol 1986:57:29H–35H.
65. Franceschini G, Sirtori M, Vaccarino V, et al. Mechanisms of HDL reduction after probucol: Changes in HDL subfractions and increased reverse cholesteryl ester transfer. Arteriosclerosis 1989;9:462–469.
66. Ying H, Saku K, Harada R, et al. Putative mechanisms of action of probucol on high-density lipoprotein apolipoprotein A-1 and its isoprotein kinetics in rabbits. Biochim Biophys Acta 1990;1047:247–254.
67. McPherson R, Hogue M, Milne RW, et al. Increase in plasma cholesteryl ester transfer protein during probucol treatment. Arterioscler Thromb 1991;11:476–481.
68. Bagdade JD, Kaufman D, Ritter MC, et al. Probucol treatment in hypercholesterolemic patients: Effects on lipoprotein composition, HDL particle size, and cholesteryl ester transfer. Atherosclerosis 1990;84:145–154.
69. Cortese C, Marenah CB, Miller NE, et al. The effects of probucol on plasma lipoproteins in polygenic and familial hypercholesterolemia. Atherosclerosis 1982;44:319–325.
70. Inazu A, Brown ML, Hesler CB, et al. Increased high-density lipoprotein levels caused by a common cholesteryl-ester transfer protein gene mutation. N Engl J Med 1990;323:1234–1238.
71. Walldius G, Carlson LA, Erikson U, et al. Development of femoral atherosclerosis in hypercholesterolemic patients during treatment with cholestyramine and probucol/placebo. Probucol Quantitative Regression Swedish Trial (PQRST): A status report. Am J Cardiol 1988;62:37B–43B.
72. Kushwaha RS. Female sex steroid hormones and lipoprotein metabolism. Curr Opin Lipidol 1992;3:167–172.

73. Knopp RH. The effects of oral contraceptives and postmenopausal estrogens on lipoprotein physiology and atherosclerosis. In: Halbe HW, Rekers H, eds. Oral Contraception into the 1990s. Lancs, U.K.: Parthenon, 1989, pp. 31–45.
74. Walsh BW, Schiff I, Rosner B, et al. Effects of postmenopausal estrogen replacement on the concentrations and metabolism of plasma lipoproteins. N Engl J Med 1991;325:1196–1200.
75. Moorjani S, Dupont A, Labrie F, et al. Changes in plasma lipoprotein and apolipoprotein composition in relation to oral versus percutaneous administration of estrogen alone or in cyclic association with utrogestan in menopausal women. J Clin Endocrinol Metab 1991;73:373–379.
76. Stampfer MJ, Colditz GA, Willett WC, et al. Postmenopausal estrogen therapy and cardiovascular disease: Ten-year follow-up from the Nurses' Health Study. N Engl J Med 1991;325:756–780.
77. Knopp RH. Estrogen replacement therapy for reduction of cardiovascular risk in women. Curr Opin Lipidol 1991;2:240–247.
78. Hong MK, Romm PA, Reagan K, et al. Effects of estrogen replacement therapy on serum lipid values and angiographically defined coronary artery disease in postmenopausal women. Am J Cardiol 1992;69:176–183.

DRUGS AFFECTING THROMBOSIS AND ATHEROSCLEROSIS

C.R. SIRTORI and S. COLLI

ABSTRACT. The effect of drugs affecting lipid metabolism on atherosclerosis development/progression may be linked to their activity on the clotting system, i.e. at the platelet, fibrinogen or fibrinolysis levels. Both resins and HMG CoA reductase inhibitors reduce, over prolonged treatments, platelet sensitivity to major aggregants. This effect seems to occur best with non-liver selective agents (e.g. simvastatin) although recent data cast doubts on the constancy of the effect. A comparative evaluation of different reductase inhibitors has never been carried out. These drugs also reduce the circulating levels of the tissue factor pathway inhibitor (TFPI) carried by LDL, this being a potentially negative effect.

Fibric acids belong to a multifaceted series of "fraudolent" fatty acids, known to interact with a liver nuclear receptor, thus activating fatty acid catabolism. A similar activity may be exerted by n-3 fatty acids, MEDICA 16, thia-fatty acids etc. Among fibric acids, all but gemfibrozil can reduce fibrinogen levels; this last compound can, however, apparently activate fibrinolysis. Bezafibrate, as well as n-3 fatty acids, also exerts a significant platelet antiaggregatory activity. Anti-oxidants may possibly play a role in controlling platelet activation. Probucol was recently shown to reduce the excretion of thromboxane metabolites in patients with homocystinuria. The complex effect of this molecule may, however, also suggest other mechanisms.

1. Introduction

Among the major complications of hyperlipoproteinemias (HLP) are thrombotic disorders, both related to the progressive alterations of the arterial walls, and to primary changes in platelet aggregation, fibrinolysis and/or fibrinogen levels, frequently detected in these patients (1-3). The major changes exerted by atherogenic lipoproteins on specific functions of cells involved in thrombosis, have been described in detail by Tremoli (this Symposium). It remains, therefore, to be discussed whether drugs affecting lipid metabolism may exert a significant activity at different steps of the clotting system, i.e. at the platelet, fibrinogen or fibrinolysis levels. In second place, it should be argued as to whether the improvement in cardiovascular risk after these drugs may be, in large or small part, related to changes in the major clotting parameters.

This review will attempt to summarize the major findings from drug trials, that have evaluated the effect of major lipid lowering medications on the thrombotic risk. In particular, in the case of drugs specifically acting on total and low density lipoprotein (LDL) cholesterol levels, major emphasis has been placed on platelet aggregation and activation of eicosanoid metabolism. In the case of "fraudolent" fatty acids (fibric acids and others) the pattern of

A. L. Catapano et al. (eds.), Drugs Affecting Lipid Metabolism, 215–229.
© 1993 Kluwer Academic Publishers and Fondazione Giovanni Lorenzini.

activity is more variable, i.e. including both platelet aggregability as well as fibrinogen levels and, in some cases, fibrinolysis.

2. Resins, HMG CoA reductase inhibitors

Anion exchange resins (cholestyramine, colestipol) and inhibitors of hydroxymethylglutaryl coenzyme A reductase (HMG CoA reductase) are drugs specifically affecting plasma total and LDL cholesterol levels. As such, they should be uniquely active on the repeatedly described "**hyperactive platelets**" typically found in type II HLP: hyperactive platelets are characterized by an enhanced sensitivity to various aggregants, e.g. collagen, ADP and adrenaline (4). Platelets from type IIA hypercholesterolemic patients also release increased amounts of thromboxane B_2 (TXB_2) during aggregation (5) the TXB_2 generation being directly related to the total or LDL cholesterol levels of examined patients (6). Moreover, platelets from hypercholesterolemic patients exhibit a reduced sensitivity to prostacyclin (PGI_2) apparently linked to a reduction of PGI_2 binding sites (7).

The evaluation of cholesterol lowering drugs, as relates to platelet reactivity, has been approached in a non systematic way. There are two possible problems in evaluating the effect of these drugs: the first is that, in our experience, platelet hyperactivity tends to undergo a slow, progressive spontaneous reduction (a "regression to the mean" phenomenon). This occurs during prolonged dietary therapy, including polyunsaturated fatty acids, eventually soybean proteins. The second problem is that hyperactivity is best detected when exposing platelets to low-dose collagen (0.3-1.2 µg/ml): at this concentration TXB_2 release is clearly raised in type II patients (8). No difference between controls and type II patients in terms of aggregation and TXB_2 generation is seen after higher doses of collagen.

Contrasting data have been provided on the response of platelets from type II patients to plasma cholesterol reduction. Part of these discrepancies relates to the above exposed problems; it may also depend on the generally poor design of studies, mainly of a retrospective nature. Initial studies by Briones et al. (9) and Zucker et al. (10) failed to show changes in platelet aggregability after cholesterol lowering medications. In the first study (9), after colestipol, there was a reduction in the number of circulating platelet aggregates, but no change in ADP induced platelet aggregation ex vivo, despite a significant decrease of total serum and LDL cholesterol. Similar negative results were reported in the Zucker et al. (10) study, investigating the effect of a combination of probucol+colestipol: no change in platelet function, TXB_2 formation or PGI_2 sensitivity were noted, despite a 30% reduction in the mean LDL cholesterol. In this study there appeared to be no enhanced baseline platelet reactivity in treated patients vs controls, thus suggesting that the first type of error (spontaneous tendency of platelets to revert to a "normal" function after a prolonged diet), may have been present.

More recently two studies were carried out by German investigators, in both cases comparing untreated type II patients with normolipidemic controls and with other type II patients treated for many months (8 or more) with either resins or the HMG CoA reductase inhibitor simvastatin. Löbel et al. (8), investigating the effect of cholestyramine (12 g/day for 8-11 months) with this protocol, did not detect changes in the platelet hyperactivity and enhanced TXB_2 release, remaining significantly higher vs untreated controls, despite a 21% reduction in total plasma and LDL cholesterol. In this study, however, the sensitivity of platelet rich plasma to the antiaggregatory effect of Iloprost, a stable PGI_2 analogue, was reduced in untreated patients, and raised back to normal after cholestyramine, thus suggesting a normalization of platelet PGI_2 receptors. In the second study, Schrör et al. (11) evaluated the effect of 8 months of simvastatin (20-40 mg/day, resulting in 25 and 24% reductions of total and LDL cholesterol). In this case both platelet aggregation and TXB_2 generation, significantly enhanced in untreated patients, were apparently normalized by simvastatin. Similar results, i.e. a progressive reduction of platelet-derived TXB_2 formation, was noted in type II patients treated for up to 24 weeks with simvastatin by Davì et al. (12).

Our experience with another HMG CoA reductase inhibitor, pravastatin, in type II patients, as part of a large multicenter study carried out in Italy (13), was somewhat disappointing and not leading to significant changes vs controls in terms of, particularly, TXB_2 generation. These unpublished data were, in our view, consistent with the well defined liver selectivity of pravastatin, a hydrophilic compound reaching in very low concentrations other tissues, e.g. the bone marrow (14).

However, more recently, Davì et al. (15) carried out an extensive study in type II patients, this time evaluating the stable urinary metabolite 11-dehydro-TXB_2, a well established marker of platelet activation. In this study, the authors could confirm a clear correlation with the logarithm of total plasma cholesterol concentration vs the logarithm of the urinary TXB_2 metabolite (TXM) (Fig. 1). However, when evaluating the effect of drug treatment in 10 type II patients (Table 1) it was clear that, in spite of a more than 25% mean reduction of cholesterolemia, TXM excretion was inconsistently reduced, 4 out of 10 patients exhibiting an increase after treatment. In order to confirm the biological significance of these observations, the authors treated 6 of the patients with a low dose of aspirin (ASA) for just one week, with no change of cholesterolemia but a dramatic reduction of TXM excretion in all.

These findings in type II patients allow, altogether, only equivocal conclusions. Platelet hyperresponsiveness/activation of eicosanoid metabolism are, as of now, well ascertained findings. However, they are prone to analytical variability (e.g. the platelet responsiveness to collagen) and they may also show a tendency to regression to the mean phenomenon. This might be particularly the case of patients with concomitant dietary management. In our experience, only the reduced sensitivity to PGI_2 or its analogues (a possible consequence of membrane receptor loss) (7) seems to be a rather stable characteristic of platelets from these patients.

Especially in view of the results from the last study with simvastatin (16), it appears that plasma cholesterol normalization may not be necessarily linked

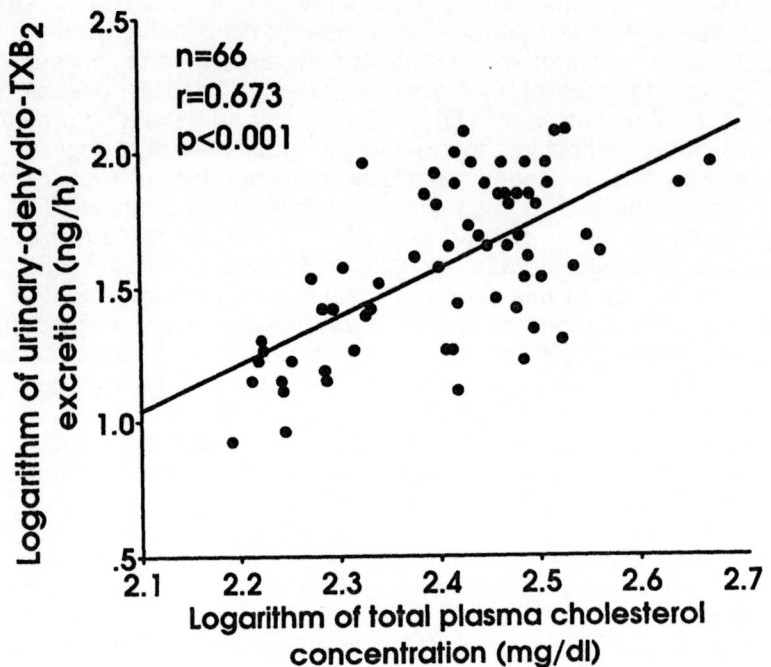

Figure 1. Correlation between urinary excretion of 11-dehydro-thromboxane-B_2 (TXM) and total plasma cholesterol in 20 controls and 46 type IIa hypercholesterolemic patients (from 15).

TABLE 1. Different effects of reductase inhibitor and ASA on plasma lipids/TXB_2 excretion in type II patients (from 15)

Simvastatin (n = 10)

	Base	6 months
Chol mg/dl	351±46	251±39**
TXM ng/hr	76±38	48±15*
	(increased in 4 out of 10)	

ASA 50 mg (n = 6)

	Base	1 week
TXM ng/hr	79±44	25±13**

to an improvement of the activated platelet/eicosanoid metabolism. A reduction of TXM excretion did not, in fact, occur in all patients, vs the case of ASA treatment. Moreover, none of the reported studies was a classical double-bind placebo controlled trial, monitoring eventual spontaneous changes of platelet reactivity over time. Future studies should also allow a re-examination of the possible issue of lipophilia vs liver selectivity in the case of HMG CoA reductase inhibitors (e.g. lovastatin-simvastatin vs pravastatin) (14). In this particular case, in fact, it would be possible to clarify whether any observed changes of platelet reactivity are secondary either to an inhibited sterol biosynthesis in the bone marrow (as postulated from animal studies investigating platelet membrane changes after different diets) (16) or to "environmental" plasma cholesterol changes.

A new area of potential interest for cholesterol lowering medications relates to the so called **tissue factor pathway inhibitor** (TFPI) (17), also named "lipoprotein associated extrinsic pathway inhibitor" (LACI) (18) and "extrinsec pathway inhibitor" (EPI) (19). This serine-type protease inhibitor, responsible for controlling the activation of factor Xa by tissue factor, is carried in plasma mostly by lipoproteins. About 50% of TFPI is associated with LDL and another 40-45% with HDL. In view of the crucial role of this protease inhibitor in starting blood clotting, it will be of interest to define the activity of drugs affecting plasma lipoproteins. In the only reported study (20), as could be theoretically postulated, the HMG CoA reductase inhibitor simvastatin dramatically reduced TFPI level, the reduction being correlated with the LDL cholesterol fall. This would be a potentially negative effect on the thrombotic risk, although the clinical consequences of this change are difficult to evaluate. An interesting hypothesis would be that of a potential activity of drugs affecting HDL cholesterol levels (see below): these, in fact, by increasing the carrier lipoprotein might elevate TFPI levels. This hypothesis should be evaluated within a clinical study.

3. Fraudulent fatty acids, fibrinogen and fibrinolysis

Drugs affecting the metabolism of very low density lipoproteins (VLDL), in turn raising HDL levels and also, in some cases, reducing LDL, belong in most cases to the series of **"fraudulent" fatty acids**. This defines molecules characterized by an abnormal fatty acid structure, either in a linear form (n-3 fatty acids, MEDICA 16, thia-fatty acids) or with an aromatic structure (fibric acids) (21). All these molecules are not directly recognized by mitochondria, but interact with a nuclear receptor (PPAR), well characterized in liver cells (22). PPAR belongs to the steroid receptor superfamily of ligand activated transcription factors, also including receptors for vitamins A and D_3, thyroid hormones and others.

The most likely hypothesis for the mode of action of fraudolent fatty acids is that, when reaching the liver, they activate the PPAR and, as a consequence, a cytochrome P450 (IV A1) (23), leading to the active metabolism of these abnormal substrates; a parallel consequence is the activation of mitochondria, responsible for the disposable of peroxidative products, coming from this metabolism and probably the key factor in the increased catabolism of the liver "natural" fatty acids. This liver operated mechanism leads in turn to a peripheral activation of lipolytic enzymes, namely lipoprotein lipase and hepatic lipase, delivering fatty acids to the liver for their enhanced catabolism (24).

The results of all these phenomena are obviously a reduction of VLDL triglycerides and also a rise of HDL cholesterol. The activation of hepatic lipase will also lead to the catabolism of HDL_2, finally resulting in increase of HDL_3 (25); a possible exception is that of n-3 fatty acids, probably weak agonists in the system, that only give rise to an increase of HDL_2 (not of total HDL) without subsequent transformation into HDL_3 (26). By this or unrelated mechanisms, fraudolent fatty acids affect particularly circulating levels of fibrinogen and may also reduce platelet sensitivity to some agonists.

Fibrinogen is a highly adhesive molecule, interacting with various tissue sites, and in particular with the platelet integrins (GP IIB, IIIA) (27). Fibrinogen levels are an established risk factor for coronary and also for cerebrovascular disease (3). On the other hand, levels of fibrinogen seem to be very strictly determined by genetics, thus apparently leaving little space for pharmacological modulation (28).

In spite of this, several reports have indicated that, particularly fibric acids may exert a potent reducing effect on fibrinogen levels. Table 2 summarizes the up to now reported activity of major fibric acids on fibrinogen levels. Data on fenofibrate have been mentioned in this Symposium (29). What is instead clear, however, is that gemfibrozil is essentially ineffective on fibrinogen levels, as shown by a variety of studies (30), whereas bezafibrate appears possibly the most effective agent. This points out to the fact that these fraudolent fatty acids, although sharing considerable similarities, are certainly different molecules.

TABLE 2. Fibrinogen levels after treatment with different fibric acids

Clofibrate	↓ 13% (up to -30%)
Bezafibrate	↓ 17% (↓43% in hyperfibrinogenemia)
Fenofibrate	↓ ? (-20%)
Gemfibrozil	→
Ciprofibrate	↓ 18%

In the case of bezafibrate, patients with elevated fibrinogen levels are the most sensitive. Niort et al. (31) showed that these may experience a more than 45% reduction from the starting levels upon bezafibrate (600 mg/d) treatment. Within a controlled investigation of patients with hypertriglyceridemias (both type IIB and IV) we could show an average reduction around 20% on bezafibrate vs placebo and, more interestingly, the fibrinogen reduction appeared to be directly related to the starting fibrinogenemia (Fig. 2) (32). Since, from our findings, as well as from those of others, it seems that fibrinogen levels in the normal range are virtually unchanged after fibric acids, whereas elevated levels tend to go back to normal, it remains to be determined as to whether this fibrinogen regulating effect is a "normalization" phenomenon or else a reduction of fibrinogenemia is correlated to changes in lipoprotein metabolism.

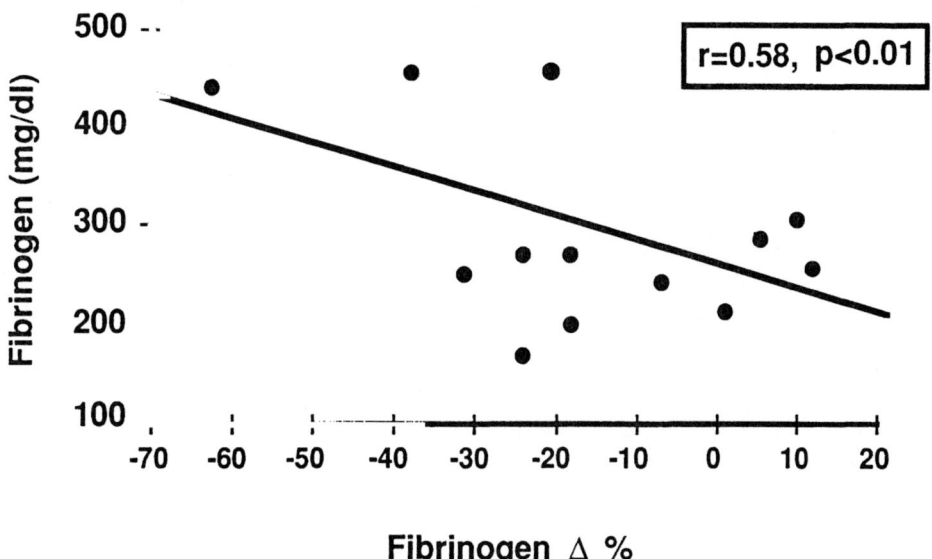

Figure 2. Correlation between fibrinogen reduction following bezafibrate and starting fibrinogenemia in hypertriglyceridemic patients (from 32).

Supportive evidence for the lipoprotein mediation of fibrinogen reduction is just indirect. In rats, hypertriglyceridemia induced by Triton WR-1339 leads to a close to doubling of fibrinogenemia, with a concomitant reduction in the α_2 plasmin inhibitor (33). Furthermore, with other lipid lowering medications, e.g. probucol (see below) changes in fibrinogen may occur, possibly related to an altered lipid metabolism. However, as of now, it cannot be clearly argued whether fibrinogen changes induced by fibric acids or other fraudolent fatty acids are related to their effects on lipoproteins. Data on n-3 fatty acids are at least inconclusive (34) and no activity of HMG CoA reductase inhibitors was reported in a previously quoted study (20).

Data pertaining to **platelet aggregation**, as related to fraudolent fatty acids, provide dyshomogeneous findings. Earlier studies had shown that clofibrate, the prototype fibric acid, can significantly reduce platelet sensitivity to various aggregants, as well as improve platelet half-life in plasma, particularly in hypercholesterolemic patients (35). These findings were not followed up by any data pertaining to eicosanoid metabolism after this type of agent. Enrichment of the diet with n-3 fatty acids is an established mode of reducing platelet aggregability, particularly when exerted by arachidonic acid or other agonists affecting the eicosanoid pathway (36).

Data on other fibric acids have, however, provided some indication that the activity on platelets, if any, may not be the direct consequence of changes in platelet eicosanoid metabolism. Gemfibrozil, in our experience, when given to hypertriglyceridemic patients somewhat reduced (the effect not reaching statistical significance) TXB_2 release from collagen activated platelets (37); in a later, above quoted study (13), we failed to see significant changes in platelet behavior in severely hypercholesterolemic patients after either gemfibrozil or pravastatin. Somewhat different results were achieved, instead, in bezafibrate treated patients, where we could show a clear reduction in platelet sensitivity to collagen (32). This was apparently not associated to any change in TXB_2 release, thus suggesting that possibly the mode of action of these molecules is not directly related to changes in the platelet eicosanoid metabolism.

Fibrinolysis is an index of thrombotic risk that has received considerable attention in recent years in the field of hyperlipidemia. Increased plasma levels of PAI-1, a stable inhibitor of fibrinolysis, be it of liver or endothelial origin, have been repeatedly described in hypertriglyceridemia (38). Elevated PAI-1 levels are directly correlated with triglyceridemia and also with plasma insulin levels (39) and this impairment of fibrinolysis may be a part of the so called "polymetabolic syndrome" or "syndrome X" (40).

While certainly an important target for drug management, elevations of PAI-1 levels have proven considerably resistant to diet and/or drug treatments. n-3 fatty acids raise, rather than reduce PAI-1 levels (41) and the activity of fibric acids is mostly insignificant. While during our controlled investigation with bezafibrate (32) we failed to see any changes in PAI-1, a possible exception might be that of gemfibrozil, where, in one study in post-myocardial infarction patients, a significant reduction of PAI-1 antigen levels (together with a rise of fibrinogen) were noted with active drug treatment (30) (Table 3).

This effect of gemfibrozil, which needs confirmation in a controlled trial, may be apparently related to a direct inhibitory effect on PAI-1 synthesis in liver cells. This was documented by an in vitro study in Hep G2 cells, where the drug reduced basal PAI-1 secretion by 43% and attenuated the rise of PAI-1 synthesis induced by different growth factors, over 35% (42). Again, an

TABLE 3. Gemfibrozil: effect on lipids and hemostasis after myocardial infarction (from 30)

	BASE	8 WEEKS
Fibrinogen g/l		
GEM	2.35	2.95
Placebo	2.60	2.90
F VII-PL%		
GEM	47.5	19.0**
Placebo	45.0	37.0
tPA Ag (ng/ml)		
GEM	35.0	37.2*
Placebo	44.8	43.8
PAI Ag (ng/ml)		
GEM	47	38**
Placebo	63	60

activity of HMG CoA reductase inhibitors on fibrinolysis has been clearly excluded (20), whereas the most effective drug on PAI-1 is metformin, an antidiabetic-hypotriglyceridemic drug, extensively evaluated by our group (43). In numerous studies in type II diabetics or hyperlipidemic patients metformin has constantly reduced PAI-1 antigen and activity levels (44).

4. Probucol: effects on clotting parameters induced by antioxidation or other mechanisms.

Probucol, a drug active on elevated cholesterol levels (45), has recently been the focus of attention, because of its capacity to apparently improve cardiovascular changes, in spite of a not marked cholesterol lowering activity and of a significant potential to lower HDL (46). Among the properties of probucol, two have been particularly underlined: one is the potential to activate the cholesteryl ester transport protein (CETP) system, thus improving the delivery of tissue cholesterol to lower density lipoproteins for subsequent disposal (47); the other is an interesting antioxidant activity, possibly in play in lipoprotein tissue deposition (48), but on the other hand not supported by studies on pharmacological agents more specifically designed as antioxidants (49). Among additional properties attributed to probucol are: a potential to reduce plasma fibrinogen levels and a selective activity on thromboxane biosynthesis.

In terms of fibrinogen levels, while only scattered reports suggest that this drug may reduce fibrinogenemia in man, an interesting study has been reported in Watanabe heritable hyperlipidemic rabbits (50). This animal strain, well known for the LDL receptor deficiency and for a stably elevated cholesterolemia with early atheromatous lesions, is among others characterized by a constant rise of fibrinogenemia throughout life. Interestingly, Mori et al. could report (Table 4) that probucol, well known to prevent the development of atherosclerotic lesions in this strain (46), without significantly changing serum cholesterol (but reducing HDL cholesterol), can prevent the age dependent increase of fibrinogenemia.

TABLE 4. Probucol reduces fibrinogen, factors IX and VIII in aging WHHL rabbits (from 50)

	(8-month old males Watanabe)	
	Control	*Probucol*
F. IX (%)	742	567**
F. VIII (%)	1052	852**
Fbg (mg/dl)	450	318**

Finally, following up earlier reports indicating that, in some hypercholesterolemic patients probucol may reduce TXB_2 excretion, Di Minno et al. (51), recently evaluated the effect of this drug in a series of patients with cystathionine β-synthase deficiency. This, the most common form of the so called homocystinuria, a frequent cause of early cardiovascular disorders, is characterized by increased TXB_2 excretion (52). In these patients, probucol, in spite of the normal cholesterol levels not changing throughout treatment,   reduced TXB_2 excretion   up to 50%, with an interesting persistence of the effect after drug withdrawal (possibly attributable to the long tissue half-life of the agent). These data provide a clear indication for the use of probucol also in conditions characterized by increased thrombotic risk, although they do not, at present, provide any clue as to mechanism of these changes.

5. References

1. Ross, R (1988) The pathogenesis of atherosclerosis, in E. Braunwald (ed), Heart Disease, WB Saunders Co, Philadelphia, pp 1135-1152.
2. Fuster, V.,   Badimon, L., Cohen, M, Ambrose, J.A., Badimon, J.J. and Chesebro, J.H. (1988) Insights into the pathogenesis of acute ischemic syndromes, Circulation 77, 1213-1220.
3. Meade, T.W., Brozovic, M., Chakrabarti, R.R., Haines, A.P., Jameson, J.D., Mellowes, S., Miller, G.J., North, W.R.S., Stirling, Y. and Thompson, S.G. (1986) Haemostatic function and ischemic heart disease: principal results of the Northwich Park heart study, Lancet II, 533-537.
4. Tremoli, E., Maderna, P., Sirtori, M. and Sirtori, C.R. (1979) Platelet aggregation   and   malondialdehyde function   in type IIa hypercholesterolemic patients, Haemostasis 8, 47-53.
5. Tremoli, E., Maderna, P., Colli, S., Morazzoni, G., Sirtori, M. and Sirtori C.R. (1984) Increased platelet sensitivity and thromboxane B_2 formation in type-II hyperlipoproteinaemic patients, Eur. J. Clin. Invest. 14, 329-333.
6. Tremoli, E., Folco, G.C., Agradi, E. and Galli, C. (1979) Platelet thromboxane and serum cholesterol, Lancet I, 106-107.
7. Oliva, D.W., Maderna, P., Accomazzo, M.R., Nicosia, S. and Tremoli, E. (1989) Iloprost binding and inhibition of aggregation in platelet rich plasma. Differences between normal and type IIa hypercholesterolemic subjects, Biochem. Pharmacol. 38, 39-45.
8. Löbel, P., Steinhagen-Thiessen, E. and Schrör, K. (1988) Cholestyramine treatment of type IIa hypercholesterolemia normalizes platelet reactivity against prostacyclin, Eur. J. Clin. Invest. 18, 256-260.
9. Briones, E.R., Steiger, D., Palumbo, P.J. and Kottke, B.A. (1984) Primary hypercholesterolemia: effect of treatment on serum lipids, lipoprotein fractions, cholesterol absorption, sterol balance and platelet aggregation, Mayo Clin. Proc. 59, 251-257.

10. Zucker, M.L., Trowbridge, C., Krehbiel, P., Jackson, B., Chernoff, S.B. and Dujovne, C.A. (1986) Platelet function in hypercholesterolaemics before and after hypolipidemic drug therapy, Haemostasis 16, 57-64.
11. Schrör, K., Löbel, P. and Steinhagen-Thiessen, E. (1989) Simvastatin reduces platelet - thromboxane formation and restores normal platelet sensitivity against prostacyclin in type IIa hypercholesterolemia, Eicosanoids 2, 39-45.
12. Davì, G., Averna, M., Novo, S., Barbagallo, C.M., Mogavero, A., Notarbartolo, A. and Strano, A. (1989) Effects of synvinolin on platelet aggregation and thromboxane B_2 synthesis in type IIa hypercholesterolemic patients, Atherosclerosis 79, 79-83.
13. Crepaldi, G., Baggio, G., Arca, M., Avellone, G., Avogaro, P., Bittolo Bon, G., Bompiani, G.D., Capurso, A., Cattin, L., D'Alò, G., Descovich, G.C., Feruglio, F.S., Gaddi, A., Gnasso, A., Liberatore, S., Lupattelli, G., Mancini, M., Miccoli R., Muggeo, M., Muntoni, S., Navalesi, R., Patrizi, G.F., Pintus, F., Querena, M., Resta, F., Ricci, G., Segato, T., Sirtori, C.R., Sirtori, M. and Ventura, A. (1991) Pravastatin vs gemfibrozil in the treatment of primary hypercholesterolemia, Arch. Int. Med. 151, 146-152.
14. Sirtori, C.R. (1990) Pharmacology and mechanism of action of the new HMG-CoA reductase inhibitors, Pharmacol. Res., 22, 555-563.
15. Davì, G., Averna, M., Catalano, I., Barbagallo, C., Ganci, A., Notarbartolo, A., Ciabattoni, G. and Patrono, C. (1992) Increased thromboxane biosynthesis in type IIa hypercholesterolemia, Circulation 85, 1792-1798.
16. Schick, B.P. and Schick, P.K. (1985) The effect of hypercholesterolemia on guinea pig platelets, erythrocytes and megakaryocytes, Biochim. Biophys. Acta 833, 291-302.
17. Nordfang, O., Bjorn, S.E., Valentin, S., Nielsen, L.S., Wildgoose, P., Beck, T.C. and Hedner, U. (1991) The C-terminus of tissue factor pathway inhibitor is essential to its anticoagulant activity, Biochemistry 30, 10371-10376.
18. Broze, G.J. jr, Warren, L.A., Novotny, W.F., Higuchi, D.A., Girard, J.J. and Miletich, J.P. (1988) The lipoprotein-associated coagulation inhibitor that inhibits factor VII - tissue factor complex also inhibits Xa: insight into its possible mechanism of action, Blood 71, 335-343.
19. Rapaport, S. (1991) The extrinsic pathway inhibitor: a regulator of tissue factor-dependent blood coagulation, Thromb. Haemost. 66, 6-15.
20. Sandset, P.M., Lund, H., Norseth, J. Abildgaard, U. and Ose, L. (1991) Treatment with hydroxymethylglutaryl-coenzyme A reductase inhibitors in hypercholesterolemia induces changes in the components of the extrinsic coagulation system, Arteriosclerosis and Thrombosis 11, 138-145.
21. Hertz, R., Bar-Tana, J., Sujatta, M., Pill, J., Schmidt, E.H. and Fahimi, H.D. (1988) The induction of liver peroxisomal proliferation by β, β'-methyl-substituted hexadecanedioic acid (MEDICA 16), Biochem. Pharmacol. 37, 3571-3577.

22.Issemann, I. and Green S. (1990) Activation of a member of the steroid hormone receptor superfamily by peroxisome proliferators, Nature 347, 645-649.
23.Aoyama, T., Hardwick, J.P., Imaoka, S., Funae, Y., Gelboin H.V. and Gonzalez, F.J. (1990) Clofibrate-inducible rat hepatic P450s IVA1 and IVA3 catalyze the ω -and (ω-1)-hydroxylation of fatty acids and the ω-hydroxylation of prostaglandins E_1 and $F_2\alpha$, J. Lipid Res. 31, 1477, 1482.
24.Sirtori, C.R. and Franceschini, G. (1988) Effects of fibrates on serum lipids and atherosclerosis, Pharmacol. Ther. 37, 167-191.
25.Patsch, J.R., Prasad, S., Gotto, A.M. jr and Bengtsson-Olivecrona, G. (1984) Postprandial lipemia. A key for the conversion of high density lipoprotein 2 into high density lipoprotein 3 by hepatic lipase, J. Clin. Invest. 74, 2017-2023.
26.Franceschini, G., Calabresi, L., Maderna, P., Galli, C., Gianfranceschi, G. and Sirtori, C.R. (1991) $\omega-3$ fatty acids selectively raise high-density lipoprotein 2 levels in healthy volunteers, Metabolism 40, 1283-1286.
27.Phillips, D.R., Charo, I.F., Parise, L.V. and Fitzgerald, L.A. (1988) The platelet membrane glycoprotein IIb-IIIa complex, Blood 71, 831-843.
28.Cook, N.S. and Ubben, D. (1990) Fibrinogen as a major risk factor in cardiovascular disease, TIPS 11, 444-451.
29.Leschke, M. (1992) Fibrinogen-pathogenetical and therapeutical implications in atherosclerosis XI Int. Symposium on "Drugs Affecting Lipid Metabolism", Florence, Italy May 13-16, pp. 4
30.Andersen, P., Smith, P., Seljeflot, I, Brataker, S. and Arnesen, H. (1990) Effects of gemfibrozil on lipids and haemostasis after myocardial infarction, Thromb. Haemost. 63, 174-177.
31.Niort, G., Bulgarelli, A., Cassader, M. and Pagano, G. (1988) Effect of short term treatment with bezafibrate on plasma fibrinogen, fibrinopeptide. A platelet activation and blood filterability in atherosclerotic hyperfibrinogenemic patients, Atherosclerosis 71, 113-119.
32.Pazzucconi, F., Mannucci, L., Mussoni, L., Gianfranceschi, G., Maderna, P., Franceschini, G., Sirtori, C.R. and Tremoli, E. (1992) Bezafibrate lowers plasma lipids, fibrinogen and platelet aggregability in hypertriglyceridemic patients, Eur.J. Clin. Pharmacol. in press.
33.Okazaki, M., Suzuki, M. and Oguchi, K. (1990) Changes in coagulative and fibrinolytic activities in Triton WR-1339 induced hyperlipidemia in rats, Japan J. Pharmacol. 52, 353-361.
34.Ernst, E., Saradeth, T. and Achhammer, G., (1991) N-3 fatty acids and acute-phase proteins, Eur. J. Clin. Invest. 21, 77-82.
35.De Carvalho, A.C., Colman, R.W. and Lees, R.S. (1974) Clofibrate reversal of platelet hypersensitivity in hyperbetalipoproteinemia, Circulation 50, 570-74.

36.von Schacky, C., Fischer, S. and Weber, P.C. (1985) Long-term effects of dietary marine ω-3 fatty acids upon plasma and cellular lipids, platelet function, and eicosanoid formation in humans, J. Clin. Invest. 76, 1626-1631.
37.Sirtori, C.R., Franceschini, G., Gianfranceschi, G., Sirtori, M., Montanari, G., Tremoli, E., Maderna, P., Colli, S. and Zoppi, F. (1987) Effects of gemfibrozil on plasma lipoprotein-apolipoprotein distribution and platelet-reactivity in patients with hypertriglyceridemia, J. Lab. Clin. Med. 110, 279-286.
38.Mehta, J., Mehta, P., Lawson, D. and Saldeen, T. (1987) Plasma tissue plasminogen activator inhibitor levels in coronary artery disease: correlation with age and serum triglyceride concentrations, J. Am. Coll. Cardiol. 9, 263-268.
39.Juhan-Vague, I., Vague, P., Alessi, M.C., Badier, C., Valadier, J., Aillaud, M.F. and Atlan, C. (1987) Relationships between plasma insulin, triglyceride, body mass index and plasminogen activator inhibitor 1, Diabete Metab. 13, 331-336.
40.Reaven, G.M. (1988) Role of insulin resistance in human disease, Diabetes 37, 1595-1607.
41.Fumeron, F., Brigant, L., Ollivier, V., de Prost, D., Driss, F., Darcet, P., Bard, J.M., Parra, H.J. Fruchart, J.C. and Apfelbaum, M. (1991) N-3 polyunsaturated fatty acids raise low-density lipoproteins, high-density lipoprotein 2, and plasminogen-activator inhibitor in healthy young men, Am. J. Clin. Nutr. 54, 118-122.
42.Satoshi, F. and Burton, E.S. (1992) Direct effects of gemfibrozil on the fibrinolytic system: diminution of synthesis of plasminogen activator inhibitor type I, Circulation 85, 1888-1893.
43.Montanari, G., Bondioli, A., Rizzato, G., Puttini, M., Tremoli, E., Mussoni, L., Mannucci, L., Pazzucconi, F. and Sirtori, C.R. (1992) Treatment with low dose metformin in patients with peripheral vascular disease, Pharmacol. Res. 25, 63-73.
44.Vague, P., Juhan-Vague, I., Alessi, M.C., Badier, C. and Valadier, J. (1987) Metformin decreases the high plasminogen inhibition capacity, plasma insulin and triglyceride levels in non-diabetic obese subjects, Thromb. Haemost 57, 326-328.
45.Buckley, M.M.T., Goa, K.L., Price, A.H. and Brogden, R.N. (1989) Probucol, a reappraisal of its pharmacological properties and therapeutic use in hypercholesterolemia, Drugs 37, 761-800.
46.Carew, T.E., Schwenke, D.C. and Steinberg, D. (1987) Antiatherogenic effect of probucol unrelated to its hypocholesterolemic effect: evidence that antioxidants in vivo can selectively inhibit low density lipoprotein degradation in macrophage rich fatty streaks slowing the progression of atherosclerosis in the WHHL rabbit, Proc. Natl. Acad. Sci. USA 84, 7725-7729.

47. Franceschini, G., Chiesa, G. and Sirtori, C.R. (1991) Probucol increases cholesteryl ester transfer protein activity in hypercholesterolaemic patients, Eur. J. Clin. Invest. 21, 384-388.
48. Parthasarathy, S., Young, S.G., Witztum, J.L., Pittman, R.C. and Steinberg, D. (1986) Probucol inhibits oxidative modification of low density lipoprotein, J. Clin. Invest. 77, 641-644.
49. Mao, S.J.T., Yates, M.T., Parker, R.A., Chi, E.M. and Jackson, R.L. (1991) Attenuation of atherosclerosis in a modified strain of hypercholesterolemic Watanabe rabbits with use of a probucol analogue (MDL 29, 311) that does not lower serum cholesterol, Arteriosclerosis and Thrombosis 11, 1266-1275.
50. Mori, Y., Wada, H., Nagano, Y, Deguchi, K., Kita, T. and Shirakawa, S. (1989) Hypercoagulable state in the Watanabe heritable hyperlipidemic rabbit, an animal model for the progression of atherosclerosis - Effect of probucol on coagulation, Thromb. Haemostas. 61, 140-143.
51. Di Minno, G., Davì, G., Margaglione, M., Cirillo, F., Ciabattoni, G., and Patrono, C. (1992) Enhanced thromboxane biosynthesis in homozygous cystathionine β-synthase deficiency, Clin. Res. 40, 202a.
52. Vesterqvist, O. and Green, K. (1984) Urinary excretion of 2,3-dinor-thromboxane B_2 in man under normal conditions, following drugs and during some pathological conditions, Prostaglandins 27, 627-644.

LIPID LOWERING: PROGRESSION AND REGRESSION OF ATHEROSCLEROTIC LESIONS

David H. Blankenhorn and the MARS and CLAS Study Groups

Abstract

Two clinical trials with identical <u>coronary</u> and <u>carotid</u> end points indicate that aggressive reduction of blood <u>lipoprotein</u> level can induce beneficial change throughout the range of the <u>atherosclerotic process</u>. The drug treatments tested were combined <u>colestipol/niacin</u> and <u>lovastatin</u>. The data are most convincing for intrusive coronary lesions. There are also clear indications of benefit to very early pre-intrusive carotid lesions in men from CLAS and encouraging results from a small number of women in MARS.

Introduction

Seven randomized clinical trials testing lipid lowering therapy have reported beneficial change by coronary angiography.
Intrusive lesions have been evaluated with a variety of end point measurements in the seven trials. Two of the seven, the Cholesterol Lowering Atherosclerosis Study (CLAS) (1) and the Program on Surgical Control of Hyperlipoproteinemia, POSCH (2), reported a global coronary score (GCS). GCS is a consensus score obtained by expert angiographers. It reflects change in the overall status of the coronary tree. GCS has been shown to predict later coronary events (3).

A. L. Catapano et al. (eds.), Drugs Affecting Lipid Metabolism, 231–239.
© 1993 Kluwer Academic Publishers and Fondazione Giovanni Lorenzini.

Other trials in progress use ultrasound imaging of the carotid
artery. The target lesions are generally in the internal carotid
artery or at the bifurcation of the common carotid. It is also
possible to study very early atheroma formation in the distal common
carotid with ultrasound measurements of wall thickness. Common
carotid lesion formation parallels that in coronary artery, but
after a lag period (4). Wall thickness measurements of the distal
common carotid artery offer an opportunity to look at treatment
effects on very early lesions which do not intrude into the vessel
lumen. Two trials, CLAS which tested colestipol\niacin treatment,
and the Mevinolin (Lovastatin) Atherosclerosis Study (MARS) have end
point data which span the range of atherosclerosis from
pre-intrusive carotid wall thickening to advanced intrusive coronary
lesions. This report on CLAS and MARS includes coronary GCS results
because this measure includes all lesions, even the most advanced
(5). It also includes ultrasound measurements of intima-media
thickness of the distal common carotid artery (6), a measure of very
early atherosclerosis.

Details of CLAS and MARS

CLAS was a randomized, controlled clinical trial in non-smoking men
with previous coronary bypass surgery (7). Target vessels were
chosen to provide as complete a survey of atherosclerosis as
possible, consistent with patient safety. Femoral, coronary, and
cervical vessel beds were visualized in 162 patients at baseline and
after two treatment years (CLAS-I), and in a subset of 101 patients
after four years (CLAS-II). Carotid B-mode images were recorded at
four month intervals. CLAS showed strong evidence for therapy
benefit in coronary arteries at two years (1) and four years (8).
Femoral angiographic results at two years have indicated therapy
benefits which are significant but less consistent than coronary
(9). Table 1 summarizes baseline-four year lipid levels in CLAS
subjects.

TABLE 1. Baseline, and On-Trial Lipid and Apolipoprotein
Levels for 101 Patients Completing CLAS-I AND CLAS-II.
(n = 56 Drug; 45 Placebo)1

Lipid/ Apo	Group	Baseline2	CLAS-I	CLAS-II P-Value5
Total-C (mmol/L)6	D	6.37 [.10]3	4.61 [.08] (-27%)4	4.77 [.10] <0.001 (-25%)
	P	6.30 [.13]	6.04 [.13] (-4%)	5.93 [.10] (-6%)
LDL-C (mmol/L)	D	4.43 [.10]	2.49 [.08] (-43%)	2.62 [.08] <0.001 (-40%)
	P	4.33 [.10]	4.17 [.10] (-4%)	4.07 [.10] (- 6%)
HDL-C (mmol/L)	D	1.14 [.03]	1.55 [.05] (37%)	1.55 [.05] <0.001 (37%)
	P	1.14 [.03]	1.17 [.03] (2%)	1.17 [.03] (2%)
Trig. (mmol/L)7	D	1.74 [.14]	1.24 [.07] (-22%)	1.28 [.09] <0.03 (-18%)
	P	1.77 [.16]	1.60 [.14] (- 5%)	1.55 [.13] (- 5%)
Apo A-I (mg/dL)	D	121 [2]	139 [2] (16%)	144 [3] <0.001 (21%)
	P	117 [3]	123 [2] (6%)	127 [3] (10%)
Apo B (mg/dL)	D	127 [4]	83 [3] (-33%)	85 [2] <0.001 (-32%)
	P	120 [4]	126 [3] (7%)	118 [3] (- 0%)

1 For apolipoproteins: n = 54 Drug; 45 Placebo. 2 All group
differences at baseline were non-significant. 3 Mean [sem].
4 Percent change (in parentheses) calculated relative to
baseline. 5 P-values are for group differences at two and
four years. 6 Conversion factor for cholesterol is 38.6 mg/dL
1 mmol/L. 7 Conversion factor for triglycerides is 87.6 mg/dL
for 1 mmol/L.

MARS is a prospective, randomized, double-blind, placebo-controlled
trial to evaluate the effect of monotherapy with lovastatin, a
HMG-CoA reductase inhibitor. Progression and regression of coronary
atherosclerosis is assessed by both computerized quantitative
coronary angiography (QCA), as well as by visual human panel reading
of angiograms at baseline and after two and four years of treatment.
In addition, ultrasound measurements of carotid, brachial, and
popliteal vessels to assess peripheral vascular disease are
performed.

Between September, 1985 and January, 1989, 270 participants of both
sexes, aged 21-67 years, were randomized at two centers to diet and
either 40 mg b.i.d. lovastatin or placebo. Subjects were considered
eligible if they had angiographically demonstrable atherosclerosis
in two or more coronary artery segments, unaltered by angioplasty,
with at least one lesion of >50% but <100% stenosis. The inclusion
range for plasma total cholesterol was between 190 - 295 mg/dL (4.9
- 7.6 mmol/L). Ninety-one percent of MARS subjects were male.
Average age was 58 years. Average blood pressure was 125/80 and 22%
were current smokers. Forty-two percent had angina, 51% previous
myocardial infarction.

Lipid, lipoprotein cholesterol and apolipoprotein at baseline and
on-trial MARS are summarized in Table 2.

TABLE 2. Baseline, On-trial, and Percent Change from Baseline in Levels of Plasma Lipids

| | | ----Repeat Angiogram---- | |
		Lovastatin (n = 123)	Placebo (n = 124)
Total Chol	Baseline	5.97 $\pm$ 0.61[1]	6.01 $\pm$ 0.59
(mmol/L)	On-Trial	4.03 $\pm$ 0.45	5.90 $\pm$ 0.68*
	% Change	-32.2 $\pm$ 7.0**	-1.8 $\pm$ 7.5*
LDL-C	Baseline	3.91 $\pm$ 0.62	4.00 $\pm$ 0.64
Friedewald	On-Trial	2.41 $\pm$ 0.42	3.96 $\pm$ 0.63*
(mmol/L)	% Change	-38.0 $\pm$ 12.3**	-0.9 $\pm$ 13.8*
LDL-C	Baseline	4.05 $\pm$ 0.63	4.07 $\pm$ 0.56
ultracent	On-Trial	2.22 $\pm$ 0.41	3.94 $\pm$ 0.61*
(mmol/L)	% Change	-44.7 $\pm$ 9.0**	-3.0 $\pm$ 10.3*
HDL-C	Baseline	1.10 $\pm$ 0.26	1.11 $\pm$ 0.25
(mmol/L)	On-Trial	1.18 $\pm$ 0.25	1.13 $\pm$ 0.24
	% Change	8.5 $\pm$ 10.3**	2.3 $\pm$ 11.9*
Triglyceride	Baseline	1.80 $\pm$ 0.83	1.80 $\pm$ 0.85
(mmol/L)	On-Trial	1.36 $\pm$ 0.25	1.82 $\pm$ 1.07*
	% Change	-21.6 $\pm$ 20.2**	3.5 $\pm$ 26.5*
Apo A-I	Baseline	133.4 $\pm$ 29.5	130.4 $\pm$ 28.9
(mg/dL)	On-Trial	132.5 $\pm$ 19.8	128.5 $\pm$ 20.8
	% Change	3.1 $\pm$ 21.8	2.2 $\pm$ 24.1
Apo B	Baseline	110.1 $\pm$ 25.1	109.0 $\pm$ 23.7
(mg/dL)	On-Trial	78.2 $\pm$ 13.5	115.6 $\pm$ 19.0*
	% Change	-26.0 $\pm$ 19.3**	11.2 $\pm$ 32.4*

1 Mean $\pm$ sd, * p <0.01, ** p <0.001

Coronary Angiographic Results in CLAS and MARS

GCS results in CLAS and MARS at two years were remarkably similar. Both trials showed a significant therapy effect. In CLAS, GCS scores were +0.3 Drug and +0.8 Placebo (p=0.007). In MARS, GCS scores were +0.4 Drug and +0.9 Placebo (p=0.002). These results are comparable to those which were obtained at three years in POSCH, where ileal bypass treated subjects progressed with a score of 0.3 and control with a score of 0.8. Table 3 breaks down the GCS scores of MARS by progression/regression categories and by entrance cholesterol level above and below 6.22 mmol/L.

TABLE 3. Analysis of Global Change Score and Change in
Panel-Read Percent Diameter Stenosis (%S)

	Lovastatin (n = 123)	Placebo (n = 123)	p
Global Change Score (GCS)			
Overall (123-L, 123-P)	0.41 ± 1.14[1]	0.88 ± 1.12	0.002[2]
# with GCS < 0 (non-progression)	65 (53%)	43 (35%)	0.053
# with GCS < 0 (regression)	28 (23%)	13 (11%)	0.05
# with GCS > 0 (progression)	58 (47%)	80 (65%)	0.007
GCS Stratified by Baseline TC			
TC < 6.22 mmol/L (82-L, 76-P)	0.39 ± 1.13	0.74 ± 1.09	0.053
TC > 6.22 mmol/L (41-L, 47-P)	0.46 ± 1.19	1.11 ± 1.15	0.01

[1] Mean ± sd

[2] Wilcoxon rank sum test (two-tailed)

Carotid Ultrasound Results from CLAS and MARS

A transducer with 9 MHz central frequency was used in both trials.
Longitudinal views were recorded in anterior and lateral positions
of near and far walls of the distal 10 mm of the common carotid
artery. This area is reported to have least measurement variability
(6). The distance between characteristic echoes arising from blood
intimal interface and medial-adventitial interface (10) was measured
with a 386/33 computer and inhouse software. Variability in
computer measurement of intima-media wall thickness in 20 subjects
showed intra-operator and inter-operator correlations of 0.97.
Coefficients of variation within operators was 3.0% and between
operators was 3.1%. Table 4 summarizes baseline, two and four year
results in 46 subjects with coronary and cervical angiograms and
matching ultrasound examinations

TABLE 4. Carotid Ultrasound Measurements in CLAS

	Drug (n=24)		Placebo (n=22)		P-value[1]
Far Wall Thickness					
Baseline (BL)	0.64	(0.10)[2]	0.60	(0.11)	0.25
Year 2	0.59	(0.08)	0.64	(0.13)	0.11
Year 4	0.58	(0.09)	0.67	(0.15)	0.03
Change					
Yr 2 − BL	−0.05	(0.05)	0.04	(0.06)	<0.0001
Yr 4 − BL	−0.05	(0.07)	0.07	(0.09)	<0.0001
Yr 4 − Yr 2	−0.01	(0.05)	0.03	(0.06)	0.06
Average Diameter					
Baseline	6.47	(0.52)	6.36	(0.74)	0.58
Year 2	6.38	(0.61)	6.56	(0.55)	0.30
Year 4	6.31	(0.70)	6.52	(0.59)	0.29
Change					
Yr 2 − BL	−0.09	(0.61)	−0.19	(0.64)	0.13
Yr 4 − BL	−0.16	(0.62)	0.15	(0.55)	0.08
Yr 4 − Yr 2	−0.07	(0.60)	−0.04	(0.44)	0.87

[1] t test, two-tailed

[2] mean (standard deviation)

These are the first controlled clinical trial results indicating
that the pre-intrusive stage of atherosclerosis can be improved with
drug therapy. Reduction of blood cholesterol level is known to
induce generalized endothelial-dependent vessel relaxation (11,12)
and this may have occurred to a greater extent in treated drug
subjects in CLAS. However, it cannot account for the reduction in
wall thickness. Table 4 indicates a nonsignificant trend in a
direction opposite to that expected if reduction in wall thickness
were due to vessel wall stretching with increase in lumen diameter.
CLAS findings are limited to non-smoking men treated aggressively
with colestipol-niacin. They do not apply to stenotic carotid
disease as imaged by ultrasound and angiography or detected by
Doppler ultrasound flow patterns.

To extend information on treatment of pre-intrusive lesions we have
examined baseline and two year ultrasound images from women in MARS.
Fifteen women were enrolled in the University of Southern California
clinic where ultrasound imaging was performed. Seven drug treated
women showed significant wall thinning (p=0.01) compared to eight
placebo treated women. Ultrasound images from male MARS subjects
have not been analyzed.

Conclusions

Together, the CLAS and MARS trials suggest that aggressive reduction
of blood lipoprotein level can induce beneficial change through out
the range of the atherosclerotic process. The data is most complete
for advanced intrusive coronary lesion. There are clear indications
of benefit to very early pre-intrusive carotid lesions from CLAS and
encouraging results from a small number of women included in MARS.

References

1.   Blankenhorn, D.H., Nessim, S.A., Johnson, R.L.,
Sanmarco, M.E., Azen S.P., Chasin-Hemphill, L. (1987) 'Beneficial
effects of combined colestipol-niacin therapy therapy on coronary
atherosclerosis and coronary venous bypass grafts', JAMA 257,
3233-3240.

2.   Buchwald, H., Varcom R.L., Matts, J.P., et al. (1990) 'Effect
of partial ileal bypass surgery on mortality and morbidity from
coronary heart disease in patients with hypercholesterolemia.
Report of the Program on the Surgical Control of the Hyperlipidemias
(POSCH)', N Engl J Med 323, 946-955.

3.   Buchwald, H., Matts, J,P., Fitch, L.L., Stamler, J., and the
POSCH Group (1991), 'Clinical prognostic significance of serial
changes in coronary angiograms: Ten year data from the Program on
the Surgical Control of the Hyperlipidemias (POSCH)', (Abstract),
Circulation 84, II-286.

4.   Solberg, L.A., McGarry, P.A., Moosy, J., Strong, J.P., Tejada,
C., Loken, A (1968) 'Severity of atherosclerosis in in cerebral
arteries, coronary arteries, and aortas', Ann NY Acad Sci 149,
956-973.

5.   Azen, S.P., Cashin-Hemphill, L., Pogoda, J., et al. (1991)
'Evaluation of human panelists in assessing coronary of human
panelists in assessing coronary atherosclerosis', Arterioscler
Thromb 11, 385-394.

6.   O'Leary, D.H., Polak, J.F., Wolfson, S.K. Jr., et al.   (1991)
'Use of sonography to evaluate carotid atherosclerosis in the
elderly.   The Cardiovascular Health Study.   CHS Collaborative
Research Group', Stroke 22, 1155-1163.

7.   Blankenhorn, D.H., Johnson, R.L., Nessim, S.A., Azen, S.P.,
Sanmarco, M.E., Selzer, R.H. (1987) 'The Cholesterol Lowering
Atherosclerosis Study (CLAS): Design, Methods, and Baseline
Results', Controlled Clinical Trials 8, 354-387.

8.   Cashin-Hemphill, L., Mack, W.J., Pogoda, J.M., Sanmarco, M.E.,
Azen, S.P., Blankenhorn, D.H. (1990) 'Beneficial effects of
colestipol-niacin on coronary atherosclerosis.   A 4-year follow-up',
JAMA 264, 3013-3017.

9.   Blankenhorn, D.H., Azen, S.P., Crawford, D.W., et al.   (1991)
'Effects of colestipol-niacin therapy on human femoral femoral
atherosclerosis', Circulation 83, 438-447.

10.   Pignoli, P., Tremoli, E., Poli, A., Oreste, P., Paoletti, R.
(1986) 'Intimal plus medial thickness of the arterial wall: a direct
measurement with ultrasound imaging', Circulation 74, 1399-1406.

11.   Farrar, D.J., Green, H.D., Wagner, W.D., Bond, M.G.   (1980)
'Reduction in pulse wave velocity and improvement of aortic
distensibility accompanying regression of atherosclerosis in the
rhesus monkey', Cir Res 47, 425-432

12.   Shimokawa, H. and Vanhoutte, P.M. (1989) 'Hypercholesterolemia
causes generalized impairment of endothelium-dependent relaxation to
aggregating platelets in porcine arteries', J Am Coll Cardiol 13,
1402-1408.

Clinical Trials of Atherosclerosis Regression

Barry Lewis

Abstract

Ten trials, employing twelve different interventions by
diets, drugs or surgery, have assessed the effects of lipid
lowering on the course of coronary atherosclerosis. The
outcomes are consistent in showing favourable effects on
serial angiography; all revealed a reduced incidence of
progression and most showed increased regression. In many,
these angiographic changes were accompanied by reduced
incidence of clinical coronary events. Underlying mechanisms
may include anatomical regression of lesions, stabilization
of plaques against fissuring and thrombotic occlusion, and
restoration of impaired endothelium-dependent
vasodilatation. The trials support the lipid hypothesis of
atherosclerosis and affirm the value of the treatments
studied.

Introduction

Complementary to the twenty-four trials of lipid-lowering on
clinical coronary heart disease end-points, ten major trials
have been completed in which serial angiography has been
employed to study effects of lipid lowering on the evolution
of coronary atherosclerosis. Further trials have employed
angiography or ultrasound to investigate femoral and carotid
artery disease. This review concerns the outcomes and
implications of several of the fully-published coronary
angiographic trials, the essential features of which are
shown in Table 1. The CLAS and MARS trials are considered
further in the accompanying contribution by Dr D.H.
Blankenhorn.

Outcome Data

The trials reviewed have been remarkably consistent in their
results (Table 1). All have indicated that lowering of the
serum cholesterol level is associated with reduced
progression of coronary artery disease. This is evident from
the randomised controlled trials [2-9], from an uncontrolled
study [1] and from one employing a non-randomised comparison
group [10]. Progression is defined as an increase in

241

A. L. Catapano et al. (eds.), Drugs Affecting Lipid Metabolism, 241–249.
© 1993 Kluwer Academic Publishers and Fondazione Giovanni Lorenzini.

narrowing at the site of a coronary lesion relative to
adjacent artery (percentage diameter stenosis or percentage
area stenosis) or as a decrease in absolute diameter of a
coronary segment or in absolute minimum diameter of a
stenosis. Both visual assessment panels and quantitative
image analysis have been employed.

In the active treatment groups of the controlled
trials, regression (angiographic change in the opposite
direction) has been almost equally consistent (Table 1),
though it did not achieve statistical significance in two
studies.

The trials, therefore, confirm the impression obtained
from numerous case reports (for review, see ref 11), and
from autopsy series during wartime nutritional deprivation
[12], that reduction of lipid and perhaps other risk factors
favourably modifies the progressive natural history of
atherosclerosis. The extent of angiographic changes
described in these trials is small, and its haemodynamic
significance has justifiably been questioned. For this
reason it is important to note (last column in Table 1) that
in several trials the favourable angiographic outcome was
associated with significant reduction in clinical coronary
events.

Evidence of benefit was consistent, too, among the
several visual and image-analysis end-points used, among
findings in native coronary arteries and in saphenous vein
bypass grafts [3,4], and among the large number of lipid-
lowering interventions employed. One plausible explanation
of the high concordance of outcomes is that lipid-lowering
therapy has been highly effective in the regression trials
(serum cholesterol reduction 14-31%, LDL-cholesterol
reduction 16-46%). This in turn is likely to be a function
of the smaller size of regression trials than clinical event
trials, permitting closer supervision of compliance.

Types Of Therapy, Lipoprotein Changes, And Outcome

In the trials tabulated (two of which [5,9], each had two
intervention groups), eleven distinct though overlapping,
treatments were used to lower plasma lipid levels. A twelfth
is reviewed in Blankenhorn's companion chapter. The
similarity in outcome between these trials makes it unlikely
that the reduction in progression and increase in regression
are treatment-specific; rather, these results were mediated
by intermediate effects common to the several interventions
employed.

Table 2 summarises the main effects of these
interventions on plasma lipids and lipoproteins. The
consistent lipoprotein change accompanying the favourable

Table 1. Main features of published coronary angiographic trials.

	Selection	Entered n	Completed n	Duration m	Design*	Treatment	ΔSC (ΔLC)	Progression	Outcome Regression	Events
								αSC:HC		
Leiden[1]	CHD	53	39	24	Uncontrolled QCA	Vegetarian diet, P:S 2.5	17(26)			→ NS
NHLBI[2]	CHD	143	116	60	RCT, DB Visual	Cholestyramine		↓	←	
CLAS[3,4]	CABG C>4.8	188	162 / 103	24 / 48	RCT, SB Visual Grafts + C.A.	Colestipol and nicotinic acid	26(43) / 25(40)	↓ ↓	← ←	
FATS[5]	CHD + family history ApoB>125	146	120	32	RCT QCA	Colestipol + lovastatin or nicotinic acid	32(46) / 22(32)	↓ ↓	← ←	→→ →
POSCH[6]	CHD C>5.7	838	696-175	116	RCT Visual	Partial ileal bypass	23(37)	↓		→
FH[7]	FH(het) CAD	126	72	26	RCT QCA	Colestipol nicotinic acid Lovastatin	31(38)	↓	←	
Lifestyle[8]	CHD	96/48	41	15	RCT QCA	Vegetarian hypocaloric diet; exercise; stress man 'gt		↓	←	→ AP
STARS[9]	CHD C>6	90	74	38	RCT QCA End-pt-blinded	Diet or Diet + cholestyramine	14(16) / 25(36)	↓ ↓	← ←	→→
Homburg[10]	CAD C>6.8	65	42	21	non-RCT QCA	Fenofibrate	19(20)	↓	←	

* QCA = quantitative coronary angiography; RCT = randomized controlled trial; DB = double-blind; CA = coronary arteries; C = cholesterol; CAD = coronary artery disease; FH = familial hypercholesterolaemia; ΔSC ΔLC = difference in serum cholesterol, LDL cholesterol.

effect on progression/regression was a decrease in LDL-
cholesterol. Serum triglyceride decreased in some studies
but increased in others; HDL-cholesterol increased in most
but not in all trials showing benefit. Estimates of
association between ambient lipoprotein levels and
angiographic progression have consistently shown significant
direct correlations with LDL-cholesterol [2-9]. Progression
has also been correlated with serum cholesterol: HDL-
cholesterol ratio [1] and was more evident in patients with
low HDL levels in the NHLBI trial [2] and in the 2-year
report of the CLAS trial [3]. Associations between
triglyceride levels and progression have not been reported,
but in the STARS trial IDL-cholesterol was directly related
to progression.

Which Lesions Respond To Lipid Lowering?

In the STARS trial, the angiographic outcome was separately
analysed in 489 coronary segments according to the extent of
stenoses present at baseline, i.e. <15%, 15-50%, and >50%
baseline stenoses. As in the CLAS and FATS trials, the

Table 2. Lipoprotein changes during trials.

	Progression	LDL-C	Triglyceride	HDL-C
Lifestyle	↓	↓	↑	→
STARS diet diet + ch'styramine	↓ ↓	↓ ↓	↓ NC →	→ →
CLAS 2y	↓	⇓	↓	↑
CLAS 4y	↓	⇓	↓	↑ NC
NHLBI	↓	↓	↑	↑
FH	↓	⇓	↓	↑
POSCH	↓	⇓	↑	↑
FATS lovastatin– colestipol nicotinic acid–colestipol	↓ ↓	⇓ ⇓	↓ NS ↓	↑ ⇑
Homburg	↓	↓	↓	↑ NS

NS = not significant
NC = no correlation with progression

greatest treatment effect was seen in segments with >50%
stenoses. However, segments with 15-50% stenoses, (which are
known to be the commonest precursors of acute coronary
events [13]) also showed reduced progression and increased
regression, by all four angiographic criteria employed, in
the treatment groups in STARS.

Diet And Atheroma Regression

A characteristic diet is an invariable feature of
populations with high CHD mortality rates, high in energy,
saturated fat and cholesterol, and relatively poor in fibre-
rich carbohydrate foods. Replacement of this diet by various
cholesterol-lowering diets has been studied in three
coronary angiographic trials, providing tests of the dietary
lipid hypothesis. In the uncontrolled Leiden Study the diet
was vegetarian and had a high P:S ratio of 2.54; it lowered
serum cholesterol 10.1% and increased serum cholesterol:HDL
cholesterol ratio by 8.5%. The Lifestyle Heart Trial [8]
diet was also almost exclusively vegetarian, had an
extremely low fat content (6.8% energy) and cholesterol
content (12.4 mg/day), and was associated with 24.3% serum
cholesterol reduction and 10.1 kg weight loss. Diet was one
of several interventions in this trial. Favourable
angiographic changes occurred in both trials.
        By contrast the regime employed in the dietary limb of
the STARS trial [9] was comparatively moderate, including
all usual food groups, providing 27% energy from fat, 100 mg
cholesterol per 1000 kcals, P:S ratio 0.8, and increased
soluble fibre-containing foods. Plasma cholesterol decreased
14.2% in the diet group (2% in control group) and body
weight changed little.
        In the STARS diet group, coronary lesions showed
significant regression by per-segment analysis; and on a
per-patient basis, 38% of subjects in the diet group showed
overall regression, (4% in the usual care group, p<0.02).
Progression occurred in 15% of the diet group subjects and
in 46% of usual care subjects. There were 10 clinical
cardiovascular events (hard end-points only) in the usual
care group, three in the diet group (p<0.06) and one in the
diet and cholestyramine group (p<0.01). The STARS results,
in a randomised controlled end-point blinded trial of diet
as the only intervention, offer strong support for the view
that a high saturated fat, high cholesterol diet plays a
powerful causal role in coronary atherosclerosis.

Conclusions From The Progression/Regression Trials

Coronary 'regression' trials have, to date, been based upon

arteriography, and are therefore studies of visual or
quantified changes in coronary lumen. Treatment effects on
atheroma volume, and especially on plaque composition and on
endothelial integrity are as yet unknown. That angiographic
benefit reflects regression or reduced progression of
atherosclerosis, at least in part, is based on the analogy
with regression, documented histopathologically, in
comparable studies of lipid lowering in atherosclerotic
primates and other animals [14,15]. Ultrasound carotid
studies, and intra-coronary luminal ultrasound, will in due
course test this inference.

There is growing evidence that a further mechanism may
contribute to angiographic benefit. Endothelium-dependent
vasodilatation responses are modulated by LDL, being
impaired by experimental hypercholesterolaemia [16] and
restored by a low fat diet [17]. The direction and magnitude
of the response of human coronary arteries to intraluminal
acetylcholine is related to LDL-cholesterol levels [18]:
with higher cholesterol levels, dilatation is attenuated and
replaced by constriction. Since angiographic change has been
documented after only 15 months, in the Lifestyle Trial, a
rapidly-acting mechanism, such as lipoprotein effects on the
EDRF response, becomes credible.

In the two regression trials in which absolute changes
in diameter have been reported (Leiden and STARS), few
coronary segments changed by more than ± 0.5 mm (in 2 or 3.2
years respectively). In STARS, the lesions with >50%
baseline stenoses become wider (Δ MinAWS) by 0.25 to 0.42
mm. The haemodynamic effects of such changes are probably
usually modest. Nevertheless, hard clinical coronary event
rates decreased, in parallel with favourable angiographic
changes, in POSCH, and in both intervention groups of FATS
and STARS, and in MARS. Speculative reasons for this
parallelism may be offered. One is that haemodynamic
improvement is indeed of benefit, mediated by regression or
restored vasomotion. Lesser thrombotic tendency is possible
although, in STARS, angiographic change was not
significantly associated with mean plasma fibrinogen. A
plausible further possibility is that regression is
associated with stabilization of the plaque against
fissuring of the fibrous cap with acute thrombotic
consequences. Lipid-rich plaques with thin fibrous caps are
most prone to this process [19]. In primates, the regression
induced by lipid lowering comprises lipid depletion, with
some reversion of endothelial changes. but at most, modest
reduction in collagen [20]. Hence angiographic improvement
may be a marker for more subtle compositional change that
reduces the risk of plaque fissuring.

Future Regression Trials: What Shall We Learn?

Direct serial assessment of arterial disease by controlled trial is informative both as a test of the lipid hypothesis (see foregoing) and in the assessment of a therapeutic intervention. For the former purpose additional trials are hardly necessary: as discussed in an earlier section the outcome was consistently favourable with twelve distinct lipid-lowering therapies, establishing a highly reproducible relation between LDL-lowering, reduced progression, and (in most) increased regression.

For the second purpose, however, increased use of quantitative coronary angiographic trials is likely. Not only is arterial disease regression an informative end-point in its own right; also, the five interventions studied in FATS, STARS, and MARS all led to parallel reductions in arterial disease progression and in clinical cardiac events. Hence regression trials (which are relatively inexpensive, rapid and small, the latter feature being also conducive to high compliance) can provide an initial assessment of the value of new lipid-lowering or artery-protective therapies.

1. Arntzenius, AC, Kromhout, D, Barth JD, et al. (1985) 'Diet, lipoproteins, and the progression of coronary atherosclerosis', N Engl J Med 312, 805-811.
2. Brensike, JF, Levy, RI, Kelsey, SF, et al. (1984) 'Effects of therapy with cholestyramine on progression of coronary atherosclerosis: results of the NHLBI type II coronary intervention study', Circulation 69, 313-324.
3. Blankenhorn, DH, Nessim, SA, Johnson, RL, Sanmarco, ME, Azen, SP, and Cashin-Hemphill L. (1987) 'Beneficial effects of combined colestipol-niacin therapy on coronary atherosclerosis and coronary venous bypass grafts', JAMA 257, 3233-3240.
4. Cashin-Hemphill, L, Mack, WJ, Pogoda, JM, et al. (1990) 'Beneficial effects of colestipol-niacin on coronary atherosclerosis. A 4-year follow-up', JAMA 264, 3013-3017.
5. Brown, BG, Albers, JJ, Fisher, ID, et al. (1990) 'Regression of coronary artery disease as a result of aggressive lipid lowering in men with high levels of apolipoprotein B', N Engl J Med 323, 1289-1298.
6. Buchwald, H, Varco, RL, Matts, JP, et al. (1990) 'Effect of partial ileal bypass surgery on mortality and morbidity from coronary heart

disease in patients with hypercholesterolemia.
Report of the Program on the Surgical Control of
the Hyperlipidemias (POSCH)', N Engl J Med 323,
946-955.

7.   Kane, JP, Malloy, MJ, Ports, TA, Phillips, NR, Diehl,
     JC, Havel, RJ. (1990) 'Regression of coronary
     atherosclerosis during treatment of familial
     hypercholesterolaemia with combined drug
     regimens', JAMA 264, 1007-1012.

8.   Ornish, D, Brown, SE, Scherwitz, LW, et al. (1990) 'Can
     lifestyle changes reverse coronary heart
     disease?', Lancet 336, 129-133.

9.   Watts, GF, Lewis, B, Brunt, JNM, Lewis, ES, Coltart,
     DJ, Smith, LDR, Mann, JI, Swan, AV. (1992)
     'Effects on coronary artery disease of lipid-
     lowering diet. or diet plus cholestyramine in the
     St Thomas' Atherosclerosis   Regression Study
     (STARS)', Lancet 339, 563-569.

10. Hahmann, HW, Bunte, T, Hellwig, N, et al. (1991)
     'Progression and regression of minor coronary
     arterial narrowings by quantitative angiography
     after fenofibrate therapy', Am J Cardiol 67, 957-
     961.

11. Malinow, MR. (1984) 'Atherosclerosis: progression,
     regression, and resolution', Am Heart J 108, 1523-
     1537.

12. Vartiainen, I, Kanerva, A. (1947) 'Arteriosclerosis and
     wartime', Ann Med Internae Fenniae 36, 748.

13. Ambrose, JA, Tannenbaum, MA. Alexopoulos, D. et al.
     (1988) 'Angiographic progression of coronary
     artery disease and the development of myocardial
     infarction', J Am Coll Cardiol 12, 56-62.

14. Armstrong, ML. (1976) 'Regression of atherosclerosis.
     in: Paoletti R, Gotto AM, eds. Atherosclerosis
     reviews, vol 1. Raven, New York, pp 137-182.

15. Wissler, RW, Vesselinovitch, D. (1976) 'Studies of
     regression of advanced atherosclerosis in
     experimental animals and men', Ann NY Acad Sci
     275, 363-378.

16. Habib, JB, Wells, C, Williams, S, Henry, PD. (1984)
     'Atherosclerosis impairs endothelium-dependent
     arterial relaxation', Circulation 70, 123-126.

17. Harrison, DG, Armstrong, ML, Freiman, PC, Heistad, DD.
     (1987) 'Restoration of endothelium-dependent
     arterial relaxation by dietary treatment of
     atherosclerosis', Circulation 80, 1808-1811.

18. Vita, JA, Treasure, CB, Nabel, EC, et al. (1990)
     'Coronary vasomotor response to acetylcholine
     relates to risk factors for coronary artery

disease', Circulation 81, 491-497.
19.   Richardson, PD, Davies, MJ, Born, GVR. (1989)
          'Influence of plaque configuration and stress
          distribution on fissuring of coronary
          atherosclerotic plaques,' Lancet ii, 941-944.
20.   Armstrong, ML. (1978) 'Connective tissue in
          regression,' Atherosclerosis Reviews 3, 147-166.

BIOCHEMICAL MECHANISMS ASSOCIATED WITH THE LIPOLYTIC EFFECTS OF CALCIUM CHANNEL BLOCKERS

KENNETH B. POMERANTZ, ANDREW C. NICHOLSON, ORLI ETINGIN, BARBARA SUMMERS, AND DAVID P. HAJJAR

ABSTRACT. Calcium channel blockers are now widely used for the treatment of hypertension and angina. However, recent evidence suggests that calcium channel blockers may also be beneficial in controlling processes leading to atherosclerosis. In these studies, we evaluated the effects of two dihydropyridine calcium channel blockers, Nifedipine and Nicardipine on cholesterol metabolism in aortic smooth muscle cells. Nicardipine increased LDL receptor activity that was paralleled by an increase in the steady state level of LDL receptor mRNA. These calcium channel blockers also increased lysosomal and cytoplasmic cholesteryl ester hydrolase activities, but did not alter ACAT activity. Since we have demonstrated that these processes are modulated by prostacyclin (PGI_2) and cyclic AMP, we evaluated the effects of calcium channel blockers on PGI_2 release and cyclic AMP levels. We found that these agents increased both PGI_2 release and cyclic AMP production. Finally, several calcium channel blockers reduced cholesterol content in cholesterol-enriched smooth muscle cells derived from atherosclerotic rabbits, and reduced cholesterol content in aortic biopsies taken from patients undergoing coronary bypass surgery. Taken together, our data demonstrate that calcium channel blockers reduce cholesterol content in vascular tissue by stimulating LDL catabolism through a process that is mediated by PGI_2 and cyclic AMP. Our results engender support for the use of calcium channel blockers as anti-atherosclerotic agents.

1. Introduction

1.1 CONTROL OF CELLULAR CALCIUM CONCENTRATION

The therapeutic efficacy of calcium channel blockers in the treatment of hypertension and angina pectoris is well established. It is believed that calcium channel blockers, which constitute a heterogeneous class of compounds, act by inhibiting or reducing metabolic events that are dependent upon elevated levels of cytoplasmic free calcium. Cytoplasmic calcium concentration is generally very low; calcium entry from the extracellular space into the cytoplasm may occur through three possible routes which are dependent on the cell type and the method of agonist stimulation. Myocardial and smooth muscle cells possess slow calcium channels of the L-type and the T-type which allow calcium entry from the extracellular space into the cytoplasm following depolarization of the cell membrane. These calcium channels may also be activated by humoral stimulation by agonists such as catecholamines and endothelin. In addition, there is a cell membrane-associated sodium/calcium exchange protein which

A. L. Catapano et al. (eds.), Drugs Affecting Lipid Metabolism, 251–260.
© 1993 Kluwer Academic Publishers and Fondazione Giovanni Lorenzini.

facilitates the removal of intracellular sodium. Finally, the smooth endoplasmic reticulum (or sarcoplasmic reticulum) is an organelle responsible for the storage of calcium. This pool is generally activated following phospholipase C activation and subsequent release of inositol phosphates, which open microsomal large calcium channels. These calcium pools are activated in response to such factors as PDGF and thrombin.

1.2 CALCIUM CHANNEL BLOCKER TYPES

There are numerous types of calcium channel blockers that are used therapeutically. Verapamil is representative of the type I group of calcium channel blockers known as phenylalkylamines, which are have a net basic charge, and prolong AV nodal conduction and refractoriness. Second generation verapamil-like compounds include anipamil and gallopamil. Diltiazem is also a member of the type I group of calcium channel blockers, and is a representative of the benzothiazepine group of compounds. The type II group of calcium channel blockers is represented by Nifedipine, which is one of the dihydropyridine group of calcium channel blockers. Second generation Nifedipine-like compounds currently in use include Nicardipine and Nisoldipine. These calcium channel blockers are potent peripheral vasodilators but do not have electrophysiologic effects in usual doses. Nicardipine and Flunarizine preferentially act on the inactivated state of the L- and T-type slow calcium channel, while verapamil and diltiazem preferentially inhibit the L-type slow calcium channel. Differences in their clinical efficacy may also be due to their relative lipophilicity and their volume of distribution.

1.3 CALCIUM CHANNEL BLOCKERS AND ATHEROGENESIS

There is an expanding body of evidence supporting the concept that calcium channel blockers inhibit the progression of atherosclerosis [1-4]. Using the cholesterol-fed rabbit, numerous investigators have demonstrated that calcium channel blockers, including Nicardipine, and Nifedipine significantly reduce the severity of plaque formation without changing plasma cholesterol levels [5,6]. However, the influence of calcium channel blockers in the Watanabe rabbit is not as clear, since calcium channel blockers do not retard the progression of atherosclerosis in this model.

There are several potential mechanisms by which calcium channel blockers are believed to inhibit the atherosclerotic process [7]. Importantly, each of these processes are regulated by the accumulation of intracellular calcium flux. Since calcium is an important mediator of vascular tone, calcium channel blockers may decrease arterial pressure and shear stress, thus reducing turbulent flow across predilected sites for atherosclerosis. Calcium channel blockers may inhibit platelet aggregation and release of other soluble mediators which promote vascular spasm and smooth muscle cell proliferation, such as thromboxane and platelet-derived growth factor, respectively. Calcium channel blockers appear to preserve endothelial cell function in an atherogenic milieu, presumably by reducing permeability of LDL and other macromolecules [7], and preserving EDRF release [7]. Next, calcium channel blockers may directly inhibit the accumulation of vascular intracellular cholesterol and cholesteryl ester content, which may or may not be secondary to decreased transendothelial LDL flux [8,9]. Finally, calcium channel blockers may prevent smooth muscle cell migration and proliferation [10]. However, it is unclear as to which calcium channel, or groups of calcium channels mediates the protective effects of calcium channel blockers on the development of atherosclerosis.

1.4 CONTROL OF CHOLESTEROL TRAFFICKING BY PROSTACYCLIN AND CYCLIC AMP

Our laboratory has been studying the role of intracellular second messengers, including PGI_2 and cyclic AMP, in the regulation of intracellular cholesterol trafficking (**Figure 1**, from [11]). Briefly, LDL is taken up into smooth muscle cells by receptor mediated endocytosis. LDL-derived cholesteryl esters are hydrolyzed in the lysosome into free cholesterol and free fatty acids by the action of acid cholesteryl

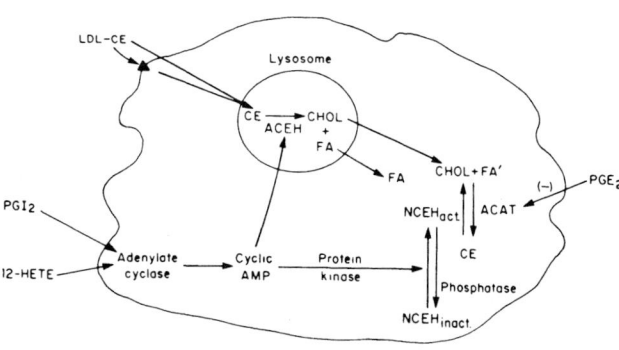

ester hydrolase (ACEH). The liberated cholesterol is a substrate for acyl CoA cholesteryl acyltransferase (ACAT) which converts the free cholesterol to a cytoplasmic cholesteryl ester pool. Hydrolysis of cytoplasmic cholesteryl esters is achieved by a neutral cholesteryl ester hydrolase (NCEH). Our laboratory has shown that exogenous or endogenously synthesized PGI_2 stimulates cyclic AMP content, which directly activates ACEH activity, and stimulates NCEH activity through a protein kinase-dependent pathway [12-14]. Thus, it is conceivable that a potential mechanism by which calcium channel blockers have anti-atherosclerotic properties may be due to their ability to influence the processes of cholesterol delivery, hydrolysis, and esterification in smooth muscle cells. These observations also suggest the possibility that calcium channel blockers may influence intracellular cholesterol trafficking through the activation of PGI_2 synthesis and subsequent accumulation of cyclic AMP.

2. METHODOLOGY

Rat, rabbit or bovine aortic smooth muscle cells were grown to confluent density and exposed to two calcium channel blockers of the dihydropyridine class, Nicardipine and Nifedipine at the indicated concentrations, followed by assays for the measurement of LDL receptor activity [15], cholesteryl ester hydrolytic activities [12,13], ACAT activity [13], PGI_2 release [16] and cyclic AMP production [13]. Cholesterol and cholesteryl ester content were measured either by microfluorometric assay [12] or by gas-liquid chromatography [16].

3. Results

3.1 NICARDIPINE STIMULATES LDL RECEPTOR ACTIVITY.

The effects of Nicardipine on the binding, internalization, and degradation of LDL to confluent monolayers of rat aortic smooth muscle cells was evaluated **(Figure 2)**. Cells were incubated with serum-free media containing Nicardipine (0-25 uM) overnight, and then incubated for an additional 5 hours in the presence of [^{125}I]-LDL at 10 ug/ml. Supernatants were assayed for degraded LDL as TCA-soluble counts. Receptor-bound LDL was measured as dextran sulfate-releasable counts, and internalized LDL was measured following solubilization in NaOH. Nicardipine increased LDL binding, internalization, and degradation in a dose-dependent fashion (* = $p < 0.05$) (from [17]).

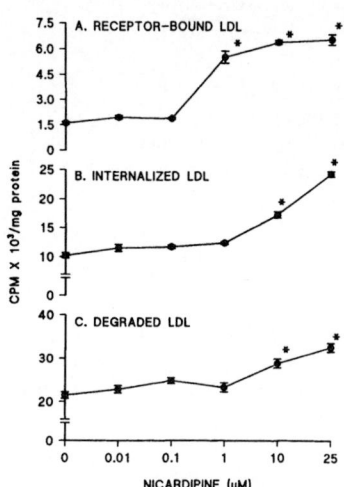

3.2. NICARDIPINE UPREGULATES LDL RECEPTOR mRNA STEADY STATE LEVELS.

To determine a potential mechanism by which Nicardipine increased LDL receptor expression, we examined the possibility that Nicardipine could alter the expression of LDL receptor mRNA steady state levels **(Figure 3)**. Smooth muscle cells were incubated in media in the absence and presence of Nicardipine. After 24 hours, total RNA was extracted, and the steady state levels of LDL receptor mRNA was measured by Northern analysis. The blots were also probed using the cDNA for a constituitively expressed gene, namely glyceraldehyde phosphate dehydrogenase or GAPDH. The data are expressed as the LDL-receptor/ GAPDH ratio, and normalized to the percent of control levels. These data demonstrate that Nicardipine increased the steady state levels of LDL-receptor mRNA by 4.0 fold (from [17]). The mechanism by

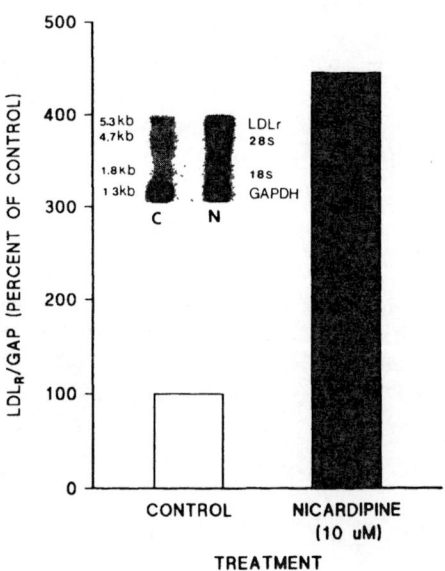

which Nicardipine stimulates LDL-receptor mRNA expression is not clear, but may be due to increased transcription rates or increased mRNA stability.

3.3. NIFEDIPINE STIMULATES CHOLESTERYL ESTER HYDROLYTIC ACTIVITIES.

The above data suggest that calcium channel blockers increase the uptake and degradation of LDL cholesteryl esters, and support the hypothesis that calcium channel blockers may also be stimulating intracellular cholesteryl ester hydrolytic activities. To examine this possibility, the influence of Nifedipine (50 ng/ml for two hours) on ACEH, NCEH, and ACAT activity was evaluated (**Figure 4**). These data demonstrate that Nifedipine stimulates ACEH and NCEH activities (* = p < 0.05), with no change in ACAT activity. Taken together, these data indicate that dihydropyridine calcium channel blockers may stimulate incorporation and degradation of LDL-derived cholesteryl esters, and promote the hydrolysis of cytoplasmic cholesteryl ester stores (from [18]).

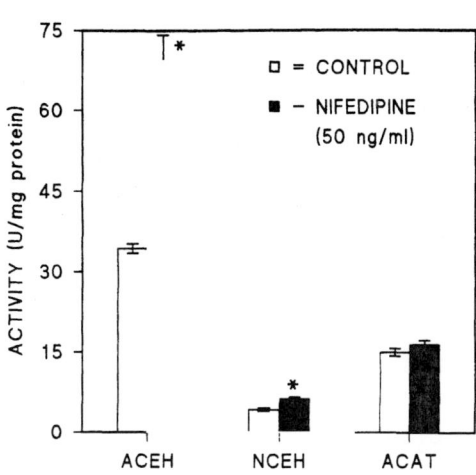

3.4. CALCIUM CHANNEL BLOCKERS STIMULATE PROSTACYCLIN SYNTHESIS.

Because ACEH and NCEH activities are stimulated by second messengers, including PGI_2 and cyclic AMP, we next determined if calcium channel blockers stimulated lipolytic enzymes by stimulating PGI_2 release. To examine this possibility, arterial smooth muscle cells were exposed to media alone, or media containing 10 or 100 uM Nicardipine for 24 hours. PGI_2 in the conditioned media was then measured by radioimmunoassay of its stable hydrolysis product, 6-keto-$PGF_{1\alpha}$. Data are expressed as ng/mg cell protein. The data summarized in **Figure 5** demonstrates that Nicardipine stimulates PGI_2 release in a dose-dependent manner (* = p < 0.05) (from [17]).

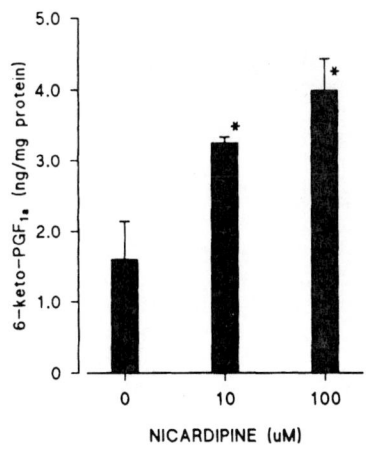

In other studies, the time-course of PGI_2 release in response to either Nifedipine or Nicardipine was evaluated. Neither of these agents acutely stimulated PGI_2 release within 30 minutes (data not shown), suggesting that calcium channel blockers do not activate phospholipases A_2 or C. To determine a potential mechanism by which calcium channel blockers increase eicosanoid generation by arterial smooth muscle cells, the influence of Nicardipine on the steady state levels of cyclooxygenase mRNA was evaluated (**Figure 6**). Total RNA was extracted from aortic smooth muscle cells grown in media alone or media containing 0.1 and 10 uM Nicardipine for 24 hours, and probed for steady state levels of cyclooxygenase mRNA. Nicardipine increased the expression of cyclooxygenase mRNA steady state level relative to GAPDH approximately 2-fold. The mechanism by which Nicardipine exerts this effect is unclear. These results suggest that Nicardipine is either increasing the transcription rate or stability of cyclooxygenase message (from [17]).

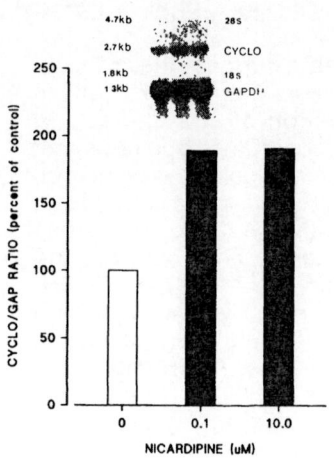

3.5 CALCIUM CHANNEL BLOCKERS STIMULATE CYCLIC AMP FORMATION.

The above data suggest that calcium channel blockers may be increasing lipolytic enzymes since PGI_2 is a well-documented agonist of cellular cholesteryl ester hydrolases. Furthermore, our data suggests that calcium channel blockers increase lipolytic enzyme activities by elevations in cyclic AMP. To directly test this hypothesis, we examined the effect of Nicardipine on the cyclic AMP levels. Cells were exposed to Nicardipine (0.1 μM) for two hours. Cell homogenates were then assayed for cyclic AMP, and normalized to cell protein. As summarized in **Figure 7**, Nicardipine increased cyclic AMP levels

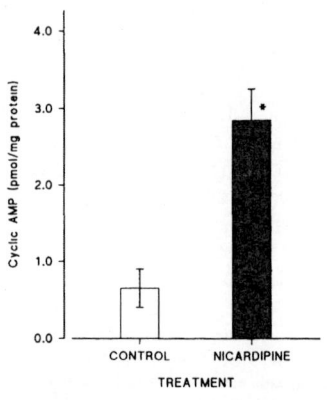

over 2-fold relative to controls (* = $p < 0.05$) (from [17]). Taken together, the above data demonstrate that Nicardipine increases cytoplasmic cholesteryl ester hydrolysis in arterial smooth muscle cells through cyclic AMP-dependent mechanisms.

3.6 CALCIUM CHANNEL BLOCKERS FACILITATE NET CHOLESTEROL REMOVAL FROM CHOLESTEROL-ENRICHED RABBIT SMOOTH MUSCLE CELLS.

We next determined if calcium channel blockers could actually decrease cellular cholesterol and cholesteryl ester content, since cellular cholesterol trafficking is enhanced by these agents. To evaluate this possibility, smooth muscle cells were cultured from the thoracic aorta from rabbits that had received either normal rabbit chow or an egg-supplemented diet, consisting of one egg per day for six months. Cells recovered by enzymatic dispersion were then exposed to Nifedipine *in vitro* at 100 ng/ml on days 0,3, and 6, in the presence of HDL and bovine serum albumin as cholesterol acceptors. Cholesterol and cholesteryl ester were then measured by microfluorometric analysis. The data summarized in **Figure 8** shows that at day 0, cells from atherosclerotic rabbits contained significantly more cholesterol and cholesteryl ester than cells isolated from normolipemic animals. Seven day exposure of these cells to Nifedipine decreased both cholesterol and cholesteryl ester content from cells derived from atherosclerotic animals (* = $p < 0.05$), but did not alter either the cholesterol or cholesteryl ester content in cells from normal animals (from [18]).

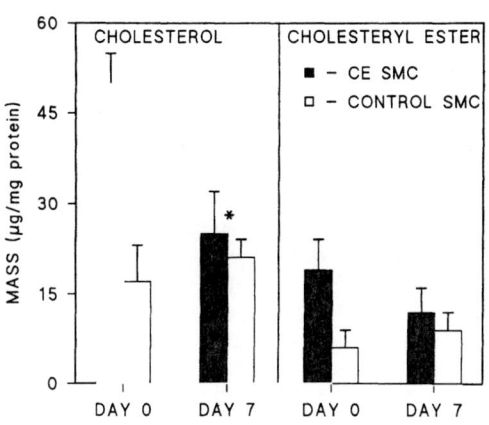

3.7 HUMAN STUDIES

In additional studies, we explored the possibility that calcium channel blockers could reduce cholesterol and cholesteryl ester content in human atherosclerotic vessels. To this end, we determined the influence of calcium channel blockers on cholesteryl ester metabolic activities, cyclic AMP content, and cholesterol and cholesteryl ester content in aortic biopsies taken at the time of coronary bypass surgery. The mean age, and the serum cholesterol levels of the patients in this study were similar, being 62 years of age, having plasma cholesterol levels of 200-210 mg/dl. The patients who were in the calcium channel blocker group received Nifedipine (10 mg three times daily), Diltiazem (30-60 mg, three or four times daily), or Verapamil (120 mg/day). The patients also received a final dose six hours prior to coronary artery bypass surgery.

3.7.1. *Calcium channel blockers stimulate cholesteryl ester hydrolases.*

Cell homogenates from aortic punch biopsies were assayed for ACEH, NCEH, and ACAT, Data illustrated in **Figure 9** demonstrates that calcium channel blockers increase ACEH and NCEH activities by approximately 2-fold (* = $p < 0.05$). Calcium channel blockers did not affect ACAT activity (data not shown) (from [19]).

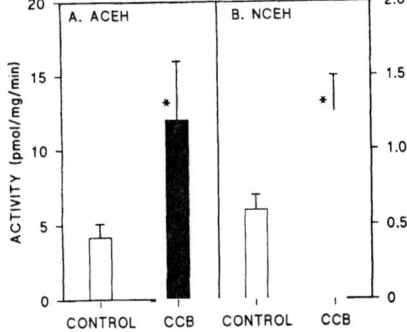

3.7.2. *Calcium channel blockers increase cyclic AMP content in human aortic tissue.*

To determine if the increased cholesteryl ester hydrolytic activities
were due to increased cyclic AMP,
the level of this nucleotide was
measured, and correlated with
ACEH activity of human aortic tissue
homogenates (**Figure 10**). These
data demonstrate that calcium
channel blockers increased cyclic
AMP content and ACEH activity.
There was also a statistically significant correlation between cyclic AMP
content and ACEH activity (open
squares, r = 0.563, p < 0.01). In
contrast, ACEH and cyclic AMP
were low and were not correlated in
aortic tissue from patients not receiving calcium channel blockers
(closed squares) (from [19]).

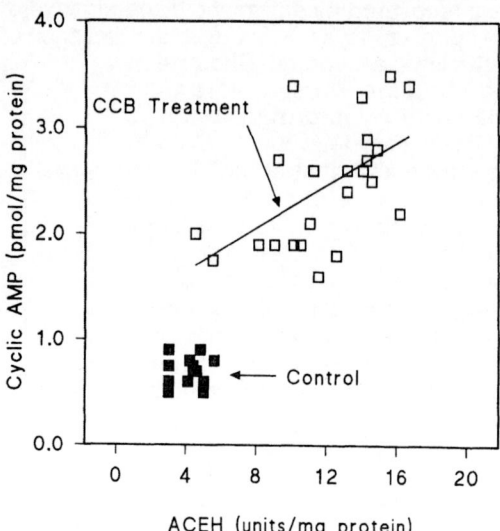

3.7.3. *Calcium channel blockers reduce cholesterol mass in human aortic tissue.*

Based on these results, we next
determined if calcium channel
blockers could reduce cholesterol
mass (**Figure 11**). Free and esterified cholesterol were measured in
aortic punch biopsies of patients
who did or did not receive calcium
channel blockers, as measured by
gas-liquid chromatography. These
results demonstrate that aortic
tissue derived from patients taking
calcium channel blockers had less
than half the content of free and
esterified cholesterol than patients
who were not taking calcium channel blockers (* = p < 0.05) (from
[19]).

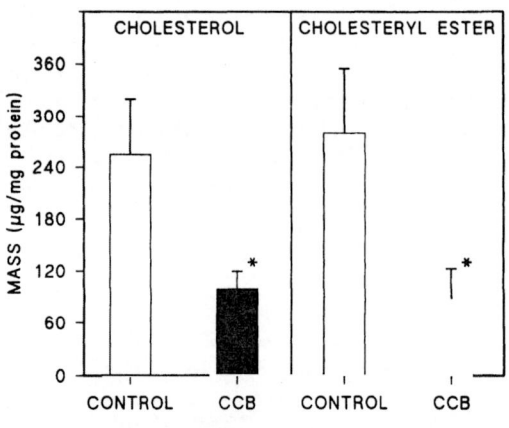

4. Discussion

Our data demonstrate that members of the dihydropyridine group of calcium channel
blockers, namely Nifedipine and Nicardipine, increase LDL receptor expression, cholesteryl ester hydrolysis, and decrease net cholesterol content from arterial smooth
muscle cells in animal models and in human atherosclerosis. While the detailed

mechanisms by which this occurs is not fully understood, these calcium channel blockers increase second messengers, including PGI_2 and cyclic AMP, which we and others have demonstrated to stimulate cholesteryl ester removal in smooth muscle cells. Our data suggest the possibility that these agents act by increasing the steady state levels of the LDL receptor, and cyclooxygenase. The mechanism by which calcium channel blockers affect the regulation of these genes is unknown, and requires further investigation. The concept that PGI_2 or related eicosanoids may mediate the protective effects of calcium channel blockers is reinforced by recent observations that cyclooxygenase inhibitors abolished the hypolipidemic actions of Isradipine, also a dihydropyridine calcium channel blocker (Sinzinger et al - this symposium).

The observation that increased LDL receptor activity is important in the mechanism of the beneficial effects of these calcium channel blockers is reinforced by observations that the Watanabe rabbit is not protected from the development of atherosclerosis by calcium channel blockers [20]. We interpret our data to suggest that calcium channel blockers increase the catabolism of LDL-cholesterol esters, and promote net free cholesterol formation by increasing the activities of lysosomal and neutral cholesteryl ester hydrolases. Although we did not directly access HDL-receptor activity, our observations that HDL/BSA-induced cholesterol efflux was increased following ex vivo calcium channel blocker administration suggests the possibility that calcium channel blockers may also increase those processes leading to cholesterol delivery to the plasma membrane and subsequent incorporation into HDL.

In summary, our data are consistent with the hypothesis that calcium channel blockers can increase LDL receptor activity [4,8], and decrease cellular cholesterol content [5,21]. Our results reinforce the prospects that calcium-channel blockers may be useful agents in the treatment of atherosclerotic vascular disease.

6. References

1. Parmley, W. (1990) "Vascular protection from atherosclerosis: potential of calcium antagonists", Amer J Cardiol, 66, 16I-22I.
2. Henry, P. (1990) "Calcium channel blockers and atherosclerosis", J Cardiovasc Pharmacol, 16 (Suppl I), S12-S15.
3. Kjeldsen, K. and Stender, S. (1989) "Minireview: Calcium antagonists and experimental atherosclerosis", Proc Soc Exptl Biol Med, 109, 219-228.
4. Paoletti, R. and Bernini, F. (1990) "A new generation of calcium antagonists and their role in atherosclerosis", Amer J Cardiol, 66, 28H-31H.
5. Henry, P. and Bentley, K. (1981) "Suppression of atherogenesis in cholesterol-fed rabbits treated with Nifedipine", J Clin Invest, 68, 1366-1369.
6. Koegh, A. and Schroeder, J. (1990) "A review of calcium antagonists and atherosclerosis", J Cardiovasc Pharmacol, 16 (Suppl.6), S28-S35.
7. Schmitz, G., Hankowitz, J. and Kovacs, E. (1991) "Cellular processes in atherogenesis: potential targets of Ca^{2+} channel blockers", Athero, 88, 109-132.
8. Stein, O., Leitersdorf, E. and Stein, Y. (1985) "Verapamil enhances receptor-mediated endocytosis of low density lipoprotein by aortic cells in culture", Arterio, 5, 35-44.
9. Paoletti, R., Bernini, F., Fumagalli, R., Allorio, M. and Corsini, A. (1988) "Calcium antagonists and LDL receptors", Ann N Y Acad Sci, 522, 390-398.

10. Jackson, L., Bush, R. and Bowyer, D. (1988) "Inhibitory effects of calcium antagonists on balloon catheter-induced smooth muscle proliferation and lesion size" , Athero, 69, 115-122.
11. Pomerantz, K. and Hajjar, D. (1989) "Eicosanoids in regulation of arterial smooth muscle cell phenotype, proliferative capacity, and cholesterol metabolism" , Arterio, 9, 413-429.
12. Hajjar, D. and Weksler, B. (1983) "Metabolic activity of cholesteryl esters in aortic smooth muscle cells is altered by prostaglandins I_2 and E_2" , J Lipid Res, 24, 1176-1185.
13. Hajjar, D., Weksler, B., Falcone, D., Hefton, J., Tack-Goldman, K. and Minick, C. (1982) "Prostacyclin modulates cholesteryl ester hydrolytic activity by its effect on cyclic adenosine monophosphate in rabbit aortic smooth muscle cells" , J Clin Invest, 70, 479-488.
14. Hajjar, D., Minick, C. and Fowler, S. (1983) "Arterial neutral cholesteryl esterase. A hormone-sensitive enzyme distinct from the lysosomal enzyme" , J Biol Chem, 258, 192-198.
15. Brown, M., Dana, S. and Goldstein, J. (1975) "Receptor-dependent hydrolysis of cholesteryl esters contained in plasma low density lipoprotein" , Proc Natl Acad Sci USA, 72, 2925-2929.
16. Pomerantz, K. and Hajjar, D. (1989) "Eicosanoid metabolism in cholesterol-enriched arterial smooth muscle cells: reduced arachidonate release with concommitant decrease in cyclooxygenase products" , J Lipid Res, 30, 1219-1231.
17. Nicholson, A., Etingin, O., Pomerantz, K., Summers, B., Friday, K., Wolff, A. and Hajjar, D. (1992) "Dihydropyridine calcium antagonist modulates cholesterol metabolism and eicosanoid biosynthesis in vascular cells" , J Cell Biochem, 48, 393-400.
18. Etingin, O. and Hajjar, D. (1985) "Nifedipine increases cholesteryl ester hydrolytic activity in lipid-laden rabbit arterial smooth muscle cells. A possible mechanism for its antiatherogenic effect" , J Clin Invest, 75, 1554-1558.
19. Etingin, O. and Hajjar, D. (1990) "Calcium channel blockers enhance cholesteryl ester hydrolysis and decrease total cholesterol accumulation in human arterial tissue" , Circ Res, 66, 185-190.
20. Van Niekerk, J., Hendricks, T., De Boer, H. and Van't Laar, A. (1984) "Does Nifedipine suppress atherogenesis in WHHL rabbits?" , Athero, 53, 91-98.
21. Willis, A., Nagel, B., Churchill, V., Whyte, M., Smith, D. and Mahmud, I. (1985) "Antiatherosclerotic effects of Nicardipine and Nifedipine in cholesterol-fed rabbits", Athero, 5, 250-255.

PRAVASTATIN REDUCES PLASMA CONCENTRATION OF A MORE ELECTRONEGATIVELY CHARGED LDL SUBFRACTION IN FH

G. BITTOLO-BON, G. CAZZOLATO, P. ALESSANDRINI
and P. AVOGARO

ABSTRACT. After a 12-week period of prudent diet, 10 patients (7 males, 3 females, mean age 42 ± 11 years) with familial hypercholesterolemia were treated with 12-weeks pravastatin 40 mg once-day at bedtime. At the beginning and at the end of each treatment period LDL (d 1.020-1.063 g/ml) were separated by ultracentrifugation. Lipid determinations and the assays of malondialdehyde and vitamin E were performed both in plasma and LDL. LDL were also subfractionated by ion exchange chromatography, using a high performance liquid chromatography apparatus, in order to evaluate the content of a more electronegatively charged LDL subfraction (LDL⁻). The drug treatment induced a significant reduction of total cholesterol (-32%), LDL cholesterol (-37%), plasma and LDL malondialdehyde (-32 % and - 39% respectively), and a significant increase in LDL vitamin E concentration (+ 38%). The LDL⁻ plasma concentration fell from 51 ± 21 to 20 ± 9. In addition to the known effect on plasma lipids, pravastatin therefore contributes to a reduction of lipid peroxidation products; this is shown by the fall of plasma and LDL malondialdehyde and LDL⁻, a small circulating LDL subfraction that behaves like a mildly oxidized LDL. Because the drug does not display antioxidant properties in vitro, the present data are likely due to an increased LDL catabolism, with a reduced LDL residence time in the circulation, induced by pravastatin.

Introduction

Several lines of evidence suggest that oxidative modification of LDL may play an important role in atherogenesis [1]. LDL can be oxidized in vitro by a variety of cultured cells (endothelial cells, monocyte-macrophages, smooth muscle cells) [2-4] or following incubation with transitional metal ions such as Cu^{++} [5]. Recent studies have shown that oxidative modifications of LDL also occur in vivo [6, 7]. It was assumed that this modification occurs primarily in the intima, in microdomains sequestered from the many plasma antioxidants [1]. There are however several evidences that a modest degree of oxidative modification of LDL occurs in the circulation [8-10], so that plasma LDL might be "primed" for more rapid cell-mediated oxidative modifications [11]. By the use of ion exchange chromatography, a more electronegative LDL subfraction (LDL⁻) has been isolated in human plasma, which displays many of the characteristics of an vivo oxidized LDL [12-14]. In this study we have investigated the effect of the hypocholesterolemic drug pravastatin, a

261

A. L. Catapano et al. (eds.), Drugs Affecting Lipid Metabolism, 261–268.
© 1993 Kluwer Academic Publishers and Fondazione Giovanni Lorenzini.

competitive inhibitor of 3-hydroxy-3-methyl-glutaryl coenzyme A (HMG-CoA) reductase, on the LDL⁻ plasma concentration. The variations induced by the drug on LDL chemical composition, vitamin E and malondialdehyde concentration in both plasma and LDL were also studied.

Material and methods

Ten patients with heterozygous familial hypercholesterolemia (FH) (7 males and 3 females; mean age 42 ± 11 years) were selected for the study. The diagnosis of FH was done by the following clinical criteria: 1) type IIa hyperlipoproteinemia in the patient (TC > 95th percentile of the population; TG < 240 mg/dl; HDL-C < 75 mg/dl); 2) tendon xantomata in the patient and/or in one first-degree or two second-degree relatives; 3) and/or one first-degree or two second-degree relatives with hyperlipoproteinemia type IIa and premature IHD. After a 12 week period during which patients followed an isocaloric diet (carbohydrate 55%, protein 15%, fat 30%: saturated 10%, monounsaturated 10%, polyunsaturated 10% and cholesterol less than 300 mg/day), they were treated with 40 mg pravastatin once day at bedtime for 12 weeks. The analyses were performed at the beginning and at the end of each treatment period. Venous blood, drawn after a 14-hr fast, was collected in test tubes containing ethylendiamine tetraacetic acid (EDTA; 1 mg/ml). The blood was immediately centrifuged at 1500 x g. LDL (d = 1.020-1.063 g/ml) were separated through preparative ultracentrifugation from freshly drawn plasma, according to Havel et al. [15]. After separation, LDL were dialyzed 24 hr under N_2 stream at 4° C in the dark against a TRIS-HCl 0.01M, pH 7.2, containing EDTA (10 μM). Total cholesterol (TC), triglycerides (TG) and high density lipoprotein cholesterol (HDL-C) were assayed enzymatically; LDL-cholesterol (LDL-C) was calculated according to the Friedwald formula. In LDL samples TC, free cholesterol (FC) TG, phospholipids (PL) were determined enzymatically with specific test kits from Menarini (Firenze-Italy); cholesterol ester (CE) concentrations were calculated as (TC - FC) x 1.68; proteins (P) were assayed by the method of Lowry et al. [16] with human albumin as standard. Malondialdehyde (MDA) was assayed as thiobarbituric acid reactive substances (TBARS) with the fluorimetric method of Yagi [17]; vitamin E was estimated in plasma and in LDL by HPLC using a fluorescence detector set at an excitation of 292 nm and an emission of 335 nm [18].

LDL subfractions were separated by analytic IE-HRLC using a 700B Bio-Rad (Milano - Italy) liquid chromatographyc system equipped with a 7.8 x 50 mm MA-7Q column, according to Cazzolato et al. [13]. The effluent was monitored at 280 nm, and the areas of the obtained peaks were integrated by IBM based workstation. The method allows the separation of two LDL subfractions: the major one shows the usual chemico-physical and biological characteristics of a normal LDL (nLDL), the minor corresponds to the more electronegative LDL⁻ subfraction [13,14].

In vitro experiments were done by incubating LDL samples from control donors, adjusted to a cholesterol concentration of 500 μg/ml, with 3 μM copper ions at 37° C according to Barnhart et al. [19]. An aliquot of 4 different LDL samples was incubated alone, or in the presence of 5 μM pravastatin, or 5 μM probucol, or 5 μM α-tocopherol. In vitro peroxidation experiments were also performed in LDL samples obtained from patients treated with pravastatin (40 mg/day), probucol (1 g/day) or vitamin E (900 mg/day) for 12 weeks. Incubation with copper ions was performed in 4 different LDL samples for each group of treatment. As a measure of lipoprotein peroxidation in vitro time-dependent changes of fluorescence intensity, assayed according to McLean and Hagaman [20], were recorded.

Results

The mean values of the various parameters assayed in the plasma are reported in table 1. After diet no significant variations were observed. The drug treatment induced a significant reduction of TC and of TG. LDL cholesterol was reduced by 37% and HDL cholesterol increased by 10%. There was also a 32% decrease of TBARS plasma concentration. Total plasma vitamin E concentration has significantly decreased after drug treatment. However a significant increase of vitamin E to total plasma cholesterol ratio was observed.

TABLE 1. Mean ($\pm$ SD) values of plasma total cholesterol (TC), triglycerides (TG), LDL and HDL-cholesterol (LDL-C and HDL-C), thiobarbituric acid reactive substances (TBARS) and of vitamin E in FH patients at baseline, after diet and after pravastatin treatment.

	BASELINE	DIET	PRAVASTATIN	diff.%
TC (mg/dl)	375 ± 84	378 ± 86	249 ± 33	-32**
TG "	154 ± 79	160 ± 74	117 ± 61	-27*
LDL-C "	295 ± 86	290 ± 83	175 ± 29	-37**
HDL-C "	46 ± 12	46 ± 11	51 ± 13	+10*
TBARS (nM/ml)	4.4 ± .8	4.6 ± .7	3.0 ± .5	-32**
Vit. E (μg/ml)	12 ± 3	11 ± 3	9.5 ± 4	-13*
Vit. E (μg/mg TC)	3.1 ± .4	2.9 ± .5	3.8 ± .4	+31**

* = $P < .05$; ** = $P < .01$ vs diet

The concentration of total LDL was reduced by 40% following the treatment with pravastatin, while the LDL⁻ plasma concentration decreased by 60% (Table 2).

TABLE 2. Mean (± SD) values of total plasma LDL and of LDL⁻ in FH patients at baseline, after diet and after pravastatin treatment.

	BASELINE	DIET	PRAVASTATIN	diff.%
total LDL (mg/dl)	702 ± 93	707 ± 96	414 ± 52	-41*
LDL⁻ "	50 ± 24	51 ± 21	20 ± 9	-27*

* = P < .01 vs diet

After drug treatment significant variations in LDL composition were recorded. There was an increase in phospholipid and a reduction of protein percentage content. A significant reduction of TBARS and an increase of vitamin E LDL content were also observed. Finally, the treatment with pravastatin induced a significant reduction of LDL⁻ to total LDL ratio (Table 3).

TABLE 3. Mean (± SD) percentage content of cholesterol esters (CE), free cholesterol (FC), triglycerides (TG), phosholipids (PL), proteins (P), thiobarbituric acid reactive substances (TBARS) and vitamin E content of LDL and mean percentage contribution of LDL⁻ to total LDL in FH patients at baseline, after diet and after pravastatin treatment.

		BASELINE	DIET	PRAVASTATIN	P
CE	%	41.5 ± 1.9	40.7 ± 2.0	41.2 ± 1.2	ns
FC	"	11.0 ± 1.6	10.7 ± 1.5	11.1 ± 1.1	ns
TG	"	5.2 ± 1.8	5.7 ± 1.6	5.7 ± 1.4	ns
PL	"	21.4 ± 1.2	21.7 ± 1.3	23.0 ± 1.1	<.05
P	"	21.4 ± 0.7	21.2 ± 0.4	19.0 ± 0.8	<.01
TBARS (mol/mol LDL)		1.83 ± 0.9	1.87 ± 0.8	1.15 ± 0.7	<.01
Vit. E (mg/mg LDL-P)		5.3 ± 1.8	5.2 ± 1.9	7.2 ± 2.4	<.01
LDL⁻ %		7.6 ± 3.5	7.9 ± 3.3	5.2 ± 2.1	<.01

The addition of 5 μM pravastatin during the incubation of LDL with 3 μM copper ions does not offer any protection to in vitro induced LDL peroxidation, while the presence of 5 μM vitamin E or probucol almost totally prevents the lipoprotein oxidation (Fig. 1).

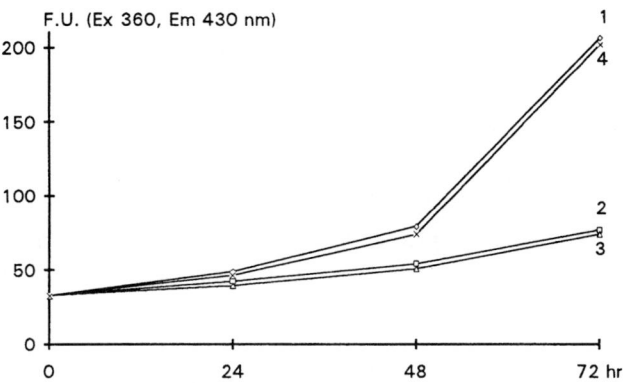

Fig. 1: variations of fluorescence intensity in LDL incubated with 3mM copper ions. Control LDL (1), LDL + 5 mM vitamin E (2), LDL + 5mM probucol (3), LDL + 5 mM pravastatin (4). Each point of the curves corresponds to the mean values of four different LDL samples.

LDL samples obtained from patients treated with vitamin E (900 mg/day for 12 weeks) or with probucol (1 g/day for 12 weeks) show resistance to peroxidation by copper ions. LDL samples obtained from the patients treated with pravastatin (40 mg/day for 12 weeks) do not display significant resistance to peroxidation, even though a tendency to a lesser extent of fluorescence than in control LDL can be detected during the incubation time with copper (Fig. 2)

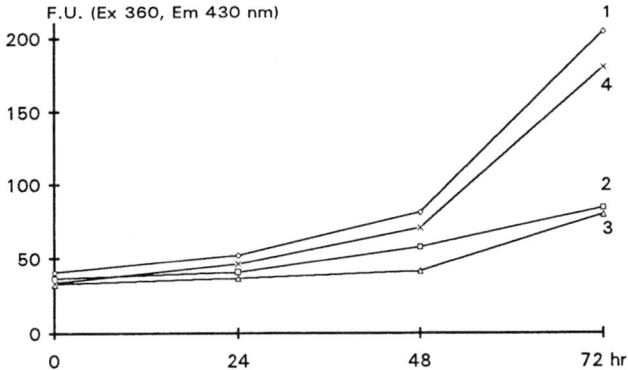

Fig. 2: variations of fluorescence intensity in LDL incubated with 3mM copper ions. Control LDL (1), LDL from patients treated with vitamin E (2), probucol (3) and pravastatin (4). Each point of the curves corresponds to the mean values of four different LDL samples.

Discussion

The reduction of plasma TC, TG, LDL-C and the increase of HDL-C, are well known effects of the HMG-CoA reductase inhibitor pravastatin [21]. The drug selectively inhibit hepatic cholesterol synthesis due to its hydrophilia and thus to its inability to enter cells other than hepatocytes [22]. Also due of its hydrophilia, the drug does not interact with LDL. This may explain the absence of in vitro antioxidant capacity, an effect observed with the more lypophilic compounds such as lovastatin (though to a lesser extent than with other antioxidants) [23]. Recently, however, LDL obtained from patients treated with pravastatin have been shown to have a slight reduction in the susceptibility to in vitro oxidation [24].

In this study LDL isolated from patients treated with pravastatin does not show a reduced susceptibility to the in vitro oxidation, thus differing from LDL obtained from patients treated with vitamin E or probucol.

A slight antioxidant effect in vivo may however be observed with pravastatin. Our experience, has recorded reduced values of total plasma MDA and of the vitamin E to total cholesterol ratio in treated patients. Moreover, decreased values of LDL MDA, increased values of LDL vitamin E and a highly significant reduction of plasmat LDL⁻. In our study pravastatin has also induced an increase of LDL-PL content and of the LDL PL/P ratio have been recorded. These latter findings seems to be of interest as a decreased amount of PL and of the PL/P ratio is a peculiar feature of LDL⁻ , a more electronegatively charged subfraction, that shows the chemico-physical and biological characterisctics of a mildly oxidized LDL [12-14].

As pravastatin does not display any effective antioxidant activity in vitro, its mild antioxidant properties recorded in vivo is likely a function of the mechanism of its hypolipidemic effect. Actually, the drug increases the expression of the LDL receptor in the liver and decreases the half life of circulating LDL. Such an effect decreases the time during which LDL is exposed to lipid peroxidation, thus explaining the apparent incoherence of the in vivo as compared to in vitro results. Furthermore, the reduced residence time of LDL in the circulation may suggest the formation of a LDL population containing less aged particles, likely less "primed" for a more rapid oxidative modification.

References

1. Steinberg, D., Parthasarathy, S., Carew, T.E., Khoo, J.C., and Witztum, J.L. (1989) 'Beyond cholesterol: modifications of low density lipoprotein that increase its atherogenicity', N. Engl. J. Med. 320, 915-924.
2. Henriksen, T., Mahoney, E.M., and Steinberg, D. (1981) 'Enhanced macrophage degradation of low density lipoprotein previously incubated with cultured endothelial cells: recognition by receptors for acetylated low density lipoproteins', Proc. Natl. Acad. Sci. USA 78, 6499-6503.

3. Heinecke, J.W., Baker, L., Rosen, H., and Chait,A. (1986) 'Superoxide-mediated modification of low density lipoprotein by arterial smooth muscle cells', J. Clin. Invest. 77, 757-763.

4. Parthasarathy, S., Printz, D.J., Boyd, D., Joy, L., and Steinberg, D. (1986) 'Macrophage oxidation of low density lipoprotein generates a form recognized by the scavenger receptor',. Arteriosclerosis 6, 505-510.

5. Heinecke, J.W., Rosen, H., and Chait, A. (1987) 'Iron and copper promote modification of low-density lipoprotein by human arterial smooth muscle cells in culture', J. Clin. Invest. 74, 1890-1984.

6. Palinsky, W., Rosenfeld, M.E., Yla-Herttula, S., Gurtner, G.C., Socher, S.S., Butler, S.W., Parthasarathy, S., Carew, T.E., Steinberg, D., and Witztum, J.L. (1989) 'Low-density lipoprotein undergoes oxidative modification in vivo', Proc. Natl. Acad. Sci. USA 86, 1372-1376.

7. Haberland, M., Fong, D., and Cheng, L. (1988), ' Malondialdehyde-altered proteins occurs in atheroma of Watanabe heritable hyperlipidemic rabbits', Science 241, 215-218.

8. Yagi, K. (1987) 'Lipid peroxides and human diseases' Chem. Phys. Lipids 45, 337-351.

9. Morel, D.W., and Chisolm, G.M. (1989) 'Antioxidant treatment of diabetic rats inhibits lipoprotein oxidation and cytotoxicity', J. Lipid Res. 30, 1827-1834.

10. Harats, D., Ben-Naim, M., Dabach, Y., Hollander, G., Havivi, E., Stein, O., and Stein, Y. (1990) 'Effect of vitamin C and E supplementation on susceptibility of plasma lipoproteins to peroxidation induced by acute smoking', Atherosclerosis 85, 47-54.

11. Witztum, J.L., and Steinberg, D., (1991) 'Role of oxidized low density lipoproteins in atherogenesis', J. Clin. Invest. 88, 1185-1192.

12. Avogaro, P., Bittolo-Bon, G., and Cazzolato, G., (1988) 'Presence of a modified low density lipoprotein in humans', Arteriosclerosis 8, 79-81.

13. Cazzolato, G., Avogaro, P., and Bittolo-Bon, G., (1991) ' Characterization of a more electronegatively charged LDL subfraction by ion exchange HPLC', Free Radical Biol. Med. 11, 247-253.

14. Avogaro, P., Cazzolato, G., and Bittolo-Bon, G., (1991) 'Some questions concerning a small, more electronegative LDL circulating in human plasma', Atherosclerosis 91, 163-171.

15. Havel R.J., Eder H.A., and Bragdon J.H., (1955) 'The distribution and chemical composition of ultracentrifugally separated lipoproteins in human serum', J. Clin. Invest. 34,1345-1351.

16. Lowry O.H., Rosenbourg N.J., Farr A.L., and Randall R.J., (1951) 'Protein measurement with the folin phenol reagent', J. Biol. Chem. 193,165-167.

17. Yagi K ., (1985) 'Assay for serum lipid peroxide level and its clinical significance', in K. Yagi (ed.), Lipid Peroxides in Biology and Medicine, Academic Press, New York, pp 223-242.

18. Lehman S., and Martin H.L., (1982) 'Improved direct determination of alpha- and gamma-tocopherol in plasma and platelets in liquid chromatography, with fluorescence detection', Clin. Chem. 28,1784-1787.

19. Barnhart G.L., Busch S.J., and Jackson R.L., (1989) 'Concentration dependent antioxidant activity of probucol in low density lipoproteins in vitro: probucol degradation precedes lipoprotein oxidation', J. Lipid. Res. 30,104-111.

20. McLean R.L., and Hagaman K.A., (1989) 'Effect of probucol on the phisical properties of low density lipoproteins oxidized by copper', Biochemistry 28, 321-327.

21. Crepaldi, G., Baggio, G., Arca, M, Avellone, G., Avogaro, P., Bittolo-Bon, G., Bompiani, G.D., et al., (1991) 'Pravastatin vs gemfibrozil in the treatment of primary hypercholesterolemia', Arc. Intern. Med. 151, 146-152.

22. Koga, T., Shimada, Y., Kuroda, M., Tsujita, Y., Hasegawa, K., and Yamasaki, M., (1990) 'Tissue-selective inhibition of cholesterol synthesis in vivo by pravastatin sodium, a 3-hydroxy-3-methyl-glutaryl coenzyme A reductase inhibitor' Biochim. Biophys. Acta 1045, 115-121.

23. Aviram, M., Dankner, G., Cogan, U., Hochgraf, E., and Brook, G., (1992) 'Lovastatin inhibits low-density lipoprotein oxidation and alters its fluidity and uptake by macrophages: in vitro and in vivo studies', Metabolism 41, 229-235.

24. Hoffman, R., Brook, G.J., and Aviram, M., (1992) 'Hipolipidemic drugs reduce lipoprotein susceptibility to undergo lipid peroxidation', Atherosclerosis 93, 105-113.

CLINICAL EXPERIENCE WITH FLUVASTATIN, THE FIRST SYNTHETIC HMG-
CoA REDUCTASE INHIBITOR

L. A. Jokubaitis, A. J. Troendle, J. M. Fattu, and R. I. Levy

ABSTRACT. Fluvastatin (FL), the first synthetic HMG-CoA reductase inhibitor, was administered to 946 hypercholesterolemic patients in four Phase III trials of 18 to 54 weeks duration. At 20 mg QPM, FL treatment resulted in a mean change in LDL-C of -20.5% (p < 0.001). At 40 mg daily, the mean LDL-C change was -24.0%. Apolipoprotein B reductions were similar to the LDL-C reductions. Small but meaningful increases in HDL-C and corresponding decreases in triglycerides were noted. No effect upon Lp(a) was found. None of the adverse complaints common to the statin class were produced in FL subjects at a rate significantly above those on placebo. Three (0.3%) FL-treated and three (0.5%) control patients had elevations of CPK to greater than ten times the upper limit of normal (>10xULN). No cases of myositis were reported. Persistent transaminase elevations to >3xULN occurred in 13 (1.4%) FL-treated patients and six (1.2%) placebo controls. The data suggest that fluvastatin is an effective agent for treating hypercholesterolemia, with tolerability comparable to placebo and a safety profile that is potentially distinct from other HMG-CoA reductase inhibitors with respect to specific parameters.

Introduction

The need for safe and effective agents to treat hypercholesterolemia has focused attention on inhibitors of 3-hydroxyl-3-methylglutaryl coenzyme A (HMG-CoA) reductase, the rate-limiting enzyme in cholesterol synthesis. Currently available first-generation HMG-CoA reductase inhibitors include lovastatin, simvastatin, and pravastatin, all of which were derived from fungal metabolites, are analogs of compactin, and are structurally similar. In clinical trials, these agents have been shown to be effective and well tolerated in lowering serum cholesterol levels (Lovastatin Study Group II, 1986; Bradford et al, 1991; Stein et al, 1990; Hunninghake et al, 1990).

Fluvastatin (XU 62-320) is the first entirely synthetic HMG-CoA reductase inhibitor. The molecule was synthesized *de novo* following an extensive program of analogue synthesis (Kathawala, 1991). Fluvastatin is structurally distinct from the currently available HMG-CoA reductase inhibitors, with its' side chain in the open dihydroxy acid form and the presence of an indole ring as well as a fluorinated phenyl group (see Figure 1).

This unique structure of fluvastatin leads to unique biopharmaceutical properties. Fluvastatin is completely absorbed from the gastrointestinal tract regardless of the presence of food. Systemic exposure is extremely short, with plasma half-lives of approximately 30 minutes. The drug is targeted to the liver, with 95% excretion through the biliary route. The open side chain renders the drug hydrophilic allowing minimal penetration of

269

A. L. Catapano et al. (eds.), Drugs Affecting Lipid Metabolism, 269–276.
© 1993 Kluwer Academic Publishers and Fondazione Giovanni Lorenzini.

the central nervous system in preclinical models. In addition, fluvastatin is the active pharmacologic moiety. There are no other circulating active metabolites demonstrated in man.

Figure 1. Comparative Structures of HMG-CoA Reductase Inhibitors

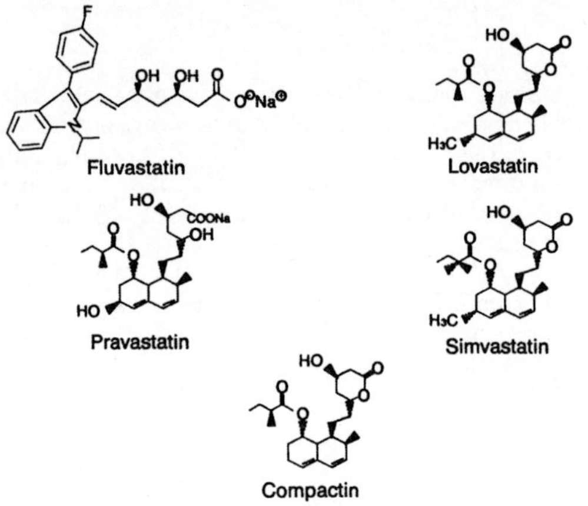

Fluvastatin is the first synthetic HMG-CoA reductase inhibitor to be submitted to the United States Food and Drug Administration (FDA) for approval. Over 2600 North American subjects were included in the studies presented in the fluvastatin New Drug Application (NDA) to the FDA. Of the 2263 subjects who received fluvastatin, 1938 received the drug in doses between 20 to 40 mg per day. This report presents a review of pooled data from controlled clinical trials with fluvastatin.

Methods

Data from four controlled Phase III trials were pooled and analyzed for efficacy determinations (data on file, Sandoz Research Institute). All four trials were of multicenter, randomized, double-blind, parallel group, and either placebo- or active-controlled design. Patients entering the studies were diagnosed with primary hypercholesterolemia, with a minimum entry low-density lipoprotein cholesterol (LDL-C) level requirement of at least 160 mg/dL after dietary intervention. One of the studies involved a higher risk patient population, with a baseline LDL-C level of at least 200 mg/dL required for entry into the study. Maximum entry triglyceride (TG) level was 350 mg/dL in two studies, and 300 mg/dL in the other two.

A six-week placebo washout period was followed by 18 to 54 weeks of treatment in these studies. The time points selected for analysis of the clinical and statistical significance of the effects of drug exposure on plasma lipids, however, were endpoints ranging from Week 8 to Week 12 of treatment across all studies prior to dose titration or combination therapy. Fluvastatin was given in dosages of 10 mg to 40 mg, and in all but one of the four studies, the drug was given once daily. In one study, patients in two of six randomized groups were given fluvastatin with randomly assigned cholestyramine. This combination was also used in an extension phase of another of the four studies.

Different databases were used for safety determinations (data on file, Sandoz Research Institute). Data from all twelve controlled clinical trials included in the NDA (Phases II and III) were analyzed for assessment of patients prematurely discontinued from trials. Adverse event assessments were based on data from two Phase III trials that were conducted solely against a placebo control. The same four Phase III controlled trials used for the assessment of efficacy provided information regarding transaminase elevations, creatine phosphokinase elevations, and myopathy, incorporating data from all time points of these studies.

Results

PATIENT POPULATION (data on file, Sandoz Research Institute)

A total of 1605 patients were randomized in the four controlled Phase III trials used to assess efficacy and safety, with 946 receiving fluvastatin. Six hundred fifty-seven patients received 20 mg of fluvastatin daily, an additional 214 received 40 mg daily, and 485 control patients received placebo (with diet controlled). In addition, 75 patients received 10 mg of fluvastatin daily, and 174 patients received an active control formulation of lovastatin. Efficacy data are presented for patients who received 20 mg to 40 mg of fluvastatin per day, focusing on the group who received 20 mg.

The mean ages of patients in the fluvastatin 20 mg (FL20), fluvastatin 40 mg (FL40), and the placebo (PBO) groups were 54, 52, and 54 years, respectively. The percentages of males in the three groups were 59%, 55%, and 57%, respectively, and the percentages of patients who were white were 93%, 95%, and 91%, respectively. The FL20 and placebo groups were quite similar in their mean age, sex distribution, baseline lipid abnormalities, and presence of coronary artery disease at baseline. The FL40 group is primarily composed of a patient population with heterozygous familial hypercholesterolemia (FH), resulting in patients with considerably higher baseline LDL-C levels and a slightly greater incidence of coronary artery disease at baseline. For an appropriate comparison, the FL40 group data is compared in this report to the corresponding placebo group derived from the same study population rather than the entire pooled placebo group.

EFFICACY (data on file, Sandoz Research Institute)

Low-Density Lipoprotein Cholesterol (LDL-C). As shown in Figure 2, at a dose of 20 mg QPM, fluvastatin treatment resulted in a pooled mean percent change in LDL-C across all studies of -20.5% (range of -18.0% to -22.2%) in 644 patients. This is a highly significant ($p < 0.001$) change compared to the negligible decrease (-0.2%) in the placebo group (n = 475). Baseline LDL-C levels were comparable for the two groups (215 mg/dL in FL20 group, and 218 mg/dL in the placebo group). At a daily dose of 40 mg, fluvastatin treatment resulted in a mean 24% reduction in LDL-C (range of -22.5% to -25.4%) for 210 patients as compared to a 0.9% increase for 105 patients in the placebo group ($p < 0.001$). Baseline LDL-C levels were comparable for the FL40 and placebo groups (269 mg/dL), but were considerably higher in this group comprising FH patients than for the FL20 and corresponding placebo groups.

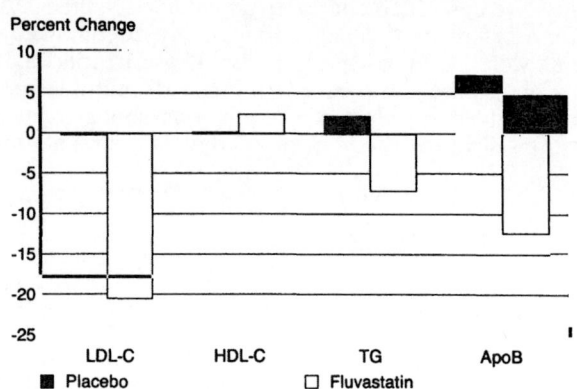

Figure 2. Lipid Changes in Fluvastatin (20 mg/day) Phase III Controlled Trials

Therapeutic LDL-C responses, defined as those reductions greater than 15% from baseline, were seen in 72% of all patients receiving 20 mg of fluvastatin daily, while only 7% of placebo patients had a similar degree of response. The categorical analysis applied to the FL40 and placebo groups demonstrated that approximately 70% of patients in the FL40 group achieved at least a 20% reduction in LDL-C levels from baseline, whereas over 90% of placebo patients demonstrated a poor response (<10% reduction or an increase).

When the LDL-C results in the FL20 and placebo groups were analyzed by patient age, the data showed a somewhat greater treatment effect in the subgroup of patients 65 years or older than in younger patients, even when adjusted for the placebo response. LDL-C was reduced by 20% in the group of patients younger than 65 years (n = 525) and 24% in the group 65 years or older (n = 119). Analysis of the response in the FL40 group demonstrates an even greater treatment effect in the group 65 years or older (n = 28) than in the group younger than 65 years (n = 180) when adjusted for placebo (-30% and -24%, respectively). In addition, females had a slightly greater LDL-C response to fluvastatin treatment than did males.

High-Density Lipoprotein Cholesterol (HDL-C). As shown in Figure 2, HDL-C increased modestly (+2.4%) in the group receiving 20 mg of fluvastatin daily (n = 648) as compared to a slight increase (+0.2%) for 477 patients in the placebo group, a finding that was nonetheless statistically significant (p < 0.01). Mean baseline HDL-C levels approximated 50 mg/dL in both groups, not considered in the high-risk range. At a daily dose of 40 mg, fluvastatin treatment resulted in a considerably greater increase (+6.6%) in HDL-C levels from baseline (n = 210), while the placebo group demonstrated a modest increase (+3.1%); the difference between groups was statistically significant (p < 0.05).

Triglycerides (TG). As shown in Figure 2, triglyceride levels decreased moderately (-7.1%) in the group receiving 20 mg of fluvastatin daily (n = 648) as compared to a small increase (+2.2%) for the 477 patients in the placebo group (p < 0.001). Baseline TG levels (151 to 153 mg/dL) were well within the normal range as expected for a predominantly type II phenotype patient population. At a daily dose of 40 mg, fluvastatin treatment (n = 210) resulted in a 11% reduction in TG from baseline as compared to an increase of 7% for 105 patients in the placebo group (p < 0.001).

Apolipoprotein B (apoB). The changes seen with apoB levels indicate a dose-related response. Changes in apoB levels for the FL20 (n = 106), FL40 (n = 208), and placebo (n = 103) groups were -12%, -17%, and +7%, respectively. The magnitudes of the apo B change in the two fluvastatin groups, when adjusted for placebo effect, parallel the degrees of LDL-C reduction in the two treatment groups.

Lp(a). Mean Lp(a) values in the two fluvastatin treatment groups were not statistically significant compared to the placebo group. Baseline and endpoint values were 30 mg/dL and 32 mg/dL, respectively, for the FL20 group; 35 mg/dL and 37 mg/dL, respectively, for the FL40 group; and 38 mg/dL and 38 mg/dL, respectively, for the placebo group. The median percent change for all three groups was 0.0.

SAFETY (data on file, Sandoz Research Institute)

A review of all Phase II and Phase III clinical trials suggests that fluvastatin was generally well tolerated in patients with primary hypercholesterolemia.

Premature Discontinuation. Of the 2263 patients exposed to fluvastatin, 1446 (64%) were involved in at least one of the 12 controlled clinical trials included in the NDA. Of these 1446 subjects, only 102 (7.1%) discontinued prematurely from these trials compared with 81 out of 899 (9.0%) control patients (placebo or lovastatin). When the reasons for premature discontinuation are grouped into five mutually exclusive categories (death, adverse events, uncooperative, lack of efficacy, other), the numbers of subjects who discontinued for each reason are comparable between the fluvastatin and control groups (see Table 1).

TABLE 1. Number (%) of Patients Discontinued in Controlled Clinical Trials

Discontinuation Reason	Fluvastatin (n = 1446)	Control (n = 899)
Mean Exposure (wks)	23	22 (placebo) 18 (lovastatin)
Death	3 (0.2%)	0 (0.0%)
Adverse Event	42 (2.9%)	32 (3.6%)
Uncooperative	18 (1.2%)	24 (2.7%)
Lack of efficacy	2 (0.1%)	2 (0.2%)
Other	37 (2.6%)	23 (2.6%)
Total	102 (7.1%)	81 (9.0%)

Three deaths were reported during controlled clinical trials. All of these were of cardiac etiology, and none were attributed to fluvastatin administration. Both the percentage of patients who discontinued due to adverse events and the total percentage of discontinued patients were greater in the control group than in the fluvastatin group.

The safety assessment of fluvastatin in Phase III controlled trials involved comprehensive evaluations of all patients, including adverse event reporting, laboratory assessment, physical examination, electrocardiograms, and ophthalmologic examination. This report focuses on three areas of safety assessment: adverse event frequencies, the incidence of transaminase elevations, and the issue of myopathy seen with other agents in this class.

Adverse Event Frequencies. In evaluating adverse events, the experience of 1031 patients in two Phase III trials is of particular interest because both were conducted solely against a placebo control, both were of three or more months duration, and both used the proposed market dosage range of 20 mg to 40 mg per day. In these studies, designated as core trials, 620 patients were exposed to fluvastatin and 411 patients were exposed to placebo.

Table 2 lists the adverse events reported in these placebo-controlled trials that were considered by the investigator to be possibly or probably attributable to fluvastatin therapy and is limited to those that occurred with a frequency greater than 2%. There was no statistical significance in the incidence of adverse events among patients taking fluvastatin when compared to the corresponding placebo control. While fatigue was seen more frequently with placebo than with fluvastatin, there was a slight increase in the frequency of dyspepsia and abdominal pain with fluvastatin treatment.

TABLE 2. Adverse Events Attributable to Fluvastatin Therapy (20 to 40 mg/day) Occurring at Frequency of >2% in Core Trials

Adverse Event	Fluvastatin, % (n = 620)	Placebo, % (n = 411)
Dyspepsia	6.6	3.6
Headache	3.5	3.6
Abdominal pain	3.9	2.4
Diarrhea	3.2	3.2
Nausea	2.7	1.5
Fatigue	2.3	2.9
Rash	2.1	2.9

Transaminase Elevations. It has been well documented that elevations of serum transaminases occur with other HMG-CoA reductase inhibitors (Tobert, 1988). The frequencies of persistent, marked elevations (defined as greater than three times the upper limit of laboratory normal) are reported as 1.9%, 1.0%, and 1.3% for lovastatin, simvastatin, and pravastatin, respectively (US Full Prescribing Information). Asymptomatic transaminase elevations have also been observed with fluvastatin therapy. These cases have rapidly reversed upon discontinuation of therapy, and all instances of transaminase elevations observed to date that are attributable to fluvastatin have occurred in the first three months of therapy. In Phase III studies, 13 (1.4%) of 946 patients receiving fluvastatin were defined as having persistent elevations, virtually indistinguishable from the 1.2% (6 of 485) incidence of elevations observed in the corresponding placebo group. Of the patients who experienced transaminase elevations, eight (0.8%) fluvastatin-treated patients were discontinued from the trials according to protocol, while 0.6% were discontinued in the placebo group. No patient treated with fluvastatin to date has been reported to have chronic transaminase elevations or other evidence of residual liver dysfunction.

Myopathy. Rhabdomyolysis with renal insufficiency secondary to myoglobinuria has been reported with all approved agents of this class, including lovastatin, simvastatin, and pravastatin (Pierce et al, 1990; US Full Prescribing Information for simvastatin and pravastatin). Frequencies reported for lovastatin and pravastatin are 0.5% and 0.1%, respectively (US Full Prescribing Information). A syndrome of myopathy, involving either muscle aching or weakness, associated with CPK elevations generally greater than ten times the upper limit of laboratory normal, has also been associated with HMG-CoA reductase inhibitors (US Full Prescribing Information for lovastatin and pravastatin).

To date, no cases of rhabdomyolysis or myopathy with elevated CPK values have been reported with fluvastatin therapy. In all Phase III controlled trials, no patients were discontinued due to a myopathic adverse event. The incidence of CPK elevations greater than 10xULN in these controlled trials was actually lower in the fluvastatin group (0.3%) than in the corresponding placebo group (0.6%).

Other Toxicities. There are other characteristic toxicities seen in preclinical models with HMG-CoA reductase inhibitors. Central nervous system vascular lesions have been noted in the beagle dog and have been reported with lovastatin, simvastatin, and pravastatin (US Full Prescribing Information). To date, these have not been described with fluvastatin. Additionally, liver tumors have been reported in rodent models associated with the other three currently available agents of this class, lovastatin, simvastatin, and pravastatin (US Full Prescribing Information). These tumors also have not been seen with fluvastatin to date.

Conclusion

Fluvastatin is the first entirely synthetic HMG-CoA reductase inhibitor and has a very favorable efficacy/side-effect ratio. Its unique structure leads to unique biopharmaceutical properties with selective targeting to the liver. The clinical data accumulated with fluvastatin to date suggest that it is an effective agent in the treatment of primary hypercholesterolemia, with tolerability over the dosage range of 20 to 40 mg daily that is comparable to placebo and a profile that is potentially distinct from other fungally derived HMG-CoA reductase inhibitors in the incidence and nature of particular key safety concerns. The safety and efficacy of fluvastatin at doses greater than 40 mg daily are currently under study.

Acknowledgements

This article is based on an oral presentation reviewing the clinical experience with fluvastatin in the treatment of hypercholesterolemia (XI Symposium on Drugs Affecting Lipid Metabolism, Florence, Italy, May 1992). The data presented have been drawn from unpublished reports (data on file, Sandoz Research Institute), which have been pooled and reported. The objective of the presentation and, hence this article, is to provide a general overview of the clinical experience, using data combined from unpublished studies, and not to serve as a thorough reporting of original data from individual studies.

The authors gratefully acknowledge the writing assistance of Martha Dwyer Hoffmann and the statistical assistance of Rachel B. Neuwirth and Kevin McCague.

References

Bradford, R.H., Shear, C.L., Chremos, A.N., et al. (1991) 'Expanded clinical evaluation of lovastatin (EXCEL) study results, I. Efficacy in modifying plasma lipoproteins and adverse event profile in 8245 patients with moderate hypercholesterolemia.' Arch Intern Med 151, 43-49.

Data on file, Sandoz Research Institute, East Hanover, NJ.

Hunninghake, D.B., Knopp, R.H., Schonfeld, G., et al. (1990) 'Efficacy and safety of pravastatin in patients with primary hypercholesterolemia, I. A dose-response study.' Atherosclerosis 85, 81-89.

Kathawala, F.G. (1991) 'HMG-CoA reductase inhibitors: An exciting development in the treatment of hyperlipoproteinemia,' Medicinal Research Reviews 11(2), 121-146.

Lovastatin Study Group II. (1986) 'Therapeutic response to lovastatin (mevinolin) in non-familial hypercholesterolemia: A multicenter study.' JAMA 256(20), 2829-2834.

Pierce, L.R., Wysowski, D.K., Gross, T.P. (1990) 'Myopathy and rhabdomyolysis associated with lovastatin-gemfibrozil combination therapy.' JAMA 264(1), 71-75.

Stein, E., Kreisberg, R., Miller, V., et al. (1990) 'Effects of simvastatin and cholestyramine in familial and nonfamilial hypercholesterolemia.' Arch Intern Med 150, 341-345.

Tobert, J.A. (1988) 'Efficacy and long-term adverse effect pattern of lovastatin.' Am J Cardiol 318, 1222.

US Full Prescribing Information for Mevacor® (lovastatin), Merck Sharp & Dohme, West Point, PA, in 1992 Physicians' Desk Reference, Medical Economics Data Inc., Montvale NJ, p 1505.

US Full Prescribing Information for Pravachol® (pravastatin), Bristol-Myers Squibb Co, Princeton, NJ, 1992.

US Full Prescribing Information for Zocor® (simvastatin), Merck Sharp & Dohme, West Point, PA, 1992.

SECONDARY PREVENTION OF CARDIOVASCULAR DISEASE:
THE ROLE OF HMG-CoA REDUCTASE INHIBITORS

John C. LaRosa, M.D.

ABSTRACT. There continues to be considerable debate about the wisdom of drug-induced cholesterol lowering in the primary prevention of coronary artery disease (CAD). There is no debate, however, that in patients with established disease, cholesterol treatment is of prime importance. Cohort studies demonstrate that LDL and HDL continue to be important predictors of both morbidity and mortality in patients with established coronary disease. Data from secondary prevention trials indicate that all-cause and CAD mortality are decreased in patients whose cholesterols are lowered. Evidence from regression studies indicates that coronary atherosclerosis can be arrested and perhaps reversed by aggressive lipid treatment. Finally, cost-benefit analyses demonstrate actual cost savings by vigorous cholesterol interventions. Current guidelines, however, do not sufficiently emphasize the importance of treatment in patients with CAD. Animal and human regression studies indicate that a desirable LDL cholesterol is one less than 100 mg/dl (2.6 meq/L). It is unlikely that such levels can be routinely obtained in most patients with hypercholesterolemia without the use of HMG-CoA reductase inhibitors. Properly used, HMG-CoA reductase inhibitors can become agents not only of prevention but also for reversal of established coronary disease.

Considerable evidence links the reduction of low density lipoprotein cholesterol (LDL-C) levels to the prevention of recurrent events in patients with established coronary artery disease (CAD). Such evidence includes observations that LDL-C and high density lipoprotein cholesterol (HDL-C) predict the risk of subsequent CAD in both those with and without established coronary disease [1]. In addition, meta-analysis of trials of cholesterol lowering in patients with established disease have demonstrated significant declines in CAD events, as well as all-cause mortality [2]. Finally, regression studies using serial angiograms have demonstrated the arrest of progression and even regression of coronary atherosclerosis with cholesterol lowering induced by

A. L. Catapano et al. (eds.), Drugs Affecting Lipid Metabolism, 277–281.
© 1993 Kluwer Academic Publishers and Fondazione Giovanni Lorenzini.

drugs [3-5], diet [6], or ileal bypass surgery [7].

All of this evidence raises the question as to whether more intensive intervention should be considered in patients with CAD than is currently recommended. Both animal [8] and human [3-7] studies suggest that LDL-C levels below 100 mg/dl (2.56 meq/L) may be associated with the best results in terms of regression or arrest of progression of coronary lesions. Such a goal would be considerably lower than the current United States goal of LDL-C below 130 mg/dl (3.33 meq/L) for those with coronary disease. Moreover, proper management of patients with coronary disease would require that all patients, regardless of total cholesterol levels, have an LDL, HDL, and triglyceride determined.

Current evidence suggests that physicians may be slow to institute cholesterol-lowering intervention in patients with established coronary disease. In fact, although it is difficult to establish a precise figure, some studies have suggested that only one third of patients with established coronary disease undergo regular cholesterol lowering with either diet or drug therapy [9-10]. The reasons for this are unclear but may include the belief that: (a) Survival after infarction is unaffected by cholesterol intervention. (b) The feeling that coronary bypass surgery or angioplasty has cured the problem and no further intervention is necessary. (c) Physician discomfort about providing nutritional counseling. (d) Lack of physician time to provide adequate counseling. (e) Patient resistance to changes in lifestyle. (f) Poor long-term compliance with drug regimens. (g) Concern that cholesterol lowering may have risks, including excess mortality from cancer, hemorrhagic stroke, and violent death. (h) Concern about the expense of long-term cholesterol lowering.

It is known from secondary prevention trials that the rate of recurrent infarction is approximately 6% annually, compared with 1% in primary prevention trials [2]. LDL-lowering, then, has the potential to prevent many more events in a population with established disease than in one without. In fact, cholesterol lowering compares favorably with other medical therapies, including aspirin [11] and beta-blockers [12], in reducing subsequent coronary events in an individual with established disease.

There is also evidence that cholesterol lowering is valuable in patients who have undergone bypass surgery [3] as well as those who have undergone angioplasty [13], although the magnitude of the benefit with these procedures is unclear and is still under investigation.

Meta-analysis of primary prevention trials has indicated a net excess mortality from violent or traumatic deaths, including suicides, homicides, and accidents, in such studies. It must be remembered that the degree of LDL-C lowering achieved in these studies was small (in the 10 to 15% range), and, in addition, that the total number of mortal events was small. Moreover, the addition of suicides, accidents, and homicides in one group is questionable since it is not clear that they have any common antecedents. Individual case audits of these trauma deaths in the two largest studies indicated that many patients were taking no cholesterol-lowering drug at the time of death [14]. While this issue should remain one for investigation, it is insufficiently developed to dictate public policy, but is, nevertheless, one of concern.

No such concern, however, should exist in secondary prevention, in which meta-analyses have not demonstrated excess mortality from non-cardiovascular deaths and, in fact, have demonstrated significant declines both in morbid and mortal coronary disease events and borderline declines in all-cause mortality [2].

Thus, the long-term safety of cholesterol lowering is and should be the subject of continued investigation. This issue, however, is far less pressing in patients with established coronary disease since over 80% of deaths in such patients are from cardiovascular disease.

Cost-effectiveness of cholesterol lowering in those with CAD also continues to be a matter of considerable debate, particularly when the alteration of cholesterol levels requires drug therapy. Cost-effectiveness analysis, however, indicates that cholesterol lowering is highly cost-effective in patients with CAD. In fact, in certain patients, for example, men less than 65 years of age and women less than 55 years of age, with cholesterols over 250 mg/dl (6.41 meq/L), cholesterol lowering actually is cost saving because of the probability of eliminating the costs of subsequent events as well as the costs of additional bypass surgery or angioplasty [15]. Thus, overall, cost considerations support cholesterol interventions in patients with established disease.

Issues that remain to be decided include the precise targets for LDL-lowering in patients with coronary disease. The role of triglyceride-lowering and HDL-increasing in patients with established disease is also unclear, although both epidemiologic and primary prevention trials support the notion that both HDL-C increases and, to a lesser extent, triglyceride-lowering may be beneficial in both primary and secondary prevention [16]. Finally, it is unclear whether there is sufficient benefit in patients with LDL-C levels within the "normal" range who also have coronary disease in lowering those levels below 100 mg/dl (2.56 meq/L). Evidence from the Cholesterol Lowering Atherosclerosis Study (CLAS) indicates that those with lower cholesterol levels had the same degree of regression as those with higher cholesterol levels [3]. This implies that there may be a population of individuals who are particularly susceptible to coronary disease, even at LDL-C levels that would otherwise be considered normal. The characteristics of such individuals is, as yet, unclear, but factors that may predispose to the progression of atherosclerosis in individuals with established disease, in addition to an elevated LDL, might include such things as a low HDL level, elevated levels of lipoprotein (a) {Lp(a)}, elevated levels of intermediate density lipoprotein, increased quantities of small, dense LDL, hyperinsulinemia, high waist-to-hip ratios, and the apoE phenotype.

If LDL-C levels below 100 mg/dl (2.56 meq/L) are required for adequate treatment of individuals with established disease to prevent recurrent events and even induce regression of atherosclerosis, then the role of HMG-CoA reductase inhibitors is clear. For many patients with coronary disease, LDL-C levels will be far too high to be lowered by any other single drug and, in fact, even in many patients, HMG-CoA reductase inhibitors alone will be insufficient. As the most powerful agents available to lower LDL-C levels, however, it is likely that reductase inhibitors alone, or in combination with bile acid sequestrants, will prove pivotal in the treatment of many patients with established disease. Bile acid sequestrants alone, or in combination, then, can not only arrest the progression of coronary disease but perhaps also induce regression. Ongoing debates about primary prevention and cost effectiveness should not interfere with the application of vigorous LDL-C lowering therapy in those with established coronary disease.

1.   Pekkanen, J., Linn, S., Heiss, G., et al. (1990) 'Ten-year mortality from cardiovascular disease in relation to cholesterol level among men with and without preexisting cardiovascular disease', N Engl J Med 322, 1700-1707.

2.   Rossouw, J.E., Lewis, B., and Rifkind, B.M. (1990) 'The value of lowering cholesterol after myocardial infarction', N Engl J Med 323, 1112-1119.

3.   Blankenhorn, D.H., Nessim, S.A., Johnson, R.L., et al. (1987) 'Beneficial effects of combined colestipol-niacin therapy on coronary atherosclerosis and coronary venous bypass grafts', JAMA 257, 3233-3240.

4.   Brown, G., Albers, J.J., Fisher, L.D., et al. (1990) 'Regression of coronary artery disease as a result of intensive lipid-lowering therapy in men with high levels of apolipoprotein B', N Engl J Med 323, 1289-1298.

5.   Kane, J.P., Malloy, M.J., Ports, T.A., et al. (1990) 'Regression of coronary atherosclerosis during treatment of familial hypercholesterolemia with combined drug regimens', JAMA 264, 3007-3012.

6.   Ornish, D., Brown, S.E., Scherwitz, L.W., et al. (1990) 'Can lifestyle changes reverse coronary heart disease?' Lancet 336, 129-133.

7.   Buchwald, H., Varco, R.L., Matts, J.P., et al. and the POSCH group (1990) 'Effect of partial ileal bypass surgery on mortality and morbidity from coronary heart disease in patients with hypercholesterolemia. Report of the Program on the Surgical Control of the Hyperlipidemias (POSCH)', N Engl J Med 323, 946-955.

8.   St. Clair, R.S.W. (1983) 'Atherosclerosis regression in animal models: Current concepts of cellular and biochemical mechanisms', Prog Cardiovasc Dis 26, 109-132.

9.   Boekeloo, B., Becker, D., Yeo, E., et al. (1987) 'Post myocardial infarction cholesterol management by primary physicians', J Am Coll Cardiol 9, 77A.

10.   Cohen, M.V., Byrne, M-J, Levine, B., et al. (1991) 'Low rate of treatment of hypercholesterolemia by cardiologists in patients with suspected and proven coronary artery disease', Circulation 83, 1294-1304.

11.   Yusuf, S., Wittes, J., and Friedman, L. (1988) 'Overview of results of randomized clinical trials in heart disease. II. Unstable angina, heart failure, primary prevention with aspirin, and risk factor modification', JAMA 260, 2259-2263.

12.   Yusuf, S., Peto, R., Lewis, J. et al. (1985) 'Beta blockade during and after myocardial infarction: An overview of the randomized trials', Prog Cardiovasc Dis 27, 335-371.

13.   Sahni, R., Maniet, A.R., Voci, G., and Banka, V.S. (1991) 'Prevention of restenosis by lovastatin after successful coronary angioplasty', Am Heart J 121 (part I), 1600-1608.

14.   Wysowski, D.K., and Gross, T.P. (1990) 'Deaths due to accidents and violence in two recent trials of cholesterol-lowering drugs', Arch Intern Med 150, 2169-2172.

15.   Goldman, L., Weinstein, M.C., Goldman, P.A., and Williams, L.W. (1991) 'Cost-effectiveness of HMG-CoA reductase inhibition for primary and secondary prevention of coronary heart disease', JAMA 265, 1145-1151.

16.   'The hypertriglyceridemias: risk and management. The International Committee for the Evaluation of hypertriglyceridemia as a vascular risk factor', Assmann, G., Gotto, A.M., Jr., and Paoletti, R., (Chairs), (1991) Am J Cardiol 68, 1A-42A.

COMBINED DRUG TREATMENT OF SEVERE HYPERCHOLESTEROLEMIA

P. SCHWANDT

Familial hypercholesterolemia and familial combined hyperlipidemia are the most threatening disorders of lipoprotein metabolism regarding premature atherosclerotic complications. Dietary and drug monotherapy often are not sufficient to control these disorders. Especially in patients with symptomatic coronary artery disease LDL-cholesterol should be lowered at least to 135 mg/dl (or even 100 mg/dl ?). This is often achieved only with combined treatment. As shown in figure 1 there are multiple options to combine lipid-regulating drugs with different sites of actions to interfere rather specifically according to the underlying defect of lipoprotein metabolism.

Figure 1:   Sites of action of lipid-lowering treatment

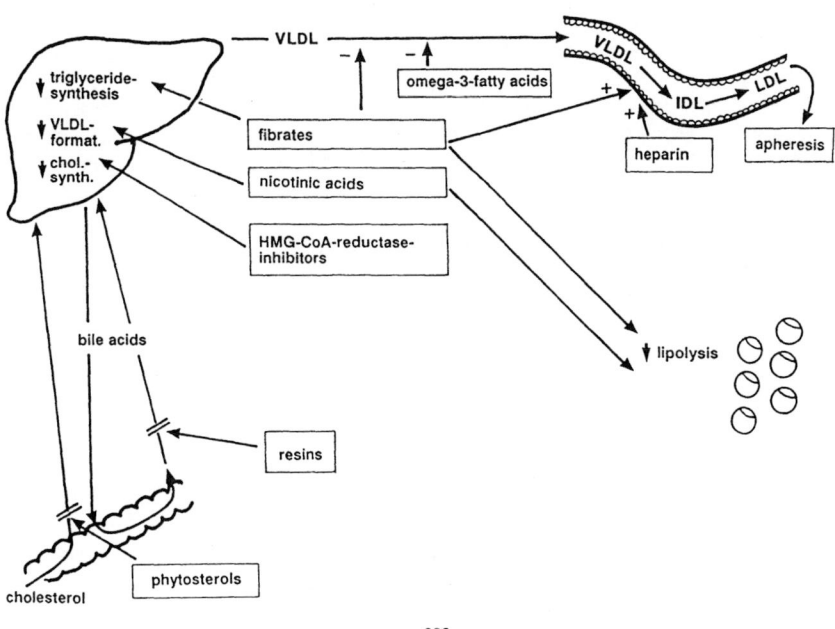

283

A. L. Catapano et al. (eds.), Drugs Affecting Lipid Metabolism, 283–292.
© 1993 Kluwer Academic Publishers and Fondazione Giovanni Lorenzini.

Elevated low density lipoprotein (LDL) cholesterol concentrations have been the main target of combined lipid lowering drug treatment. The bile acid sequestrants cholestyramine and colestipol lower LDL cholesterol plasma concentrations by stimulating their receptor related uptake into the liver cell which is depleted from cholesterol by an increased degradation of cholesterol into bile acids due to the sequestrant-interrupted bile acid recirculation from the gut to the liver. Since the resins are not absorbed they do not cause major systemic side effects.

The second possibility to reduce the cellular cholesterol level and thereby to stimulate the LDL receptor is to inhibit cholesterol synthesis. This is achieved specifically by the HMG-CoA-reductase (CSE) inhibitors Lovastatin, Pravastatin and Simvastatin. A combination of resins and CSE inhibitors seems ideal, since they stimulate the expression of the LDL receptor on the liver cell maximally by two separate mechanisms.

Nicotinic acid as well as the fibrates do not interfere directly with synthesis and biliary elimination of cholesterol. However, they are ideal partners for the combination with resins: not only to compensate their unwanted stimulating effect on VLDL (very low density lipoproteins) secretion from the liver but in addition to interfere beneficially with the metabolism of VLDL and of high density lipoproteins (HDL).

1. Bile acid sequestrants plus nicotinic acid

As demonstrated in table 1 the LDL cholesterol lowering effect of this combination was between 32-47 %. This effect and all the others are no true comparative data, since the baseline values were as different as the dosage, the time of application and the underlying disorders.

The Cholesterol-Lowering-Atherosclerosis-Study (CLAS) demonstrates that after two (8) and four (9) years this drug combination has not only a beneficial longterm effect on serum lipoproteins (table 1) but even more important also on coronary artery disease (CAD) in coronary bypass subjects (figure 2).

Figure 2:   CLAS: Coronary global change score

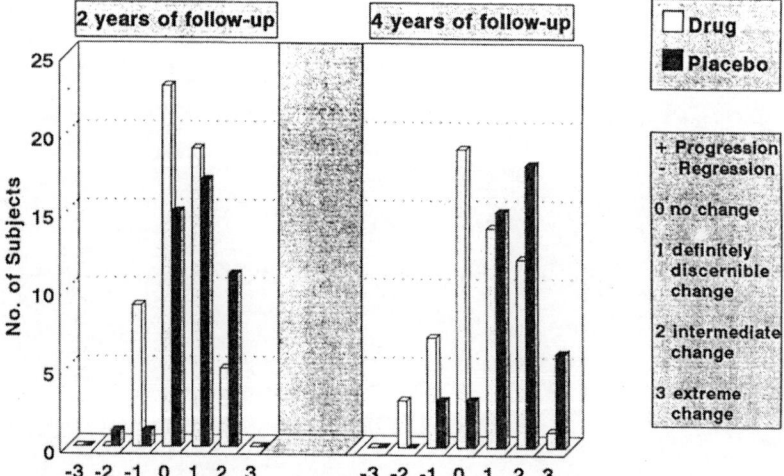

Cashin-Hemphill et al., 1990

A comparable regression of CAD together with a decrease of LDL cholesterol by 39 % and an increase of HDL cholesterol by 25 % has been demonstrated after 26 months in a trial with 72 patients with heterozygous familial hypercholesterolemia. Fourty subjects (22 women) have been treated with drug combinations partly consisting of resins plus nicotinic acid (11). One arm of the Familial Atherosclerosis Treatment Study (FATS) did also use the combination of bile acid sequestrants and nicotinic acid for 2.5 years with comparable effects om CAD (39 % regression) and lipoproteins (table 1).

Table 1: **Effects of bile acid sequestrants (Cx, Co) plus nicotinic acid (Ns) and analogue (Ac) on serum lipoproteins**

| Drug regimen | n | % change of | | | | Initial | Ref |
		Chol	LDL	HDL	TG	LDL (mg/dl)	
Cx (16 g) + Ns (3 g)	6	- 41	- 48	+25	- 37	360	1
Cx (16 g) + Ns (2-12 g)	10	- 26	- 32	+23	- 20	373	2
Cx (12 g) + Ac (750 mg)	28	- 27	- 32	+ 6	- 13	285	3
Cx ((12 g) + Ac (750 mg)	9	- 29	- 39	+31	- 8	320	4
Co (20 g) + Ns (6-7,5 g)	11	-	- 45	+17	-	278	5
Co (30 g) + Ns (3-8 g)	13	- 40	- 47	+32	- 35	337	6
Co (30 g) + Ns (3-7 g)	32	- 34	- 45	+22	- 34	263	7
Co (30±4 g) + Ns (4,3±1,3 g)	80	- 26	- 43	+37	- 22	171	8
Co (30±6 g) + Ns (4,2±2 g)	56	- 25	- 40	+37	- 18	171	9
Co (30 g) + Ns (4 g)	36	- 23	- 32	+43	- 29	190	12
Co (30 g) + Ns (1,5-7,5 g)	21	- 30	- 36	+25	- 20	326	13
Co (30 g) + Ns (3-6 g)	154	- 28	- 46	+40	- 31	175	30

Cx = Cholestyramine	Ac = Acipimox	TG = Triglycerides
Co = Colestipol	Ns = nicotinic acid	n = number of patients

2. Bile acid sequestrants plus fibrates

"The potential clinical usefulness of the combination of bile acid sequestrant resin plus clofibrate in the treatment of hyperlipidemia seems clear." DeWitt S. Goodman (14) and his coworkers suggested further that clofibrate does not "block the increased rate of cholesterol synthesis and turnover resulting from bile acid sequestrant treatment." The two bile acid sequestrants cholestyramine and colestipol both have been investigated in combination with bezafibrate, fenofibrate and gemfibrozil with comparable LDL cholesterol lowering effects. Clofibrate seems to be less effective (table 2).

Table 2:   **Effects of bile acid sequestrants plus fibrates on serum lipoproteins**

| Drug regimen | n | % change of | | | | Initial LDL (mg/dl) | Ref |
		Chol	LDL	HDL	TG		
Co (12 g) + Cl (2 g)	4*	- 23	- 29	-	- 24	192	15
Co (12 g) + Cl (2 g)	11**	- 5	+14	-	- 41	109	15
Co (15 g) + Cl (2 g)	20	- 25	-	-	- 29	-	16
Co (20 g) + Cl (2 g)	14	- 11	- 12	+25	- 22	197	17
Co (20 g) + Cl (2 g)	7***	- 21	- 14	+30	- 35	146	18
Cx (24 g) + Be (600 mg)	18	- 35	- 39	+ 2	- 19	278	19
Cx (16 g) + Be (400 mg)	21	- 28	- 36	+22	- 39	228	20
Cx (24 g) + Be (400 mg)	47	- 24	- 36	+31	- 33	227	21
Cx (20 g) + Ge (1,2 g)	12	- 41	- 44	- 11	-	347	22
Co (15 g) + Fe (250 mg)	6	- 36	- 41	+14	- 30	380	25
Cx (20 g) + Fe (300 mg)	10	- 28	- 36	+ 8	- 20	357	26
Co (20 g) + Ge (1,2 g)	9*	- 22	- 20	+11	- 44	229	23
Co (20 g) + Ge (1,2 g)	8**	- 17	- 15	+14	- 17	148	23

Cx = Cholestyramine	Ge = Gemfibrozil	* = Type IIb
Co = Colestipol	Cl = Clofibrate	** = Type IV
Be = Bezafibrate	TG = Triglycerides	*** = Type III
Fe = Fenofibrate	n = number of patients	

3. Bile acid sequestrants and probucol

This combination effectively lowers LDL cholesterol. However, it also decreases HDL cholesterol substantially together with a slight increase of plasma triglycerides (table 3). The HDL cholesterol lowering effect of probucol is well known and seems to be investigated by colestipol (24, 27). In 19 patients treated with 30 g/day colestipol plus 1 g/day probucol for 3.4 to 4.1 years coronary arteriographic follow-up investigations "showed that combined treatment stabilized the progression of established lesions and prevented the formation of new ones." (29).

Table 3:   **Effects of bile acid sequestrants plus probucol on serum lipoproteins**

| Drug regimen | n | % change of | | | | Initial LDL (mg/dl) | Ref. |
		Chol	LDL	HDL	TG		
Co (20 g) + Pr (1 g)	47	- 28	- 29	- 29	+11	242	24
Co (10 g) + Pr (1 g)	22	- 29	- 29	- 40	+14	239	27
Cx (16 g) + Pr (1g)	18	- 26	- 32	- 18	+ 1	300	28
Co (30 g) + Pr (1 g)	44	- 49	- 53	- 30	+15	341	29
Co (8 g) + Pr (1 g)	6	- 29	-	- 7	-	-	10

| Cx = Cholestyramine | Pr = Probucol | n = number of patients |
| Co = Colestipol | | TG = Triglycerides |

4. HGM CoA-reductase (CSE) inhibitors plus bile acid sequestrants

This drug combination seems to be the most effective way to decrease the cholesterol concentration in the liver cell as a consequence of increased degration of cholesterol to bile acids as well as of decreased synthesis of cholesterol. As shown in table 4 the result is a decrease of plasma LDL cholesterol concentrations by more than 50 %. In addition, HDL cholesterol levels are increased by about 10-15 % together with a tendency of triglycerides to decrease.

Table 4:   Effects of HMG-CoA-reductase inhibitors plus bile acid sequestrants on serum lipoproteins

Drug regimen	n	% change of Chol	LDL	HDL	TG	Initial LDL (mg/dl)	Ref
Cp (90 mg) + Cx (12 g)	10	- 39	- 52	+44	- 34	263	31
Lo (80 mg) + Co (20 g)	10	- 45	- 54	- 2	+ 7	409	32
Lo (40 mg) + Co (20 g)	7	- 37	- 46	+10	- 17	361	32
Lo (40 mg) + Co (20 g)	8	- 43	- 52	+29	+ 1	321	33
Lo (40 mg) + Co (20 g)	10	- 36	- 48	+17	+ 8	196	34
Lo (80 mg) + Cx (8 g)	19	- 47	- 56	+22	- 28	391	35
Lo (80 mg) + Cx (16 g)	19	- 51	- 61	+22	- 25	391	35
Lo (40 mg) + Co (20 g)	16	- 42	- 52	± 0	- 12	325	36
Lo (80 mg) + Co (20 g)	13	- 43	- 54	+ 6	- 13	325	36
Lo (80 mg) + Cx (8 g)	12	- 33	- 40	+18	- 23	303	37
Pra (40 mg) + Cx (8 g)	13	- 30	- 39	+ 6	+12	306	37
Pra (40 mg) + Cx (24 g)	9	- 33	- 53	+18	+ 8	209	38
Pra (10 mg) + Cx (24 g)	11	- 38	- 56	+11	+ 5	194	38
Pra (20 mg) + Cx (24 g)	7	- 32	- 47	+15	+13	206	38
Si (40 mg) + Cx (24 g)	5	- 43	- 55	+12	- 8	319	40
Si (40 mg) + Cx (16 g)	19	- 42	- 43	+ 9	- 8	355	42
Si (40 mg) + Cx (8 g)	43	- 42	- 49	+13	- 19	352	43
Si (20-40 mg) + Cx (8-24 g)	20	- 47	- 56	+ 7	+ 4	320	44

Cx = Cholestyramine   Pra = Pravastatin   n = number of patients
Co = Colestipol   Si = Simvastatin   TG = Triglycerides
Lo = Lovastatin   Cp = Compactin

5. HMG CoA-reductase (CSE) inhibitors plus fibrates or nicotinic acid

As shown in table 5 most studies with this combination have been performed with Lovastatin plus Gemfibrozil in subjects who do not seem to be optimal candidates for such a combination (Diabetes mellitus, Type IV HLP and Type III HLP). Since "the Food and Drug Administration documents the receipt of 12 case reports of severe myopathy or rhabdomyolosis" (48) the conclusion of Illingworth (41) seems acceptable: "We conclude that the combination of lovastatin plus gemfibrozil does not provide significant further LDL lowering as compared with monotherapy with lovastatin alone in patients with heterozygous familial hypercholesterolemia and that this combined drug regimen may be associated with an increased risk of myopathy". The combination CSE inhibitors plus nicotinic acid seems to be more effective (table 5), however caution should be exercised regarding hepatic function, uric acid and diabetes mellitus.

Table 5:   **Effects of HMG-CoA reductase inhibitors plus fibrates or nicotinic acid on serum lipoproteins**

Drug regimen	n	% change of				Initial LDL (mg/dl)	Ref
		Chol	LDL	HDL	TG		
Lo (40 mg) + Ge (1,2 g)	9*	- 29	- 27	+27	- 55	204	23
Lo (40 mg) + Ge (1,2 g)	8**	- 25	- 14	+36	- 56	146	23
Lo (40 mg) + Ge (1,2 g)	10****	- 40	- 7	+19	- 52	89	39
Lo (40 mg) + Ge (1,2 g)	6****	- 24	- 17	+14	- 35	124	39
Lo (80 mg) + Ge (1,2 g)	12	- 34	- 40	+ 7	- 45	194	41
Lo (20-80 mg + Ge (1,2 g)	25	- 20	- 23	± 0	- 18	155	45
Lo (40 mg) + Cl (2 g)	6***	- 68	- 24	+37	- 75	127	46
Pra (40 mg) + Be (600 mg)	19	- 32	-	+15	- 26	-	47
Pra (40 mg) + Ac (750 mg)	8	- 25	- 36	+26	- 34	299	47
Lo (80 mg) + Ns (3 g)	8	- 38	- 49	+25	- 43	327	49

Lo = Lovastatin	Cl = Clofibrate	*	= Type IIb
Pra = Pravastatin	Fe = Fenofibrate	**	= Type IV
Si = Simvastatin	Ac = Acipimox	***	= Type III
Nc = Nicotinic acid	n = number of patients	****	= Diabetes
Ge = Gemfibrozil	TG = Triglycerides		

6. Triple drug therapy

As shown in figure 1 even more options for ternary or quarterly combinations might be promizing though the experience with those combinations is limited yet. Again it is reasonable to reduce the dose of either drugs to reduce side effects and possibly costs. While the addition of probucol to the very effective combination lovastatin plus colestipol (52 % decrease of LDL cholesterol) (36) nicotinic acid as the third drug might add benefit (table 6).

Table 6:   **Effects of the ternary combination of Lovastatin (Lo), Colestipol (Co) and nicotinic acid (Ns) on serum lipoproteins**

Drug regimen	n	% change of				Initial LDL (mg/dl)	Ref
		Chol	LDL	HDL	TG		
Lo (80 mg) + Co (20 g) + Ns (3 g)	3	- 53	- 62	+46	- 57	372	49
Lo (40-60 mg) + Co (30 g) + Ns (1,5-7,5 g)	6	- 56	- 68	+28	- 48	323	13

n = number of patients   TG = Triglycerides

Literatur

1. Packard, C.J., Stewart J.M., Morgan H.G., Lorimer A.R. and Shepherd J. (1980) 'Combined drug therapy for familial hypercholesterolemia', Artery 7:281-289

2. Angelin, B., Eriksson M. and Einarsson K. (1986) 'Combined treatment with cholestyramine and nicotinic acid in heterozygous familial hypercholestrolemia: effects on biliary lipid composition', Europ J Clin Invest 16:391-396

3. Series, J.J., Gaw A., Kilday C., Bedford D.K., Lorimer A.R., Packard C.J. and Shepherd J. (1990) 'Acipimox in combination with low dose cholestyramine for the treatment of type II hyperlipidaemia', Br J clin Pharmac 30:49-54

4. Gylling, H., Vanhanen H. and Miettinen T.A. (1989) 'Effects of acipimox and cholestyramine on serum lipoproteins, non-cholesterol sterols and cholesterol absorption and elimination', Eur J Clin Pharmacol 37:111-115

5. Kane, J.P., Malloy M.J., Tun P., Phillips N.R., Freedman D.D., Williams M.L., Rowe J.S. and Havel R.J. (1981) 'Normalization of low-density-lipoprotein levels in heterozygous familial hyperchoelsterolemia with a combined drug regimen', New Engl J Med 304:251-258

6. Illingworth, D.R., Rapp J.H., Phillipson B.E. and Connor W.E. (1981) 'Colestipol plus nicotinic acid in treatment of heterozygous familial hypercholesterolaemia', Lancet I:296-298

7. Kuo, P.T., Kostis J.B., Moreyra A.E. and Hayes J.A. (1981) 'Familial type II hyperlipoproteinemia with coronary heart disease', Chest 79:286-291

8. Blankenhorn, D.H., Nessim S.A., Johnson R.L., Sanmarco M.E., Azen S.P. and Cashin-Hemphill L. (1987) 'Beneficial effects of combined Colestipol-Niacin therapy on coronary atherosclerosis and coronary venous bypass grafts', JAMA 257:3233-3240

9. Cashin-Hemphill, L., Mack W.J., Pogoda J.M., Sanmarco M.E., Azen S.P. and Blankenhorn D.H. (1990) 'Beneficial effects of Colestipol-Niacin on coronary atherosclerosis', JAMA 264:3013-3017

10. Pasquali, R., Biso P., Parenti M. and Melchionda N. (1981) 'Combined effects of probucol and cholestyramine in familial type II hyperlipoproteinaemia', Lancet I:1368

11. Kane, J.P., Malloy M.J., Ports T.A., Phillips N.R., Diehl J.C. and Havel R.J. (1990) 'Regression of coronary atherosclerosis during treatment of familial hypercholesterolemia with combined drug regimens', JAMA 264:3007-3012

12. Brown, G., Albers J.J., Fisher L.D., Schaefer S.M., Lin J.T., Kaplan C., Zhao X.Q., Bisson B.D., Fitzpatrick V.F. and Dodge H.T. (1990) 'Regression of coronary artery disease as a result of intensive lipid-lowering therapy in men with high levels of apolipoprotein B', New Engl J Med 323:1289-1298

13.   Malloy, M.J., Kane J.P., Kunitake S.T. and Tun P. (1987) 'Complementarity of Colestipol, Niacin, and Lovastatin in treatment of severe familial hypercholesterolemia', Ann Intern Med 107:616-623

14.   Goodman, D.S., Noble R.P. and Dell R.B. (1973) 'The effects of colestipol resin and of colestipol plus clofibrate on the turnover of plasma cholesterol in man', J Clin Invest 52:2646-2655

15.   Rose, H.G., Haft G.K. and Juliano J. (1976) 'Clofibrate-induced low density lipoprotein elevation therapeutic implications and treatment by colestipol resin', Atherosclerosis 23:413-427

16.   Fellin, R., Baggio G., Briani G., Baiocchi M.R., Manzato E., Baldo G. and Crepaldi G. (1978) 'Long-term trial with colestipol plus clofibrate in familial hypercholesterolemia', Atherosclerosis 29:241-249

17.   Hunninghake, D.B., Bell C. and Olson L. (1981) 'Effects of Colestipol and Clofibrate, singly and in combination, on plasma lipid and lipoproteins in type IIb hyperlipoproteinemia', Metabolism 30:610-615

18.   Hoogwerf, B.J., Peters J.R., Frantz I.D. and Hunninghake D.B. (1985) 'Effect of clofibrate and colestipol singly and in combination on plasma lipids and lipoproteins in type III hyperlipoproteinemia', Metabolism 34:978-981

19.   Curtis, L.D., Dickson A.C., Ling K.L.E. and Betteridge J. (1988) 'Combination treatment with cholestyramine and bezafibrate for heterozygous familial hypercholesterolaemia', Brit Med J 297:173-175

20.   Series, J.J., Caslake M.J., Kilday C., Cruickshank A., Demant T., Lorimer A.R., Packard C.J. and Shepherd J. (1989) 'Effect of combined therapy with bezafibrate and cholestyramine on low-density lipoprotein metabolism in type IIa hypercholesterolemia', Metabolism 38:153-158

21.   Fischer, S., Hanefeld M., Lang P.D., Fücker K., Bergmann S., Gehrisch S., Leonhardt W. and Jaroß W. (1990) 'Efficacy of a combined bezafibrate retard-colestyramine treatment in patients with hypercholesterolemia', Arzneim.-Forsch./Drug Res. 40:469-472

22.   Jones, A.F., Hughes E.A. and Cramb R. (1988) 'Gemfibrozil plus cholestyramine in familial hypercholesterolaemia', Lancet I:776

23.   East, C., Bilheimer D.W. and Grundy S.M. (1988) 'Combination drug therapy for familial combined hyperlipidemia', Ann Intern Med 109:25-32

24.   Dujovne, C.A., Krehbiel P., DeCoursey S., Jackson B., Chernoff S.B., Pittermann A. and Garty M. (1984) 'Probucol with colestipol in the treatment of hypercholesterolemia', Ann Intern Med 100:477-482

25.   Weisweiler, P. and Schwandt P. (1986) 'Colestipol plus fenofibrate versus synvinolin in familial hypercholesterolaemia', Lancet II:1212-1213

26. Malmendier, C.L., Delcroix C. and Lontie J.F. (1987) 'The effect of combined fenofibrate and cholestyramine therapy on low-density lipoprotein kinetics in familial hypercholesterolemia patients', Clin Chim Acta 162:221-227

27. Dujovne, C.A., Chernoff S.B., Krehbiel P., Jackson B., DeCoursey S. and Taylor H. (1984) 'Low-dose colestipol plus probucol for hypercholesterolemia', Am J Cardiol 53:1514-1518

28. Sommariva, D., Bonfiglioli D., Tirrito M., Pogliaghi I., Branchi A. and Cabrini E. (1986) 'Probucol and cholestyramine combination in the treatment of severe hypercholesterolemia', Int J Clin Pharm Ther Toxicol 24:505-510

29. Kuo, P.T., Wilson A.C., Kostis J.B. and Moreyra A.E. (1986) 'Effects of combined probucol-colestipol treatment for familial hypercholestrolemia and coronary artery disease', Am J Cardiol 57:43H-48H

30. Cashin-Hemphill, L., Spencer C.A., Nicoloff J.T., Blankenhorn D.H., Nessim S.A., Chin H.P. and Lee N.A. (1987) 'Alterations in serum thyroid hormonal indices with colestipol-niacin therapy', Ann Intern Med 107:324-329

31. Mabuchi, H., Sakao T., Sakai Y., Yoshimura A., Watanabe A., Wakasugi T., Koizumi J. and Takeda R. (1983) 'Reduction of serum cholesterol in heterozygous patients with familial hypercholesterolemia', New Engl J Med 308:609-613

32. Illingworth, D.R. (1984) 'Mevinolin plus colestipol in therapy for severe heterozygous familial hypercholesterolemia', Ann Intern Med 101:598-604

33. Grundy, S.M., Vega G.L. and Bilheimer D.W. (1985) 'Influence of combined therapy with mevinolin and interruption of bile-acid reabsorption on low density lipoproteins in heterozygous familial hypercholesterolemia', Ann Intern Med 103:339-343

34. Vega, G.L. and Grundy S.M. (1987) 'Treatment of primary moderate hypercholesterolemia with lovastatin (Mevinolin) and colestipol)', JAMA 257:33-38

35. Leren, T.P., Hjermann I., Berg K., Leren P., Foss O.P. and Viksmoen L. (1988) 'Effects of lovastatin alone and in combination with cholestyramine on serum lipids and apolipoproteins in heterozygotes for familial hypercholesterolemia', Atherosclerosis 73:135-141

36. Witztum, J.L., Simmons D., Steinberg D., Beltz W.F., Weinreb R., Young S.G., Lester P., Kelly N. and Juliano J. (1989) 'Intensive combination drug therapy of familial hyperchoelsterolemia with lovastatin, probucol, and colestipol hydrochloride', Circulation 79:16-28

37. Jacob, B.G., Möhrle W., Richter W.O., Schwandt P. (1992) 'Short- and long-term effects of lovastatin and pravastatin alone and in combination with cholestyramine on serum lipids, lipoproteins and apolipoproteins in primary hypercholesterolaemia', Eur J Clin Pharmacol 42:353-358

38.   Pan, H.Y., DeVault A.R., Swites B.J., Whigan D., Ivashkiv E., Willard D.A. and Brescia
        D. (1990) 'Pharmacokinetics and pharmacodynamics of pravastatin alone and with
        cholestyramine in hypercholesterolemia', Clin Pharmacol Ther 48:201-207

39.   Garg, A. and Grundy S.M. (1989) 'Gemfibrozil alone and in combination with
        lovastatin for treatment of hypertriglyceridemia in NIDDM', Diabetes 38:364-372

40.   Ytre-Arne, K. and Nordoy A. (1989) 'Simvastatin and cholestyramine in the long-term
        treatment of hypercholesterolaemia', J Int Med 226:285-290

41.   Illingworth, D.R. and Bacon S. (1989) 'Influence of lovatatin plus gemfibrozil on
        plasma lipids and lipoproteins in patients with heterozygous familial
        hypercholesterolemia', Circulation 79:590-596

42.   Emmerich, J., Aubert I., Bauduceau B., Dachet D., Chanu B., Erlich D., Gautier D.,
        Jacotot B. and Rouffy J. (1990) 'Efficacy and safety of simvastatin (alone or in
        association with cholestyramine). A 1-year study in 66 patients with type II
        hyperlipoproteinaemia', Europ Heart J 11:149-155

43.   Geisel, J., Oette K. and Burrichter H. (1990) 'HMG-CoA-Reduktase-Inhibitoren bei
        familiärer Hypercholesterinämie', Fortschr Med 108:69-72

44.   Mölgaard, J., Lundh B.L., von Schenck H. and Olsson A.G. (1991) 'Long-term
        efficacy and safety of simvastatin alone and in combination therapy in treatment of
        hypercholesterolaemia', Atherosclerosis 91:S21-S28

45.   Glueck, C.J., Speirs J. and Tracy T. (1990) 'Safety and efficacy of combined
        gemfibrozil-lovastatin therapy for primary dyslipoproteinemias', J Lab Clin .Med
        115:603-609

46.   Illingworth, D.R. and O'Malley J.P. (1990) 'The hypolipidemic effects of lovastatin and
        clofibrate alóne and in combination in patients with type III hyperlipoproteinemia',
        Metabolism 39:403-409

47.   Lintott, C.J., Scott R.S., Nye E.R., Robertson M.L. and Sutherland W.H.F. (1991) 'The
        hypolipidaemic effects of pravastatin (CS-514) alone and in combination with
        bezafibrate or acipimox in patients with primary hypercholesterolaemia', Diab Nutr
        Metab 4:117-122

48.   Pierce, L.R., Wysowski D.K. and Gross T.P. (1990) 'Myopathy and rhabdomyolysis
        associated with lovastatin-gemfibrozil combination therapy', JAMA 264:71-75

49.   Illingworth, D.R. and Bacon S. (1989) 'Treatment of heterozygous familial
        hypercholestrolemia with lipid-lowering drugs', Arteriosclerosis (Suppl I) 9:I-121-134

REGRESSION OF CORONARY ATHEROSCLEROSIS BY LDL-APHERESIS

A. YAMAMOTO*, Y. GOTO, Y. NAKASHIMA, T. YASUGI, Y. OKAMURA, Y. SAITO,
T. NISHIDE, N. INOUE, N. KOGA, B. KISHINO, H. ITO, T. TERAMOTO, and
R. TATAMI for LDL-Apheresis Regression Study (LARS) Group

A. YAMAMOTO

ABSTRACT.

Lowering cholesterol by the treatment with LDL-apheresis using dextran
sulfate-cellulose beads affinity column resulted in a regression of
coronary atherosclerosis in 38% of the patients including 7 cases of
homozygous familial hypercholesterolemia (FH), 25 cases of heterozygous
FH, and 5 other cases of mild to severe hypercholesterolemia. In
heterozygous FH and others, regression took place in 7 out of 15 cases
where plasma cholesterol was reduced more than 120 mg/dl by apheresis
treatment, but in only 3 out of 14 cases, where cholesterol reduction was
less than 120 mg/dl. Regression was also observed in 4 out of 7 cases of
homozygous FH and there was no case with progression in this group.

1. Introduction

Plasma exchange or plasmapheresis was first introduced by J.L. DeGennes
followed by G.R. Thompson in this field about 20 years ago for the
treatment of severe cases of hypercholesterolemia which is resistant to
drug therapy[1]. At an early stage, the indication was almost conclusively
limited to the treatment of homozygous familial hypercholesterolemia
(homozygous FH). As excellent devices being developed and the efficacy
and the safety of the whole procedure being approved, heterozygous FH and
even more common types of hyperlipidemia also became the target of this
therapy[2].

Epidemiological studies and also some clinical observations have shown
that the rate of the increase in incidence of coronary artery disease
markedly accelerates following the elevation of plasma cholesterol levels.
Such phenomenon is observed world-wide; not only in U.S. and Europe, but
also in Japan on the same scale[3-5]. It is now widely approved by
cardiologists that the ideal level of plasma cholesterol is below 180
mg/dl; LDL-cholesterol below 120 mg/dl. For the purpose of prevention of
atherosclerosis, especially among the people at high risk, it is
recommended to reduce cholesterol to this level. Regression of
atherosclerotic vascular lesions was observed by lowering serum
cholesterol to such a low level by use of antilipidemic drugs[6-8]. But
in many patients with hereditary hyperlipidemias like FH, it is difficult
to keep plasma cholesterol at such a low level even by using two or three
drugs in combination and plasmapheresis is the only practical therapeutic
method, besides surgical operation like partial ileal bypass or liver
transplantation.

The assessment of LDL-apheresis has been done extensively in these 10
years on short and relatively long-term basis[9]. In addition to the
regression of cutaneous and tendon xanthomas, remarkable regression of
atheromatous plaques in renal artery, cervical arteries, aorta, and even
the stenosing lesions of the coronary arteries has been reported by
several groups. It is especially important to note that the regression
took place in such patients with homozygous FH, even though the integral
average of plasma cholesterol level between two apheresis operations was
still as high as 250 mg/dl or more owing to the severe rebound of

293

A. L. Catapano et al. (eds.), Drugs Affecting Lipid Metabolism, 293–297.

cholesterol after apheresis.

It is still not clear at this moment, to what extent the apheresis therapy is effective with heterozygous FH and more common types of hyperlipidemia and also, to what extent we have to lower cholesterol to achieve regression. There is a hypothesis that, for the purpose of achieving the regression, a much lower cholesterol level is required than is necessary for the prevention of atherosclerosis.

Our LDL-apheresis Regression Study (LARS) Group conducted a multicenter study at 13 institutions in Japan, to evaluate the effect of LDL-apheresis on regression of coronary atherosclerosis in 37 patients. We used the same type of adsorption system and the same technique. The coronary angiograms were assessed by visual judgement first at each institution and then by 3 expert cardiologists in this group, followed by the computerized analysis with edge detection method operated by Hashizume at Koga Hospital.

2.Subjects and Methods

The 37 patients registered in LARS included 7 homozygous FH patients, 25 heterozygous FH, and 5 others, including 3 essential hypercholesterolemia suspicious but not confirmed to be FH and 2 familial combined hyperlipidemia. Dextran sulfate-cellulose beads collumm[10] was commonly used in this group for LDL-apheresis. An apparatus (Liposorber system, Kanegafuchi Chemical Industries, Co., Osaka) equipped with either one large (LA-40, 400ml) column or two small (LA-15, 150 ml) columns for alternate use was used.

All patients had been treated with LDL-apheresis for at least one year, mostly more than 2 years, with the mean period of 83 (±31) months in homozygous FH and 37 (±17) months in heterozygous FH and others. Coronary angiography had been undergone, at least twice more than one year apart, to determine the change in patency of stenosed segments. Mean intervals between two angiograms were 49 (±26) months in homozygotes and 32 (±13) months in heterozygotes and others.

Most patients had been treated with cholesterol-lowering drugs such as pravastatin, probucol, and cholestyramine in combination with LDL-apheresis. Total cholesterol levels before the start of the apheresis therapy, which are mean baseline total cholesterol levels, were 627 (±91) mg/dl in FH homozygotes, and 388 (±86) mg/dl in FH heterozygotes and others. During the LDL-apheresis treatment period, these values fluctuated between a pretreatment level of 440 (±76) mg/dl and a posttreatment level of 149 (±40) mg/dl on average in homozygotes, and between 247 (±60) and 105 (±27) mg/dl in the heterozygotes and others.

The angiograms were reviewed by 3 expert cardiologists and the extent of stenosis was visually evaluated based on the criteria recommended by American Heart Association. Changes by at least two degrees were judged as to be significant. Determination of the extent of stenosis was further performed by computerized analysis using the automated edge detection method with Mypron I System. Criterion for definite change was a difference of at least 3 times standard deviation; that is 11.2% based on computer analysis. At the lesions near the branching part or accompanying ectasia, computer analysis was not possible. Such places occupied about 40% of the total lesions.

3. Results

In a typical case (a 30-year-old female with receptor-defective type homozygous familial hypercholesterolemia, Kyoto-Daiichi Red Cross Hospital), lesions in both right and coronary arteries showed marked regression; (right) Segment 1: from 75 to 25%, Segment 2: from 75 to 25%, Segment 3: from 90 to 25%, (left) Segment 8: from 51 to 34% on the visual interpretation[11].

On angiograms, cases with at least one segment showing definite regression without a progression in other segments were defined as "regression". Those cases with at least one segment showing definite progression with no regression in other segments were judged as "progression". Cases listed as "no change" had either no definite regression or definite progression.

Regression took place in 14 cases (37.8%) out of 37 patients. Only 5 patients (13.5%) showed progression. In one of them, angiography carried out after further 2 years revealed that the occlusion at the first two years of the treatment was probably due to the spasm. No patient had both regressed and progressed segments. It is especially noteworthy that, in FH homozygotes, there was no case with progression and 4 cases out of seven showed regression. These data suggest that the characteristic and beneficial effects of LDL-apheresis can be obtained even in severe hypercholesterolemia by depression of LDL-cholesterol.

Definite regression was observed angiographically in 21 segments in 14 patients out of total number of 106 segments assessed in 37 patients. There was very good agreement in the results obtained by the two methods. For example, in case E.K., RCA segment 4 was regressed from 95 to 25% by visual interpretation, and from 78% to 30% by computer analysis.

The distribution of regression, no change, and progression was investigated in different groups of patients according to their backgrounds. There was no correlation between regression and sex nor age. Of particular interest was that 3 cases of regression were observed in 6 FH patients over 70 years of age. Regression was observed even in patients with two or more vessel disease; 4 cases out of 5 homozygotes and 7 cases out of 23 heterozygotes and others. The data indicate that the regression can take place even in patients with severe coronary artery disease by LDL-apheresis as in patients with slight to moderate coronary involvement.

The influence of the extent of cholesterol extraction on the change in coronary atherosclerosis was analyzed in FH heterozygotes and others. FH homozygotes were excluded, because of the difference in the rebound of cholesterol after the apheresis operation. A higher frequency of regression was observed in the patient group with a larger difference in total cholesterol levels between pre- and post-treatment. There was also a tendency toward a higher frequency of regression in cases where posttreatment total cholesterol level was maintained below 100 mg/dl (Table 1).

A summary of progression-regression data according to the posttreatment cholesterol level in FH homozygotes was shown in Fig. 1. It is interesting to note that the regression took place frequently when the cholesterol level was brought down below 150 mg/dl after the apheresis operation. In the other cases, where cholesterol stayed at a higher level, there was a progression and almost no regression. There was also a case, in which the remarkable improvement could not be expressed by the standard judgment. In one patient, there was almost complete occlusion at the stem of the right coronary artery. Collaterals were supplying blood from left to right. After two years of the treatment, a short segment of the stem of the right coronary artery was visualized, and after another 2 years, we could follow the right coronary artery on angiogram down to the region where collaterals were joining.

4. Conclusion

Our present results strongly suggest that regression of coronary atherosclerosis can be induced by the aggressive cholesterol-lowering therapy with LDL-apheresis in combination with drugs. We expect that LDL-apheresis treatment will be beneficial for primary and secondary prevention of cardiovascular events in FH patients who are refractory to diet and cholesterol-lowering drugs, who have advanced stenosing

Table 1.   Influence of cholesterol levels on coronary atherosclerosis excluding homozygotes.

			Total		Regression		No change		Progression	
			No.of cases	%	No.of cases	%	No.of cases	%	No.of cases	%
			30	100	10	33.3	15*	50.0	5	16.7
TC (mg/dl)	Pre- treatment	≥230 <230	16 13	100 100	7 3	43.8 23.1	7 7	43.8 53.8	2 3	12.5 23.1
	Post- treatment	≥100 <100	14 15	100 100	4 6	28.6 40.0	7 7	50.0 46.7	3 2	21.4 13.3
	Difference	≥120 <120	15 14	100 100	7 3	46.7 21.4	6 8	40.0 57.1	2 3	13.3 21.4
LDL-C (mg/dl)	Pre- treatment	≥170 <170	15 14	100 100	7 3	46.7 21.4	6 8	40.0 57.1	2 3	13.3 21.4
	Post- treatment	≥70 <70	14 15	100 100	5 5	35.7 33.3	7 7	50.0 46.7	2 3	14.3 20.0
	Difference	≥95 <95	15 14	100 100	7 3	46.7 21.4	6 8	40.0 57.1	2 3	13.3 21.4

* Plasma cholesterol levels are not available in 1 of 15 patients with unchanged segments.

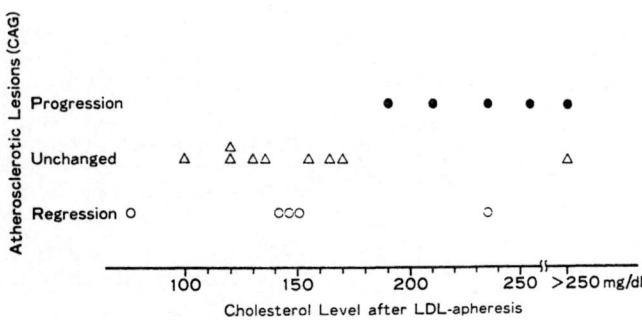

Fig. 1.   Progression-Regression of coronary atherosclerosis by LDL-apheresis in patients with homozygous familial hypercholeterolemia.

lesions, with or without previous myocardial infarction.

5. References

1) Thompson, G.R., Lowenthal, R. and Myant, N.B. (1975) 'Plasma exchange in the management of homozygous familial hypercholesterolemia.' Lancet, 1, 1208.
2) Yamamoto, A., Yokoyama, S., Satani, M., Kikkawa, T. and Kishino, B.(1988) 'Evaluation of selective LDL-removal in the treatment of familial hypercholesterolemia: Double membrane filtration and adsorption system In: K. Widhalm and H. Naito (Eds.), Recent Aspects of Diagnosis and Treatment of Lipoprotein Disorders: Impact on Prevention of Atherosclerotic Diseases.' Alan R. Liss, Inc., New York, pp.357-366.
3) Castelli, W.P. (1988) 'Cholesterol and lipids in the risk of coronary artery disease: The Framingham Heart Study.' Can. J. Cardiol., 4 (suppl A), 5A.
4) Assmann, G., Schulte, H., Funke, H., von Edkardstein, A., Schmitz, G. and Robnek, H. (1989) 'High density lipoproteins and atherosclerosis.' in : G. Crepaldi, A.M. Gotto, E. Manzato, G. Baggio (Eds.), Atherosclerosis VIII, Excerpta Medica, Amsterdam, pp 341-351.
5) Tarui, S. for the Study Group on Essential Hyperlipidemia in Japan (sponsored by Ministry of Health and Welfare) (1990) 'Hyperlipidemia and its complication among Japanese.' J. Jap. Atherosclerosis Soc., 18, 1 (in Japanese).
6) Cashin-Hemphill, L., Mack, W.J., Pogoda, J.M., Sanmarco, M.E., Azen, S.P. and Blankenhorn, D.H. (1990) 'Beneficial effects of colestipol-niacin on coronary atherosclerosis: A 4-year follow-up.' JAMA, 264, 3013.
7) Brown, G., Albers, J.J., Fisher, L.D., Schaefer, S.M., Lin, J.T., Kaplan, C., Zhao, X.Q., Bisson, B.D., Fitzpatrick, V.F. and Dodge, H.T. (1990) 'Regression of coronary artery disease as a result of intensive lipid-lowering therapy in men with high levels of apolipoprotein B.' N. Engl. J. Med., 323. 1289.
8) Kane, J.P., Malloy, M.J., Ports, T.A., Phillips, N.R., Diehl, J.C. and Havel, R.J. (1990) 'Regression of coronary atherosclerosis during treatment of familial hypercholesterolemia with combined drug regimens.' JAMA, 264, 3007.
9) Yamamoto, A. (1991) 'Regression of atherosclerosis in humans by lowering serum cholesterol.' Atherosclerosis 89, 1.
10) Yokoyama, S., Hayashi, R., Kikkawa, T., Tani, N., Takada, S., Hatanaka, K. and Yamamoto, A. (1984) 'Specific adsorbent of apolipoprotein B-containing lipoproteins for plasmapheresis: Characterization and experimental use in hypercholesterolemic rabbits.' Arteriosclerosis, 4, 276.
11) Yamazaki, S., Ono, T., Kondo, M., Iwamoto, N., Wada, S. and Inoue, N. (1990) 'A case of homozygous familial hypercholesterolemia which showed a remarkable regression of the coronary stenosing lesions by LDL-apheresis.' Therapeutic Plasmapheresis, 9, 261.

PARTIAL ILEAL BYPASS - RESULTS OF THE PROGRAM ON THE SURGICAL CONTROL OF THE HYPERLIPIDEMIAS (POSCH)

C. T. CAMPOS, H. BUCHWALD, and the POSCH GROUP

ABSTRACT. The Program on the Surgical Control of the Hyperlipidemias (POSCH) was a prospective, randomized, secondary, atherosclerosis intervention trial designed to examine the effects of lipid lowering by the partial ileal bypass (PIB) operation on overall and coronary heart disease morbidity and mortality. POSCH enrolled 838 hypercholesterolemic survivors of a single myocardial infarction (417 randomized to a diet-treated control group and 421 randomized to a diet plus PIB-treated surgery group) with a mean follow-up of 9.7 years. Compared to the control group, the surgery group had a 23.3% lower total plasma cholesterol level, a 37.7% lower low density lipoprotein (LDL) cholesterol level, and a 4.3% higher high density lipoprotein (HDL) cholesterol level at five-year follow-up. Overall and coronary heart disease mortality were reduced, but these reductions did not achieve statistical significance. In patients with a left ventricular ejection fraction $\geq 50\%$, overall mortality was 36% lower in the surgery group (p=0.021). The occurrence of the combined endpoint of coronary heart disease death or confirmed nonfatal myocardial infarction was reduced by 35% (p<0.0001). Comparison of baseline coronary arteriograms with studies performed 3, 5, 7, or 10 years after randomization consistently demonstrated decreased coronary artery disease progression and increased coronary artery disease regression in the surgery group. The principal side effects of partial ileal bypass included diarrhea, kidney stones, gallstones, and intestinal obstruction. The POSCH trial results clearly demonstrate the beneficial effects of aggressive, non-pharmacologic lipid lowering and carefully document the long-term results of partial ileal bypass in hypercholesterolemic patients with atherosclerosis.

1. Partial Ileal Bypass

1.1. EXPERIMENTAL BASIS AND METABOLIC RATIONALE

Between 1962 and 1964, the initial experiments establishing the metabolic basis for partial ileal bypass were performed.[1,2] These studies demonstrated that both cholesterol absorption from the intestinal tract and the blood cholesterol level were significantly reduced, without concomitant weight loss, after bypass or resection of substantial lengths of the distal small bowel. Although the entire small intestine is capable of cholesterol absorption, preferential cholesterol uptake occurs in the distal one-half of the small bowel. Intestinal transit time strongly influences quantitative cholesterol absorption.

Localization of bile acid absorption sites has proven more difficult and the results have often been contradictory. We have shown that bypass of the distal one-third of the small bowel interferes with the enterohepatic bile acid cycle and leads to a three-fold increase in fecal

299

A. L. Catapano et al. (eds.), Drugs Affecting Lipid Metabolism, 299–307.
© 1993 Kluwer Academic Publishers and Fondazione Giovanni Lorenzini

bile acid loss. Thus, partial ileal bypass alters body cholesterol dynamics through:

(1) a direct drain on the body cholesterol pool from increased fecal loss of normally absorbed exogenous (dietary) and endogenous (biliary and intestinally secreted) cholesterol, and

(2) an indirect drain on the body cholesterol pool resulting from increased hepatic conversion of body cholesterol stores to bile acids in order to replenish the depleted bile acid reservoir.

Evaluation of cholesterol dynamics after partial ileal bypass in man has been accomplished using radioisotope techniques. [3] Cholesterol absorption from the intestine is reduced by 60 percent after partial ileal bypass. This reduction has been maintained up to 10 years after operation. A 3.8-fold increase in total fecal steroid excretion, with a greater increase in bile acid excretion (4.9-fold) than in neutral steroid excretion (2.7-fold), has been observed. This increased steroid excretion has also been maintained for up to 10 years post-operatively. Compensatory cholesterol and bile acid absorptive adaptation by the non-bypassed small intestine was not observed. Thus, the effects of partial ileal bypass on cholesterol dynamics and on the enterohepatic bile acid circulation appear to remain unchanged over time.

Other cholesterol homeostatic mechanisms are altered in response to the increased fecal loss of cholesterol and bile acids. A 5.7-fold increase in the cholesterol synthesis rate occurs after partial ileal bypass. This effect is also maintained for as long as 10 years after operation. The cholesterol turnover rate increased greatly. One year after partial ileal bypass, the total exchangeable cholesterol pool was reduced by about one-third. This reduction was reflected in both the freely miscible cholesterol pool (plasma, red blood cells, liver, intestinal mucosa) and in the less freely miscible cholesterol pool (fat stores, muscle, organs). The less freely miscible pool also includes cholesterol deposited in arterial walls. Loss of cholesterol from the less freely miscible pool may reflect removal of cholesterol from atherosclerotic plaques.

1.2. OPERATIVE TECHNIQUE

Partial ileal bypass has been performed for the reduction of elevated cholesterol levels by our group since 1963. Over 600 partial ileal bypass procedures have been performed in the United States and abroad. [4] Briefly, under general anesthesia, the small bowel length is measured along the mesenteric border, allowing 25 cm for the duodenal length. The small intestine is divided 200 cm proximal to the ileocecal valve or at a distance one-third the total small bowel length from the ileocecal valve if the total length is greater than 600 cm. The distal end of the divided ileum is closed, and the proximal end is anastomosed, in end-to-side fashion, into the anterior taenia of the cecum. The appendix is removed routinely. The closed end of the bypassed ileum is sutured to the anterior taenia of the cecum, between the anastomosis and the appendiceal stump, to prevent intussusception of this segment, and the mesenteric defects are closed to prevent internal herniation. The partial ileal bypass procedure is illustrated in Figure 1.

1.3. OPERATIVE MORTALITY AND SIDE EFFECTS

In the University of Minnesota experience,[5,6] partial ileal bypass can be performed with an operative mortality of less than 1 percent, even though the majority of operative candidates have overt atherosclerotic cardiovascular disease. Wound infections, pneumonia, pulmonary emboli, or other serious postoperative complications requiring hospitalization for more than 1 week have occurred in only 2 percent of patients. Intussusception of the bypassed segment and bowel obstruction resulting from internal herniation due to inadequate closure of the mesenteric defects have not occurred in this series and appear to be entirely avoidable. The incidences of late bowel obstruction secondary to adhesions (2 percent) and late development of incisional hernia (less than 2 percent) are similar to those observed after any abdominal

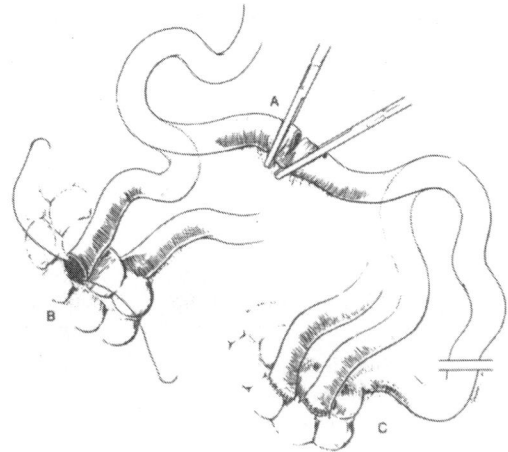

Figure 1. Partial Ileal Bypass. A. Division of the ileum 200 cm proximal to the ileocecal valve or one-third of the total small bowel length proximal to the ileocecal valve if the total small intestinal length is greater than 600 cm. B. End-to-side anastomosis of the proximal segment into the anterior taenia of the cecum, 6 cm distal to the appendiceal stump.
C. Tacking of the closed distal segment to the anterior taenia of the cecum midway between the anastomosis and the appendiceal stump.

surgical procedure.

Diarrhea is the most frequent side effect after partial ileal bypass. Generally, it is not persistent. One year after operation, 86 percent of patients have fewer than five bowel movements per day without bowel-controlling medications. Further intestinal adaptation occurs, and most patients experience an additional increase in the firmness and consistency of their stools over time. Fewer than 5 percent of patients in the University of Minnesota series have had operative restoration of intestinal continuity because of intractable diarrhea.

After partial ileal bypass, vitamin B_{12} absorption is either severely impaired or totally lost. After several years, absorptive adaptation for vitamin B_{12} occurs in approximately 50 percent of patients. Nevertheless, it is prudent to prescribe 1,000 micrograms of vitamin B_{12} intramuscularly every 4 to 6 weeks for the lifetime of the patient after partial ileal bypass.

An increased incidence of calcium oxalate renal calculi has been observed after partial ileal bypass. The incidence rate of renal calculi, detected clinically or by radiographic techniques, was 4 percent per year in patients following partial ileal bypass. This rate was nearly six times higher than the rate (0.7 percent per year) observed in a comparable group of hypercholesterolemic patients following a fat and cholesterol restricted diet. Oral calcium was prescribed at one time to reduce intestinal oxalate absorption without appreciable effect. Patients are currently advised to avoid dietary oxalate, to maintain an adequate daily fluid intake, and to take oral potassium citrate (20 mEq three times daily) to alkalize their urine. It is not clear whether this latter treatment decreases renal stone formation. The use of potassium citrate after partial ileal bypass is currently being evaluated in a randomized, placebo-controlled clinical trial. No case of nephrocalcinosis leading to renal function impairment or loss has been noted after partial ileal bypass.

The incidence of gallstone formation is increased three- to four-fold after partial ileal bypass. In 320 operated patients free of gallstones at the time of operation, 14 subsequently required cholecystectomy and an additional 40 developed gallstones during a five-year follow-up period. In 286 comparable, hypercholesterolemic patients following a fat and cholesterol restricted diet, four required cholecystectomy and ten additional patients developed documented gallstones.

Excessive, foul-smelling flatus and the gas-bloat syndrome are occasionally encountered after partial ileal bypass. These symptoms generally respond to a two-week course of oral metronidazole (250 mg three times daily). If these symptoms recur, patients are placed on oral metronidazole indefinitely (250 mg daily).

Although variable in occurrence, gastric hypersecretion after massive intestinal resection or the jejunoileal bypass for morbid obesity has been documented. However, laboratory and clinical studies of gastric volume and acid output after partial ileal bypass have demonstrated no similar hypersecretory effect.

A small loss of weight can occur following partial ileal bypass. In the Program on the Surgical Control of the Hyperlipidemias (POSCH) trial, the average baseline weight of partial ileal bypass patients and control patients following a fat and cholesterol restricted diet was 82.6 kg. At the five-year follow-up visit, the average weight in the control group was 84.6 kg and was 79.5 kg in the surgery group. This 5.1 kg difference in weight attributable to partial ileal bypass certainly does not approach the weight loss observed following the more extensive jejunoileal bypass formerly performed for the treatment of morbid obesity.

Contrary to the experience frequently encountered after jejunoileal bypass for morbid obesity, no significant changes in serum electrolytes follow partial ileal bypass. Specifically, the potassium, calcium, and magnesium values remain within normal limits. Need for electrolyte supplementation after partial ileal bypass has not been reported. Nutrient malabsorption has not been described after partial ileal bypass. Finally, and of considerable importance in clearly distinguishing partial ileal bypass from the jejunoileal bypass, hepatic fatty infiltration or fibrosis leading to hepatic insufficiency has not occurred after partial ileal bypass.

2. Results from the Program on the Surgical Control of the Hyperlipidemias (POSCH)

The Program on the Surgical Control of the Hyperlipidemias (POSCH) was a multi-centered, prospective, randomized, controlled, clinical trial designed to ascertain whether reductions in total plasma cholesterol and LDL cholesterol induced by the partial ileal bypass operation would reduce overall mortality and the mortality and morbidity due to coronary heart disease in survivors of a single myocardial infarction. Detailed descriptions of the design and methodology of POSCH have been published.[7,8]

Between 1975 and 1983, 838 survivors of a single enzyme- and electrocardiographically-documented myocardial infarction were entered into POSCH - 417 randomly assigned to treatment with American Heart Association (AHA) Phase II diet instruction only (control group) and 421 randomly assigned to treatment with identical dietary instruction plus a partial ileal bypass (surgery group). Patients were males or females between 30 and 64 years of age. After at least six weeks on the AHA Phase II diet, they were required to have a total plasma cholesterol level of at least 220 mg/dl or a LDL cholesterol level of at least 140 mg/dl if their total plasma cholesterol level was between 200 and 219 mg/dl. Potentially confounding major atherosclerosis risk factors such as hypertension (systolic blood pressure $\geq$ 180 mm Hg or diastolic blood pressure $\geq$ 105 mm Hg), obesity, or diabetes were causes for exclusion. Other exclusion criteria included: greater than 75 percent stenosis of the left main coronary artery, no measurable coronary artery stenosis on the pre-randomization arteriogram, and previous coronary artery bypass surgery or percutaneous coronary angioplasty. Cigarette smokers were eligible and were distributed by the randomization process.

All patients were followed by means of clinic visits and telephone contacts according to a uniform protocol. Serial lipid analyses were performed at the POSCH Central Lipid Laboratory at baseline, three months after randomization, and at every clinic visit (annual visits during the first five years and one visit at either seven or ten years). Coronary arteriograms were obtained at baseline, three years, five years, and at either seven years (for patients enrolled on or after June 1, 1980) or ten years (for patients enrolled before June 1, 1980). The formal POSCH trial ended, with the vital status of all 838 patients known, in July of 1990 with an average follow-up of 9.7 years (range: 7 - 14.8 years).

Determination of the specific cause of death was based upon a blinded review of all available records by the POSCH Mortality Review Committee. The diagnosis of myocardial infarction during the trial was made following a blinded review of all available records by a POSCH cardiologist. The sequential coronary arteriography assessments were performed by two-member teams from the POSCH Arteriography Review Panel. No team member was from the clinic from which the arteriograms originated. The films were interpreted in pairs, with the reviewers blinded to the patient's treatment assignment and to the temporal sequence of the films. With use of an evaluation protocol virtually identical to that employed by the Cholesterol Lowering Atherosclerosis Study (CLAS), a global evaluation of the severity of the coronary artery disease was derived by consensus. An eight-point scale was used to grade the change between two sets of films (-3, -2, -1, -0, +0, +1, +2, and +3; -3=much worse and +3=much better).

2.1. LIPID AND LIPOPROTEIN RESULTS

Five years after randomization, [6] the surgery group, as compared with the control group, had a 23.3 ± 1.0 (mean ± S.E.) percent lower total plasma cholesterol level (p<0.0001), a 37.7 ± 1.2 percent lower LDL cholesterol level (p<0.0001), a 4.3 ± 1.8 percent higher HDL cholesterol level (p=0.02), an 18.3 ± 7.5 percent higher very low density lipoprotein (VLDL) cholesterol level (p=0.02), and a 19.8 ± 6.5 percent higher triglyceride level (p=0.003). The five-year total plasma cholesterol and LDL cholesterol results are presented in Figures 2 and 3. The ratio of HDL cholesterol to total plasma cholesterol was 37.8 ± 2.8 percent higher, and the ratio of HDL cholesterol to LDL cholesterol was 71.8 ± 4.3 percent higher in the surgery group. Determinations of apolipoprotein and HDL subfraction levels were added to the POSCH protocol in June of 1985. In the subset of patients with five-year apolipoprotein and HDL subfraction determinations, a significantly higher HDL subfraction 2 level (10.4 ± 6.6 mg/dl versus 8.1 ± 5.8 mg/dl; p<0.0001), a significantly higher apolipoprotein A-I level (118.7 ± 22.4 mg/dl versus 106.0 ± 20.5 mg/dl; p<0.0001), and a significantly lower

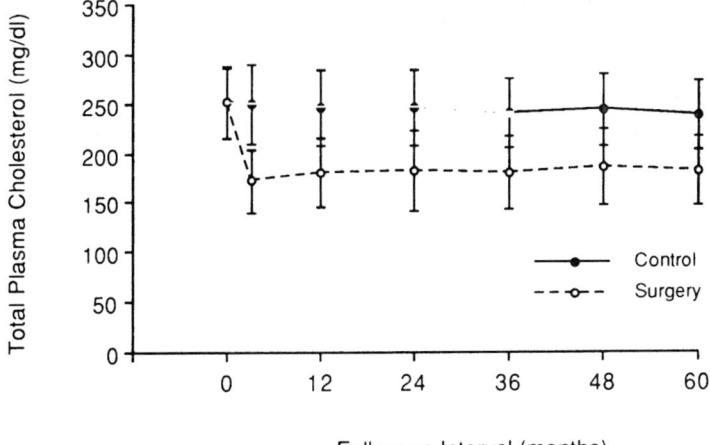

Figure 2. Five-year total plasma cholesterol results presented as mean ± S.D. The differences between groups were statistically significant (p<0.0001) at each follow-up interval.

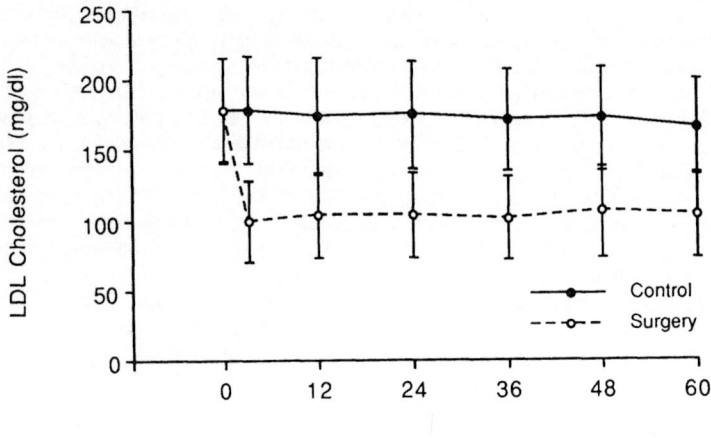

Follow-up Interval (months)

Figure 3. Five-year LDL cholesterol results presented as mean ± S.D.The differences between groups were statistically significant (p<0.0001) at each follow-up interval.

apolipoprotein B-100 level (92.8 ± 20.5 mg/dl versus 123.4 ± 21.7 mg/dl; p<0.0001) were observed in the surgery group.

2.2 OVERALL AND CAUSE-SPECIFIC MORTALITY

During the mean 9.7-year follow-up period of POSCH, there were 62 deaths in the diet-treated control group and 49 deaths in the partial ileal bypass-treated intervention group.[6] This 21.7 percent reduction in overall mortality in the surgery group did not, however, achieve statistical significance (two-sided p = 0.164). The mortality due to atherosclerotic coronary heart disease was reduced by 28 percent (p = 0.113), with 44 atherosclerotic coronary heart disease deaths among controls and 32 similar deaths in the surgery group patients.

In a subgroup analysis dividing the POSCH population into two groups: patients with a left ventricular ejection fraction ≥ 50 percent and patients with a left ventricular ejection fraction < 50 percent, no significant difference in overall mortality between the control and surgery group patients with a depressed resting left ventricular ejection fraction (< 50 percent) was observed. However, in the patients with a normal left ventricular ejection fraction following a myocardial infarction (≥ 50 percent), there were 39 deaths in the control group and only 24 deaths in the partial ileal bypass group, a reduction of 36 percent (p = 0.052 by Mantel-Haenszel test, and p = 0.021 by Gehan test). This result suggests that aggressive lipid modification may be of benefit in increasing survival in hypercholesterolemic survivors of a myocardial infarction with preserved resting left ventricular function. This is the first demonstration of a significant overall mortality effect from lipid intervention observed during a clinical trial of the lipid-atherosclerosis theory.

2.3. ATHEROSCLEROSIS ENDPOINTS COMBINED WITH OVERALL MORTALITY

Analysis of the combined endpoint of death due to coronary heart disease and definite nonfatal myocardial infarction[6] disclosed 125 such events in the control group and 82 occurrences in

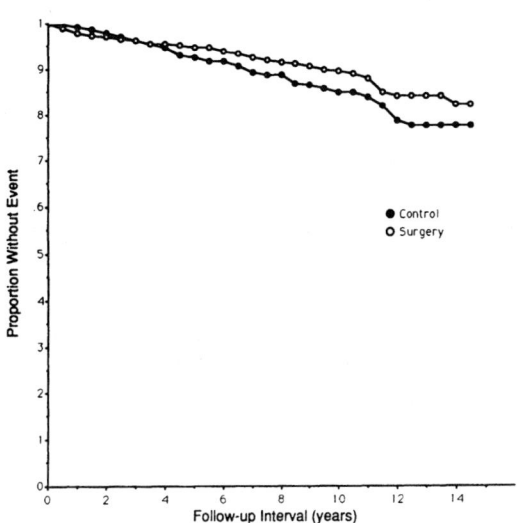

Figure 4. Combined atherosclerotic coronary heart disease death or definite, non-fatal myocardial infarction results in the POSCH control and surgery groups. The difference between groups was statistically significant (two-sided p < 0.001).

the surgery group (Figure 4), a 35 percent risk reduction (p < 0.001). This is the endpoint employed by the Lipid Research Clinics Coronary Primary Prevention Trial (LRC-CPPT) and several other trials of the lipid-atherosclerosis theory. Rather than relying on a one-sided test of significance to demonstrate a statistically significant result as in the LRC-CPPT, the POSCH results were statistically significant at the p < 0.001 level using a more rigorous two-sided test of statistical significance. All combinations of overall mortality with other clinical atherosclerosis events (definite nonfatal myocardial infarction, suspected nonfatal myocardial infarction, or the occurrence of unstable angina) demonstrated highly significant reductions (p < 0.001) in the group undergoing partial ileal bypass compared with the group receiving dietary therapy alone as treatment for hypercholesterolemia.

2.4. SEQUENTIAL CORONARY AND PERIPHERAL ARTERIOGRAPHY

In POSCH, the percentage of patients with angiographic progression of coronary artery disease increased in both groups as follow-up continued.[6] However, the percentage of patients with progression (global change score = -3, -2, or -1) was consistently greater in the diet-treated control group compared with the partial ileal bypass-treated intervention group: 41 percent versus 28 percent at three years, 65 percent versus 38 percent at five years, 77 percent versus 48 percent at seven years, and 85 percent versus 55 percent at ten years (p < 0.001 for all comparisons). These decreases in the rate of angiographic coronary artery disease progression were associated with a marked decline in the occurrence of clinical atherosclerotic coronary artery disease events. This is the first such demonstration by a lipid-atherosclerosis intervention trial. Furthermore, statistically significant evidence (p < 0.01) for angiographic coronary artery disease regression was observed at five- and seven-year follow-up. The proportion of POSCH patients free of peripheral vascular disease assessed angiographically was consistently higher in the surgery group compared with the control group, a difference that approached statistical significance after 10 years of follow-up (p = 0.09).

2.5. CORONARY ARTERY BYPASS SURGERY, ANGIOPLASTY, AND HEART
     TRANSPLANTATION

One of the important observations in the POSCH trial was the demonstration that aggressive
lipid modification can limit the clinical progression of coronary atherosclerosis to the point
requiring interventional therapy.[6] In POSCH, all clinical decisions were made by the
patients' primary physicians functioning independently of the trial. Coronary artery bypass
grafting was performed in 137 control group patients and in 52 surgery group patients, a
reduction of 62.4 percent (p < 0.0001). Repeat coronary artery bypass operations were
required in nine control patients and in two surgery patients. In addition, 33 control patients
underwent percutaneous transluminal coronary angioplasty with or without concomitant
coronary artery bypass grafting versus 15 patients in the surgery group, a reduction of 55
percent (p = 0.005). Three control group patients underwent cardiac transplantation for end-
stage coronary atherosclerosis versus two patients in the surgery group. The total number of
interventional cardiac procedures was 2.6 times greater in the diet-treated control group
compared with the partial ileal bypass-treated surgery group during the POSCH trial.

3. SUMMARY AND CONCLUSIONS

The clinical and arteriographic results of the Program on the Surgical Control of the
Hyperlipidemias (POSCH) have provided clear and convincing evidence supporting the
beneficial effects of cholesterol lowering in hypercholesterolemic survivors of a myocardial
infarction.[6] Even though overall mortality as a single endpoint was not significantly
reduced, a favorable trend toward improved overall survival in patients undergoing aggressive
lipid modification was observed, and in the post hoc subgroup of patients with preserved
ejection fractions (≥ 50%) following a myocardial infarction, a statistically significant
improvement in overall survival was noted. For the combined endpoint of atherosclerotic
coronary heart disease mortality and subsequent confirmed nonfatal myocardial infarction, the
POSCH results clearly demonstrate a significant reduction in the intervention group. In
POSCH, the 35% reduction in atherosclerotic coronary heart disease mortality or definite
nonfatal myocardial infarction was significant at the p < 0.001 level using a two-sided test of
significance. Thus, the POSCH clinical results provide the strongest evidence to-date
supporting the beneficial effects of lipid modification in reducing clinical atherosclerosis event
rates in hypercholesterolemic patients with clinically evident coronary heart disease.
     With more than a quarter century of clinical experience, most of which has been
accumulated within POSCH, an independently monitored, diet-controlled, randomized,
clinical trial, partial ileal bypass has moved beyond the experimental stage and can be
performed confidently and safely. Partial ileal bypass is indicated in hypercholesterolemic
patients at high risk following the NCEP guidelines[9] in lieu or in addition to pharmacologic
therapy. Standard dietary restriction of daily fat, cholesterol, and caloric intake appears to be
safe and is the appropriate initial recommendation when commencing treatment of
hypercholesterolemia. Many high risk patients, however, fail to achieve adequate total plasma
cholesterol or LDL cholesterol lowering from dietary intervention alone. In these high risk
patients, particularly those with overt atherosclerotic cardiovascular disease or those who have
previously undergone coronary artery bypass or coronary angioplasty, partial ileal bypass
should be considered at the same time as pharmacologic therapy. Randomized, controlled,
clinical trial data clearly demonstrate that partial ileal bypass as a single intervention modality,
is as effective as, or even more effective than, single-, double-, or triple-drug regimens.[10]
The treatment effect of partial ileal bypass is substantial, is durable, is independent of the
vicissitudes of patient compliance, and can be achieved at a fraction of the cost of life-long
single or multi-drug therapy. Partial ileal bypass and pharmacologic agents need not be
regarded as competing treatment modalities. The combination of partial ileal bypass and

pharmacologic therapy can lead to substantial total plasma cholesterol and LDL cholesterol lowering, bringing even the most severely elevated total plasma cholesterol and LDL cholesterol levels into acceptable ranges to maximally reduce atherosclerosis risk.

3. References

1. Buchwald, H. and Gebhard, R. L. (1964) 'Effect of interstinal bypass on cholesterol absorption and blood levels in the rabbit', Am J Physiol 207, 567-572.
2. Buchwald, H. and Gebhard, R. L. (1968) 'Localization of bile salt absorption in vivo   in the rabbit', Ann Surg 167, 191-198.
3. Moore, R. B., Frantz, I. D., Jr., and Buchwald, H. (1969) 'Changes in cholesterol pool size, turnover rate, and fecal bile acid and sterol excretion after partial ileal bypass in hypercholesterolemic patients', Surgery 65, 98-108.
4. Buchwald, H. and Campos, C. T. (1990) 'Partial ileal bypass for control of hyperlipidemia and atherosclerosis', in: D. C. Sabiston Jr. and F. C. Spencer (eds.), Surgery of the Chest, 5th ed., W. B. Saunders, Philadelphia, pp. 1799-1820.
5. Buchwald, H., Moore, R. B., and Varco, R. L. (1974) 'Ten years clinical experience with partial ileal bypass in management of the hyperlipidemias', Ann Surg 180, 384-392.
6. Buchwald, H., Varco, R. L., Matts, J. P., et al. (1990) 'Effect of partial ileal bypass surgery on mortality and morbidity from coronary heart disease in patients with hypercholesterolemia', N Engl J Med 323, 946-955.
7. Buchwald, H., Matts, J. P., Fitch, L. L., et al. (1989) 'Program on the Surgical Control of the Hyperlipidemias (POSCH): design and methodology', J Clin Epidemiol 42, 1111-1127.
8. Matts, J. P., Buchwald, H., Fitch, L. L., et al. (1991) 'Program on the Surgical Control of the Hyperlipidemias (POSCH): patient entry characteristics', Controlled Clin Trials 12, 314-339.
9. The Expert Panel. (1988) 'Report of the National Cholesterol Education Program Expert Panel on detection, evaluation, and treatment of high blood cholesterol in adults', Arch Intern Med 148, 36-69.
10. Buchwald, H., Fitch, L. L., and Campos, C. T. (1992) 'Partial ileal bypass in the treatment of hypercholesterolemia', J Fam Pract 35, 69-76.

HYPERCHOLESTEROLEMIA: NEGOTIATING THE ISSUES

John C. LaRosa, M.D.

ABSTRACT. Current U.S. guidelines for the treatment of hypercholesterolemia in adults have been widely accepted. Criticisms of these guidelines, however, define the issues now emerging as important in the management of lipid disorders. On the one hand, there are those who say that the guidelines miss those with low cholesterols who also have low HDL levels. On the other hand, the guidelines have been criticized for being too inclusive and have been criticized by health economists who feel that treatment of hypercholesterolemia in younger individuals may not be cost-beneficial. Finally, it has been pointed out that in primary (but not secondary) prevention trials total mortality has been unaffected and higher rates of traumatic death observed. On the other hand, secondary prevention trials and regression studies indicate considerable benefit on both mortality and morbidity in those with established disease. This debate has been misunderstood and has led to undertreatment of hypercholesterolemia, particularly in those with coronary disease. Issues to be settled include the benefit of drug intervention in women, in the elderly, and in young adults without established coronary disease, as well as the role of newer risk factors, including Lp(a), small, dense LDL, and truncal obesity. The cause-effect relationship between cholesterol and coronary disease is accepted. Debate continues about the proper level for cholesterol cutpoints, and the potential value of new lipoprotein risk factors.

In the last few years, several issues involving the relationships between circulating lipoproteins and atherosclerosis has emerged. It has become clear that the importance of lipoprotein-altering treatment in patients with established coronary disease has been underestimated. Meta-analyses of secondary prevention trials have revealed consistent declines in all-cause cardiovascular and coronary artery disease (CAD) morbidity and mortality [1]. Regression studies in humans [2-6] have demonstrated that drug, surgical, and dietary therapy, all resulting in low density lipoprotein cholesterol

309

A. L. Catapano et al. (eds.), Drugs Affecting Lipid Metabolism, 309–315.
© 1993 Kluwer Academic Publishers and Fondazione Giovanni Lorenzini.

(LDL-C) lowering and/or high density lipoprotein cholesterol (HDL-C) increasing, are associated with arrest of progression and even regression of atherosclerosis on serial coronary angiography. Studies have indicated that patients with established coronary disease are undertreated and that as many as two thirds of patients with established disease are receiving no lipoprotein-altering therapy [7,8]. This, despite the fact that cost-benefit analyses indicate that actual cost savings may be achieved with such treatments [9].

The issue of primary prevention, however, has become, in many ways, less clear. Meta-analysis of primary prevention trials has shown no effect on total mortality and an apparent excess mortality from cancer and trauma [10]. It must be remembered that these trials are generally of only a few years duration, have few mortal events, and show significant excess mortality in non-cardiovascular groups only if combinations of groups are made that are not necessarily epidemiologically sound. For example, cancer mortality has increased only if all forms of cancer are counted. Traumatic mortality is only increased if suicides, accidents, and homicides are counted in one category. Moreover, many patients dying with traumatic death have been found on case audit to be taking no cholesterol-lowering medication [11]. Nevertheless, these results have refocused attention on dietary intervention as well as weight reduction and fitness as a means of achieving primary prevention.

A recent study of fitness and mortality, which has been a difficult area to understand, has been reported [12]. Individuals characterized by exercise level at the beginning of the study were followed for mortality over the ensuing ten years. Relatively modest forms of exercise were associated with substantial declines in mortality in both men and women. More vigorous exercise did not appear to have additional effects on declining mortality. Whatever the benefits of exercise, the effects appear to be associated with only modest changes in circulating lipoproteins. Meta-analyses of 27 longitudinal studies of exercise indicated only small changes in LDL-C and HDL-C, probably too small to account for the rather substantial effects of fitness on mortality [13].

Another issue that has been raised concerning lipoprotein-altering is the value of such therapy in those who are not male and not middle-aged. It is important to remember in this context that the most common cause of death, in women as well as in men in Western society, is CAD [14]. In an unpublished meta-analysis of three secondary prevention trials, which involved both men and women, cholesterol lowering was associated with the same decline in coronary death rates in women as in men [15]. In a recent regression study, which involved both men and women with familial hypercholesterolemia, the same degree of LDL-C lowering and HDL-C increasing were achieved in both men and women, but women had somewhat better results in terms of regression than men in the study [4].

Another issue of growing importance in women is the effect of endogenous gonadal hormones. Menopause at any age is a risk factor for the development of CAD [16]. Estrogen replacement therapy, on the other hand, has been associated with approximately 50% decline in coronary and all-cause mortality in epidemiologic cohort studies [17]. Some but not all of this benefit is explained by the fact that exogenous estrogen has favorable effects on circulating lipoproteins, raising HDL-C and lowering LDL-C levels [18]. This effect, however, can be partly or completely blocked by the addition of progestins that are needed to protect the uterine mucosa from hyperplasia from unopposed estrogen [18]. An unsolved medical question at this point is what combination of estrogen and progestin in postmenopausal hormone replacement regimens would be both beneficial in terms of preventing coronary atherosclerosis and also in protecting the uterus against the effects of unopposed estrogen.

Another large population group about which questions have been raised concerning cholesterol lowering are those over 65 years of age [19]. Coronary artery disease mortality attributable to high cholesterol actually goes up as individuals age into their sixties and seventies. Although studies are still incomplete, involve mostly total cholesterol measurements, and are less certain for women than for men, the relative risk of recurrent infarction in cholesterols over 275 mg/dl (7.5 meq/L) is over four times as great than if cholesterols are less than 200 mg/dl (5.13 meq/L). Thus, there is considerable circumstantial evidence of the importance of cholesterol in older patients. However, data are limited to epidemiologic observational studies; there are no clinical trials. One such study, the Cholesterol Reduction in Senior Persons Study (CRISP) has been completed in pilot form but has not yet begun a study large enough to demonstrate effects on coronary morbidity and mortality.

Still another set of issues that have been raised recently involve two forms of LDL that appear to be particularly atherogenic. LDL appears to be most atherogenic after it has been oxidized. Oxidation not only increases LDL's direct atherogenicity, but also its' direct uptake by macrophages. In addition, oxidized LDL is a chemotactic agent for monocytes, inhibits macrophage migration from the arterial wall, and itself is cytotoxic [20].

Some individuals have genetic tendencies to have a particular form of small, dense LDL, which may be aggravated by hypertriglyceridemia and which may also be associated with low HDL-C levels. This syndrome may also predispose to atherosclerosis [21].

Lipoprotein abnormalities may also be associated in both men and women to increases in waist-to-hip ratio [22,23]. This forms a part of a larger complex of findings that include hyperinsulinemia, hypertension, high HDL-C, low LDL-C, and hypertriglyceridemia [24]. The precise way in which these are inter-related is, at this point, not entirely clear, but a good working hypothesis is that circulating gonadal hormones determine the distribution of weight gain and that individuals, both male and female, with higher levels of testosterone are more likely to gain weight around the middle [25]. The mesenteric fat thus produced is drained directly by the portal vein into the liver and may in turn result in hyperinsulinemia, hypertriglyceridemia, and the chain of events that lead to atherosclerosis. Support for this hypothesis is also found in a study that indicates that women who take estrogen during the peri and postmenopausal period do not gain weight and specifically do not gain central adiposity compared to non-estrogen users [26].

A concept that has been growing in recent years is that of individual "susceptibility" to atherosclerosis. Such susceptibility may include a variety of genetically inherited factors including high lipoprotein (a) {Lp(a)} levels, which have been shown in a variety of populations to be associated with increased risk of coronary disease [27]. In addition, ApoE phenotype [28], and presence of the small, dense LDL pattern may be additional predictors. Thus, different individuals with the same LDL-C and HDL-C levels, because of differences in these less well-appreciated genetic factors may have very different levels of cardiovascular risk.

Finally, an underappreciated risk factor is that of socioeconomic status. In Western societies, individuals of all races studied are more likely to have coronary disease if they are in lower socioeconomic levels than if they are in higher levels [29]. This, in turn, is related to the higher level of coronary risk factors in individuals who are in the lower socioeconomic levels [30].

In summary, secondary prevention is a beneficial but still underutilized concept. Primary prevention with drugs, on the other hand, has recently again come into question and should be undertaken more conservatively than secondary prevention. Attention to diet, weight gain, and regular exercise should be re-emphasized in primary prevention. Cholesterol lowering appears to be as beneficial in women as it is in men, although there is less data in women. On the other hand, data justifying the importance of cholesterol lowering in those over 65 is limited, and no clinical trials have been completed. Drug treatment should probably be limited to those with demonstrated coronary disease.

Finally, there is a growing concept that susceptibility to CAD may be defined by factors other than simply circulating lipoprotein levels, including the presence of small, dense LDL, increased waist-to-hip ratio, increased levels of lipoprotein (a), and apoE phenotype. In all of this, another forgotten risk factor for CAD is low socioeconomic status that is, in turn, associated with higher levels of traditional risk factors and higher levels of coronary atherosclerosis.

1.   Rossouw, J.E., Lewis, B., and Rifkind, B.M. (1990) 'The value of lowering cholesterol after myocardial infarction', N Engl J Med 323, 1112-1119.

2.   Blankenhorn, D.H., Nessim, S.A., Johnson, R.L., et al. (1987) 'Beneficial effects of combined colestipol-niacin therapy on coronary atherosclerosis and coronary venous bypass grafts', JAMA 257, 3233-3240.

3.   Brown, G., Albers, J.J., Fisher, L.D., et al. (1990) 'Regression of coronary artery disease as a result of intensive lipid-lowering therapy in men with high levels of apolipoprotein B', N Engl J Med 323, 1289-1298.

4. Kane, J.P., Malloy, M.J., Ports, T.A., et al. (1990) 'Regression of coronary atherosclerosis during treatment of familial hypercholesterolemia with combined drug regimens', JAMA 264, 3007-3012.

5. Ornish, D., Brown, S.E., Scherwitz, L.W., et al. (1990) 'Can lifestyle changes reverse coronary heart disease?', Lancet 336, 129-133.

6. Buchwald, H., Varco, R.L., Matts, J.P., et al. and the POSCH group (1990) 'Effect of partial ileal bypass surgery on mortality and morbidity from coronary heart disease in patients with hypercholesterolemia. Report of the Program on the Surgical Control of the Hyperlipidemias (POSCH)', N Engl J Med 323, 946-955.

7. St. Clair, R.S.W. (1983) 'Atherosclerosis regression in animal models: Current concepts of cellular and biochemical mechanisms', Prog Cardiovasc Dis 26, 109-132.

8. Boekeloo, B., Becker, D., Yeo, E., et al. (1987) 'Post myocardial infarction cholesterol management by primary physicians', J Am Coll Cardiol 9, 77A.

9. Goldman, L., Weinstein, M.C., Goldman, P.A., and Williams, L.W. (1991) 'Cost-effectiveness of HMG-CoA reductase inhibition for primary and secondary prevention of coronary heart disease', JAMA 265, 1145-1151.

10. Muldoon, M.F., Manuck, S.B., and Matthews, K.A. (1990) 'Lowering cholesterol concentrations and mortality: A quantitative review of primary prevention trials', BMJ 301, 309-314.

11. Wysowski, D.K., and Gross, T.P. (1990) 'Deaths due to accidents and violence in two recent trials of cholesterol-lowering drugs', Arch Intern Med 150, 2169-2172.

12. Blair, S.N., Kohn, H.W.,3d., Paffenbarger, R.S.,Jr., et al. (1989) 'Physical fitness and all-cause mortality. A prospective study of healthy men and women', JAMA 262, 2395-2401.

13. Lokey, E.A., and Tran, Z.V. (1989) 'Effects of exercise training on serum lipid and lipoprotein concentrations in women: A meta-analysis', Int J Sports Med 10, 424-429.

14. Vital Statistics of the U.S., (1988) Vol. II, Mortality, Part A: pp 256, 258, 274.

15.   Rossouw, J. 'Coronary heart disease and total cholesterol in three clinical trials: Newcastle, Edinburgh, Finnish Mental Hospitals' (unpublished).

16.   Adapted from Framingham Study, DHEW, No. 74 (1974) 'Annual incidence of cardiovascular disease per 1000 women, by menopause status'.

17.   Bush, T.L., Barrett-Connor, E., Cowan, L.D., et al. (1987) 'Cardiovascular mortality and noncontraceptive estrogen use in women: Results from the Lipid Research Clinics Program Follow-up Study', Circulation 75, 1102-1109.

18.   Lobo, R.A. (1991) 'Effects of hormonal replacement on lipids and lipoproteins in postmenopausal women', J Clin Endocrinol Metab 73, 925-930.

19.   Rubin, S.M., Sidney, S., Black, D.M., et al. (1990) 'High blood cholesterol in elderly men and the excess risk for coronary heart disease', Ann Intern Med 113, 916-920.

20.   Luc, G., and Fruchart, J.C. (1991) 'Oxidation of lipoproteins and atherosclerosis', Am J Clin Nutr 53(1 Suppl), 206S-209S.

21.   Austin, M.A. (1988) 'Epidemiologic associations between hypertriglyceridemia and coronary heart disease', Semin Thromb Hemost 14, 137-142.

22.   Larsson, B., Svärdsudd, K., Welin, L., et al. (1984) 'Abdominal adipose tissue distribution, obesity, and risk of cardiovascular disease and death: 13 year follow up of participants in the study of men born in 1913', BMJ 288, 1401-1404.

23.   Lapidus, L., Bengtsson, C., Larsson, B., et al. (1984) 'Distribution of adipose tissue and risk of cardiovascular disease and death: a 12 year follow up of participants in the population study of women in Gothenburg, Sweden', BMJ 289, 1257-1261.

24.   Krauss, R.M. (1991) 'The tangled web of coronary risk factors', Am J Med 90(2A Suppl), 36S-41S.

25.   Hauner, H., Ditschuneit, H.H., Pal, S.B., et al. (1988) 'Fat distribution, endocrine and metabolic profile in obese women with and without hirsutism', Metabolism 37, 281-286.

26.   Haarbo, J., and Marslew, U. (1991) 'Postmenopausal hormone replacement therapy prevents central distribution of body fat after menopause', Metabolism 40, 1323-1326.

27.   Schreiner, P., Smith, R., Morrisett, J., and Samsa, G. (1991) 'The association of lipoprotein(a) with arterial wall thickening in a biracial cohort: The ARIC Study', Circulation 84 (II Suppl), 118.

28.   Miettinen, T.A. (1991) 'Impact of apo E phenotype on the regulation of cholesterol metabolism', Ann Med 23, 181-186.

29.   Kraus, J.F., Borhani, N.O., and Franti, C.E. (1980) 'Socioeconomic status, ethnicity, and risk of coronary heart disease', Metabolism 111, 407-414.

30.   Stern, M.P., Rosenthal, M., Haffner, S.M., et al. (1984) 'Sex difference in the effects of sociocultural status on diabetes and cardiovascular risk factors in Mexican Americans. The San Antonio Heart Study', Am J Epidemiol 120, 834-851.

ANTIATHEROSCLEROTIC DRUGS: A CRITICAL ASSESSMENT

M. RAITERI, A. CORSINI, M.R. SOMA, E. DONETTI,
F. BERNINI, R. FUMAGALLI, and R. PAOLETTI

ABSTRACT. The increasing knowledge on the processes specific to atherogenesis occurring in the arterial wall and on the physiology of lipid transport, suggest that the antiatherosclerotic pharmacological targets should not be limited to plasma lipids or blood pressure control but should involve a direct effect on the arterial wall. Pivotal roles are played by arterial smooth muscle cells (myocyte, SMC) migration and proliferation, as well as by cholesterol esterification and deposition in arterial macrophages. The importance of mevalonate and of cholesterol biosynthesis in cell growth prompted us to investigate inhibitors of HMGCoA reductase, with in vitro and in vivo models, on SMC proliferation. The results show that fluvastatin (F), simvastatin (S), but not pravastatin (P), decreased the rate of vascular SMC growth and prevented neointimal formation induced by perivascular manipulation of rabbit carotid artery. F and S displayed an inhibitory activity on cholesterol esterification induced by acetylated LDL in mouse peritoneal macrophages. These effects might represent components, along with the inhibition of cholesterol synthesis, of the antiatherosclerotic action of these drugs. Calcium antagonists (CA) may also affect major processes of atheroma formation such as cholesteryl esters metabolism and cell proliferation. Verapamil completely inhibited the ability of acetylated LDL to stimulate cholesterol esterification in macrophages. The dihydropyridine nifedipine was ineffective at this regard. However, the new nifedipine–like derivative lacidipine inhibited esterification in macrophages very efficiently. We also observed that lacidipine and isradipine, another nifedipine–like CA, inhibited proliferation of cultured myocytes. This effect was paralleled by the ability of these compounds to prevent neointimal formation of rabbit carotid artery.

In conclusion, a pharmacological control of atherosclerosis may be achieved by directly affecting the processes involved in the atheroma formation. This effect may be obtained with compounds already able to modify major risk factors of atherosclerosis such as hypertension and hypercholesterolemia, or in the future, with new compounds specifically designed as direct antiatherosclerotic drugs.

A. L. Catapano et al. (eds.), Drugs Affecting Lipid Metabolism, 317–331.
© 1993 Kluwer Academic Publishers and Fondazione Giovanni Lorenzini.

INTRODUCTION

Atherosclerosis is a complex multifactorial process. It is not surprising that multiple risk factors are involved, interact, and promote atherogenesis. Hence, preventive management as well as risk estimation in individuals should be multifactorial with the goal to improve the cardiovascular risk profile, thus retarding or preventing the onset of heart or vascular disease (1). This is accomplished, ultimately, by causing existing lesions to regress, become stable, or progress more slowly and also by preventing the formation of new lesions.

At the present time knowledge of the role of lipids in atherosclerosis still greatly exceeds that of any other factors involved (2). A relation between abnormalities in plasma lipids and lipoproteins and coronary heart disease (CHD) is well established (2,3). Aggressive manipulation and normalization of lipid profiles by pharmacological means and for a relatively long period of time (2 years or more), induces regression of vascular atherosclerotic lesions and decreases the incidence of coronary events (4–6). The reduction in LDL–cholesterol has been most closely associated with lesion regression, but other potential predictor of arteriosclerosis progression, such as HDL, Apo B, Apo C–III, and Lp (a) are emerging (4–7). These studies indicate that a therapy directed at atherogenic hyperlipidemia of diverse origins is effective, validating the lipid hypothesis.

With the increasing knowledge on the pathogenesis of atherosclerosis (8) it appears that the prevention of CHD in the future will involve not only the correction of the plasma lipid profile, but also the direct pharmacological control of atherogenic processes occurring in the arterial wall.

Major process involved in the formation of atherosclerotic lesions are deposition of lipids, mainly cholesteryl esters, and arterial smooth muscle cell (myocyte, SMC) migration and proliferation (8). The atheroma contains two main cell types, macrophages and SMC.

Macrophages derive from circulating monocytes and represent the predominant lipid – loaded cells in the lesions. The mechanism by which they accumulate lipoprotein cholesterol and develop into foam cells depends mainly upon receptor – mediated processes involving the so called "scavenger receptor" that recognizes chemically and biologically modified LDL, such as acetyl LDL (acLDL) and oxidized LDL (9,10). The scavenger receptor, unlike LDL receptor, does not undergo feed–back regulation allowing a massive accumulation of cholesterol in cells. Cholesterol accumulates in macrophages in esterified form by a process involving the enzyme acyl–CoA–cholesterol acyltransferase (ACAT) which catalyzes the cholesterol esterification in cytoplasm (11).

Arterial myocytes migrate from the media layer to and proliferate in the intima layer under the effect of various mitogens: both migration and proliferation are critical events in the development of atheromatous plaques (8). Factors controlling these processes are thought to be important in the development of atherosclerotic disease. Several data indicate the role played by calcium ion, mevalonate and cholesterol biosynthetic pathway in stimulating both cell growth and cellular lipid deposition.

Based on these findings, drugs able to modulate these processes have received increasing attention as pharmacological tools for controlling abnormal cell growth, such as myocyte proliferation, and cholesterol ester deposition in macrophages under atherogenic conditions. In the present study we have evaluated with in vitro and in vivo models, the effect of calcium antagonists (CA) and hydroxymethylglutaryl coenzyma A (HMGCoA) reductase inhibitors (vastatins) on these processes involved in atherogenesis.

MATERIALS AND METHODS

Eagle's Minimum Essential Medium (MEM), Dulbecco's minimum essential medium (DMEM), fetal calf serum (FCS), trypsin–EDTA, penicillin (10000 U/ml), streptomycin (10 mg/ml), tricine buffer (1 M, pH 7.4) and non–essential amino acid solution (100 x) were purchased from Gibco (Madison, WS, USA). Disposable culture flasks and petri dishes were from Corning, Glassworks (Amedfield, MA, USA), and from Nune (Roskilde, Denmark) Filters were from Millipore (Bedford, MA, USA).

Simvastatin in the lactone form, kindly provided by Merck Sharp & Dohme Research Laboratories (Woodbridge, MJ, USA), was brought into solution by 0.1 M NaOH (MSD file) to give the active form, and the pH was adjusted to 7.4 by adding 0.1 M HCL. Pravastatin, kindly provided by Brystol Myers Squibb Pharmaceutical Research Institute (Priceton, NJ, USA), was dissolved in 0.15 M NaCl. Solutions were sterilized by filtration. Racemic fluvastatin and isradipine were kindly provided by Sandoz Prodotti Farmaceutici (Milan, Italy) and lacidipine by Glaxo (Verona, Italy). Fluvastatin and lacidipine were dissolved in ethanol; isradipine was solubilized in a H_2O/Ethanol mixture (70/30 v/v).

$2[^{14}C]$–acetate, sodium salt (58.9 mCi/mmole) 1, 2 (n)$[^3H]$–cholesterol, (43.7 Ci/mmole) and $1[^{14}C]$–oleic acid (54 mCi/mmol), were from Amersham (Amersham, UK). Isoton II was purchased from Coulter Instruments (Milan – Italy).

"In vitro" studies.

Cell cultures. Smooth muscle cells were cultured, according to Ross (12), from intima–media layers of aorta of male Sprague–Dawley rats (200–250 g). Cells were grown in monolayers at 37°C in a humidified atmosphere of 5% CO_2 in MEM supplemented with 10% (v:v) FCS, 100 U/ml penicillin, 0.1 mg/ml streptomicin, 20 mM tricine buffer and 1% (v:v) non–essential amino acid solution (13). The medium was changed every third day. Cells were used between the 4th and 10th passages. Smooth muscle cells were identified for growth behaviour, morphology and using monoclonal antibodies techniques (14). The cell grew out of explants after 12–16 days, piled up after confluency and contained numerous myofilaments and dense bodies, as observed by transmission electron microscopy (8,12). Human vascular myocytes (A617 from human femoral artery) were grown in the same culture conditions (15).

Mouse peritoneal macrophages (MPM) were obtained from mice (Balb/C Charles River, Calco, Italy) after intraperitoneal injection of thioglycollate. Cells ($3 \cdot 10^6$/35mm dish) were plated in Dulbecco's minimum essential medium containing 10% FCS. After 3 h, the dishes were washed to eliminate unattached cells and maintained in DMEM plus FCS until use. Cell viability was evaluated by tripan blue exclusion test and by measuring lactate dehydrogenase activity (LDH) in the culture medium (Merck LDH, Danmstadt, Germany). Protein was measured according to Lowry et al. (16).

AcLDL preparation. Human LDL (d= 1.019 – 1.063 g/ml) was isolated from plasma of healthy volunteers by sequential ultracentrifugation (Beckman L5–50, Palso Alto, CA, USA) (17). AcLDL was prepared by repeated additions of acetic anhydride (18).

Cell proliferation was evalutated by cell count after trypsinization of the SMC monolayers using a Coulter Counter model ZM from Coulter Instruments (Milan, Italy) (13,15). Cell viability was assessed by trypan blue exclusion, and found to be higher than 95% at the drug concentrations used. In a separate set of petri dishes cholesterol synthesis was estimated in the same experimental conditions, by measuring the incorporation of [^{14}C]–acetate into cellular sterols (19). The concentrations of drugs required to inhibit 50% of cholesterol synthesis and cell proliferation (IC$_{50s}$) were computed by linear regression analysis of the logarithm of the concentrations (uM) vs probits and read from a probit transformation table (20).

Experimental protocol. Cells were seeded at density of $2 \cdot 10^5$ per petri dish (35mm), and incubated with MEM supplemented with 10% FCS. Twenty–four hours later the medium was changed to one containing 0.4% FCS to stop cell growth, and the cultures were incubated for 48 h (21). At this time (time 0) the medium was replaced by one containing 10% FCS and the incubation was continued for 48 h or 72 h at 37°C in the presence of CA or vastatins respectively. At time zero, just before the addition of the drugs to be tested, few petri dishes were used for cell counting.

Synthesis of cholesterol was determined by measuring the incorporation of radioactive acetate into cellular sterols (19). Cell monolayers, after incubation with 2[^{14}C]–acetate (1 µCi/ml, sp.act. 0.9 µCi/nmole) for 72 h were washed with phosphate–buffer saline (PBS) and digested with 0.1 NaOH. Aliquots were saponified at 60°C for 1 h in alcoholic NaOH after the addition of 1, 2 (n)– [^{3}H]–cholesterol as internal standard (0.02 µCi/sample). The unsaponifiable material was extracted with low–boiling petrol ether and counted for radioactivity. To evaluate the incorporation of labelled acetate into cellular sterols, these were separated from the unsaponifiable fraction by TLC (22). Radioactivity was measured with lipoluma scintillator (Lumal, Olen, Belgium).

Determination of cholesterol esterification. MPM were incubated for 24 h in lipoprotein–free medium and compounds under investigation, followed by 24 h in the same medium plus 50 µg of acLDL protein/ml. The rate of cholesterol esterification was measured after addition of   1[^{14}C]–oleic acid–(Amersham, Buckinghamshire,

England; 0.68 uCi/sample, 54 mCi/mmol) albumin complex during the last 2 h of incubation, by determining the incorporation of radioactivity into cellular cholesteryl esters (23). To evaluate the cellular content of free and esterified cholesterol, the incubation medium was discarded, cells were washed with PBS, and the lipids were extracted with hexane: isopropanol (3:2). Free and esterified cholesterol were partitioned by TLC.

"In vivo" studies.

New Zealand White male rabbits (1.8–2 kg) (Charles River) were employed for the study. All animals had free access to food and water and were allowed to acclimatize for at least 2 weeks before undergoing any experimental manipulation. Surgery to insert the collar was performed essentially as described by Booth et al. (24) and Soma et al. (25). Rabbits were anesthetized by intramuscular injection of 5 mg/kg xylazine and 35 mg/kg ketamine. Animals were then placed in dorsal recumbency. A neck midline incision was made and both carotid arteries were surgically exposed. A non occlusive, biologically inert, soft, and hollow silastic collar was positioned around both carotids. The collar was 1.5 cm in length and it touched the artery circumference at two points 1.0 cm apart. In the sham arteries the collar was removed just before carotids were replaced and the wounds were sutured. Experimental protocol is described in the results session.

RESULTS AND DISCUSSION

Effect of vastatins on arterial myocyte proliferation and on cholesterol ester formation in macrophages.

In view of the important role of mevalonate and cholesterol biosynthesis in stimulating the proliferation of arterial smooth muscle cells, the "in vitro" effect of potent HMG–CoA reductase inhibitors, simvastatin, pravastatin, and fluvastatin on the proliferation of rat aorta myocytes was investigated. Proliferation was evaluated by direct counting after exposure of cell to drugs for 72 h; all the tested compounds were used in the active hydroxyacid form (not lactone).

Simvastatin decreased the replication of rat arterial myocytes (13,15). This inhibitory effect, already detectable at the lowest concentration tested, became statistically significant at 0.1 uM (the reported therapeutic concentration), and was dose dependent with an IC_{50} of 2.8 uM. Myocytes cultured in the presence of simvastatin and fluvastatin had longer doubling times than controls (Table I). By contrast, pravastatin failed to reduce arterial myocyte proliferation even at the highest not toxic concentration used (500 uM). When tested on the proliferation of human myocytes, simvastatin and fluvastatin inhibited cell growth in a dose–dependent manner with IC_{50} values of 0.5 and 0.6 uM, respectively: pravastatin was inactive (26).

The addition of mevalonate restored rat and human cell proliferation to control levels (Fig. 1). These results demonstrate that arterial myocytes require mevalonate itself

TABLE I

MEAN DOUBLING TIMES FOR MUSCLE CELLS CULTURED FROM RAT AORTA: EFFECT OF SIMVASTATIN, PRAVASTATIN AND FLUVASTATIN

DRUGS	µM	DOUBLING TIME (h) Mean (SD)
SIMVASTATIN	---	44.8 (1.6)
	0.01	48.1 (1.5)
	0.1	50.3 (0.5)*
	1	54.4 (1.1)*
	5	72.8 (0.6)**
PRAVASTATIN	---	44.8 (1.6)
	0.01	45.7 (0.5)
	0.1	45.5 (1.2)
	1	46.5 (2.0)
	10	46.0 (0.5)
	50	45.1 (3.2)
FLUVASTATIN	---	37.7 (1.9)
	0.5	39.7 (1.2)
	1	40.2 (0.3)
	2	50.6 (4.3)*
	5	62.9 (1.4)**

Doubling times were measured after 72h of incubation; each point was run in triplicate. Drug versus control: *$p < 0.01$; **$p < 0.001$ (Student's t–test).

or some of its non–sterol metabolites, in addition to a source of cholesterol (fetal calf serum), for their proliferation. All the tested vastatins inhibited the incorporation of [^{14}C]–acetate into cholesterol. The results suggest that conditions producing 80–90% inhibition of cholesterol synthesis correlate with approximately 50% inhibition of cell growth.

The in vivo activity of different HMGCoA reductase inhibitors was investigated on neointimal formation induced by insertion of a flexible collar around one carotid artery of normocholesterolemic rabbits (24,25). The contralateral carotid served as sham. Pravastatin, simvastatin, and fluvastatin were given mixed with food, at daily doses of 20 mg/kg for 2 weeks, starting from the day of collar placement. The treatment with vastatins did not modify rabbit plasma cholesterol concentrations. The neointimal formation was assessed by measuring with light microscopy the cross–sectional thickness of intimal (I) and media (M) tissue of fixed arteries. Fourteen days after the insertion the process of intima hyperplasia, mostly cellular, was pronounced in carotid arteries with collar: the I/M tissue ratio was 12 fold higher than in the arteries without collar (0.36±0.04 vs 0.03±0.02). The animals treated with simvastatin (n = 12) and fluvastatin

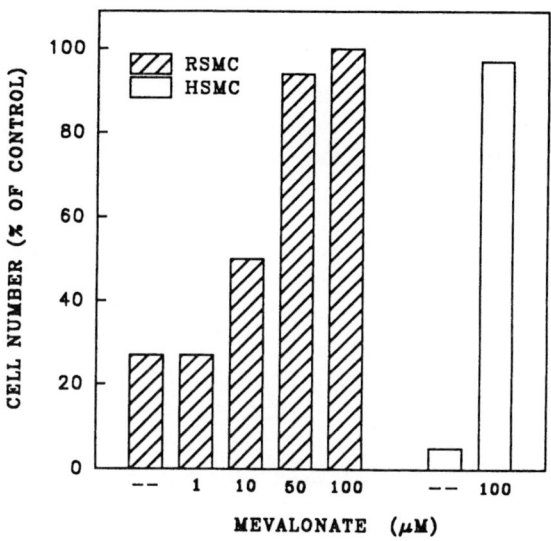

FIGURE 1 – Ability of mevalonate to prevent cell growth inhibition by simvastatin in rat and human myocytes.

Cells were seeded (2·10⁵/dish for rat myocytes and 5·10⁴/dish for human myocytes) and incubated with MEM supplemented with 10% FCS; 24h later the medium was changed with one containing 0.4% FCS to stop cell growth, and the cultures were incubated for 48h. At this time (time 0) the medium was replaced with one containing 10% FCS, simvastatin (3.5μM and 2μM for rat and human myocytes, respectively) and the reported concentrations of mevalonate. The incubation was continued for further 72h at 37°C. Each point represent the average of three different experiments that did not differ more than 10%.

(n = 12) showed significant reduction of the neointimal formation: I/M tissue ratios were 0.20±0.03, and 0.17±0.03, respectively. The inhibition elicited by pravastatin (0.32±0.03) did not reach statistical significance (25).

These results are of interest in the contest of suggestions that interference with myocyte proliferation represents a component of a direct antiatherosclerotic effect. The ability of simvastatin and fluvastatin to inhibit myocyte proliferation at the reported therapeutic concentration (0.1μM) may be of potential clinical importance (28). Accelerated proliferation of SMC appears to be a cause of early coronary occlusion in patients undergoing heart transplantion, coronary artery bypass graft and percutaneous transluminal coronary angioplasty (PTCA) (28). Pharmacological approaches including heparin, calcium antagonists, and angiotensin converting enzyme inhibitors have been tried with variable success in preventing restenosis after PTCA.

Simvastatin and fluvastatin may decrease the incidence of coronary occlusion by simultaneously reducing serum cholesterol levels and preventing myocytes proliferation. To address this issue, Gellman et al. (29), have recently shown that lovastatin, reportedly active as inhibitor of vascular SMC proliferation "in vitro" (30), reduces intimal hyperplasia after balloon angioplasty of the femoral artery in the hypercholesterolemic rabbits; the beneficial effect appears to be unrelated to cholesterol lowering. Similarly Zhu et al. (31) have shown that lovastatin can halt the progression of the aortic plaque in experimental atherosclerosis in rabbits independently of cholesterol levels. On the other hand the lack of effect of pravastatin on SMC proliferation provides an unique tool to evaluate the importance of reduction of plasma lipids on atherosclerosis. Preliminary results in patients undergoing coronary angioplasty have shown a significant reduction in the incidence of short term restenosis with lovastatin (32) but not with pravastatin (33).

In summary, the "in vivo" data in accordance with the "in vitro" observations show that vastatins, with different potency, may affect an early event of atherogenesis by mechanisms other than or beyond changes in serum lipoprotein levels by retarding or inhibiting arterial myocyte proliferation, possibly through local inhibition of mevalonic acid synthesis. Moreover, vastatins by depleting the endogenous pool of mevalonate, represent a pharmacological tool to evaluate the role of mevalonate products in other cellular functions.

Recently it has been reported that vastatins are able to inhibit cholesterol esterification induced by acLDL in human macrophages (34).

This action of vastatins was not due to a direct inhibition of ACAT activity and was independent of intracellular cholesterol formation (34). We confirmed the inhibitory activity of simvastatin on ac–LDL induced cholesterol esterification in MPM and demonstrated a similar activity of the new HMG–CoA reductase inhibitor fluvastatin (Table II). Our preliminary results indicate that the inhibition of cholesterol esterification in MPM by vastatins are fully reversed by low concentrations (<100μM) of exogenous mevalonate suggesting that the production of mevalonate play an essential role in the process of esterification of excess cholesterol delivered to macrophages by modified LDL. This observation may be of importance in understanding the cellular mechanisms of cholesteryl ester accumulation in these cells.

Effect of calcium antagonists on arterial myocyte proliferation and on cholesterol ester formation in macrophages.

Several calcium antagonists (CA) are effective in reducing the severity of experimentally induced atherosclerosis in cholesterol–fed animals without affecting plasma lipid levels (35–37). Two randomized placebo controlled studies have reported on the action of calcium antagonists on atheroma in the coronary arteries (38,39). In these studies the inhibitory effect on progression of new lesions, with no effect on the preexisting lesions, was accomplished without interfering with blood lipid levels. Thus, it seems that some as yet unidentified biological processes in the early development of atheromatous lesions is sensitive to calcium antagonists. The ability of these drugs to act as antiatherosclerotic agents is complex. Several calcium dependent processes

TABLE II

EFFECT OF SIMVASTATIN AND FLUVASTATIN ON [^{14}C]-OLEATE
INCORPORATION INTO CHOLESTERYL ESTERS IN MOUSE PERITONEAL
MACROPHAGES INCUBATED WITH acLDL

VASTATINS	(μM)	% OF ACAT INHIBITION (SD)
FLUVASTATIN	0.1	17.7 (3.4)*
"	0.5	44.2 (1.9)**
"	1	64.2 (7.8)**
"	5	84.3 (1.0)***
SIMVASTATIN	0.5	20.7 (4.1)*
"	1	32.0 (5.0)***
"	5	77.5 (14.0)***

Cells were incubated with the indicated concentrations of drugs for 24h, followed by a 24h incubation in the same medium added with acLDL (50μg protein/ml). Data are the mean ± SD of triplicate samples.
Drug versus control: *p< 0.05; **p< 0.01; ***p< 0.001 (Student's t–test)

contribute to atherogenesis, including lipid infiltration and oxidation, endothelial injury, action of chemotactic and growth factors, smooth muscle cells migration and proliferation (40).

In the present study we evaluated the effect of CA on two processes involved in the formation of atherosclerotic plaque: a) arterial myocyte proliferation; b) cholesterol esterification.

a) The potential antiproliferative action of the dihydropyridine derivatives isradipine and lacidipine was studied in rat aortic myocytes at drug concentrations ranging between 1 and 20 μM and was compared with that of verapamil, a CA reportedly active on this parameter (41). Lacidipine and isradipine decreased SMC proliferation in a concentration–dependent manner and treated cells had longer doubling times than controls (Table III). The effect, already detectable at the lowest concentration tested, became statistically significant at 5 μM. Verapamil was less potent in this respect.

Preliminary data in our laboratory indicate that lacidipine (3 mg/kg/die) and isradipine (1 mg/kg/die) were able to inhibit neointimal proliferation induced "in vivo" in hypercholesterolemic and normocholesterolemic

TABLE III

DOUBLING TIMES FOR SMOOTH MUSCLE CELLS CULTURED FROM RAT AORTA: EFFECT OF LACIDIPINE, ISRADIPINE AND VERAPAMIL

DRUGS	(μM)	DOUBLING TIME (h)
NONE		21.7 (0.1)
VERAPAMIL	50	31.0 (0.6)**
LACIDIPINE	1	23.3 (1.1)
"	5	23.7 (0.6)*
"	10	31.5 (2.6)*
"	20	70.4 (11.4)*
NONE		19.5 (0.5)
ISRADIPINE	5	21.8 (0.6)*
"	7.5	24.2 (0.3)**
"	10	33.2 (0.2)**

Doubling times were measured the second day of culture growth; each point is the mean (SD) of triplicate dishes.
*p< 0.01; **p< 0.001 (Student's t–test)

rabbits, respectively. The neointimal/media ratio was reduced about 50% as compared to control.

b) The activity of lacidipine on cholesterol esterification induced by acLDL was compared to that of nifedipine, verapamil and progesterone, an ACAT inhibitor, in MPM incubated with the drug (50μM) for 7h in the presence of acLDL. Addition of acLDL to culture medium stimulated about 30 times [^{14}C]–oleate incorporation into cholesteryl esters. In the presence of lacidipine cholesterol esterification induced by acLDL was almost abolished (Table IV). As expected (11,42) both verapamil and progesterone completely inhibited [^{14}C]–oleate incorporation into cholesteryl esters. According to previous data of our laboratory nifedipine had a minor effect on cholesterol esterification (43).

The results reported herein provide experimental support to a possible antiatherosclerotic action of lacidipine and isradipine through effects on mechanisms involved in atherogenesis.

TABLE IV

EFFECTS OF LACIDIPINE, VERAPAMIL, NIFEDIPINE AND
PROGESTERONE ON THE CHOLESTEROL ESTERIFICATION IN MOUSE
PERITONEAL MACROPHAGES LOADED WITH acLDL

DRUGS (μM)		[^{14}C]–OLEATE INCORPORATION INTO CHOLESTERYL ESTER (ng/mg Cell prot · h)	% OF CONTROL
BASAL		54.9 (0.6)	----
CONTROL	+ acLDL	1555.2 (77.4)	100.0 (4.9)
LACIDIPINE (50)	+ acLDL	6.6 (0.5)*	0.4 (0.03)
VERAPAMIL (50)	+ acLDL	10.2 (0.2)*	0.7 (0.3)
NIFEDIPINE (50)	+ acLDL	1399.2 (50.4)	89.9 (3.2)
PROGESTERONE (30)	+ acLDL	32.1 (7.9)*	2.1 (0.5)

Cells were preincubated in DMEM containing Essentially Fatty Acid Free Albumin (EFAF) 0.1% and drugs for 2h. Monolayers underwent a second incubation (5 h) in the presence of acLDL (50 μg/ml), [^{14}C]–oleate–albumin complex and drugs.
Each point is the mean (SD) of triplicate dishes.
*p< 0.001 (Student's t–test)

In conclusion, a pharmacological control of atherosclerosis and prevention of CHD can be achieved by correcting plasma lipid disorders as well as by directly affecting atheroma formation. While the former approach is now definitely demonstrated in man, the latter still represent a "therapeutic hope" which deserves larger experimental and clinical studies.

ACKNOWLEDGEMENTS

This research was partially supported by MURST and CNR (Italian

Government).

The Authors are grateful to Prof. G. Gabbiani (University of Geneva, Switzerland) for providing the human femoral artery cell line A617. Mrs Monica Zamati is acknowledged for typing the manuscript.

REFERENCES

1.   Anderson K.M., Wilson P.W.F., Odell P.M. and Kannel W.B. (1991) "Coronary risk profile. A statement for health professionals", Circulation, 83, 356–362.
2.   Lerner D.J. and Kannel W.B. (1986) "Patterns of coronary heart–disease morbidity and mortality in the sexes. A 26 years follow–up of the Framingham population", Am. Heart J., 111, 383–390.
3.   Consensus Conference. (1985) "Lowering blood cholesterol to prevent heart disease", J. Am. Med. Assoc., 253, 2980–3086.
4.   Kane J.P., Malloy M.J., Ports T.A., Phillips N.R., Diehl J.C. and Havel R.J. (1990) "Regression of coronary atherosclerosis during treatment of familial hypercholesterolemia with combined drug regimens", J. Am. Med. Assoc. 264, 3007–3012.
5.   Brown G., Alberts J.J., Fisher L.D., Schaefer S.M., Lin J.T., Kaplan C., Zhao X.Q., Bisson B.D., Fitzpatrick V.F. and Dodge H.T. (1990) "Regression of coronary artery disease as a result of intensive lipid–lowering therapy in men with high levels of apolipoprotein B", N. Eng. J. Med., 323, 1289–1298.
6.   Blankenhorn D.H. (1992) "Lipid lowering: progression and regression of atherosclerotic lesions", Abstract book XI Int. Symp. on: Drugs affecting lipid metabolism, Florence, May 13–16.
7.   Utermann G. (1989) "The mysteries of lipoprotein (a)", Science 246, 904–910.
8.   Ross R. (1986) "The pathogenesis of atherosclerosis. An update", N. Engl. J. Med., 314, 488–500.
9.   Brown M.S. and Goldstein J.L. (1983) "Lipoprotein metabolism in the macrophage: implications for cholesterol deposition in atherosclerosis" Annu. Rev. Biochem., 52, 223–261.
10.   Kurhara Y., Matsumoto A., Itakura H. and Kodama T. (1991) "Macrophage scavenger receptors", Curr. Opin. Lipid. 2, 295–300.
11.   Brown M.S., Ho Y.K. and Goldstein J.L. (1980) "The cholesteryl ester cycle in macrophage foam cells: continual hydrolysis and reesterification of cytoplasmic cholesteryl esters", J. Biol. Chem., 255, 9344–9352.
12.   Ross R. (1971) "The smooth muscle cell. II. Growth of smooth muscle

in culture and formation of elastic fibers", J. Cell. Biol., 50, 172–186.

13. Corsini A., Raiteri M., Soma M., Fumagalli R. and Paoletti R. (1991) "Simvastatin but not pravastatin inhibits the proliferation of rat aorta myocytes", Pharmacological Research, 23, 173–180.

14. Skalli O., Ropraz P., Trezciak A., Benzonana G., Gillessen D. and Gabbiani G. (1986) "A monoclonal antibody against alfa–smooth muscle actin: a new probe for smooth muscle differentiation", J. Cell. Biol., 103, 2787–2796.

15. Corsini A., Raiteri M., Soma M.R., Gabbiani G. and Paoletti R. (1992) "Simvastatin but not pravastatin has a direct inhibitory effect on rat and human myocyte proliferation", Clinical Biochemistry, 25, 399–400.

16. Lowry O.H., Rosebrough N.J., Farr A.L. and Randall R.J. (1951) "Protein reagent with the Folin phenol reagent", J. Biol. Chem., 193, 265–275.

17. Havel R.J., Eder H.A. and Bragdon J.H. (1955) "The distribution and chemical composition of ultracentrifugally separated lipoproteins in human serum", J. Clin. Invest., 34, 1345–1354.

18. Goldstein J.L., Ho Y.K., Basu S.K. and Brown M.S. (1979) "Binding site on macrophages that mediates uptake and degradation of acetylated low density lipoprotein producing massive cholesterol deposition", Proc. Natl. Acad. Sci., USA, 76, 333–337.

19. Corsini A., Bernini F., Cighetti G., Soma M., Galli G. and Fumagalli R. (1987) "Lipophilic beta–adrenoceptor antagonists stimulate cholesterol biosynthesis in human skin fibroblasts", Biochem. Pharmacol., 36, 1901–1906.

20. Fisher R.A. and Yates F. (1953) "Statistical tables for biological agricultural and medical research", 4th edn, Oliver and Boyd, Edinburgh, 60.

21. Hoover R.L., Rosemberg R., Haerling W. and Karnovsky M.J. (1980) "Inhibition of rat arterial smooth muscle cell proliferation by heparin. II. In vitro studies", Circulation Res., 47, 578–583.

22. Fumagalli R. and Paoletti P. (1971) "Sterol test for human brain tumors: relationship with different oncotypes", Neurology, 21, 1149–1156.

23. Via D.P., Plant A.L., Craig I.F., Gotto A.M.Jr. and Smith L.C. (1985) "Metabolism of normal and modified low–density lipoprotein by macrophage", Biochimica et Biophysica Acta, 833, 417–428.

24. Booth R.G.F., Martin J.F., Honey A.C., Hassall D.G., Beesley J.E. and Moncada S. (1989) "Rapid development of atherosclerotic lesions in the rabbit carotid artery induced by perivascular manipulation", Atherosclerosis, 76, 257–268.

25. Soma M.R., Donetti E., Parolini C., Mazzini G., Ferrari C., Fumagalli R. and Paoletti R. (1993) "HMG CoA reductase inhibitors: in vivo effects on carotid intimal thickening in normocholesterolemic rabbits", Arteriosclerosis and Thrombosis, in press.

26. Soma M.R., Corsini A. and Paoletti R. (1992) "Cholesterol and mevalonic acid modulation in cell metabolism and multiplication", Toxicology Letters, 64/65, 1–15.

27. Pentikainen P.J., Saraheimo M., Schwartz J.I., Amin R.D., Schwartz M.S., Brunner–Ferber F. and Rogers J.D. (1992) "Comparative pharmacokinetics of lovastatin, simvastatin and pravastatin in human", J. Clin. Pharmacol., 32, 136–140.

28. Ip J.H., Fuster V., Badimon L., Badimon J., Taubman M.B. and Chesebro J.H. (1990) "Syndromes of accelerated atherosclerosis: role of vascular injury and smooth muscle cell proliferation", Am. J. Coll. Cardiol., 15, 1667–1687.

29. Gellman J., Ezekowitz M.D., Sarembock I.J., Azarin M.A., Nochomowitz L.E., Lerner E. and Haudenschild C.C. (1991) "Effect of lovastatin on intimal hyperplasia after balloon angioplasty: a study in an atherosclerotic hypercholesterolemic rabbit", J. Am. Coll. Cardiol., 17, 251–259.

30. Falke P., Mattiasson I., Stavenow L. and Hood B. (1989) "Effect of a competitive inhibitor (mevinolin) of 3–hydroxy–3–methylglutaryl coenzyme A reductase on human and bovine endothelial cells, fibroblasts and smooth muscle cells in vitro", Pharmacol. Toxicol., 64, 173–176.

31. Zhu B.Q., Sievers R.E., Sun Y.P., Isenberg W.M. and Parmley W.W. (1992) "Effect of lovastatin on suppression and regression of atherosclerosis in lipid–fed rabbits", J. Cardiovasc. Pharmacol., 19, 246–255.

32. Sahni R., Maniet A.R., Voci G. and Banka V.S. (1992) "Prevention of restenosis by lovastatin after successful coronary angioplasty", Am. Heart J., 121, 1600–1608.

33. Lee Y.J., Daida H., Yokoi H., Miyano H., Takaya J., Sakurai H., Yamaguchi H., Abe A. and Noma A. (1991) "Does lipid lowering therapy prevent early restenosis after coronary angioplasty?", 9th International Symposium on Atherosclerosis, 206.

34. Kempen H.J.M., Vermeer M., De Wit E. and Havekes L.M. (1991) "Vastatins inhibit cholesterol ester accumulation in human monocyte-derived macrophages", Arteriosclerosis and Thrombosis, 11, 146–153.

35. Jackson C.L., Bush R.C. and Bowyer D.E. (1989) "Mechanism of antiatherogenic action of calcium antagonists", Atherosclerosis, 80, 17–26.

36. Henry P.D. (1990) "Calcium channel blockers and atherosclerosis", J. Cardiovasc. Pharmacol., 16 (suppl. 1), S12–S15.

37. Bernini F., Catapano A.L., Corsini A., Fumagalli R. and Paoletti R. (1989) "Effects of calcium antagonists on lipids and atherosclerosis", Am. J. Cardiol., 64, 1291–1331.

38. Lichtlen P.R., Hugenholtz P.G., Rafflenbeul W., Hecker H., Jost S. and Deckers J.W. (1990) "Retardation of angiographic progression of

coronary artery disease by nifedipine. Results of international nifedipine trial on antiatherosclerotic therapy (INTACT)", Lancet, 335, 1109–1113.

39.   Waters D., Lespérance J., Francetich M., Causey D., Theroux P., Chiang Y.K., Hudon G., Lemarbre L., Reitman M., Joyal M., Gosselin G., Durda I., Macer J. and Havel R.J. (1990) "A controlled clinical trial to assess the effect of a calcium channel blocker on the progression of coronary atherosclerosis", Circulation, 82, 1940–1953.

40.   Schmitz G., Hankowitz J. and Kovacs E.M. (1991) "Cellular processes in atherogenesis: potential targets of Ca^{2+} channel blockers", Atherosclerosis, 88, 109–132.

41.   Stein O., Halpern G. and Stein Y. (1987) "Long–term effect of verapamil on aortic smooth muscle cells cultured in the presence of hypercholesterolemic serum", Arteriosclerosis, 7, 585–592.

42.   Stein O. and Stein Y. (1987) "Effect of verapamil on cholesteryl ester hydrolysis and reesterification in macrophages", Arteriosclerosis, 7, 578–584.

43.   Bernini F., Bellosta S., Didoni G. and Fumagalli R. (1991) "Calcium antagonists and cholesteryl ester metabolism in macrophages", J. Cardiovascular Pharmacol., 18 (suppl. 10), S42–S45.

Experimental and Clinical Evidence for a Protective Role of High-Density Lipoprotein in Coronary Heart Disease

A. M. GOTTO, JR.,[1] W. PATSCH,[1] and J. R. PATSCH[2]

An inverse relation between high-density lipoprotein (HDL) cholesterol and the incidence and/or prevalence of coronary heart disease (CHD) has been firmly established in numerous epidemiologic studies. Data from the Framingham Heart Study, the Lipid Research Clinics (LRC) Prevalence Mortality Follow-up Study, the LRC Coronary Primary Prevention Trial, and the Multiple Risk Factor Intervention Trial have all suggested a 2% to 3% decrease in CHD risk for each 1 mg/dl (0.026 mmol/L) increase in HDL cholesterol after correction for other risk factors [1]. In man, limited information is available as to whether increasing HDL cholesterol would reduce the risk of CHD. However, animal experiments support the notion that increasing HDL may be beneficial. Infusion of HDL into rabbits fed an atherogenic diet was associated with reduced severity and extent of atherosclerotic lesions in comparison with control animals fed the same diet [2]. Similar conclusions were reached in transgenic mice in that overexpression of human apolipoprotein (apo) A-I decreased the severity of diet-induced atherosclerosis [3].

The mechanisms whereby HDL provides protection from CHD are not fully understood. The two major hypotheses, not exclusive of each other, are that certain HDL particles directly interfere with the atherogenic process, and that high levels of HDL cholesterol are indicative of a metabolic state that confers protection from CHD.

The first hypothesis—that HDL plays a causal role in preventing atherogenesis—relates to HDL's role in reverse cholesterol transport [4]. Since cholesterol cannot be metabolized by peripheral tissues, it must be transported to the liver for excretion. Small, discoidal particles that contain apo A-I as the sole apoprotein may be secreted by the liver or generated as a result of intravascular remodeling of HDL during the metabolism of triglyceride-rich lipoproteins (TGRL). These discoidal particles, which are also termed pre-ß-HDL, may attract cholesterol from extrahepatic cells and acquire phospholipids generated during lipolysis of TGRL. The cholesterol is esterified by lecithin:cholesterol acyltransferase (LCAT). Cholesteryl esters formed provide an apolar core that is required for transition of the discoidal particles into spherical HDL particles, and particles are enlarged with continued LCAT activity and lipolysis of TGRL, so that HDL_3 particles are converted into HDL_2. Cholesteryl ester transfer protein (CETP) transfers

333

A. L. Catapano et al. (eds.), Drugs Affecting Lipid Metabolism, 333–338.
© 1993 Kluwer Academic Publishers and Fondazione Giovanni Lorenzini.

cholesteryl esters from the core of HDL to the core of TGRL, and transfers triglyceride from TGRL to HDL. As a result of this transfer, cholesteryl esters accumulate in chylomicron remnants and in intermediate-density and low-density lipoproteins (IDL and LDL). Through the LDL-receptor pathway and/or a putative remnant pathway, cell-derived cholesterol can be eliminated from the body by biliary excretion or redistributed to peripheral cells. The triglyceride-rich HDL particles are acted on by hepatic lipase, which hydrolyzes surplus phospholipids and core triglyceride. Hence, HDL becomes smaller and competent for acceptance of cellular cholesterol to undergo another cycle of cholesteryl ester delivery to TGRL. This pathway has been termed the reverse cholesterol transport pathway.

Biochemical studies support the importance of HDL in the initial step of the reverse cholesterol pathway. HDL particles enhance the net removal of cellular cholesterol from a variety of cells such as aortic smooth muscle cells, fibroblasts, and macrophages loaded with cholesterol [5,6]. However, the ability to promote cholesterol efflux from cholesterol-loaded macrophages is not specific for HDL since other plasma proteins may serve as effective cholesterol acceptors as well [6].

Besides participation in reverse cholesterol transport, a number of other mechanisms by which HDL could directly protect against atherosclerosis have been suggested. These include stimulation of endothelial cell proliferation [7], inhibition of smooth muscle cell proliferation [8], and interference with macrophage uptake of oxidized LDL by macrophages [9]. A recent study in Japanese subjects showed that apo A-I binds and stabilizes prostacyclin, which would result in reduced thrombus formation and vasoconstriction [10]. However, another group was unable to confirm the result [11].

There are marked differences in association with CHD among the number of rare genetic defects in the production and catabolism of HDL. While premature CHD is a characteristic feature of familial apo A-I/C-III deficiency, apo A-I/C-III/A-IV deficiency, and some forms of isolated apo A-I deficiency, the prevalence of CHD is not strikingly increased in other inherited forms of HDL deficiency such as apo A-I$_{Milano}$, fish-eye disease, and Tangier disease [12]. In Tangier disease, retro-endocytosis and removal of cellular cholesterol by HDL is thought to be defective and HDL is degraded in lysosomes [13]. This argues against the hypothesis that removal of cellular cholesterol is key to the "protective" function of HDL.

Various subfractions of HDL can be distinguished by differences in physical, chemical, and functional properties. Subfractionation of HDL into HDL$_2$ and HDL$_3$ has been shown to be of clinical relevance. Compared with HDL$_3$, HDL$_2$ particles are larger and less dense, contain more lipid, and exhibit a higher molar ratio of apo A-I to apo A-II [14]. There is evidence to suggest that the protective effect of HDL is better reflected by plasma levels of HDL$_2$ than HDL$_3$ or total HDL. While not all epidemiologic studies support this view [15], clinicopathological studies [16,17] and the relation between HDL$_2$ plasma levels and CHD incidence as observed in both males and females [18] point to the importance of HDL$_2$. A beneficial effect of HDL$_2$ is also suggested by a striking association of high levels of HDL$_2$ and increased life expectancy in familial hyperalphalipoproteinemia, an autosomal inherited condition [19,20].

Studies in experimental animals and of the postprandial state in human subjects have provided evidence that the metabolism of TGRL is a main determinant of HDL$_2$ and total HDL cholesterol levels in plasma. Effective catabolism of TGRL as reflected by high activity of lipoprotein lipase is associated with transfer of surface components from TGRL to HDL, leads to the anabolic formation of HDL$_2$, and is correlated with plasma levels of HDL cholesterol [21]. Conversely, elevated levels of TGRL resulting from defective clearance or from partial saturation of the clearance pathway by overproduction of TGRL lead to redistribution of triglyceride into

HDL at the expense of cholesteryl ester via lipid-transfer proteins. Hepatic lipase may then convert the triglyceride-rich HDL into smaller, denser HDL particles, which contain less cholesteryl ester [22,23]. Importantly, an imbalance in triglyceride transport may not be apparent in the fasting state, but may be detected in the postprandial state as the buffering capacity for maintaining lipid homeostasis is exhausted [22]. A series of experiments support this metabolic relationship. Injection of anti–lipoprotein lipase antibodies into chicken leads to the expected increase in plasma TGRL concentration, but also to a reduction in HDL size and HDL mass [24]. Primary and secondary hypertriglyceridemias, including lipoprotein lipase deficiency, are typically associated with very low levels of HDL cholesterol [12]. Overexpression of apo C-III in transgenic mice causes triglyceride levels to rise and HDL cholesterol levels to fall [25]. In contrast, elevated levels of plasma triglyceride are not a hallmark of disorders in which the primary abnormality lies in the structure and metabolism of HDL.

Translocation of triglyceride from TGRL to HDL in exchange for cholesteryl esters that is mediated by CETP assumes a pivotal role in the inverse relation between plasma triglyceride and HDL cholesterol. Immunologic blockage of the enzyme in rabbits increases the cholesteryl ester content of HDL and delays HDL clearance from the circulation [26]. Overexpression of CETP in transgenic mice reduces HDL cholesterol [27]. Furthermore, the inverse association between plasma triglyceride and HDL cholesterol breaks down in inherited CETP deficiency, in which HDL cholesterol levels are high irrespective of plasma triglyceride concentrations [28]. According to this view, the inverse relation between HDL cholesterol and risk of CHD is a secondary phenomenon that reflects effective clearance of TGRL.

This second hypothesis is not mutually exclusive of the notion that HDL per se is anti-atherogenic. Effective clearance of TGRL may enhance the initial step of reverse cholesterol transport, i.e., the removal of cholesterol from cell membranes, as surface phospholipids become redundant during lipolysis and may associate with apo A-I in the circulation. Such nascent HDL particles are very efficient acceptors of cholesterol [29] and may in fact represent the pre-ß-HDL that has been identified by in vitro studies as the principal acceptor of cholesterol [30]. In this metabolic scenario, triglyceride catabolism would play an important role in establishing type and quantity of HDL particles that may have specific interactive properties with peripheral cells, including those of the arterial wall, with an outcome of protection against atherogenesis. However, in lipoprotein lipase deficiency, plasma triglyceride is extremely elevated and HDL cholesterol is very low, but the risk of CHD is not increased. In this condition, TGRL are not processed into particles that are amenable for endocytosis or deposition into the arterial wall. Thus, the inverse association of HDL cholesterol and risk of CHD may in reality reflect a positive association of TGRL and CHD, provided that TGRL can be processed into remnants. This hypothesis is also supported by two studies comparing the postprandial metabolism of TGRL in patients with CHD and in controls [31,32]. In both studies, markers of postprandial TGRL metabolism were at least as accurate as HDL cholesterol level in identifying cases and controls.

Recently, subclassification of HDL particles on the basis of apolipoprotein composition has become a research focus. HDL can be separated into particles containing both apo A-I and apo A-II (Lp A-I/A-II) and particles containing apo A-I but devoid of apo A-II (Lp A-I) [33]. A number of studies indicate that Lp A-I and Lp A-I/A-II are metabolically distinct and may perform different functions. The well-established male–female difference in plasma levels of HDL_2 was shown to result from increased concentrations of Lp A-I in the HDL_2 fraction of females [34]. Lp A-I represents a much larger proportion of the HDL_2 than of the HDL_3 fraction. Furthermore, the molar ratio of apo A-I to apo A-II in HDL_2—most likely reflecting different proportions of Lp A-I to Lp A-I/A-II—was positively correlated with lipoprotein lipase activity and HDL_2 levels, but inversely correlated with the magnitude of postalimentary lipemia [22]. Particles containing only apo A-I may be the physiologic acceptor of cellular cholesterol [30] and HDL_2 particles containing apo A-I and apo A-II represent a better substrate for hepatic lipase than HDL_2 particles containing only apo A-I [35]. Studies have shown lower Lp A-I levels in patients with angiographically verified CHD than in control subjects [36]. Transgenic mice overexpressing human apo A-I exhibit enhanced protection against diet-induced atherosclerosis when compared with mice overexpressing both human apo A-I and apo A-II [37]. Nevertheless, the clinical utility of measuring Lp A-I and Lp A-I/A-II awaits more comprehensive evaluation.

References

1. Gordon DJ, Probstfield JL, Garrison RJ, Neaton JD, Castelli WP, Knoke JD, Jacobs DR Jr, Bangdiwala S, Tyroler HA. High-density lipoprotein cholesterol and cardiovascular disease. Four prospective American studies. Circulation 1989;79:8–15.
2. Badimon JJ, Badimon L, Fuster V. Regression of atherosclerotic lesions by high density lipoprotein plasma fraction in the cholesterol-fed rabbit. J Clin Invest 1990;85:1234–1241.
3. Rubin EM, Krauss RM, Spangler EA, Verstuyft JG, Clift SM. Inhibition of early atherogenesis in transgenic mice by human apolipoprotein AI. Nature 1991;353:265–267.
4. Glomset JA. The plasma lecithin:cholesterol acyltransferase reaction. J Lipid Res 1968;9:1551–1567.
5. Stein Y, Glangeaud MC, Fainaru M, Stein O. The removal of cholesterol from aortic smooth muscle cells in culture and Landschutz ascites cells by fractions of human high-density apolipoprotein. Biochim Biohys Acta 1975;380:106–118.
6. Ho YK, Brown MS, Goldstein JL. Hydrolysis and excretion of cytoplasmic cholesteryl esters by macrophages: Stimulation by high density lipoprotein and other agents. J Lipid Res 1980;21:391–398.
7. Tauber JP, Cheng J, Gospodarowicz D. Effect of high and low density lipoproteins on proliferation of cultured bovine vascular endothelial cells. J Clin Invest 1980;66:696–708.
8. Burkey BF, Vlasic N, France D, Hughes TE, Drelich M, Ma X, Stemerman MB, Paterniti JR Jr. Elevated apolipoprotein A-I (apo A-I) pools in human apo A-I transgenic rats decrease aortic smooth muscle cell proliferation following balloon angioplasty [Abstract]. Abstracts submitted to the Council on Arteriosclerosis for the 65th Scientific Sessions of the American Heart Association, November 16–19, 1992;38. Unpublished abstracts book.
9. Parthasarathy S, Barnett J, Fong LG. High-density lipoprotein inhibits the oxidative modification of low-density lipoprotein. Biochim Biophys Acta 1990;1044:275–283.
10. Yui Y, Aoyama T, Morishita H, Takahashi M, Takatsu Y, Kawai C. Serum prostacyclin stabilizing factor is identical to apolipoprotein A-I (apo A-I). A novel function of apo A-I. J Clin Invest 1988;82:803–807.
11. Tsai AL, Hsu MJ, Patsch W, Wu KK. Regulation of PGI_2 activity by serum proteins: Serum albumin but not high density lipoprotein is the PGI_2 binding and stabilizing protein in human blood. Biochim Biophys Acta 1991;1115:131–140.
12. Breslow JL. Genetic basis of lipoprotein disorders. J Clin Invest 1989;84:373–380.

13. Schmitz G, Assmann G, Robenek H, Brennhausen B. Tangier disease: A disorder of intracellular membrane traffic. Proc Natl Acad Sci USA. 1985;82:6305–6309.
14. Patsch W, Schonfeld G, Gotto AM Jr, Patsch JR. Characterization of human high density lipoproteins by zonal ultracentrifugation. J Biol Chem 1980;255:3178–3185.
15. Stampfer MJ, Sacks FM, Salvini S, Willett WC, Hennekens CH. A prospective study of cholesterol, apolipoproteins, and the risk of myocardial infarction. N Engl J Med 1991;325:373–381.
16. Miller NE, Hammett F, Saltissi S, Rao S, van Zeller H, Coltart J, Lewis B. Relation of angiographically defined coronary artery disease to plasma lipoprotein subfractions and apolipoproteins. Br Med J 1981;282:1741–1744.
17. Breier C, Patsch JR, Muhlberger V, Drexel H, Knapp E, Braunsteiner H. Risk factors for coronary artery disease: A study comparing hypercholesterolaemia and hypertriglyceridaemia in angiographically characterized patients. Eur J Clin Invest 1989;19:419–423.
18. Nichols AV. Human serum lipoproteins and their interrelationships. Adv Biol Med Phys 1967;11:109–158.
19. Glueck CJ, Gartside P, Fallat RW, Sielski J, Steiner PM. Longevity syndromes: Familial hypobeta and familial hyperalpha lipoproteinemia. J Lab Clin Med 1976;88:941–957.
20. Patsch W, Kuisk I, Glueck C, Schonfeld G. Lipoproteins in familial hyperalphalipoproteinemia. Arteriosclerosis 1981;1:156–161.
21. Patsch JR, Gotto AM Jr, Olivecrona T, Eisenberg S. Formation of high density lipoprotein$_2$-like particles during lipolysis of very low density lipoproteins in vitro. Proc Natl Acad Sci USA. 1978;75:4519–4523.
22. Patsch JR, Prasad S, Gotto AM Jr, Patsch W. High density lipoprotein$_2$. Relationship of the plasma levels of this lipoprotein species to its composition, to the magnitude of postprandial lipemia, and to the activities of lipoprotein lipase and hepatic lipase. J Clin Invest 1987;80:341–347.
23. Patsch JR, Prasad S, Gotto AM Jr, Bengtsson-Olivecrona G. Postprandial lipemia. A key for the conversion of high density lipoprotein$_2$ into high density lipoprotein$_3$ by hepatic lipase. J Clin Invest 1984;74:2017–2023.
24. Behr SR, Patsch JR, Forte T, Bensadoun A. Plasma lipoprotein changes resulting from immunologically blocked lipolysis. J Lipid Res 1981;22:443–451.
25. Ito Y, Azrolan N, O'Connell A, Walsh A, Breslow JL. Hypertriglyceridemia as a result of human apo CIII gene expression in transgenic mice. Science 1990;249:790–793.
26. Whitlock ME, Swenson TL, Ramakrishnan R, Leonard MT, Marcel YL, Milne RW, Tall AR. Monoclonal antibody inhibition of cholesteryl ester transfer protein activity in the rabbit. Effects on lipoprotein composition and high density lipoprotein cholesteryl ester metabolism. J Clin Invest 1989;84:129–137.
27. Agellon LB, Walsh A, Hayek T, Moulin P, Jiang XC, Shelanski SA, Breslow JL, Tall AR. Reduced high density lipoprotein cholesterol in human cholesteryl ester transfer protein transgenic mice. J Biol Chem 1991;266:10796–10801.
28. Inazu A, Brown ML, Hesler CB, Agellon LB, Koizumi J, Takata K, Maruhama Y, Mabuchi H, Tall AR. Increased high-density lipoprotein levels caused by a common cholesteryl-ester transfer protein gene mutation. N Engl J Med 1990;323:1234–1238.
29. Stein OJ, Vanderhoek J, Stein Y. Cholesterol content and sterol synthesis in human skin fibroblasts and rat aortic smooth muscle cells exposed to lipoprotein-depleted serum and

high density apolipoprotein/phospholipid mixtures. Biochim Biophys Acta 1976;431:347–358.

30. Castro GR, Fielding CJ. Early incorporation of cell-derived cholesterol into pre-beta-migrating high-density lipoprotein. Biochemistry 1988;27:25–29.

31. Groot PH, van Stiphout WA, Krauss XH, Jansen H, van Tol A, van Ramshorst E, Chin-On S, Hofman A, Cresswell SR, Havekes L. Postprandial lipoprotein metabolism in normolipidemic men with and without coronary artery disease. Arterioscler Thromb 1991;11:653–662.

32. Patsch JR, Miesenböck G, Hopferwieser T, Mühlberger V, Knapp E, Dunn JK, Gotto AM Jr, Patsch W. Relation of triglyceride metabolism and coronary artery disease. Arterioscler Thromb 1992;12:1336-1345.

33. Cheung MC, Albers JJ. Characterization of lipoprotein particles isolated by immunoaffinity chromatography. Particles containing A-I and A-II and particles containing A-I but no A-II. J Biol Chem 1984;259:12201–12209.

34. Ohta T, Hattori S, Nishiyama S, Matsuda I. Studies on the lipid and apolipoprotein compositions of two species of apoA-I–containing lipoproteins in normolipidemic males and females. J Lipid Res 1988;29:721–728.

35. Mowri HO, Patsch W, Smith LC, Gotto AM Jr, Patsch JR. Different reactivities of high density lipoprotein₂ subfractions with hepatic lipase. J Lipid Res 1992;33:1269–1279.

36. Luc G, Parra HJ, Zylberberg G, Fruchart JC. Plasma concentrations of apolipoprotein A-I containing particles in normolipidaemic young men. Eur J Clin Invest 1991;21:118–122.

37. Schultz JR, Verstuyft JG, Gong EL, Nichols AV, Rubin EM. ApoAI and apoAI + apoAII transgenic mice: A comparison of atherosclerotic susceptibility [Abstract]. Abstracts submitted to the Council on Arteriosclerosis for the 65th Scientific Sessions of the American Heart Association, November 16–19, 1992;38. Unpublished abstracts book.

HDL AS A RISK FACTOR FOR CORONARY HEART DISEASE: AN UPDATE ON THE HELSINKI HEART STUDY

V. MANNINEN AND M. MÄNTTÄRI

INTRODUCTION

Since the original observations (1,2) four decades ago that low level of serum high density lipoprotein cholesterol (HDL cholesterol) has an adverse effect on coronary heart disease (CHD) occurence, longitudinal and cross-sectional studies have provided substantial confirmation (3,4). In the Helsinki Heart Study (HHS) we employed the placebo grouplacebo group to explore HDL cholesterol/CHD relationships (5,6). This short report derives from subgroup analyses of the significance of low HDL cholesterol.

SUBJECTS AND METHODS

The initial screening and selection process (7) and the principal outcome of the HHS (8,9) have been reported earlier in detail. The participants were selected from 23 531 men aged 40-55 years. For inclusion, they needed a non-HDL cholesterol (total cholesterol - HDL cholesterol) of $\geq$ 5.2 mmol/l at two successive measurements. A history or sign of heart disease or any major illness were exclusion criteria. The men were allocated randomly to either gemfibrozil therapy (n = 2046) or placebo (n = 2035), and were monitored for 5 years.

HDL was measured from the supernatant by an enzymatic method, following precipitation of very low density (VLDL) and low density lipoprotein (LDL) cholesterol with dextran sulphate-magnesium chloride. Triglycerides (TG) were measured as glycerol after enzymatic hydrolysis with lipase/esterase. LDL cholesterol was calculated from the formula: LDL cholesterol = total cholesterol - HDL cholesterol - TG/2.2.

That the data on the HDL cholesterol/CHD relationships are applicable to middle-aged caucasian males in general is demonstrated by the almost identical distributions of

339

A. L. Catapano et al. (eds.), Drugs Affecting Lipid Metabolism, 339–342.
© 1993 Kluwer Academic Publishers and Fondazione Giovanni Lorenzini.

baseline HDL in the study participants (n = 4081) and the screened men
(n = 18 966). Compared to the screened individuals, the distribution of total
cholesterol in the study participants was shifted to the right, which classified them as
hypercholesterolemic. After eliminating the seasonal variation of HDL cholesterol by
calculating annual mean values, HDL cholesterol remained highly stable throughout the
entire 5-year follow-up period in the placebo group.

The HDL cholesterol tertile limits (baseline values) were < 1.08, 1.08-1.32, and >
1.32 mmol/l. The LDL cholesterol tertiles were < 4.5, 4.5-5.2, and > 5.2 mmol/l.
The lipid values were dichotomized in some analyses, the cut-off points being: LDL
cholesterol 5.0 mmol/l, TG 2.3 mmol/l, HDL cholesterol 1.08 mmom/l, and
LDL/HDL cholesterol ratio 5. Smokers were categorized as non-smokers or current
smokers, and age as above or below the median of 47 years. The cut-off value for
dichotomizing blood pressure was 130/90. Cox proportional hazard
models (10) were also used to study the risk patterns, with age, smoking and systolic
blood pressure as covariates.

RESULTS

Both total and LDL cholesterol turned out to be unsatisfactory indicators of CHD risk
in this selected dyslipidemic population (data not presented), while low HDL
cholesterol and high TG were much more satisfactory predictors. In fact in both these
subgroups the relative CHD risk grew significantly, by about 80% (Table 1).

TABLE 1
Relative risk of CHD in relation to baseline HDL cholesterol and TG

		Risk
HDL cholesterol		
	≥ 1.08 mmol/l	1
	n = 1384	
	< 1.08 mmol/l	1.73
	n = 651	(1.12-2.66)
TG		
	≤ 2.3 mmol/l	1
	n = 1529	
	> 2.3 mmol/l	1.81
	n = 506	(1.16-2.81)

Cox regression model estimates, with age, smoking and systolic bloodpressure as
covariates. The risk was set at unity for individuals with high HDL cholesterol and low
TG. 95% confidence intervals in parentheses.

Analysis of the HDL/LDL cholesterol interrelationship revealed the CHD risk to be low in the highest HDL tertile, irrespective of the LDL cholesterol level. Increased LDL cholesterol had its clearest impact in the lowest tertile of HDL cholesterol. When analysed with respect to age, smoking and blood pressure, relationships between CHD incidence and HDL and LDL cholesterol demonstrated much more obvious gradients.

TABLE 2
Relative risk of CHD in relation to baseline HDL cholesterol and TG combined and to LDL/HDL ratio and TG combined

	Risk
HDL cholesterol ≥ 1.08 mmol/l and TG ≤ 2.3 mmol/l n = 1166	1
HDL cholesterol < 1.08 mmol/l and TG > 2.3 mmol/l n = 218	2.43 (1.43-4.12)
LDL/HDL ratio ≤ 5.0 and TG ≤ 2.3 mmol/l n = 1262	1
LDL/HDL ratio > 5.0 and TG > 2.3 mmol/l n = 138	3.82 (2.20-6.63)

The lipid combinations with lowest CDH risk were set at 1. Cox regression models with age, smoking and blood pressure as covariates. 95% confidence intervals in parentheses.

A special subgroup with exceptional risk to emerge from the analysis of the joint effects of lipid levels consisted of men with baseline LDL/HDL cholesterol ratio above 5 and TG above 2.3 mmol/l (Table 2).

DISCUSSION

The men of the Helsinki Heart Study were selected from the upper end of the serum total cholesterol distribution, with only a limited number of individuals at the lower end of the distribution curve. For this reason the HHS study population was not well suited for a risk factor analysis over the entire distribution range of total cholesterol and LDL cholesterol. However, it was suitable for analysing the importance of low

HDL cholesterol. The negative influence of low HDL cholesterol is clearly revealed in both the univariate and multivariate analyses. In the special subgroup of men with LDL/HDL cholesterol ratio above 5 and TG above 2.3 mmol/l, gemfibrozil therapy led to a very considerable (75%) reduction in CHD incidence (11). On this basis, the present criteria for lipid-lowering therapy in lipid disorders (12) fail to take sufficient account of the role of low HDL cholesterol. 'Low HDL cholesterol' is arbitrarily set at below 35 mg/dl (0.91 mmol/l), while in fact much higher values app· · r associated with elevated CHD risk. In our population, the lowest tertile was set below 1.08 mmol/l (42 mg/dl) and revealed a considerably increased risk as compared to the higher tertiles (Table 1). The impact of this was even more obvious when it was jointly analysed with LDL and TG (Table 2). Only in the two lowest tertiles of HDL cholesterol distribution did the adverse influence of increased LDL cholesterol expose itself. LDL cholesterol played no role in CHD incidence among men of the highest HDL cholesterol tertile. On this basis it seems that LDL/HDL ratio appears to be the most valid cholesterol criterion for assessing CHD risk. More recent analysis of the HHS data on the joint effects of various lipid fractions (11) suggests that TG should be incorporated into such risk assessments.

REFERENCES

1   Barr DP, Russ EM, Eder HA. Am J Med 1951; 11: 480-485.
2   Nikkilä E. Scand J Clin Lab Invest 1953; 5: suppl 8.
3   Miller GJ, Miller NE. Lancet 1975; 1: 16-19.
4   Abbott RD, Wilson PWF, Kannel WB, Castelli WP. Atherosclerosis 1988; 8: 207-211.
5   Manninen V, Huttunen JK, Tenkanen L, Heinonen OP, et al. In: Miller NE, ed. High Density Lipoproteins and Atherosclerosis II. Amsterdam: Elsevier, 1989; 35-42.
6   Frick MH, Manninen V, Huttunen JK, Heinonen OP, et al. Drugs 1990; 40: Suppl. 1: 7-12.
7   Mänttäri M, Elo O, Frick MH, Haapa K, et. al. Eur Heart J 1987; 8: Suppl. 1: 1-29.
8   Frick MH, Elo O, Haapa K, Heinonen OP, et al. N Engl J Med 1987; 317: 1237-1245.
9   Manninen V, Elo O, Frick MH, Haapa K, et al. JAMA 1988; 260: 641-651.
10 Cox DR, Oakes D. In: Monographs on Statistics and Applied Propability. London: Chapman & Hall Ltd, 1984.
11 Manninen V, Tenkanen L, Koskinen P, Huttunen JK, et al. Circulation 1992; 85: 37-45.
12 National Cholesterol Education Program. National Heart, Lung, and Blood Institute publication No (NIH) 1988; 88-2925.

RELATIONSHIP OF HDL CHOLESTEROL TO INCIDENCE OF ATHEROSCLEROTIC CORONARY HEART DISEASE: THE PROCAM EXPERIENCE

Gerd Assmann[1,2], Arnold von Eckardstein , Helmut Schulte

ABSTRACT

The incidence of atherosclerotic coronary heart disease (CHD) was assessed in 4559 male partecipants of the Prospective Cardiovascular Munster (PROCAM) study, aged 40 to 64 years, over a 6 year follow-up period. In this time, 186 study partecipants developed atherosclerotic CHD (134 definite nonfatal myocardial infarctions and 52 definite atherosclerotic CHD deaths including 21 sudden cardiac deaths and 31 fatal myocardial infarctions). Univariate analysis revealed a significant association between the incidence of atherosclerotic CHD, and high density lipoprotein (HDL) cholesterol (p<0.001), which remained after adjustment for other risk factors.

INTRODUCTION

Over the past three decades, great progress has been made in identifying and correcting risk factors for cardiovascular disease (CVD), such as smoking, high blood pressure, and elevated total and low-density-lipoprotein (LDL) cholesterol. In several countries, this has led to a significant reduction in the incidence of CVD.

Despite this encouraging result, CVD is still the leading cause of death in many Western nations. A further decline in cardiovascular morbidity and mortality could be achieved by a wider, multiple-risk-factor approach, with attention paid to lipid risk factors other than hypercholesterolemia. Low high-density-lipoprotein (HDL) cholesterol levels, often associated with elevated plasma triglycerides, may play a significant role in cardiovascular risk.

At a NIH Consensus Conference on HDL and triglycerides held in Washington DC last february [l] the panel concluded that levels of HDL cholesterol below 35 mg/dl constitute a high risk for developing coronary heart disease. The group noted the importance of measuring HDL whenever cholesterol is measured to assess CHD risk.

To further investigate the relation between HDL cholesterol, and the risk of CHD some results of the Prospective Cardiovascular Munster (PROCAM) study are demonstrated.

METHODS

Description of the PROCAM study: In the PROCAM study, people at work (employees of 52 companies and authorities) were examined for cardiovascular risk factors and then kept under observation to record mortality, as well as cardiovascular events including

A. L. Catapano et al. (eds.), Drugs Affecting Lipid Metabolism, 343–355.

myocardial infarction and stroke. The examination at study entry included case history using standardized questionnaires, measurement of blood pressure and anthropometric data, a resting electrocardiogram and collection of a blood sample after a 12-hour fast for the determination of >20 laboratory parameters. The examination was carried out during paid working hours. Participation was voluntary (between 40 and 80% took part, average 60%), and free of charge both to the volunteers and to their employers (apart from loss of work). All findings were reported to the participant's general practitioner, and the volunteer was told whether the results of the examination were normal, or whether a check-up by the general practitioner might be necessary. The investigators neither carried out nor arranged for any intervention.

Total cholesterol, triglycerides and HDL cholesterol were measured using enzymatic assays and (for HDL cholesterol) a precipitation method from Boehringer Mannheim, FRG on a Hitachi 737 autoanalyzer [2]. Low density lipoprotein (LDL) cholesterol was calculated by the Friedewald formula, if triglycerides were <400 mg/dl [3]. Further methods used for the examinations and the laboratory tests are described in detail elsewhere [4].

Follow-up: Questionnaires were sent to the participants every 2 years to determine the occurence of myocardial infarction, stroke or death. At the initial examination, participants were told that they would obtain a questionnaire every 2 years. The response rate to these questionnaires was 96% after 2 reminders each by mail and phone if necessary. The death certificate was reviewed if death occurred in a study participant. For all mortality and morbidity data obtained from the questionnaire, we requested hospital records and records from the attending physician, as well as an eyewitness account of deaths, so that a Critical Event Committee (Prof. Dr. K. Kochsiek, Wurzburg, Prof. Dr. B.E. Strauer, Dusseldorf, Prof. Dr. U. Gleichmann, Bad Oeynhausen, Priv.-Doz. Dr. Uebis, Aachen) could verify the diagnosis or cause of death. The initial examination was repeated after 6 to 7 years.

For the following analyses 2 endpoints were considered: definite nonfatal myocardial infarction and definite atherosclerotic CHD death including sudden cardiac death and fatal myocardial infarction. The definition of the endpoints are described in detail elsewhere [5].

Statistics: An explorative analysis was performed using the statistical package for the social sciences (SPSS-X) [6] and the statistical analysis system (SAS) [7]. Comparisons between groups were done with the Mann-Whitney U-test for continuous variables and with the chi-square test for discrete variables. The relationship between a variable and risk of atherosclerotic CHD was described by dividing the patient series into tertiles of the studied variable and then calculating the incidence rate for each tertile. As is usual in prospective studies of CHD the simultaneous contributions of several factors to the risk of major ischemic heart disease were analyzed using a multiple logistic model.

RESULTS

Distribution of HDL cholesterol: The study began in 1979 and the recruitment phase was completed at the end of 1985. Full data records are held on a total of 19,698 participants in the PROCAM study aged range 16 to 65 years. 13,737 men in the study had an average age of 41.4 ± 11.2 years and the 5,961 women were 36.6 ± 12.5 years (p<0.001).

Unlike all the other risk factors investigated, HDL cholesterol and the prevalence of decreased HDL cholesterol levels are almost independent of age (table 1, fig. 1) in adults. On average, HDL cholesterol levels are 12 mg/dl higher in men than in women. Factors influencing plasma HDL cholesterol are hypertriglyceridemia, cigarette smoking, overweight, physical inactivity, diabetes mellitus, and anabolic hormones, all of which have a lowering effect. By contrast, moderate alcohol consumption and oral contraceptives have a raising effect [8].

Table 1 : Distribution parameters of HDL cholesterol according to age

MALES

age	n	mean	SD	median	5th percentile	95th percentile
15-24	1649	45.4	10.7	44	30	64
25-34	4113	45.6	11.5	44	29	65
35-44	4861	45.8	12.6	44	29	67
45-54	4741	46.1	11.9	45	29	68
55-64	2073	46.4	12.6	45	29	68

FEMALES

age	n	mean	SD	median	5th percentile	95th percentile
15-24	1947	56.9	14.3	56	36	82
25-34	2170	58.1	14.8	57	36	84
35-44	1662	57.4	14.6	56	35	83
45-54	1614	58.0	14.9	57	36	84
55-64	672	58.4	15.0	57	36	85

CHD incidence: An adequate incidence of atherosclerotic CHD in the PROCAM study occurred only in men ≥40 years and the analysis described below was confined to 4,559 male participants aged between 40 and 65 years, without a prior history of myocardial infarction or stroke, with a follow-up period of 6 years [5]. In this time, 134 definite nonfatal myocardial infarctions and 52 definite atherosclerotic CHD deaths were recorded including 21 sudden cardiac deaths and 31 fatal myocardial infarctions (group CHD+), 10 suspect CHD deaths occurred and 119 men died from causes other than CHD (11 from other diseases of the circulatory system, 54 from malignant neoplasms, 24 from other diseases and 30 from accidents and violence). The number of non-fatal strokes was 23 while 4,221 subjects survived the 6 years after initial examination without definite nonfatal myocardial infarction or stroke (CHD-), including 38 with suspect nonfatal myocardial infarction. The age-standardized mean values for risk factors within the groups CHD+ and CHD- are given in table 2.

The 4,221 subjects in the CHD- group had an age-standardized mean HDL cholesterol level of 45.2 ± 11.8 mg/dl, whereas in the CHD+ group the mean HDL cholesterol level was significantly (p<0.001) lower 39.5 ± 10.6 mg/dl. In the CHD+ group, 45.2 % of participants had HDL cholesterol levels <35 mg/dl; in the CHD- group only 16.1 % of subjects had levels below this limit. The numbers of observed definite events per tertile of the HDL cholesterol distribution were 77, 27 and 26 per 1000 subjects within 6 years, respectively. Individuals with HDL cholesterol levels <35 mg/dl had a nearly 4-fold increased CHD risk within 6 years compared to men with HDL cholesterol levels ≥35 mg/dl, while the difference between men with HDL cholesterol concentrations of 35-55 mg/dl and >55 mg/dl was "only" 50 % (fig. 2). A breakdown of the CHD incidence-

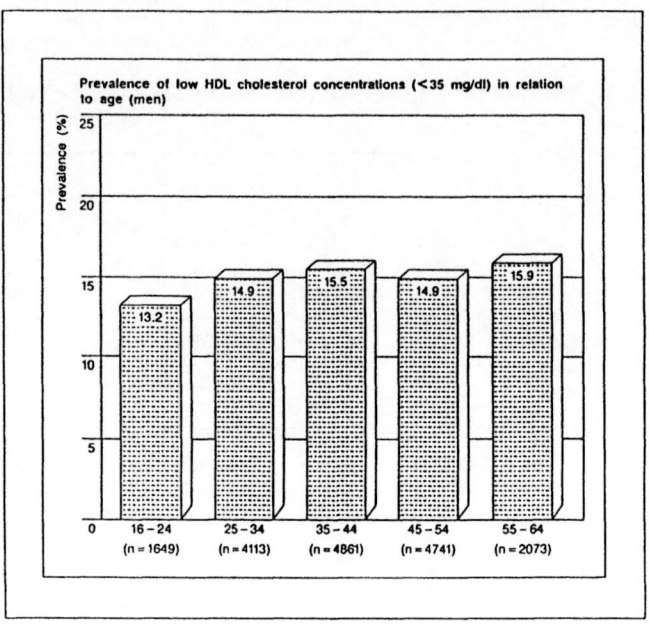

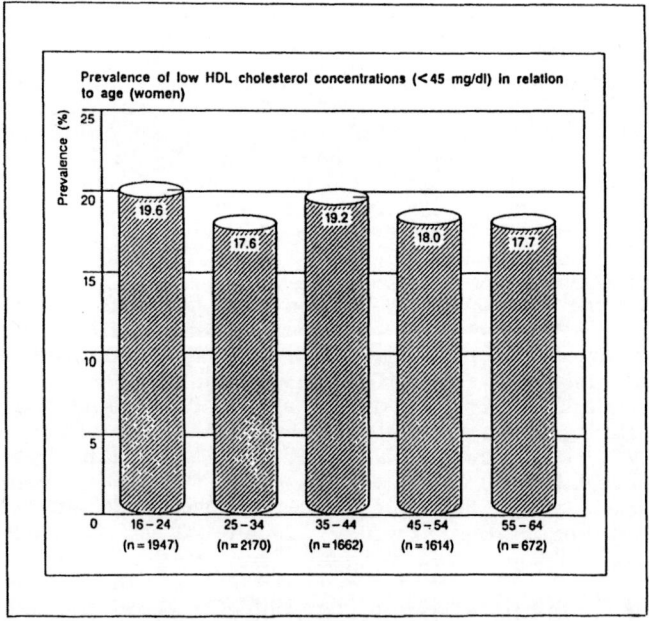

Figure 1.   Prevalence of low HDL cholesterol concentrations in relation to age
HDL = high density lipoprotein.

rates by the concentrations of HDL cholesterol and total cholesterol (fig. 3) showed a steep increase with increasing total cholesterol within each subgroup of HDL cholesterol. Low HDL cholesterol levels (<35 mg/dl) led to a 5-fold increased risk of CHD compared to normal values, if cholesterol levels ranged between 200 and 300 mg/dl, while the increase was 2.5-fold, if cholesterol concentration was <200 mg/dl or >300 mg/dl.

The breakdown of CHD risk by HDL cholesterol and LDL cholesterol (fig. 4) showed a large degree of correspondence to that of HDL cholesterol and total cholesterol. The CHD rate increased with increasing LDL cholesterol and decreasing HDL cholesterol. HDL cholesterol and LDL cholesterol are independent risk factors for the incidence of CHD.

Hypertriglyceridemia (≥200 mg/dl) was associated with markedly higher incidence rates of definite events in subgroups with lower HDL cholesterol levels (fig. 5).

In a logistic function analysis HDL cholesterol showed a significant association with CHD incidence (p<0.001), which remained after adjustment for other risk factors.

Table 2: Mean value of age-standardized factors for male partecipants in the PROCAM Study aged 40 to 65 years with (CHD+) and without (CHD-) development of atherosclerotic CHD within 6 years

Variable	CHD- (n=4,221)		CHD+ (n=186)		p
Cholesterol (mg/dl)	222.9	(41.0)	251.8	(47.3)	<0.001
HDL cholesterol (mg/dl)	45.2	(11.8)	39.5	(10.6)	<0.001
LDL cholesterol (mg/dl) *	147.1	(35.9)	176.2	(39.5)	<0.001
HDL cholest/LDL cholest ratio *	3.44	(1.20)	4.73	(1.51)	<0.001
Triglycerides (mg/dl) **	134.5		163.0		<0.001
Systolic blood pressure (mm Hg)	132.7	(18.9)	139.4	(21.2)	<0.001
Diastolic blood pressure (mm Hg)	86.3	(11.1)	89.5	(12.7)	<0.01
Body Mass Index (kg/m^2)	26.3	(3.0)	26.7	(2.9)	<0.05
Fasting blood glucose (mg/dl)	102.0	(21.1)	108.2	(33.7)	<0.02
Uric acid (mg/dl)	5.7	(1.2)	5.8	(1.3)	n.s.

* n=4,086 in CHD-, n=177 in CHD+ subjects
** geometric mean
Values are mean and standard deviation (in brackets) unless otherwise indicated.

DISCUSSION

The level of HDL cholesterol in plasma has been shown to be inversely related to the incidence of CHD in several prospective epidemiological studies [9-17]. In accordance with our f ndings, in 6 of these studies [9-14] this inverse association was statistically significant and remained so after adjustment for other risk factors.

The data of the Helsinki Heart Study (HHS) [18] showed that in both groups, placebo and subjects treated with gemfibrocil, within each low density lipoprotein (LDL) cholesterol tertile the risk of coronary heart disease increased with decreasing concentration of HDL [19]. This risk patterns remained essentially similar after adjustment for age, smoking and systolic blood pressure.

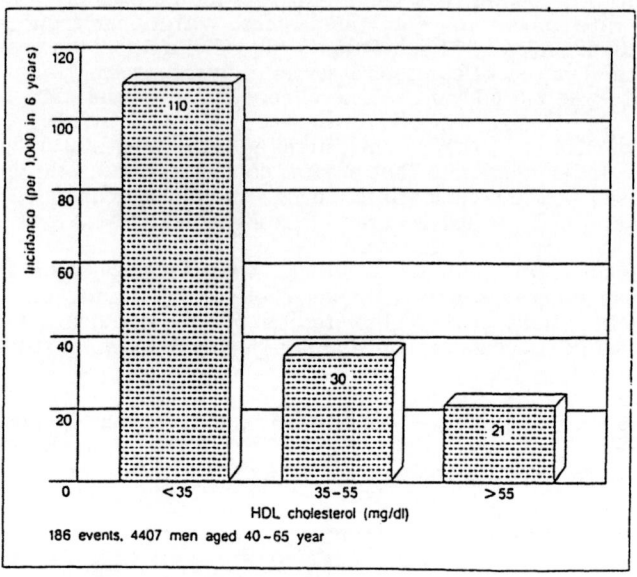

**Figure 2.   Incidence of coronary heart disease (CHD) per 1000 subjects over a 6-
year period according to HDL cholesterol levels.**
CHD = coronary artery disease;
HDL = high density lipoprotein.

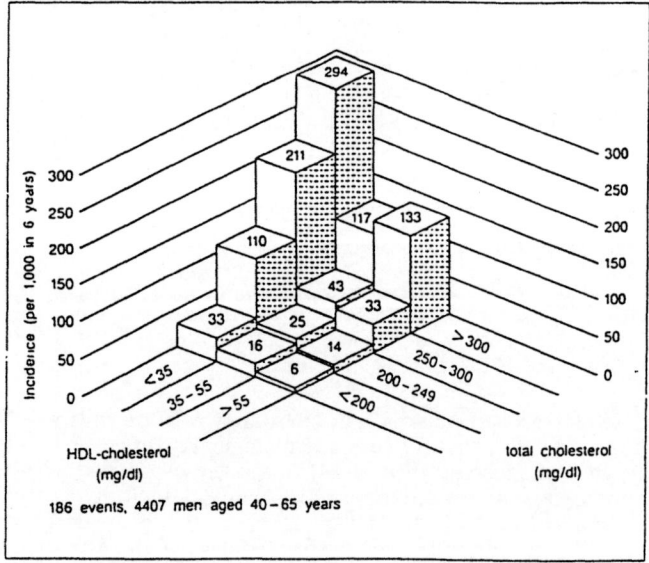

**Figure 3.   Incidence of coronary heart disease (CHD) per 1000 subjects over a 6-
year period according to total cholesterol and HDL cholesterol levels.**
CHD = coronary artery disease;
HDL = high density lipoprotein.

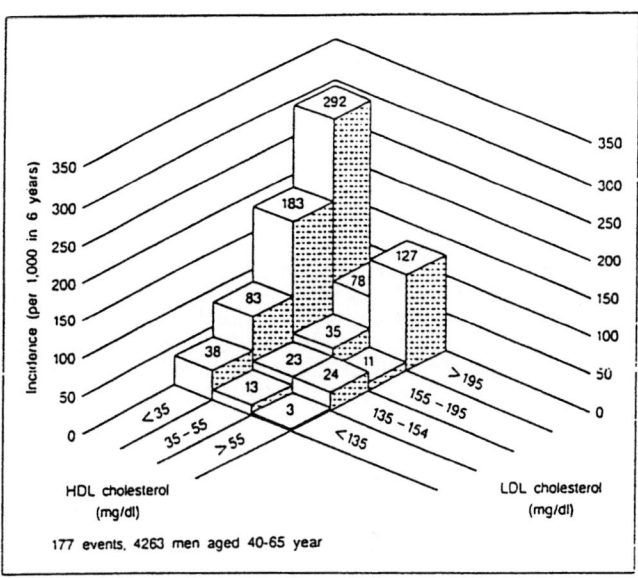

Figure 4. **Incidence of coronary heart disease (CHD) per 1000 subjects over a 6-year period according to HDL cholesterol levels.**
CHD = coronary artery disease;
LDL = low density lipoprotein;
HDL = high density lipoprotein.

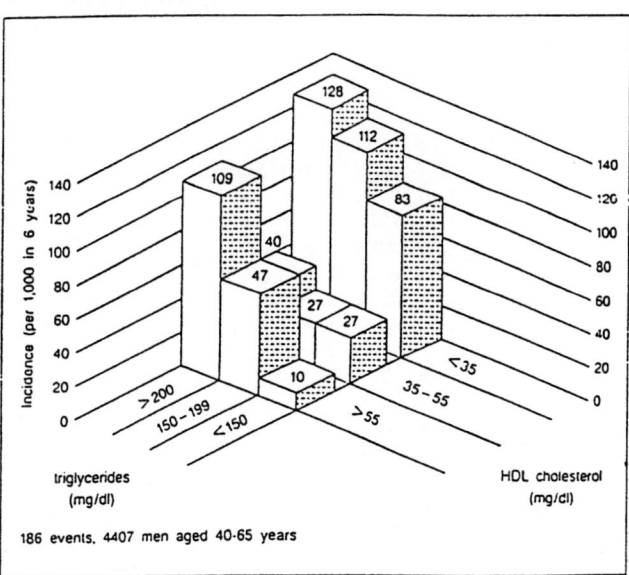

Figure 5. **Incidence of coronary heart disease (CHD) per 1000 subjects over a 6-year period according to triglycerides and HDL cholesterol levels.**
CHD = coronary artery disease;
HDL = high density lipoprotein.

Although, the HHS did not test the specific hypothesis that raising low HDL cholesterol will reduce CHD risk, a post hoc analysis of the data strongly suggest that the risk reduction observed in subjects treated with gemfibrozil was a result of simultaneous changes in the amount of LDL cholesterol and HDL cholesterol [20]. "When the relationship between the serum lipids changes during treatment and the CHD incidence was studied using Cox proportional hazard models, the increase in the concentration of serum HDL cholesterol (p<0.01) and the fall in that of LDL cholesterol (p<0.05) were both associated with reduced risk, whereas the changes in the amounts of total cholesterol and triglycerides in the serum were not" [21]. The patient group with low HDL cholesterol was most likely to benefit from gemfibrocil treatment.

Family and twin studies suggested partial heredity of low HDL cholesterol levels and have put the influence of genes at 35 to 50%. Frequently, familial HDL cholesterol-deficiency was paralleled with a family history of premature coronary heart disease [22-25]. The patho-physiological relationship between decreased serum concentrations of HDL cholesterol and the development of coronary heart disease has still remained obscure. The reverse cholesterol transport model [26] is most widely used to explain the role of HDL in lipid metabolism and in atherogenesis. In this model, HDL mediates the flux of excess cholesterol from peripheral cells to the liver. It was therefore generally hypothesized that genetic defects which interfere with the regular structure of HDL, or with processes important for the generation or removal of HDL would be disadvantageous for their carriers' health.

HDL precursors, so-called nascent HDL or HDL discs, are generated through lipolysis of chylomicrons and VLDL as well as by direct secretion of the liver (reviewed in [27,28]). Different subpopulations of HDL that can be differentiated either upon their mobility in agarose gel electrophoresis or isotachophoresis or upon their apolipoprotein composition (reviewed in [29]) were shown to take up excess cellular cholesterol by a stepwise process: It is generally accepted now that unesterified cholesterol diffuses from the cell membrane to HDL through mostly unspecific lipid-lipid interactions and that HDL apolipoproteins are not necessary for this step (reviewed in [30-32]). However, in adipocytes, macrophages and fibroblasts, the mobilization of intracellular cholesterol pools and their translocation to the cell membrane is much facilitated after the binding of some HDL apoliproteins to a specific recognition site on the cell surface (reviewed in [30-32]). The binding of HDL putatively releases diacylglycerol and thereby activates protein kinase C which in turn starts the translocation of intracellular cholesterol to the membrane (reviewed in [30-32]). The nature of the cellular HDL binding site is still a matter of debate since ligand blotting studies identified putative HDL receptors of various molecular masses ranging from 70 to 120 kDa [30-32]. Once in plasma, unesterified cholesterol from cell membranes is taken up by nascent, solely apo A-I containing HDL particles with preβ mobility on agarose gel electrophoresis. These small, discoidal, and lipid-poor particles have been termed preβ–HDL [33]. In these particles, a proportion of cell derived cholesterol is esterified by the plasma enzyme lecithin: cholesterolacyltransferase (LCAT), the remainder is transferred unesterified to LDL, which serves as a transitory storage pool before it is transferred to α-HDL for esterification [34]. α-HDL also serve as acceptors of remnants resulting from lipoprotein lipase (LPL) mediated hydrolysis of chylomicrons and VLDL [27,28]. From α-HDL, CE can be removed by at least four mechanisms to be directed to the liver where cholesterol is utilized for bile acid synthesis (reviewed in [28-30]): (i) A subpopulation of HDL acquires apo E and can be recognized by hepatic apoE receptors. (ii) HDL without apo E can also be endocytosed by hepatocytes. (iii) Hepatic triglyceride lipase (HTGL) mediates the uptake of cholesterol esters into liver cells. (iv) Cholesterol ester transfer protein (CETP) catalyzes the net transfer of HDL cholesterol esters to LDL, IDL and VLDL which are taken up via hepatic apo B,E receptors.

Genetic variations causing structural defects of HDL apolipoproteins (A-I, A-II, A-IV, and C-III) or of lipid transfer enzymes (LCAT, CETP) should importantly affect plasma concentration of HDL cholesterol and the effectiveness of reverse cholesterol transport

[35-38]. Actually, to date, a large variety of molecular defects has been established in the genes of apoA-I and LCAT that are associated with low HDL cholesterol (reviewed in [35-37]). Several defects are the molecular basis of HDL-deficiency syndromes including LCAT deficiency, fish-eye disease and apo A-I deficiency [35-37,39,40]. In other disorders, e.g. in Tangier disease, alterations in the plasma lipid metabolism possibly are secondary to disturbances in the intracellular lipid metabolism [41]. However these forms of familial HDL deficiency are very rare and cannot explain the frequent association in the population of low HDL cholesterol and coronary risk [35,36]. Moreover and surprisingly, in most cases both homozygous HDL-deficient patients and their heterozygous relatives, who exhibit HDL cholesterol levels otherwise found in CHD-patients, were not at increased risk of premature CHD. In view of nearly absent HDL cholesterol in these conditions, the discrepancy with the epidemiological findings addresses the question of the proposed causative role of HDL in preventing premature atherosclerosis. Possibly the epidemiologic data need other interpretations than provided by the reverse cholesterol transport model, and low HDL cholesterol only indicates other atherogenic disturbances, e.g. in the metabolism of triglyceride rich particles.

Metabolism of HDL and triglyceride-rich lipoproteins are closely linked, since lipolysis of chylomicrons and VLDL produces surface remnants which are one precursor pool of HDL [28,29]. Furthermore, cholesteryl ester transfer protein (CETP) catalyses the exchange of triglycerides and cholesteryl esters between HDL and triglyceride-rich lipoproteins [29,42]. Hence, the presence of high amounts of triglyceride-rich lipoproteins depletes HDL from cholesteryl esters and, since triglycerides in HDL are easily hydrolysed by hepatic lipase, leads to the reduction of larger HDL_2 and the predominance of HDL_3 [43]. On the other hand, triglyceride-rich lipoproteins become more atherogenic by the accumulation of cholesteryl esters. In this concept, the effectivity of postprandial lipid metabolism becomes crucial and actually several investigators demonstrated that the extent of postprandial hypertriglyceridemia is strongly correlated with the concentration of HDL_2 cholesterol in plasma [44,45]. Furthermore, case-control studies revealed that postprandial clearance of triglycerides is significantly retarded in CHD-patients as compared to healthy controls [46]. Another indication for the importance of postprandial lipid clearance comes from the regression study CLAS, in which the relative concentrations of apo C-III in HDL and in complete plasma was the most powerful predictor for the progression of angiographically assessed CHD. Since total apo C-III remained constant, any increase of apo C-III in HDL indicates the reduction of other lipoproteins carrying apo C-III, namely chylomicrons, VLDL and remnants [47].

In clinical and epidemiological studies triglyceride levels are correlated with the activity or concentration in plasma of factors regulating coagulation and fibrinolysis, e.g. fibrinogen, factor VII, plasminogen or plasminogen activator inhibitor type 1 (PAI-l). Hence, hypertriglyceridemia and low HDL cholesterol may indicate not only atherogenic disturbances but also a thrombophilic situation [48].

The genetic and non-genetic determinants of postprandial lipid catabolism are not fully understood. One obvious candidate is lipoprotein lipase. Its gene is highly polymorphic and many of its alleles code for dysfunctional enzymes. Actually, lipoprotein lipase activity in post-heparin plasma is positively correlated with HDL_2 cholesterol [49] and members of families with familial combined hyperlipidemia exhibit relatively low lipoprotein lipase activity [50]. However, to date it has not consistently been shown that heterozygosity for defined molecular defects in lipoprotein lipase is associated with lower HDL cholesterol and higher triglyceride or even increased risk for myocardial infarction [51]. Other candidate factors regulating postprandial triglyceride clearance are the LDL-receptor and the apo E receptor as well as their ligands apolipoproteins B, C-II, C-III, and E. Actually both familial hypercholesterolemia and type III hyperlipidemia are frequently associated with low HDL cholesterol levels. Another factor influencing the clearance of triglycerides is insulin, which regulates lipoprotein lipase activity and the production of VLDL, either directly or via free fatty acids. Thus, insulin resistance and hyperinsulinemia in type II diabetes mellitus are correlated positively with VLDL triglycerides and negatively with HDL cholesterol [52,53]. Vice versa hyperinsulinemia is frequently found in patients with coronary risk factors like hypercholesterolemia, hypoalphalipoproteinemia, hypertriglyceridemia, abdominal obesity and arterial hypertension. The clustering of this risk factors has been summarized as "syndrome X", "metabolic syndrom" or "dyslipidemic hypertension". It is hence possible that the low HDL/hypertriglyceridemia syndrome is part of a general metabolic disorder that is caused by dysregulated insulin action [54,55].

ACKNOWLEDGMENT

This work is supported by the Bundesministerium fur Forschung und Technologie, Ministerium fur Wissenschaft und Forschung NRW, Deutsche Forschungsgemeinschaft, and Landesversicherungsanstalt (LVA) Westfalen.

REFERENCES

1.   NIH Consensus Conference, Washington February 1992.
2.   Assmann G., Oberwittler W., Schulte H., Schriewer H., Funke H., Epping P.H., Hauss W.H.: Pradiktion und Fruherkennung der koronaren Herzkrankheit. Internist 1980;21:446-459.
3.   Friedewald W.T., Levy J., Fredrickson D.S.: Estimation of the concentration of low-density-lipoprotein cholesterol in plasma, without use of the preparative ultracentrifuge. Clin. Chem. 1972;18:499-509.
4.   Assmann G., Schulte H.: PROCAM Trial. Panscientia publishing house, Hedingen-Zurich 1986.
5.   Assmann G., Schulte H.: Relation of High Density Lipoprotein Cholesterol and Triglycerides to Incidence of Atherosclerotic Coronary Artery Disease (The PROCAM Experience). Am. J. Cardiol. 1992;70:733-737.
6.   Nie N.H.: SPSSX User's Guide. McGraw-Hill, New York, 1983.
7.   Ray A.A.: SAS User's Guide: Basics. Cary, NC, SAS Institute, 1982.
8.   Assmann G., Schulte H.: Results and Conclusions of the Prospective Cardiovascular Munster (PROCAM) Study. In: Assmann G. (ed.) Lipid Metabolism Disorders and Coronary Heart Disease (completely revised second edition). MMV Medizin Verlag, Munchen, 1993 (in press).
9.   Gordon T., Castelli W.P., Hjortland M.C., Kannel W.B., Dawber T.R.: High-density lipoprotein as a protective factor against coronary heart disease: The Framingham Study. Am. J. Med. 1977;62:707-714.
10. Jacobs D.R. (for Lipid Research Clinics Follow-up Study): High density lipoprotein cholesterol and coronary heart disease cardiovascular disease and all-cause mortality, abstract. Circulation 1985;72 (suppl III): 185.
11. Watkins L.O., Neaton J.D., Phillips A.N. (for the MRFIT Research Group): High-density lipoprotein cholesterol and coronary heart disease incidence in black and white MRFIT usual care men. Am. J. Cardiol. 1986;57:538-545.
12. Miller N.E., Forde O.H., Thelle D.S., Mjos O.D. The Tromso Heart Study: High-density lipoprotein as a protective factor against coronary heart disease: A prospective case-control study. Lancet 1977;i:965-970.
13. Goldbourt U., Medalie J.H.: High-density lipoprotein cholesterol and incidence of coronary heart disease: The Israeli Ischaemic Heart Disease Study. Am. J. Epidemiol. 1979;109:296-308.
14. Enger S.C., Hjermann I., Foss O.P., Helgeland A., Holme I., Leren P., Norum K.R.: High-density lipoprotein cholesterol and myocardial infarction or sudden coronary

death: A prospective case-control study in middle-aged men of the Oslo study. Artery 1979;5:170-181.

15. Shestov D.B. Results of four years of follow-up of USSR populations. In USA-USSR First Lipoprotein Symposium, Bethesda, 1982. Us Department of Health and Human Services, National Institutes of Health, Publication (NIH) 83-1966, 391-407.

16. Keys A., Karvonen M.J., Punsar S., Menotti A., Fidanza F., Farchi G.: HDL serum cholesterol and 24-year mortality of men in Finland. Int. J. Epidemiol. 1984;13:428-435.

17. Pocock S.J., Shaper A.G., Phillips A.N., Whitehead T.P.: High density lipoprotein cholesterol is not a major risk factor for ischemic heart disease in British men. Br. Med. J. 1986;292:515-519.

18. Frick H.M., Elo O., Haapa K., Heinonen O.P., Heinsalmi P., Helo P., Huttunen J.K.,Kaitaniemi P., Koskinen P., Maenpaa H., Malkonen M., Manttari M., Norola S., Pasternack A., Pikkarainen J., Romo M., Sjoblom T., Nikkila E.A.: The Helsinki Heart Study- primary prevention trial with gemfibrozil in middle aged men with dyslipidaemia. Safety of treatment, Changes in risk factors, and incidence of coronary heart disease. N. Engl. J. Med. 1987; 317:1237-1245.

19. Manninen V., Huttunen J.K., Heinonen O.P., Tenkanen L., Frick M.H.: Relation between baseline lipid and lipoprotein values and the incidence of coronary heart disease in the Helsinki Heart Study. Am. J. Cardiol. 1989; 63:42H-47H.

20. Manninen V., Elo O., Frick M.H., Haapa K., Heinonen O.P., Heinsalmi P., Helo P.,Huttunen J.K., Kaitaniemi P., Koskinen P., Maenpaa H., Malkonen M., Manttari M., Norola S., Pasternack A., Pikkarainen J., Romo M., Sjoblom T., Nikkila E.A.: Lipid alterations and decline in the incidence of coronary heart disease in the Helsinki Heart Study. J. AMA 1988; 260:641-651.

21. Huttunen J.K., Manninen V., Manttari M., Koskinen P., Romo M., Tenkanen L., Heinonen O.P., Frick M.H.: The Helsinki Heart Study: Central Findings and Clinical Implications. Annals of Medicine 1991; 23: 155-159.

22. Hunt S.C., Hasstedt S.J., Kuida H., Stults B.M., Hopkins P.N. and Wiliams R.R.: Genetic heritability and common environmental components of resting and stressed blood pressures, lipids and body mass index in Utah pedigrees and twins. Am. J. Epidemiology 1989;129:625-638.

23. Christian J.G., Carmelli D., Castelli W.P., Fabsitz R., Grim C.E., Meaney F.J., Norton J.A., Reed T., Williams C.J. and Wood P.D.: High Density Lipoprotein Cholesterol. A 16 year longitudinal study in aging male twins. Arteriosclerosis 1990;10:1020-1027.

24. DeBacker G., Hulstaerdt F., DeMunck, Rosseneu M., Van Parijs L. and Dramaix M.: Serum lipids and apoproteins in students whose patients suffered prematurely form myocardial infarction. Am. Heart J. 1986;112:478-484.

25. Pometta D., Micheli H., Suenram A., Jornot C.: HDL lipids in close relatives of coronary heart disease patients. Atherosclerosis 1979;34:419-429.

26. Glomset J.A.: The plasma lecithin:cholesterol acyltransferase reaction. J. Lipid Res. 1968;9:155-163.

27. Eisenberg S.: High Density Lipoprotein Metabolism. J. Lipid Res. 1984;25:1017-1058.

28. Tall A.R.: Plasma high density lipoproteins. Metabolism and relationship to atherogenesis. J. Clin. Invest. 1990;86:379-384.

29. Schmitz G.,Bruning T., Williamson E. and Nowick G.: The role of reverse cholesterol transport and its disturbances in Tangier disease and HDL deficiency with xanthomas. Eur. Heart. J. 1990;11 (Suppl. E):197-207.

30. Johnson W.J., Mahlberg F.H., Rothblat G.H., Phillips M.C.: Cholesterol transport between cells and high density lipoproteins. Biochim. Biophys. Acta 1991;1085:273-298.

31. Oram J.: Cholesterol traffiking in cells. Curr. Opin. Lipidol. 1990;1:416-421.

32. Ailhaud G.: Cellular signal transductans: a new role for HDL. Curr. Opin. Lipidol. 1992;2:222-226.
33. Castro G.R. and Fielding C.J.: Early incorporation of cell-derived cholesterol into pre-β-migrating high density lipoprotein. Biochemistry 1988;27:25-29.
34. Huang Y., von Eckardstein A., Assmann G.: Cell derived unesterified cholesterol is cycled betweeen high density lipoproteins and low density lipoproteins for its effective esterification. Arteriosclerosis Thromb. 1993; in press.
35. Assmann G., Schmitz G., Funke H., von Eckardstein A.: Apolipoprotein A-I and HDL Deficiency. Curr. Opin. Lipidol. 1990;1:110-115.
36. Assmann G., von Eckardstein A. and Funke H.: Lecithin:cholesterol acyltransferase deficiency and fish eye disease. Curr. Opin. Lipidol 1991;2:110-117.
37. Assmann G., von Eckardstein A., Funke H.: The role of Apolipoprotein mutants in HDL metabolism. in Rosseneu, M.Y. (ed.): Structure and function of apolipoproteins. CRC Reviews in Biochemistry, CRC Press, Boca Raton, 1992; pp 85-121.
38. Brown M.L., Hesler C. and Tall A.R.: Lecithin:cholesterol Aclytransferase and cholestery ester transfer protein. Curr. Opin. Lipidol. 1991;1:123-127.
39. Breslow J.L.: Familial Disorders of High Density Lipoprotein Metabolism. in Scriver, C.R., Beaudet A.L., Sly W.S. and Valle D. (eds.): The Metabolic Basis of Inherited Disease. 6th edition. McGraw-Hill Information Services. New York. 1989; pp 1251-1266.
40. Norum K.R., Gjone E. and Glomset J.A.: Familial lecithin:cholesterol acyltransferase deficiency including fish-eye disease. in Scriver C.R., Beaudet A.L., Sly W.S. and Valle D. (eds.): The Metabolic Basis of Inherited Disease. 6th edition. McGraw-Hill Information Services, New York, 1989; pp 1181-1194.
41. Assmann G., Schmitz G. and Brewer H.B.: Familial High Density Lipoprotein Deficiency:Tangier Disease. in Scriver C.R., Beaudet A.L., Sly W.S. and Valle D. (eds.): The Metabolic Basis of Inherited Disease. 6th edition. McGraw-Hill Information Services. New York. 1989; pp 1267-1282.
42. Swenson T.L.: Transfer proteins in reverse cholesterol transport. Curr. Opin. Lipidol. 1992;3:67-74.
43. Patsch J.R., Prasad S., Gotto A.M.: Postprandial lipemia: A key for the conversion of high density lipoproteins$_2$ into high density lipoproteins$_3$ by hepatic lipase. J. Clin. Invest. 1984;74:2017-2023.
44. Patsch J.R., Karlin J.B., Cott L.W., Smith L.C., Gotto A.M.: Inverse relationship betweeen blood levels of high density lipoprotein subfraction 2 and magnitude of postprandial lipemia. Proc. Natl. Acad. Sci. USA 1983;80:1449-1453.
45. Patsch J.R., Prasad S., Gotto A.M., Patsch W.: High density lipoproteins$_2$: reletionship of the plasma levels of this lipoprotein species to its composition, to the magnitude of postprandial lipemia, and to the activities of lipoprotein lipase and hepatic lipase. J. Clin. Invest. 1987;30:341-347.
46. Patsch J.R., Miesenbock G., Hopferwieser T., Muhlberger V., Kanapp E., Dunn J.K., Gotto A.M., Patsch W.: The relationship of triglyceride metabolism and coronary artery disease: Studies in the postprandial state. Arteriosclerosis Thromb. 1992;12.
47. Blankenhorn D.H., Alaupovic P., Wickham E., Chin H.P., Azen S.P. : Prediction of angiographic change in native human coronary arteries and aortocoronary bypass grafts. Circulation 1990;81:470-476.
48. Nachman R.L.: Thrombosis and atherogenesis: molecular connections. Blood 1992;79:1897-1906.
49. Kuusi T., Ehnholm C., Viikari J., Harkonen R., Vartiainen E., Puska P;, Taskinen M.R.: Postheparin plasma lipoprotein and hepatic lipase determinants of hypo- and hyper-alphalipoproteinemia. J. Lipid Res. 1989;30:117-1126.

50. Babirak S.P., Brown G., Brunzell J.D.: Familial combined hyperlipidemia and abnormal lipoprotein lipase. Arteriosclerosis Thromb. 1992;12:1176-1183.
51. Laloue J.M., Wilson D.E., Iverius P.H.: Lipoprotein lipase and hepatic triglyceride lipase: molecular and genetic aspects. Curr. Opin. Lipidol. 1992;3:86-95.
52. Laws A., King A.C., Haskell W.L., Reaven G.M.: Relation of fasting plasma insulin concentration to high density lipoprotein cholesterol and triglycerides in men. Arteriosclerosis Thromb 1991;11:1636-1642.
53. Laakso M., Sarlund, Mykkanen L.: Insulin resistance is associated with lipid and lipoprotein abnormalities in subjects with varying degrees of glucose tolerance. Arteriosclerosis 1990;10:223-231.
54. Williams R.R., Hunt S.C., Hopkins P.N., Stults B.M., Wu L.L., Hasstedt S.J., Barlow G.K., Stephenson S.H., Lalouel J.M., Kuida H.: Familial dyslipidemic hypertension. J AMA 1988;259 3579-3586.
55. Reaven G.M.: Role of insulin resistance in human disease. Diabetes 1988;37:1595-1607.

THE CLINICAL APPROACH TO THE PATIENTS WITH LOW HDL AND ELEVATED PLASMA TRIGLYCERIDE

A. NOTARBARTOLO, M.R. AVERNA, C.M. BARBAGALLO

ABSTRACT. High triglyceride/low HDL-C syndrome has been discussed in this report. Primary and secondary causes have been reviewed and relationships with cardiovascular disease evaluated. Finally useful advices for the clinical approach to this kind of patients have been suggested.

Hypertriglyceridemia (HTG) associated with low HDL derives from many genetic and/or acquired metabolic alterations, and is very common in the general population.

According to the recent classification of 1991 International Commitee for the Evaluation of HTG as a Vascular Risk Factor, triglyceride (TG) levels between 200-400 mg/dl should be considered "moderately elevated" and require a careful clinical and laboratory evaluation; when a "mixed hyperlipidemia" is present (total cholesterol, CHO, between 200-300 mg/dl, TG between 200-400 mg/dl) lifestyle modifications are required and, if coronary heart disease (CHD) risk remain high (high TG and/or CHO levels or low HDL-cholesterol levels, HDL-C), drug treatment may be considered; TG levels > 400 mg/dl are considered "severe", while levels > 1000 mg/dl "very severe" and usually associated with chylomicronemia and high risk of pancreatitis.

In a patient with HTG, clinicians aims are to determine patient's phenotype and, as far as possible, underlying causes (including genetic ones).

Familial HTG is symptomless and most frequently observed during screening for other diagnosic purpose, but may also be diagnosed during the clinical evaluation of a patient with CHD or pheripheral artery disease.

With only one exception, in every case-control study a

A. L. Catapano et al. (eds.), Drugs Affecting Lipid Metabolism, 357–364.

univariate, and sometimes multivariate, association
between triglyceride and myocardial infarction has been
reported. In 77 patients undergoing aorto-coronaric
bypass surgery, we have found significant higher levels
of triglyceride and apo B and lower levels of HDL-
cholesterol and apo A-I in comparison with sex, age and
body weight non CHD controls.

TABLE 1: Lipid and apoprotein levels in 77 subjects
undergoing aorto-coronary bypass surgery (BP) and in 77
controls (C). Mg/dl. Mean ± ES.

	CHO	TG	HDL-C	LDL-C	A-I	B
BP	204.1± 4.9	154.3± 8.1	37.9± 1.2	134.9± 4.0	122.4± 2.4	132.8± 3.7
p <	ns	0.001	0.001	ns	0.0001	0.001
C	200.4± 4.7	115.6± 7.9	45.4± 1.2	131.9± 3.9	148.8± 2.9	114.3± 3.6

Like Familial HTG, Familial Combined Hyperlipidemia
(FCH) is a common disorder (approximately 1-2% of the
general population) frequently do not manifest itself
until adulthood. It is typified by findings of multiple
patterns of hyperlipoproteinemia; overall roughly 50 to
80% of relatives of affected individuals are
hyperlipidemic (1/3 hypercholesterolemia, 1/3
hypertriglyceridemia, 1/3 with both abnormalities, in a
single family). FCH differs from Familial
Hypercholesterolemia because affected children never show
type IIa phenotype, but present high TG levels as the
earliest manifestation of the disorder, and it differs
from Familial HTG because this is never associated with
type IIa or IIb phenotypes.
About 15% of patients with myocardial infarction before
the age of 60 derives from families with FCH; as type IV
hyperlipoproteinemia is a phenotypic expression of this
disorder, it could be suggested that these patients are
at risk of CHD.
In HTG patients with Familial Combined Hyperlipidemia
an increase of VLDL-apo B synthesis and elevated LDL-apo
B levels, despite normal serum LDL-cholesterol levels,
have been described. Therefore in HTG patients with
manifest CHD or a family hystory of CHD may be suggested
the routinely assay of apo B plasma levels, a relatively
simple tecnique in a Lipid Research Clinic. This approach
may not give any better predictability than LDL-

cholesterol (LDL-C) levels in hypercholesterolemic
patients with normal TG levels, but it could be useful
for patients with HTG, FCH and diabetic dyslipidemia.

Nearly all the HTG conditions are associated with HDL
modifications. When HDL particles are overloaded with TG,
their efficiences as acceptors of tissue cholesterol may
be reduced. An HDL-C level below 35 mg/dl (0.91 mmmol/l)
is defined as abnormal or low; however the risk for CHD
increase as HDL-C fall. Familial Hypoalphalipoproteinemia
(HypoalfaLP) is a rare autosomal dominant disorder
characterized by a primary depression of HDL-C levels
below the 10th percentile of age and sex normal values,
without other lipoprotein abnormalities. Subjects with
genetic hypoalfaLP often have HDL-C levels into the range
of 20-29 mg/dl; they do not have remarkable findings on
physical examination despite developing premature CHD,
even in absence of other known risk factors.

Either in isolated HTG with or without low HDL-C
levels, or in combined hyperlipidemia many secondary
causes of altered lipoprotein pattern (enviromental,
iatrogenic or endogenous) could be found. Smokers show
HDL-C levels lower than general population; comparison of
active and sedentary people have shown generally lower
fasting TG and higher HDL-C levels in exercisers. Among
the drugs that usually cause a lipoprotein derangement,
selective ß-blockers and thiazides are commonly used. In
type II diabetes mellitus, obesity, excess of caloric
intake and combined hyperlipidemia there is a high
prevalence of hypertension. High blood pressure needs
particular attention; it is good practice to avoid, when
possible, ß-blockers and diuretics, and to use calcium
channel blockers and coverting enzyme inhibitors.

Clinically the most important forms of secondary HTG
are those found in diabetes mellitus, obesity and chronic
renal failure (CRF). NIDDM patients frequently show mild
to moderate HTG due to overproduction of VLDL in the
liver and decreased HDL-C levels associated with
defective TG-rich particles (TRL) catabolism. When
metabolic control occur, patients usually present mild
HTG and low HDL-C and apo A-I levels, but normal or low
LDL-C levels. Diabetics with CHD show significant
differences in plasma lipid and apoprotein profile in
comparison with subjects without CHD.

More than 80% of NIDDM are obese or overweighted;
obesity of central type may be calculated by waist-to hip
ratio (WHR), that is highly correlated with the
tomographic evaluation of visceral fat. IGT and high WHR
are very common findings of Familial HTG, FCH and type
III hyperlipoproteinemia. This is true for both, men and
women; recent studies have documented positive

correlations between splanchnic fat deposition and CHO and TG levels. It is reasonable to conclude that WHR is a useful clinical test for the diagnosis of the HTG/low HDL-C syndrome.

In Ventimiglia di Sicilia, a little rural town near to Palermo (Sicily) where we have screened more than 75% of the whole population, we have found 29 subjects with the HTG/low HDL-C syndrome out of 1150 total subjects with age of 20 or more, without any secondary cause of increase of lipids, except obesity. TG and apo B values were higher and HDL-C and apo A-I levels lower in comparison with controls (Table 2).

TABLE 2: Lipid and apoprotein levels in 29 subjects with HTG/low HDL-C syndrome (HTG) and in 1121 controls (C) in Ventimiglia di Sicilia population. Mg/dl. Mean ± SD.

	CHO	TG	HDL-C	LDL-C	A-I	B
HTG	200.6± 25.0	306.1± 84.6	28.6± 4.0	110.7± 22.6	122.1± 13.5	144.9± 24.0
p <	ns	0.0001	0.0001	ns	0.0001	0.0001
C	197.6± 41.3	107.3± 62.1	45.3± 10.8	130.8± 34.6	145.1± 24.1	111.0± 33.8

Also BMI, WHR, hematocrit, uric acid, systolic and dyastolic blood pressure values were significantly more elevated in patients than in controls; prevalence of the syndrome was about 2.5%, five-fold increased in males (4.4%) than in females (0.9%). All these alterations are included in the Polymetabolic Syndrome or X Syndrome.

In CRF, HTG has been reported as the main cause of the accelerated atherosclerosis of these patients. Prevalence of HTG in an our population of CRF patients on hemodialysis was about 50%, similar to those reported by other authors. Metabolic defect of HTG in CRF is the consequence of diminished lipolytic activity and all lipoprotein fractions show an abnormal content of TG. The HTG in uremia and/or in patients on hemodialysis is always "moderate" (Table 3) and the atherogenic impact could be due to the presence of low HDL-C levels and, probably, to abnormal apoprotein profile. We have demonstrated that apoprotein pattern in subjects with uremic HTG in comparison with age, weight, sex and TG matched HTG controls is characterized by low levels of apo A-I, A-II and B and apo C-II/apo C-III and TG/apo C-III ratios and high levels of apo C-III. These serum abnormalities could reflect lipoprotein structural changes; VLDL altered in their apoprotein composition could represent defective substrate for lipolytic enzymes or, on the contrary, apoprotein changes could be a consequence of LPL and HL impaired activities. These data suggest that HTG could be relevant to atherogenesis when, such as in uremia, it is associated to changes of size, lipid and apoproten composition of lipoprotein particles.

TABLE 3: Lipid and apoprotein levels in 40 CRF patients on hemodialysis (CRF) and in 40 normolipidemic controls (C). Mg/dl. Mean ± SD.

	CHO	TG	HDL-C	LDL-C	A-I	B
CRF	175.8±	220.8±	28.5±	103.1±	108.5±	110.7±
	40.9	115.9	8.2	34.2	19.7	32.2
p <	ns	0.0001	0.0001	ns	0.01	0.01
C	177.0±	83.5±	44.8±	115.6±	145.8±	95.9±
	16.7	33.5	9.2	15.0	23.7	16.0

To summarize, the diagnosis of this syndrome is based on a careful examination of the patient (Table 4). In particular:
- The familial and individual history is necessary to find out other cases of myocardial infarction and hypertension before the age of 60, cases of diabetes or obesity;
- It is important to detect causes of secondary hyperlipoproteinemia and adverse effects of drug administration;
- The WHR evaluation (> 0.8 in men and > 1.0 in women) may exclude or include a polymetabolic syndrome, and the blood pressure record is important because hypertension is highly prevalent in obesity, diabetes, hyperinsulinemic states and, of course, in FCH. In this form hypertension is the expression of a genetic deviation called "Familial Dyslipidemic Hypertension".
- Of course a careful physical and cardiovascular examination must be carried out.

In the blood (Table 5), beside CHO, TG, HDL-C assays and LDL-C calculation by the Friedewald Formula (if TG levels < 350 mg/dl), fasting and 2-hours after glucose load glycemia and uric acid measurements are useful because they are associated with an hyperinsulinemic condition. Total plasma apo B levels should also be detected, because when LDL-C values are normal, they are predictable of CHD in patients with HTG, FCH and diabetic dyslipidemia. Moreover epidemiological studies showed that fibrinogen is a predictor of atherosclerotic diseases and its predictive power seems to be as high as higher than accepted risk factor. There is emerging evidences that TRL affect both blood coagulation and fibrinolytic function, activating coagulation Factor VII and increasing plasma levels of plasminogen activator inhibitor-1 (PAI-1), the fast-acting inhibitor of tissue-type plasminogen activator (t-PA). Finally it seems that Lp(a) compete with plasminogen for binding to the plasminogen receptor; these property may explain the association of high Lp(a) concentrations with myocardial infarction. Actually results of PROCAM and other longitudinal studies seem to indicate an independent predictive power of Lp(a) for CHD and cerebrovascular disease.

TABLE 4: Clinical evaluation of the HTG/low HDL-C syndrome
----
1. Familial and individual history
2. Drugs administration history
3. Secondary hyperlipidemias screening
4. Alimentary and physical activity inquires
5. Physical examination (Blood Pressure, BMI and WHR)
6. Cardiological evaluation

TABLE 5: Lipids and other blood tests in the HTG/low HDL-C syndrome
----
1. CHO, TG, HDL-C, LDL-C
2. Apo B
3. Glycemia
4. Fibrinogen
5. Lp(a)
6. Uric acid

REFERENCES

Assmann G, Betteridge DJ, Gotto AM, Steiner G (1991) 'Management of hypertriglyceridemic patients. A. Treatment classification and goals', Am J Cardiol 68, 30A-34A.

Austin MA, Goto Y, Lenfant C, Tyroler HA (1991) 'Epidemiology', Am J Cardiol 68, 22A-25A.

Averna MR, Barbagallo CM, Galione A et al (1989) 'Serum apolipoprotein profile of hypertriglyceridemic patients with chronic renal failure on hemodialytic therapy:a comparison with type IV hyperlipoproteinemic patients', Metabolism 38, 601-2.

Averna MR, Barbagallo CM, Galione A et al (1990) 'Lipids and lipo-apoproteins in patients with chronic renal failure on hemodialytic therapy', in Crepaldi G, Tiengo A, Enzi G (Eds), Diabetes, Obesity and Hyperlipidemias - IV, Elsevier Science Publishers B.V., Amsterdam, pp. 41-44.

Averna MR, Barbagallo CM, Ocello S et al (1992) 'Lp(a) levels in patients undergoing aorto-coronary bypass surgery', Eur Heart J in press.

Barbagallo CM, Averna MR, Amato S et al (1990) 'Apo-lipoprotein profile in type II diabetic patients with and without coronary heart disease', Acta Diab Lat 27, 371-7.

Barbagallo CM, Averna MR, Cavera G et al (1992) 'Lipidi ed apoproteine plasmatiche: influenza del fumo di sigaretta', Rec Prog Med 83, 127-30.

Barbir M, Wile D, Trayner I, Aber VR, Thompson GR (1988) 'High prevalence of hypertriglyceridemia and apolipoprotein abnormalities in coronary artery disease', Br Heart J 60, 397-403.

Betteridge DJ (1989) 'Lipids, diabetes, and vascular disease: the time of act', Diab Med 6, 195-218.

Carlson LA, Bottinger LE (1985) 'Risk factors for ischemic heart disease in men and in women. Results of the 19-year follow-up of the Stockholm Prospective Study', Acta Med Scand 218, 207-11.

Depres JP, Moorjani S, Ferland M et al (1989) 'Adipose
tissue distribution and plasma lipoprotein levels in
obese women. Importance of intra-abdominal fat',
Arteriosclerosis 9, 203-10.

Gordon DJ, Probstfield JL, Garrison RJ et al (1989)
'High-Density Lipoprotein cholesterol and
cardiovascular disease', Circulation 79, 8-15.

Kannel WB, Wolf Pa, Castelli WP, D'Agostino R (1987)
'Fibrinogen and risk for cardiovascular disease', JAMA
258, 1183-6.

Murai A, Miyahara T, Fujimoto N, Matsuda M, Kameyama M
(1986) 'Lp(a) lipoprotein as a risk factor for coronary
heart disease and cerebral infarction', Atherosclerosis
59, 199-204.

Notarbartolo A, Averna MR, Barbagallo CM (1991)
'Secondary hyperlipoproteinemias ang aging', Arch
Gerontol Geriatr suppl 2, 569-74.

Reaven GM (1988) 'Role of insulin resistance in human
disease', Diabetes 37, 1595-607.

Sandkamp M, Funke H, Schulte H, Kohler E, Assmann G
(1990) 'Lipoprotein(a) is an indipendent risk factor
for myocadial infarction at a young age', Clin Chem 36,
20-23.

Williams RR, Hunt SC, Hasstedt SJ et al (1992) 'Are there
interactions and relations between genetic and
enviromental factors predisposing to high blood
pressure?', Hypertension 18, suppl I, I29-I37.

Vergani C, Bettale G (1981) 'Familial hypo-alpha-
lipoproteinemia', Clin Chim Acta 114, 45-52.

FAMILIAL LIPOPROTEIN DISORDERS IN PATIENTS WITH PREMATURE CORONARY ARTERY DISEASE

Ernst J. Schaefer, MD, Jose M. Ordovas, PhD; Peter W. F. Wilson, MD; Deeb N. Salem, MD; and Jacques J. Genest Jr., MD

ABSTRACT

The prevalence of familial lipoprotein disorders was assessed in 102 kindreds with a total of 603 subjects in whom the proband had angiographically documented significant (>50% narrowing) coronary artery disease. Kindreds were classified as abnormal if the proband and at least one first degree relative had fasting triglyceride, low density lipoprotein (LDL) cholesterol, apolipoprotein (apo) B, or lipoprotein (a) values >90th percentile or their high density lipoprotein (HDL) cholesterol or apoA-I value were <10th percentile of age and gender adjusted control values. The following prevalence of familial disorders was noted: Lp(a) excess 18.6%, dyslipidemia (elevated triglycerides and low HDL cholesterol) 14.7%, combined hyperlipidemia (11.7% with low HDL cholesterol) 13.7%, hyperapobetalipoproteinemia 5%, hypoalphalipoproteinemia 4%, and hypercholesterolemia 3%.

INTRODUCTION

Family history of myocardial infarction or sudden death is a frequent finding in patients with premature coronary artery disease (CAD) and is considered a risk factor for the development of CAD (1). Several familial lipid disorders, including familial hypercholesterolemia (FH) (2), familial combined hyperlipidemia (FCH) (3-5) and familial hypoalphalipoproteinemia (FHA) (6), have been associated with an increased risk of premature CAD. The role of plasma lipids and lipoproteins in the development of CAD has been shown in large prospective (7,8) and case-control studies (9,10). The protein content of low density lipoproteins (LDL) and the main apolipoproteins of high density lipoproteins (HDL), i.e., apolipoprotein (apo) B and apo A-I (11-14), as well as lipoprotein(a) [Lp(a)] and apo(a) (15,16) have been shown in some studies, but not all, to be better makers for the presence of CAD than elevated LDL cholesterol or decreased HDL cholesterol levels. Elevation of LDL apo B with normal (or near-normal) lipid values (hyperapobetalipoproteinemia) is associated with premature CAD and has been shown to segregate in family members (11). Lp(a) excess also is associated with premature CAD and is present in families of affected individuals. The modes of inheritance for many of these disorders is thought to be autosomal dominant or polygenic, with varying degrees of penetrance and/or expression in adulthood. With the exception of FH (2), familial defective apo B-100 (17), familial dysbetalipoproteinemia (type III hyperli-poproteinemia) (18), and rare disorders of the apo AI-CIII-AIV gene cluster (19,20) the molecular defects of most familial lipoprotein disorder associated with premature CAD are unknown. In FH, multiple disorders of the LDL receptor gene have been identified, and the disease is transmitted in a Mendelian dominant fashion (21,22).

A. L. Catapano et al. (eds.), Drugs Affecting Lipid Metabolism, 365–374.
© 1993 Kluwer Academic Publishers and Fondazione Giovanni Lorenzini.

The prevalence of lipid disorders is increased in patients with premature CAD. However, the type and prevalence of familial dyslipidemia have not been well characterized since the description of FCH in CAD patients (3-5), which was based on measurements of total cholesterol and triglyceride concentrations and lipoprotein electrophoresis pattern. The purpose of the present study was to determine the type and prevalence of dyslipidemia in patients with premature coronary disease. The genetic contribution of lipoprotein and apolipoprotein levels was assessed by comparing parental with offspring plasma levels of various lipid parameters.

METHODS

Patients

Two hundred and fifty nine consecutive patients referred to our hospital for coronary angiography were included in the study if they were Caucasian and less than 60 years of age at the time of angiography and had significant CAD, defined as >50% stenosis of one or more epicardial coronary artery. Patients with <50% stenosis were excluded (n=25), as were patients older than 60 years and those receiving lipid-lowering medications (n=1). Information on use of lipid lowering drugs, adrenergic blocking agents, and diuretics and history of hypertension, diabetes mellitus, and cigarette smoking was obtained. Information on the presence of coronary disease was gathered on first-degree relatives, parents, and grandparents by history. We attempted to study all kindreds consisting of patients who had a minimum of two offspring and a genetically unrelated spouse available for blood sampling.

Of 259 patients with premature CAD, 36 were unmarried or had insufficient children for this study. Of the remaining 223 families, 50 (22%) did not wish to take part in the study; 44 (20%) volunteered but were unable to participate; 21 (9%) were lost to follow-up; and 108 families (49%) were sampled. In six families, not enough first-degree relatives were available for analysis, and these kindreds were excluded from the phenotype analysis. There were 87 men (85.3%) and 15 women (14.7%) identified as probands, with 382 first-degree relatives (3.75 per proband, including 16 parents), 23 second-degree relatives, and 96 genetically unrelated spouses; 88.6% of offspring identified were sampled. A total of 603 subjects were studied.

Controls

To classify values of probands and first-degree relatives, we used the Lipid Research Clinics (LRC) data base's 90th percentile age- and sex-specific values for total cholesterol, triglycerides, and LDL cholesterol and the 10th percentile values for HDL cholesterol as cutoff points (23). No age or sex norms for apo A-I, apo B, and Lp(a) are available from the LRC study; apo A-I and apo B were measured on a sample of 3,541 participants in cycle 3 of the Framingham Offspring Study. Age and sex distribution were used for the cutoff points (<10th percentile for apo A-I and >90th percentile for apo B) in the present study. Lp(a) was determined on 1,240 men and 1,309 women, free of cardiovascular disease, from the Framingham Offspring cohort. The 90th percentile was determined to be 39 mg/dl in men and 39.5 mg/dl in women at a mean age of 50 years. As comparison groups for the probands, we used 901 healthy men aged 40-60 years (mean ± SD age, 49 ± 6 years) and 1,125 healthy women aged 40-60 years (mean ± SD age, 49 ± 6 years) from the Framingham Offspring Study who had no evidence of cardiovascular disease. Triglycerides and Lp(a) were log_{10} transformed to approximate the normal distribution.

Lipid, Lipoprotein, and Apolipoprotein Measurements

All patients and relatives were sampled in the free-living state at least 1 month after their diagnostic catheterization and at least 6 weeks after major surgery or myocardial infarction. Subjects were sampled after a 12-14 hour overnight fast. Subjects were asked to refrain from alcohol consumption for 24 hours before the sampling. Thirty milliliters of blood was drawn from an antecubital vein in EDTA-containing tubes to a final concentration of 1.2 mg/ml and put on ice. Plasma was isolated by centrifugation (2,500 rpm for 20 minutes at 4°C), and multiple aliquots were stored immediately at -80°C for later apo A-I, apo B, and Lp(a) determinations. Plasma total cholesterol and triglyceride concentrations were determined enzymatically, HDL cholesterol also was measured enzymatically after dextran-Mg^{2+} precipitation (24,25). Our laboratory meets the performance criteria of the Centers of Disease Control-National Heart, Lung, and Blood Institute Lipid Standardization program. In most subjects, LDL cholesterol was estimated with the Friedwald formula (24-26). However, in cases where the plasma triglyceride levels were >400 mg/dl, cholesterol was measured in the density >1.006 g/ml infranate plasma after ultracentrifugation; LDL cholesterol was then calculated by subtracting HDL cholesterol from infranate cholesterol (23). Apo A-I and apo B were determined by noncompetitive ELISAs (27,28). These assays were standardized using amino acid analysis of purified protein standards. Lp(a) was measured using a commercially available ELISA (Terumo Medical Corp., Elkton, Md.), which uses two antisera, one monoclonal antibody that does not cross react with plasminogens, and a polyclonal antibody that is specific for the apo (a) protein of Lp(a). The assay is standardized with respect to the total Lp(a) particle. Results are expressed in milligrams per deciliter of Lp(a). Coefficient of variance for this assay were 2.46% for interrun and 3.33% for interrun variations, respectively, and <10% for other apolipoprotein assays.

Lipoprotein Abnormalities
To classify lipid disorders, we defined hypertriglyceridemia as a plasma triglyceride level >90th percentile value of age- and sex-matched control subjects. Similarly, hypercholesterolemia was defined as a plasma level of LDL cholesterol >90th percentile, and hypoalphalipoproteinemia was defined as a plasma level of HDL cholesterol <10th percentile, based on the LRC population study (23). The LRC data for lipid and lipoprotein levels were used rather than the Framingham Study data base because the former includes data on children. However, cutoff-point values for either sample were very similar. We have avoided defining hyperlipoproteinemias by types I-V (29); rather, we have used the terms as defined above.
The criteria used to define a familial dyslipidemia are as follows: Abnormalities found in probands alone and not in any first-degree relatives were called "sporadic" and the family was considered "normal." In cases where the spouse was affected and the proband was not and segregation was found in the children, the family was labeled "normal" for the purposes of this study. If the proband was affected with a lipoprotein or apolipoprotein abnormality and at least one first-degree relative had a lipoprotein or apolipoprotein abnormality, the kindred was considered to have a familial lipoprotein abnormality. FH was defined as elevated LDL cholesterol only, regardless of the presence of xanthomas or xanthelasmas and the finding of this same abnormality in one or more first-degree relatives. Familial hypertriglyceridemia was defined as an elevated triglyceride level and the presence of the same abnormality in at least one first-degree relative. FHA was defined as low HDL cholesterol only and the presence of the same abnormality in at least one first-degree relative. FHA was defined as low HDL cholesterol only and the presence of the same abnormality in at least one first-degree relative. Familial Lp(a) excess was defined as an elevated Lp(a) level (>39 mg/dl for men, >39.5/dl for women) in the proband and at least one first-degree relative. Familial hyperapo B was defined as apo B >90th percentile in the proband and at least one first-degree relative, with normal lipid and lipoprotein levels. Familial apo A-I deficiency was defined as apo A-I levels <10th percentile with normal lipid values, including HDL cholesterol. FCH was defined as the finding of an elevated triglyceride level and/or an elevated LDL cholesterol level (>90th percentile) in the proband and at least one first-degree relative, with the stipulation that both abnormalities had to be present in the kindred. Familial hypertriglyceridemia with hypoalphalipoproteinemia was defined as an

elevated triglyceride level and/or a low HDL cholesterol level (<10th percentile) in the proband and at least one first-degree relative, with the stipulation that both abnormalities had to be present within the kindred. We call this entity familial dyslipidemia.

RESULTS
The mean age of the probands was 51 ± 6 years (age range, 34-59 years). When the CAD cases were compared with Framingham controls, prevalence rates for smoking (within the past 2 years; 44% versus 28%, p<0.01), diabetes (11% versus 3%, p<0.001), and hypertension (45% versus 20%, p<0.01) were significantly higher in the CAD group than in the control group. Mean age in men with CAD was 51 ± 6 years compared with 49 ± 6 years in the male controls (p<0.05), and mean age in women with CAD was 51 ± 3 years compared with 49 ± 6 years in the female controls (p=NS). Lipid, lipoprotein, and apolipoprotein levels in men and women with CAD were compared with levels of male and female controls from the Framingham Offspring Study, cycle 3.
The data on lipids, lipoproteins, and apolipoproteins were adjusted for sex, age, body mass index, smoking status, use of beta-blockers, and hypertension. The analysis revealed that triglycerides, LDL cholesterol, and apo B were no longer statistically different in the CAD probands after adjusting for covariates, while Lp(a) were significantly higher (p<0.005) and HDL cholesterol and apoA-I levels were significantly lower (p<0.001) in CAD probands than controls.
With the criteria outlined in "Methods", the prevalence of lipoprotein and apolipoprotein abnormalities was determined in probands alone (Table 1) and within the familial context (Table 2).

Table 1 LIPOPROTEIN AND APOLIPOPROTEIN DISORDERS* IN PROBANDS WTH PREMATURE CORONARY ARTERY DISEASE

Disorder	No. of patients (%)	
Hypoalphalipoproteinemia	40	(39.2)
Hyper apo B †	31	(30.4)
Decreased apo A-I	29	(28.4)
Hypertriglyceridemia	23	(22.5)
Lp(a) excess	19	(18.6)
Hypercholesterolemia (elevated LDL cholesterol)	11	(10.8)
Normal	24	23.5)

Apo, apolipoprotein; Lp(a), lipoprotein (a); LDL, low density lipoprotein.
* Not mutually exclusive groups.
† Based on total plasma apo B.

Table 2 PREVALENCE OF FAMILIAL LIPID DISORDERS IN 102 FAMILIES IN WHICH THE PROBAND HAS PREMATURE CORONARY ARTERY DISEASE

Familial lipid disorder	No. of families (%)	
Lp(a) (includes 5.9% with dyslipidemias)	19	(18.6)
Combined hyperlipidemia	14	(13.7)
Hyperapo B	5	(5.0)
Hypertriglyceridemia with hypoalphalipoproteinemia*	15 *	(14.7)
Hypoalphalipoproteinemia	4	(4.0)
Apo A-I deficiency	1	(1.0)
Hypercholesterolemia*	3	(3.0)
Hypertriglyceridemia	1	(1.0)
Genetic dyslipidemia †	55	(53.9)
Unclassifiedt ††	3	(3.0)
Normal	44	(43.1)

*One patient has both familial hypercholesterolemia (LDL receptor gene defect) and familial dyslipidemia (hypertriglyceridemia with hypoalphalipoproteinemia).
† Of the kindreds, 6.9% had two abnormalities; however, each case was counted only once, and the overlaps are indicated.
†† Both proband and spouse were dyslipidemic and children were affected; therefore, the type of lipid disorder could not unequivocally be assigned to the proband.

A lipoprotein or apolipoprotein abnormality was identified in 75 probands (73.5%). In 20 of these patients (19.6% of all CAD index cases), no clear familial segregation was identified, and the proband was classified as having a sporadic lipid disorder (see "Methods"). Therefore, 53.9% of the CAD probands were documented as having a familial lipoprotein or apolipoprotein disorder as previously defined. In the probands, the prevalence of lipoprotein and apolipoprotein abnormalities were hypoalphalipoproteinemia, 39.2%; elevated apo B, 30-40%; reduced apo A-I, 28.4%; elevated triglyceride levels, 22.5%; Lp(a) excess, 18.6%; and hypercholesterolemia, 10.8% (these groups were not mutually exclusive). Our assay for apo B measures total plasma apo B. When family members were considered, the prevalence of familial lipoprotein abnormalities did not always follow the proband's phenotype (Table 3).

Table 3 LIPOPROIEIN LEVELS IN PROBANDS (MEN ONLY) WITH COMMON DYSLIPIDEMIAS (mg/dl)

	n	Total Cholesterol	Triglycerides	LDL Cholesterol	HDL Cholesterol	Apo B	Apo A-I	Lp(a)
T+H	12	178±32 *	225±128 *	107±42 *	29±6 *	130±34†	99±20 *	9±12†
T+L±H	11	213±29	233±104 *	135±31	32±6 *	140±28 *	113±17†	24±20†
Lp(a)	12	189±32†	168±142	117±37†	39±10†	105±18	121±20†	47±9 *
Apo B	4	222±23	226±135†	141±30	36±4	176±32 *	120±12	11±15
HDL	4	196±28	130±61	141±16	28±3 *	127±28	90±11 *	20±26
Control	901	214±36	141±104	138±35	45±12	108±33	136±32	15±17

T, Triglycerides >90th percentile; H, high density lipoprotein (HDL) cholesterol <10th percentile; L, low density lipoprotein (LDL) >90th percentile; Lp(a), lipoprotein(a) >38 mg/dl.
*$p<0.005$, †$p<0.05$.

Isolated lipid disorders were infrequent; combined lipoprotein disorders were frequent. The majority of probands with low HDL cholesterol also had first-degree relatives with elevated triglycerides; similarly, many probands with a lipoprotein abnormality were part of families with combined disorders. The most common familial dyslipidemia were Lp(a) excess, seen in 19 families (18.6%), including 13 (12.7%) with no other lipid abnormalities hypertriglyceridemia with low HDL cholesterol, 15 families (14.7%); FCH (elevated triglycerides and/or LDL cholesterol), 14 families (13.7%) with (11.7%) or without (2%) low HDL cholesterol, and FHA, four families (4%). FH was seen in three families, two of whom had classic FH with tendinous xanthomas. Another family had hypercholesterolemia without tendinous xanthomas. One family had isolated familial hypertriglyceridemia (1%).
Levels of apo A-I and apo B further refined the analysis; five kindreds (4.9%) had elevated apo B as the sole abnormality, and one kindred (1%) had decreased apo A-I only. An additional three (3%) had an unclassifiable lipoprotein disorder. When Lp(a), apo B, and apo A-I were included in the analysis, 55 kindreds (53.9%) manifested a familial lipoprotein disorder, and 6.9% of all kindreds had more then one disorder (Table 2).
There were 20 patients (19.6% with dyslipidemia in whom no familial segregation was observed; these cases were defined as "sporadic" dyslipidemias. In 24 patients (23.5%), no lipid disorder was identified. Thus, of 44 probands with no familial lipoprotein disorder, 20 (43%) had a sporadic dyslipidemia. Ten of these index cases were diabetic. In two, a pattern consistent with FCH was found; in two other subjects, Lp(a) excess was identified; in two additional subjects, sporadic hyperlipoproteinemia was found

(both with low HDL cholesterol); and in the remaining four subjects, no lipoprotein abnormality was identified.

The lipoprotein and apolipoprotein levels in male probands with the most common disorders are shown in Table 4 (there were too few women in each category for meaningful comparison).

Table 4   LIPOPROTEIN CORRELATIONS *

	Total Cholesterol	Tri- glycerides	VLDL	LDL	HDL	Apo B	Apo A-I	Lp(a)†
Parents-offspring	0.271††	0.160	0.134	0.289††	0.284††	0.252††	0.276††	0.614††
Proband-spouse	0.017	0.111	0.087	-0.158	0.127	0.138	0.077	-0.050
Proband-offspring	0.236††	0.146	0.109	0.228	0.255††	0.148	0.137	0.434††
Spouse-offspring	0.285††	0.074	0.090	0.323††	0.174	0.217††	0.130	0.322

*Corrected for age and sex, Z score.
†Not corrected for age and sex.
††$p < 0.005$, $p < 0.05$.

It is noteworthy that patients with FHA as well as those with familial hypertriglyceridemia with hypoalphalipoproteinemia and familial Lp(a) excess had mean total cholesterol levels below 200 mg/dl. Familial Lp(a) excess without other lipoprotein abnormalities occurred in 13 kindreds. In those families, lipoprotein cholesterol levels were not significantly different from those of the control group.

The genetic relations of the various lipid and apolipoprotein parameters were assessed by calculating correlation coefficients for lipid, lipoprotein cholesterol, and apolipoprotein levels in proband offspring, mid-parent-mid-offspring, and spouse-offspring combinations and comparing them with proband-spouse pairs. An index of environmental influence, such as shared household or diet, on lipid parameters can be gleaned from proband- spouse correlations. There was a significantly positive correlation for HDL cholesterol (r=0.127, p<0.05) and apo B (r=0.138, p<0.05) and an inverse correlation for LDL cholesterol (r=0.158, p<0.01) in proband-spouse comparisons. The correlation in triglyceride concentrations between probands and spouses did not reach statistical significance (r=0.111 p>0.05). There was a significant correlation for total cholesterol (r=0.271, p<0.001), triglycerides (r=0.160, p<0.01), very low density lipoprotein (VLDL) cholesterol (r=0.134, p<0.05), LDL cholesterol (r=0.289, p<0.001), HDL cholesterol (r=0.284, p<0.001), apo B (r=0.252, p<0.001), apo A-I (r=0.276, p<0.001), and Lp(a) (r=0.614, p<0.001) between parents and offspring. The correlation coefficients were somewhat less for proband-offspring or spouse-offspring but were still significant for cholesterol, LDL cholesterol, HDL cholesterol, apo B, apo A-I, and Lp(a) (Table 6). There were no significant differences in Lp(a) levels between men and women in the control groups, nor were there significant correlations between age and Lp(a) levels in the control groups (men and women) or in the group of patients with CAD, their spouses, and their relatives.

DISCUSSION
The characterization of most familial lipid disorders has been fraught with difficulties; in FCH, the phenotypic expression of the disease may very between siblings and the proband; FHA has been described frequently, but in many families, elevated triglycerides were present. (30,31). The expression of these lipid disorders may not be evidence until adulthood. The lack of specificity in biochemical or molecular markers for each disorder has added to the difficulty in differentiating patients with various lipoprotein disorders. Plasma apo B or VLDL apo B may be a marker for FCH, whereas elevated LDL apo B may be a marker for a normolipidemic subset of FCH, i.e., familial hyperapobetalipoproteinemia (32). Single-gene disorders leading to extreme levels of lipoproteins are rare and do not account for much of the variability in plasma lipoprotein levels within a populations. These disorders account for a small fraction of lipid disorders within a group of patients with CAD (33). Single-gene effects that lead to moderate variation in lipoprotein parameters remain an important area of investigation. In the present study, the most common disorders are those in which there is combined elevation of apo B- containing particles (VLDL cholesterol, LDL cholesterol, or both), often with decreased HDL cholesterol.

REFERENCES
1.   Slack J, Evans KA: The increased risk of death from ischemic heart disease in first degree relatives of 121 men and 96 women with ischemic heart disease. JMed Genet 1966;3:329
2.   Goldstein JL, Hazzard WR, Schrott WR, Bierman EL, Motulsky AG, Levinski MJ, Campbell ED: Hyperlipidemia in coronary heart disease: I. Lipid levels in 500 survivors of myocardial infarction. J Clin Invest 1973;52:1533-1543
3.   Goldstein JL Schrott HG, Hazzard WR, Bierman EL, Motulsky AG, Campbell ED, Levinski MJ: Hyperlipidemia in coronary heart disease: II. Genetic analysis of lipid levels in 176 families and delineation of a new inherited disorder, combined hyperlipidemia. J Clin Invest 1973;52:1544-1568
4.   Nikkila EA, Aro A: Family study of serum lipids and lipoproteins in coronary heart- disease. Lancet 1973;1:954-958
5.   Rose HG, Kranz P, Weinstock M, Juliano J, Haft JI: Inheritance of combined hyperlipoproteinemia: Evidence for a new lipoprotein phenotype. Am J Med 1973;54:148-160
6.   Vergani C, Bettale G: Familial hypo-alpha-lipoproteinemia. Clin Chim Acta 1981;114:45-5
7.   Martin MJ, Hulley SB, Browner WS, Kuller LH, Wentworth D: Serum cholesterol, blood pressure, and mortality: Implications from a cohort of 361,662 men. Lancet 1986;2:933-936
8.   Castelli WP, Garrison RJ, Wilson PWF, Abbott RD, Kalousdian S, Kannel WB: Incidence of coronary heart disease and lipoprotein cholesterol levels: The Framingham Heart Study. JAMA 1986;256:2835-2838
9.   Papadapoulos NM, Bedynek JL: Serum Lipoprotein patterns in patients with coronary atherosclerosis. Clin Chim Acta 1973;44:153-156
10.   Frick MH, Dahalen G, Berg K, Valle M, Hekali P: Serum lipids in angiographically assessed coronary atherosclerosis. Chest 1978;73:62-65
11.   Sniderman AD, Shapiro S, Marpole D, Skinner B, Teng B, Kwiterovich PO: Association of coronary atherosclerosis with hyperapobetalipoproteinemia. Proc Natl Acad Sci U S A 1980;77:604-608
12.   Maciejko JJ, Holmes DR, Kottke BA, Zinsmeister AR, Dinh DM, Mao SJT: Apolipoprotein A-I as a marker of angiographically assessed coronary-artery disease. N Engl J Med 1983;309:385-389

13. Durrington PN, Hunt L, Ishola M, Kane J, Stephens WP: Serum apolipoproteins AI and B and lipoproteins in middle aged men with and without previous myocardial infarction. Br Heart J 1986;56:206-212

14. Kottke BA, Zinsmeister AR, Holmes DR Jr, Kneller RW, Hallaway BJ, Mao SJT: Apolipoproteins and coronary artery disease. Mayo Clin Proc 1986;61:313-320

15. Dhalen GH, Guyton JR, Attar M, Farmer JA, Kautz JA, Gotto Am Jr: Association of levels of lipoprotein Lp(a), plasma lipids, and other lipoproteins with coronary artery disease documented by angiography. Circulation 1986;74:758-765

16. Murai A, Miyahara T, Fujimoto N, Matsuda M, Kameyama M: Lp(a) lipoprotein as a risk factor for coronary heart disease and cerebral infarction. Atherosclerosis 1986;59:199-204

17. Soria LF, Ludwig EG, CLarke HRG, Vega Gl, Grundy SM, McCarthy BJ: Association between a specific apolipoprotein B mutation and familial defective apolipoprotein B-100. Proc Natl Acad Sci U S A 1989;86:587-591

18. Rall SC Jr, Weisgraber KH, Inneratity TL, Mahely RH: Structural basis for receptor binding heterogeneity of apolipoprotein E from type III hyperlipoproteinemia subjects. Proc Natl Acad Sci U S A 1982;79:4696-4700

19. Karathanasis SK, Ferris E, Haddad IA: DNA inversion within the apolipoproteins AI/CIII/AIV-encoding gene cluster of certain patients with premature atherosclerosis. Proc Natl Acad Sci U S A 1987;847198-7202

20. Ordovas JM, Cassidy DK, Civiera F, Bisgaier CL, Schaefer EJ: Familial apolipoprotein AI, C-III, and A-IV deficiency and premature atherosclerosis due to a deletion of a gene complex on chromosome 11. J Biol Chem 1989;28:16342-16349

21. Russell DW, Esser V, Hobbs HH: Molecular basis of familial hypercholesterolemia. Arteriosclerosis 1989;9(suppl I):I-8-I-13

22. Brown MS, Goldstein JL: A receptor-mediated pathway for cholesterol homeostasis. Science 1986;232:34-47

23. The Lipid Research Clinics: Population Studies Data Book: Vol I: The Prevalence Study. Washington, DC, US Department of Health and Human Services, NIH publication No. 80-1527, 1980

24. McNamara JR, Schaefer EJ: Automated enzymatic stadardized lipid analyses for plasma and lipoprotein fractions. Clin Chim Acta 1987;166:1-8

25. Warnick GR, Benderson J, Albers JJ: Dextran sulfate-Mg^{2+} precipitation procedure for quantitation of high-density lipoprotein cholesterol. Clin Chem 1982;28:1379-1387

26. Friedewald WT, Levy RI, Frederickson DS: Estimation of the concentration of low density lipoprotein cholesterol in plasma without use of the preparative ultracentrifuge. Clin Chem 1972;18:499-502

27. Schaefer EJ, Ordovas JM: Metabolism of apolipoproteins A-I, A-II and A-IV. Meth Enzymol 1986;129:420-443

28. Ordovas JM, Peterson JP, Santaniello P, Cohn JS, Wilson PWF, Schaefer EJ: Enzyme-linked immunosorbent assay for human plasma apolipoprotein B. J Lipid Res 1987;28:1216-1224

29. Frederickson DS, Levy RI, Lees RS: Fat transport in lipoproteins: An integrated approach to mechanisms and disorders. N Engl J Med 1967;276:34-44, 94-103, 215- 225, 273-281

30. Third JLHC, Montag J, Flynn M, Freidal J, Laskarzewski P, Glueck CJ: Primary and familial hypoalphalipoproteinemia. Metabolism 1984;33:136-146

31. Borecki IB, Rao DC, Third JLHC, Laskarzewski PM, Glueck CJ: A major gene for primary hypoalphalipoproteinemia. Am J Hum Genet 1986;38:373-381

32. Brunzell JD, Sniderman AD, Albers JJ, Kwiterovich PO Jr: Apoproteins B and A-I and coronary artery disease in humans. Arteriosclerosis 1984;4:79-83

33. Hopkins PN, Williams RR: Human genetics and coronary heart disease: A public health perspective. Annu Rev Nutr 1989;9:303-345

34. Schaefer EJ, Lery RI, Anderson DW, Danner RN, Brewer HB Jr, Blackwelder WC: Plasma triglycerides in the regulation of HDL. Lancet 1978;2:391-393
35. Chait A, Albers JJ, Brunzell JD: Very low density lipoprotein overproduction in genetic forms of hypertriglyceridemia. Eur J Clin Invest 1980;10:17-22
36. Sane T, Nikkila EA: Very low density lipoprotein triglyceride metabolism in relatives of hypertriglyceridemic probands: Evidence for genetic control of triglyceride removal. Arteriosclerosis 1988;8:217-226
37. Kissebah AH, Alfarsi S, Evans DJ: Low density lipoprotein metabolism in familial combined hyperlipidemia: Mechanisms of the multiple phenotype lipoprotein phenotypic expression. Atherosclerosis 1984;4:614-624
38. Schaefer EJ: Clinical, biochemical, and genetic features in familial disorders of high density lipoprotein deficiency. Arteriosclerosis 1984;4:303-322
39. Grundy SM, Vega GL: Causes of high blood cholesterol. Circulation 1990;81:412-427
40. Utermann G: The mysteries of lipoprotein(a). Science 1989;246:904-910
41. Genest J Jr, Ordovas JM, Robbins AM, Salem DN, Wilson PWF, Masherain U, Frossard PM, Meade T, Cohn S, Schaefer EJ: DNA polymorphisms of the apolipoprotein B gene in patients with premature coronary artery disease. Atherosclerosis 1990;82:7-17
42. Ordovas JM, Civeira F, Genest J Jr, Craig S, Robbins AM, Meade T, Pocovi M, Frossard PM, Masherain U, Wilson PWF, Salem DN, Ward RH, Schaefer EJ: Restriction fragment-length polymorphisms of the apolipoprotein AI-CIII-AIV gene locus, relationships with lipids, apolipoproteins, and premature coronary artery disease. Atherosclerosis 1991;87:75-86
43. Breslow JL: Genetic basis of lipoprotein disorders. J Clin Invest 1989;84:373-380
44. Genest J Jr, McNamara JR, Ordovas JM, Jenner JL, Silberman SR, Anderson KM, Wilson PWF, Salem DN, Schaefer EJ: Lipoprotein cholesterol, apolipoprotein A-I and B, and lipoprotein (a) abnormalities in men with premature coronary artery disease. J Am Coll Cardiol 1992;19:792-802
45. Genest J Jr, McNamara JR, Upson B, Salem DN, Ordovas JM, Schaefer EJ, Malinow MR: Prevalence of familial hyperhomocyst(e)inemia in men with premature coronary artery disease. Arterio Thromb 1991;11:1129-1136
46. Genest J Jr, Corbett HM, McNamara Jr, Schaefer MM, Salem DN, Schaefer EJ: Effect of hospitalization on high-density lipoprotein cholesterol in patients undergoing elective coronary angiography. Am J Cardiol 1986;61:998-1000
47. Genest J Jr, Martin Munley SS, McNamara JR, Ordovas JM, Lerner J, Myers RH, Silberman SR, Wilson PWF, Salem DN, Schaefer EJ: Familial lipoprotein disorders in patients with premature coronary artery disease. Circulation 1992;85:2025-2033

EFFICACY OF FENOFIBRATE ON PLASMA CHOLESTEROL IN SWINE WITH SPONTANEOUS HYPERCHOLESTEROLEMIA

J. RAPACZ, J. HASLER-RAPACZ, A.D. EDGAR

ABSTRACT: Ten pigs, 4 months of age, expressing spontaneous hypercholesterol-emia (SHC), characterized by highly elevated buoyant LDL- and low HDL-cholesterol levels, were fed three different levels of fenofibrate for 56 days (0.5 g from 1-14 days, 1 g from 15-28 days and 2 g from 29-56 days). Mean serum cholesterol for the fenofibrate fed and control groups on day 0 were 280 ± 36 and 272 ± 4 mg/dl; LDL-cholesterol 243 ± 38 and 231 ± 1 mg/dl; HDL-cholesterol 30 ± 6 and 31 ± 4 mg/dl and triglycerides 38 ± 7 and 44 ± 0 mg/dl, respectively. On day 57 total cholesterol was 209 ± 51 and 338 ± 0 mg/dl; LDL-cholesterol 184 ± 50 and 304 ± 0 mg/dl; HDL-cholesterol 19 ± 2 and 25 ± 0 mg/dl and triglycerides 28 ± 4 and 45 ± 0 mg/dl, respectively. This study showed that supplementation of fenofibrate resulted in lowering TC, LDL-C, HDL-C and triglycerides by 39% (p<0.001), 39%, (p<0.001), 22% and 38%, respectively. The most significant finding was revealed by analysis of plasma lipoprotein subfractions, showing a 68% (p<0.001) decrease of cholesterol in the buoyant LDL subfraction, which is known to be atherogenic.

Introduction

Since the introduction of fenofibrate to European clinical practice in 1975, a large number of patients with hyperlipidemias were treated. Cholesterol was lowered by 20-25% in type IIa and IIb patients and triglycerides by 40-60% in type IIb and IV patients. Intake of fenofibrate by patients with high plasma cholesterol levels caused a significant reduction in LDL-cholesterol. In instances where total cholesterol was lower at the baseline, HDL-cholesterol increased (Blane, 1989).

Of laboratory animals, the rat is the most frequently used animal model for testing fibrates. In this species fibrates were effective in lowering plasma cholesterol and occasionally plasma triglyceride concentrations. Results of a recent study in rats by Staels et al. (1992) showed that fenofibrate provoked a dose-dependent decrease in plasma cholesterol, in liver apoA-I and apoA-IV mRNA as well as a decrease in plasma apoA-I, apoA-IV and apoE, whereas plasma apoB increased with feeding very high doses (320 and 190 mg/kg, corresponding to 0.5 and 0.3% of food intake) along with unchanged liver and intestinal apoB mRNA levels. These effects are the opposite of what happens in man, thus the rat is an inappropriate model in which to investigate the mechanism of action of fenofibrate.

375

A. L. Catapano et al. (eds.), Drugs Affecting Lipid Metabolism, 375–382.
© 1993 Kluwer Academic Publishers and Fondazione Giovanni Lorenzini.

Normolipidemic pigs have about one half the cholesterol and one third the
triglyceride levels when compared to humans. We are not aware of any studies that use
swine as a model to study the effect of fenofibrate on plasma lipids or lipoproteins. As
a result of long-term studies on immunogenetically identified LDL polymorphism in
swine (Rapacz, 1978; Rapacz et al. 1978), we have developed a genetic strain that
exhibits spontaneous hypercholesterolemia (IHCL-inherited hyper-LDL-cholesterol-
emia) and slightly elevated triglycerides, when fed a low cholesterol, low fat diet
(Rapacz and Hasler-Rapacz, 1984). The IHLC phenotype, now referred to as
"spontaneous hypercholesterolemia" or SHC, is very complex, showing cholesterol
variations from 130-490 mg/dl and involves at least three alleles (Rapacz et al., 1986).
Low density lipoproteins from IHLC pigs are cholesterol-ester enriched and buoyant
compared to LDL of normolipidemic pigs (Checovich et al., 1988; Lee et al., 1990).
Metabolic and *in vitro* studies revealed that the hypercholesterolemia is accompanied by
defective binding of the buoyant LDL to the LDL receptor, which seems to be
functionally normal, as well as by a defect in LDL catabolism (Checovich et al., 1988;
Lowe et al., 1988). The most recent information shows that the plasma of IHLC pigs
exhibit decreased LCAT activity (Lacko et al., 1992).

Our recent study showed that by 2-4 years of age the SHC pigs develop complicated
atherosclerotic plaques that closely resemble advanced atherosclerotic lesions found in
humans (Prescott et al., 1991), thus the IHLC pig is the first animal model shown to
develop spontaneous hypercholesterolemia and lesions ranging from fatty streaks to
advanced plaques containing necrotic cores, calcification, neovascularization,
hemorrhage and rupture (Rapacz et al., 1986; Prescott et al., 1991). Generally at 3.5
months of age the SHC pigs reach a mean of 300 mg/dl cholesterol level, with high
LDL-cholesterol (>260 mg/dl), found primarily in the buoyant LDL fraction, and with
low HDL-cholesterol (<28 mg/dl). In SHC pigs, apolipoproteinA-I occurs in two
subspecies migrating as α– and pre-β HDL in agarose gel. The ratio of LDL-C : HDL-
C is 10 in the SHC pigs, while in the normolipidemic it is only 2.2. Their diet is low
in fat (<6%) and low in cholesterol (100 mg/day) and they have normal functioning
LDL receptors (Rapacz et al., 1986). For the study reported here we selected pigs at
4.5 months of age when cholesterol levels resemble those of humans that require lipid-
lowering treatment.

Material and Methods

Animals: Pigs used in this study were all hypercholesterolemic obtained from specific
matings and were derived from the Immunogenetic Project Herd, University of
Wisconsin. The herd is routinely lipoprotein phenotyped by 16 apoB, two apoU and
two apo-R epitope-specific alloantibodies (Rapacz, 1978). The experimental animals
were selected on the basis of their apoB and apoU genotypes and total cholesterol
levels. The study included 12 male pigs, of which 10 were fed three different doses of
fenofibrate, mixed with the standard diet, during a 56 day feeding trial. Initially the pigs
were given 500 mg/day of fenofibrate for the first 14 days, followed by 1 gram from
day 15-28, and 2 grams from day 29 to 56. Two pigs served as controls, of which one
had to be eliminated after 31 days due to sickness. All pigs were derived from 4 litters.
Fenofibrate was mixed with 1/4 the amount of the daily ration (2 kg per day) and fed
individually. The animals were treated according to the standards set in "Guide for
Care and Use of Laboratory Animals" (NIH publication No. 85-23). Animals were
fasted overnight and blood was collected prior to feeding at day 0 and every 2-3 days
during the feeding trial.

Since plasma of the SHC pigs is characterized by elevated buoyant LDL-cholesterol and apolipoprotein-B, the plasma of all pigs was separated into 5 lipoprotein subfractions (Ly1-5) by density gradient ultracentrifugation (Lee and Downs, 1986; Lee et al., 1990) with density of d <1.019 g/ml for layer-1; d 1.021-1.028 g/ml for layer-2; d 1.032-1.043 g/ml for layer-3; d 1.054-1.073 g/ml for layer-4 and d >1.073 g/ml for layer-5. Layers 2, 3 and 4 represent low density lipoproteins.

Lipid measurements: Total cholesterol, HDL-cholesterol and triglyceride concentrations in serum and plasma subfractions were measured by enzymatic techniques using Sigma Diagnostic Kits (Sigma, St. Louis, MO); LDL-cholesterol was estimated according to Friedewald (1972);
LDL-cholesterol = total cholesterol - HDL-cholesterol - triglycerides/5.

Results

Serum total cholesterol concentrations in both the fenofibrate fed and control groups during the 56 day feeding trial are shown in figure 1. On day 0 the experimental group had a mean value of 280 ± 36 mg/dl and the control group 272 ± 4.0 mg/dl. The first significant decrease in cholesterol was observed after 4 days (p<0.05). On day 56 the experimental group had a plasma cholesterol of 209 ± 51 mg/dl and the control group 338 ± 0 mg/dl.

Figure 2 shows the LDL-cholesterol levels during 56 days of feeding fenofibrate and patterns are very similar to that of total cholesterol. On day 0 the experimental group had a mean value of 243 ± 38 mg/dl and the control group 231 ± 1 mg/dl. Again the first significant decrease in LDL-cholesterol was observed on day 4 (p<0.05). On day 56 the experimental group had a LDL-cholesterol of 184 ± 50 mg/dl and 304 ± 0 mg/dl for the control.

The HDL-cholesterol patterns are shown in Figure 3. On day 0 the experimental group had a mean value of 30 ± 6 mg/dl and the control group 31 ± 4 mg/dl. On day 56 the mean values were 19 ± 2 mg/dl and 25 ± 0 mg/dl for the experimental and control groups, respectively. Fenofibrate lowered HDL-cholesterol, reaching significant lower levels (*p*<0.05) on day 8, which lasted until day 52 of feeding.

The effect of fenofibrate on triglycerides are shown in Figure 4. The mean values on day 0 were 38 ± 6 mg/dl and 44 ± 0 mg/dl and on day 56 they were 28 ± 4 mg/dl and 45 ± 0 mg/dl, respectively. There were variations, up and down with a decreasing trend in the experimental but not in the control pigs. A significant difference (*p*<0.01) between the groups was found at 4 days of feeding and also at the last bleeding.

Figure 5 shows the combined data from plasma and layers on the effect of fenofibrate on total cholesterol, LDL-cholesterol, HDL-cholesterol and triglycerides and on cholesterol in the 5 lipoprotein subfractions. The most dramatic decrease of cholesterol was observed in total and low density lipoprotein cholesterol and especially in the most buoyant subfraction of LDL (Layer-2).

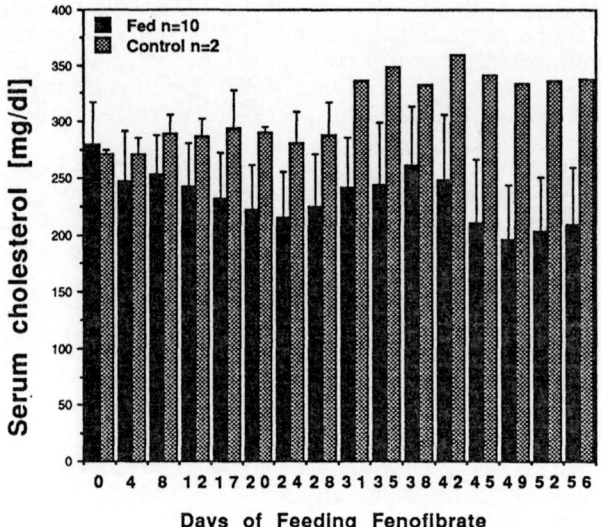

Figure 1. Efficacy of fenofibrate on changes of mean total serum cholesterol in pigs with spontaneous hypercholesterolemia.

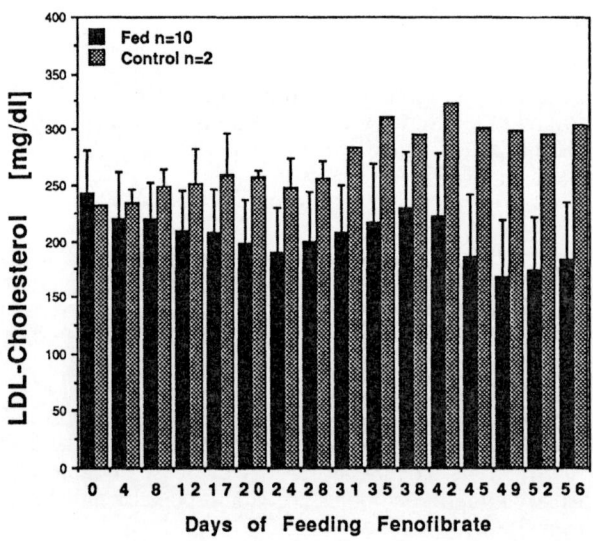

Figure 2. Efficacy of fenofibrate on changes of mean LDL-cholesterol in pigs with spontaneous hypercholesterolemia.

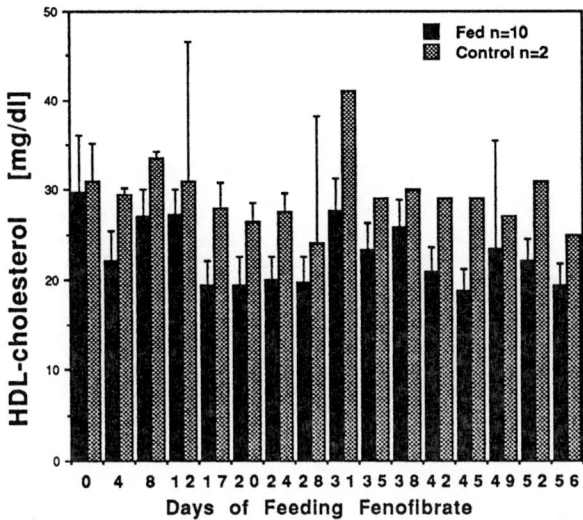

Figure 3. Efficacy of fenofibrate on changes in mean HDL-cholesterol in pigs with spontaneous hypercholesterolemia.

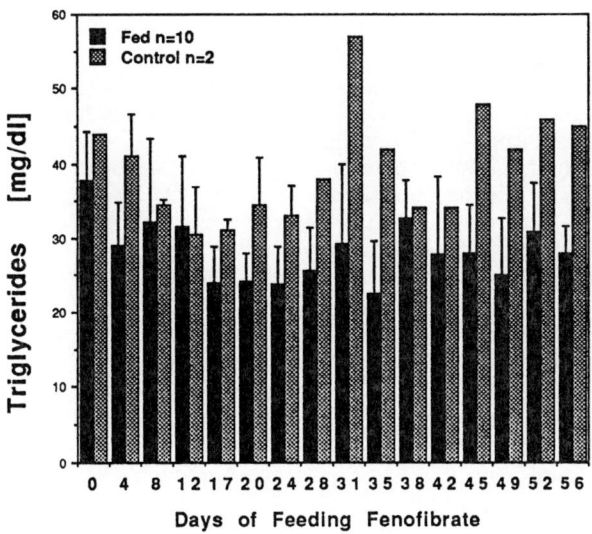

Figure 4. Efficacy of fenofibrate on changes of mean triglycerides in pigs with spontaneous hypercholesterolemia.

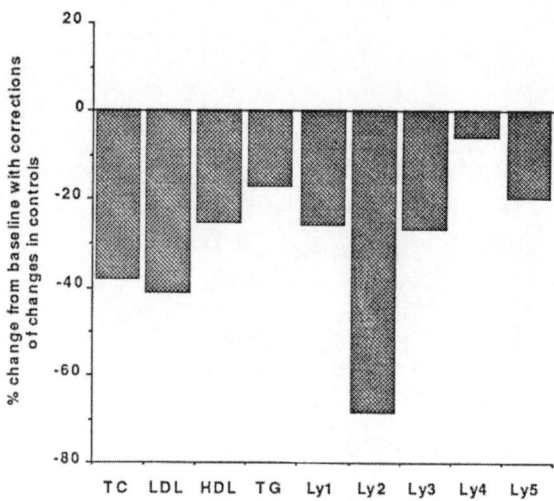

Figure 5. Effects of fenofibrate on lipids in plasma and lipoprotein subfractions (Ly1-5) in swine exhibiting spontaneous hypercholesterolemia.

Discussion

Our studies represent the first reported investigations in swine on the effect of fenofibrate on plasma lipid concentrations. The results are favorable regarding total cholesterol, LDL-cholesterol and triglycerides and comparable to humans with elevated cholesterol (Balfour et al., 1990). Unfavorable was the effect on HDL-cholesterol, which is small in comparison to other species, especially rats (Staels et al., 1992). In our pigs with spontaneous hypercholesterolemia the average cholesterol level is at least three-fold higher than in normolipidemic swine (300 vs 100 mg/dl). With this range in humans there is no effect of fenofibrate on lowering HDL-cholesterol (Balfour et al., 1990). It may be that in pigs with plasma cholesterol between 150-200 mg/dl, fenofibrate may have the same effect on HDL-C, as was observed in humans. Furthermore, the decrease in HDL-cholesterol is commonly observed in animals with low cholesterol transfer protein (CETP) (unpublished observations). We cannot exclude a possibility that in this strain of pigs where apolipoprotein A-I and the LCAT activity are lower than in normal pigs, and the pre-β-HDL (HDL3) to α–HDL ratio is higher than in humans with hypercholesterolemia (Ishida et al., 1987), there is a defective conversion of pre-β–HDL (HDL3) into α-HDL (HDL2), which may reflect on the response to fenofibrate. We recently have obtained, by specific matings of the SHC strain, several animals that have HDL-cholesterol > 40 mg/dl; however, these animals have not yet been challenged with fenofibrate.

In this first study, the most positive observation seems to be in the effect of fenofibrate on the change of the cholesterol profile in the LDL subfractions, showing a highly favorable effect on lowering the most buoyant LDL by 68%. This change in the LDL cholesterol profile, from highly abnormal to almost normolipidemic, with a shift to the intermediate LDL density is highly significant. This is an important phenomenon since in this model we demonstrated that the buoyant LDL is associated with the severity of atherosclerosis in pigs (Rapacz et al., 1986). With the exception of the decrease in HDL, which may be related to CETP activity, the effects of fenofibrate in SHC swine mirrors the results obtained in clinical use of the drug, making this an appropriate model in which to explore the mechanism of action of this drug and possibly other lipid-lowering drugs.

Acknowledgements

We appreciate the help of Buell and Gordon Gunderson for feeding and Zhi-Liang Hu for bleeding the animals. We thank J. Busby for typing and editing the manuscript. The research was supported in part by the College of Agricultural and Life Sciences, University of Wisconsin, Madison, WI, U.S.A., and Fournier Laboratories, S.A., Daix, France.

References

Balfour, J.A. (1990) 'Fenofibrate: A review of its pharmacodynamic and pharmacokinetic properties and therapeutic use in dyslipidemia', Drugs 40, 260-290.

Blane, G.F. (1989) 'Review of European clinical experience with fenofibrate' in R.I. Levy (ed.), A New Era of Lipid-Lowering Drug Alternatives, Cardiology 76 (suppl.1):1-13.

Checovich, W.J., Fitch, W.L., Krauss, R.M., Smith, M.P., Rapacz, J., Smith, C.L. and Attie, A.D. (1988) 'Defective catabolism and abnormal composition of low density lipoproteins from mutant pigs with hypercholesterolemia', Biochemistry 27, 1934-1941.

Friedewald, W.T., Levy , R.I. and Fredrickson, D.S. (1972) 'Estimation of the concentrations of low-density lipoprotein cholesterol in plasma without use of the preparative ultracentrifuge'. Clinical Chemistry 18, 499-502.

Ishida, B.Y., Frohlich, J. and Fielding, C.J. (1987) 'Prebeta-migrating high density lipoprotein: quantitation in normal and hyperlipidemic plasma by solid phase radioimmunoassay following electrophoretic transfer', J. Lipid Research 28, 778-786.

Lacko, A.G., Lee, S-M., Mirshahi, I., Hasler-Rapacz, J., Kudchodkar, B.J. and Rapacz, J. (1992) 'Decreased activity of lecithin:cholesterol acyltransferase in the plasma of hypercholesterolemic pigs', Lipids 27, 4, 266-269.

Lee D.M. and Downs, D. (1982) 'A quick and large-scale density gradient subfractionation method for low density lipoproteins'. J. Lipid Research 23, 14-27.

Lee, D.M., Mok, T., Hasler-Rapacz, J. and Rapacz, J. (1990) 'Concentrations and compositions of plasma lipoprotein subfractions of Lpb^5-Lpu^1 homozygous and heterozygous swine with hypercholesterolemia'. J. Lipid Research 31, 839-847.

Lowe, S.W., Checovich, W.J., Rapacz, J. and Attie, A.D. (1988) 'Defective receptor binding of low density lipoproteins from pigs possessing mutant Apolipoprotein B alleles'. J. Biological Chemistry. 263.30, 15467-15473

Prescott, M.F., McBride, C.H., Hasler-Rapacz, J., Von Linden, J. and Rapacz, J. (1991) 'Development of complex atherosclerotic lesions in pigs with inherited hyper-LDL cholesterolemia (IHLC) bearing mutant alleles for apolipoprotein B'. American Journal of Pathology 139, 139-147.

Rapacz, J. (1978) 'Lipoprotein immunogenetics and atherosclerosis', American Journal Medical Genetics 1:377-405.

Rapacz, J., Hasler-Rapacz, J. and Kuo, W.H. (1978) Immunogenetic polymorphism of lipoproteins in swine. 2. Five new allotypic specificities (Lpp^6, Lpp^{11}, Lpp^{12}, Lpp^{13} and Lpp^{14}) in the Lpp system. Immunogenetics 6, 405-424.

Rapacz, J. and Hasler-Rapacz, J. (1984) 'Investigations on the relationship between immunogenetic polymorphism of ·β–lipoproteins and the ·β-lipoprotein and cholesterol levels in swine', in S. Lenzi and G.D. Descovich (eds.), Atherosclerosis & Cardiovascular Diseases, Editrice Composition, Bologna, Italy, pp. 99-108.

Rapacz, J., Hasler-Rapacz, J., Taylor, K.M., Checovich, W.J. and Attie, A.D. (1986) 'Lipoprotein mutations in pigs are associated with elevated plasma cholesterol and atherosclerosis', Science 234, 1573-1577.

Staels, B., van Tol, A., Andreu, T. and Auwerx, J. (1992) 'Fibrates influence the expression of genes involved in lipoprotein metabolism in a tissue-selective manner in the rat', Arteriosclerosis and Thrombosis 12, 286-294.

LIPOPROTEIN PARTICLES HETEROGENEITY : CLINICAL AND PHARMACOLOGICAL IMPLICATION

J. C. FRUCHART

Although an increase in the number of LDL particles, as seen in familial hypercholesterolemia or hyperapobetalipoproteinemia, is strongly associated with the development of CAD (1, 2), elevations of triglyceride-rich lipoproteins (TRL) have not been established clearly as a cardiovascular risk factor in prospective studies. However, in case-control studies, triglycerides are often, on univariate analysis, a risk factor for the presence of CAD (3). The heterogeneity within TRL and the different metabolic fates of the various TRL particles may, in part, explain those findings.

It has been demonstrated previously that apo B-containing lipoproteins consist of four major lipoprotein families, those containing only apo B (Lp B), those containing apo B and apo C (Lp B:C), those containing apo B and apo E (Lp B:E), and those containing all of these three apolipoproteins (Lp B:C:E) (4).
All those lipoproteins are distributed throughout the entire density spectrum. Although the major part of Lp B occurs in LDL, this lipoprotein particle has also been detected in very low density (VLDL) and intermediate density-lipoproteins (IDL) (5). Lp B:C and Lp B:C:E represent the major component of VLDL and IDL but may also be present in significant amounts in LDL. Lp B appears to be cholesteryl ester-rich while the complex particles seem to be enriched in triglycerides. In the latter, the apo C and apo E content decreases with increasing densities (6).
The binding properties of these lipoproteins toward the LDL receptor appears to be very much dependent on the apolipoprotein composition. Apo E with phenotype E3 and E4 increases the affinity of the particle for the LDL receptor but decreases the apparent number of binding sites. In contrast, Lp B:E isolated from subjects bearing the E2/E2 phenotype do not bind to the receptor, indicating that Lp B:E isolated from subjects bearing the E3 and/or E4 phenotypes bind to the receptor through apo E and not apo B. These results suggest that apo E may mask the receptor binding site of apo B. Also, Lp B:C-III, free of apo E, do not bind to the receptor (7).

A recent work indicating that C apolipoproteins are located near residue 3249 of apolipoprotein B100 on VLDL suggests that apo C-III may impair the binding probably by the same mechanism as we hypothesized for apo E (8).

An enzyme-linked immunosorbent assay (ELISA) method has been recently described for the measurement of Lp B:C-III and Lp B:E. in this procedure, lipoproteins containing apo C-III or apo E are retained on a microtiter plate coated with a polyclonal

A. L. Catapano et al. (eds.), Drugs Affecting Lipid Metabolism, 383–389.

antibody recognizing apo C-III or apo E. In a second step, an antibody raised against apo B and labeled with peroxidase allows the quantification of lipoproteins containing both C-III or E and apo B (6).

We have studied the distribution of Lp B:C-III and Lp B:E among lipoprotein density classes. Lp B:C-III and Lp B:E were found in all major lipoprotein density classes. The distribution of Lp B:C-III seems to be uniform across density classes. However, this particle mainly accumulated in VLDL of hypertriglyceridemic subjects and represents 92% of apo B (6).

The highest concentration of Lp B:E for the three analysed groups, was found in VLDL, and this concentration decreased with increasing density. Most apo B, if not all, in normolipidemic VLDL was bound to apo E and 45% to apo C-III, suggesting the existence of a least two apo B containing particles : Lp B:E:C-III and Lp B:E. In the latter, apo B represents 55% of VLDL apo B. In hypertriglyceridemic VLDL, most apo B was bound to both apo E and apo C-III.

Although, the distribution of Lp C-III:B and Lp B:E across the density classes was different, the percentage of apo B bound to apo C-III and apo B bound to apo E decreases with increasing density (with the exception in the HDL), generating the simple form of apo B (Lp B) (6).

Comparisons of apo B containing particles, between normolipidemic and hyperlipidemic subjects show significantly elevated plasma concentrations of both Lp C-III:B and Lp B:E in all hyperlipidemic groups.

Hypercholesterolemic patients have higher levels of apo B, Lp B:C-III and Lp B:E and slightly elevated levels of apo C-III and apo E. However, it was interesting to note the elevated amount of apo B without apo C-III and without apo E. Thus the significant increase of apo B levels in hypercholesterolemic patients could reflect the increase of Lp B, a simple lipoprotein characterized by the presence of apo B as sole apolipoprotein constituent (6).

Patients with hypertriglyceridemia have an elevated level of apo B, apo C-III, apo E, Lp C-III:B and Lp B:E, but apo B without apo E and without apo C-III concentrations remain normal, indicating that the increased concentration of total apo B was due to the accumulation in the plasma of Lp C-III:B and Lp B:E (6).

Type III hyperlipoproteinemia is characterized by significantly higher levels of Lp B:E. Apo B for these patients was mainly associated with apo E ; about 59% of total apo B (ranging between 30% and 92%) (9).

We assessed Lp B:C-III and Lp B:E in 145 men with angiographically diagnosed coronary artery disease (3). Patients with CAD had higher triglyceride, apo B, Lp B:E levels than controls but no significant differences were observed for Lp B:C-III. A case control study of triglyceride rich particles in three populations with contrasting risks for CAD confirmed that Lp B:E concentration in CAD patients is higher than in controls for the three populations. Morever, while similar levels of triglycerides and VLDL cholesterol were observed in the groups, Lp B:E values were higher in Belfast than in the French centers. These results could explain in part the large excess of cases observed in Northern Ireland as compared to France (Table 1) (10).

Lipid parameters in the different groups of the ECTIM study
- subjects treated with hypolipidemic drugs excluded -

	N Ireland		France		Tests of Differences*		
	Cases (n=109)	Controls (n=180)	Cases (n=224)	Controls (n=432)	Cases vs Controls	N Ireland vs France	Interaction
	means (SD) (mg/100ml)				F values and significance		
VLDL Cholesterol	34.5 (14.5)	27.5 (15.9)	26.4 (15.7)	25.8 (16.5)	12[b]	29[c]	8[a]
Triglycerides	199.5 (87.1)	159.0 (88.9)	159.4 (77.0)	153.1 (83.1)	14[c]	24[c]	7[a]
Lp C-III:B	23. 4(15.5)	17.8 (15.9)	17.7 (13.0)	16.1 (13.3)	11[b]	23[c]	-
Lp E:B	56.0 (28.9)	48.2 (32.5)	45.2 (26.0)	39.6 (25.4)	12[b]	35[c]	-

* Two way analysis of covariance. The tests are adjusted on age, BMI, cigarettes and alcohol consumption.
- : non significant ; a : $p < 0.01$; b : $p < 0.001$; c : $p < 0.0001$.

Considering the preliminary results obtained in clinical and epidemiological studies, it is obviously interesting to study the effect of drug therapy on lipoprotein particles defined by their apolipoprotein composition. Two main questions may be raised concerning the effect of drugs : (1) Do compounds with various mechanisms of action lead to different effect on apo B-containing particles ? (2) Is there any relationship between the pharmacological modulation of a particular lipoprotein family and the change in cardiovascular morbidity and mortality ? We now have some information to answer the former but further investigation is certainly needed to answer the latter.

We did a study comparing the effects of fenofibrate and simvastatin in primary hypercholesterolemia, with particular regard to lipoprotein particles, Lp E:B, Lp C-III:B (11) (figure 1 and 2). This was a double-blind study in which patients were randomized to 2 groups, one receiving simvastatin 20 mg once daily and the other receiving fenofibrate 200 mg b.i.d., if their total cholesterol and their LDL cholesterol remained above 7.60 mmol/l (300 mg/dl) and 4.95 mmol/l (195 mg/dl) after a 4-week placebo period. Simvastatin dosage was doubled at the end of 6 weeks of therapy if the LDL-cholesterol level remained above 3.55 mmol/l (140 mg/dl). Analyses were done after 6 and 10 weeks of therapy.

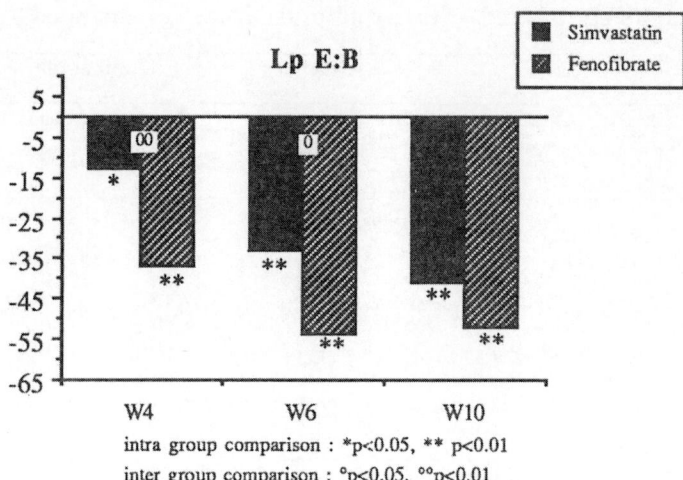

intra group comparison : *p<0.05, ** p<0.01
inter group comparison : °p<0.05, °°p<0.01

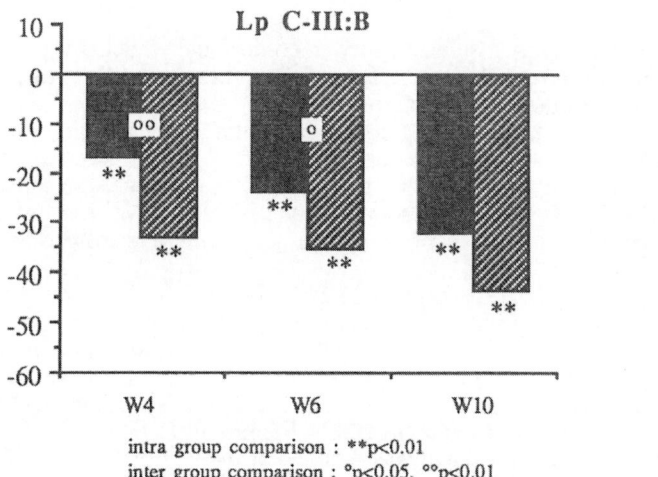

intra group comparison : **p<0.01
inter group comparison : °p<0.05, °°p<0.01

Figure 1 : Changes in apo B-containing lipoprotein particles on simvastatin or fenofibrate therapy

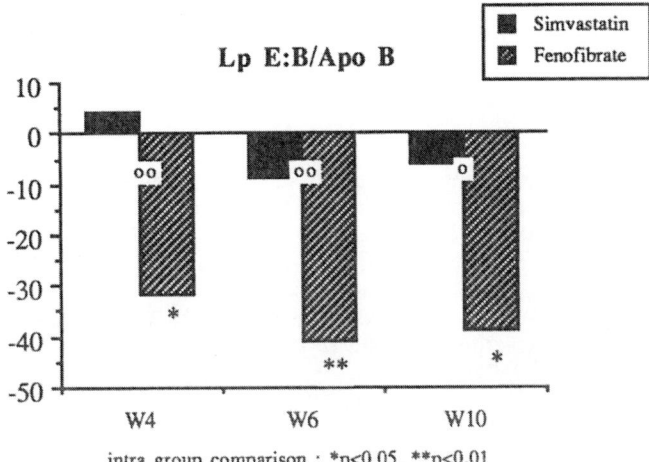

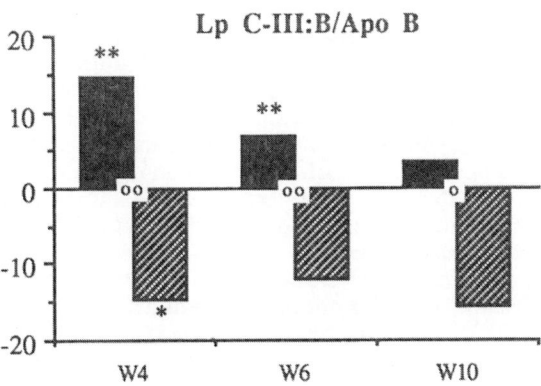

Figure 2 : Changes in the ratios between Lp E:B or Lp C-III:B and total apo B on
simvastatin or fenofibrate therapy

Simvastatin had a more pronounced effect than fenofibrate on apolipoprotein B. Lp E:B (-33.0 and -40.8% with simvastatin ; -53.8 and -52.2% with fenofibrate) and Lp C-III:B (-23.8 and -31.8M with simvastatin ; -35.1 and -43.5% with fenofibrate) were decreased by both drugs, but fenofibrate was significantly more effective in reducing these particles than simvastatin at week 6.

The decrease in apolipoprotein B may be easily related to the activation of the receptor-specific pathway, which leads to an increased catabolism of apo B-containing lipoproteins. The better effect of simvastatin on this parameter when compared with fenofibrate may reflect a more pronounced activation of this pathway with the former than with the latter. Since higher apolipoprotein B levels have been reported in patients with coronary artery disease, this apolipoprotein-B-lowering effect suggests that both drugs may demonstrate some antiatherogenic properties.

However, apolipoprotein-B-containing particles may be grossly distinguished in Lp B:E, containing both apo B and apo E, but free of apo C-III ; Lp B:C-III, containing both apo B and C-III, but free of apo E ; and Lp B:C-III:E, containing alle these 3 apolipoproteins. It should be kept in mind that our methodology measures the pool of particles containing both apo B and apo E (Lp B:E), or both apo C-III and apo B (Lp B:C-III). Activation of the receptor-specific pathway through the depletion of the cellular content may lead to an accelareted clearance of Lp B:C-III:E and Lp B:E. Since we have already shown that Lp B:C-III does not bind to the receptor, the increased receptor activity should not change the Lp B:C-III level. Thus, with our quantification method, the activation of the receptor pathway should lead to a decrease in Lp E:B and, to a lesser extent, in Lp C-III:B. Nevertheless, these tendencies could be potentiated by the inhibition of synthesis inhibition. The combination of these two phenomena may probably explain the effects of both drugs on Lp E:B and Lp C-III:B. In addition, fenofibrate activates the lipolytic system and this could be a third way to decrease the number of these complex apo B-containing particles. Thus, the combination of these three mechanisms probably explains why fenofibrate has a more pronounced effect on these particles than simvastatin. The hypothesis that simvastatin acts basically on apo B-containing particles through receptor activation and inhibition of synthesis seems to be reinforced by the increase in the ratio Lp B:C-III/apo B, while the ratio Lp B:E/apo B does not change. This fits perfectly with the hypothesis that activation of the receptor pathway would lead to a decrease in Lp E:B and, to a lesser extent, in Lp C-III:B. In contrast, if fenofibrate decreases these particles through the combination of the three mechanisms described above, it is logical to observe a decrease in both ratios with this drug.

REFERENCES

1   Anderson, K.M., Castelli, W.P. and Levy, D. (1987) "Cholesterol and mortality. 30 years of follow-up from the Framingham Heart Study", J. Am. Med. Assoc. 257, 2176.

2   Sniderman, A., Shapiro, S., Marpole, D., Skinner, B., Teng, B. and Kwiterovich, P.O. (1980) "Association of coronary atherosclerosis with hyperapobetalipoproteinemia. Increased protein but normal cholesterol levels in human plasma low density lipoproteins", Proc. Natl. Acad. Sci. USA 77, 604.

3   Genest Jr, J.J., Bard, J.M., Fruchart, J.C., Ordovas, J.M., Wilson, P.F.W. and Schaefer, E.J. (1991) "Plasma apolipoprotein A-I, A-II, B, E and C-III containing particles in men with premature coronary artery disease", Atherosclerosis 90, 149-157.

4   Alaupovic, P., McConathy, W.J., Fesmire, J., Tavella, M. and Bard, J.M. (1988) "Profiles of apolipoproteins and apolipoprotein B containing lipoprotein particles in dyslipidemia", Clin. Chem. 34, B13.

5   Bard, J.M., Candelier, L., Agnani, G., Clavey, V., Torpier, G., Steinmetz, A. and Fruchart, J.C. (1991) "Isolation oand characterization of human Lp B lipoprotein containing apolipoprotein B as the sole apolipoprotein", Biochim. Biophys. Acta 1082, 170-176.

6   Kandoussi, A., Cachera, C., Parsy, D., Bard, J.M. and Fruchart, J.C. (1991) "Quantitative determination of different apolipoprotein B containing lipoproteins by an enzyme linked immunosorbent assay : apo B with apo C-III and apo B with apo E", J. Immunoassay 12 (3), 305-323.

7   Agnani, G., Bard, J.M., Candelier, L., Delattre, S., Fruchart, J.C. and Clavey, V. (1991) "Interaction of Lp B, Lp B:E, Lp B:C-III and Lp B:C-III:E lipoproteinbs with the low density lipoprotein receptor on HeLa cells", Arteriosclerosis 11/4, 1021-1029.

8   Yang, C.Y., Lee, B., Yang, M., Guyton, J.R., Fruchart, J.C., Gotto, A.M. (1992) "Structure of human very low density lipoprotein (VLDL) subfractions : C apolipoproteins are located near residue 3249 of apolipoprotein B100 on VLDL", 59th European Atherosclerosis Society Congress, Nice, 17-21 May.

9   Lussier-Cacan, S., Bard, J.M., Boulet, L., Nestruck, A.C., Grothé, A.M., Fruchart, J.C. and Davignon, J. (1989) "Lipoprotein composition changes induced by fenofibrate in dysbetalipoproteinemia type III", Atherosclerosis 78, 167-182.

10   Parra, H.J., Arveiler, D., Evans, A.E., Cambou, J.P., Bingham, D., McMaster, P., Schaffer, P., Douste-Blazy, P., Luc, G., Ducimetière P., fruchart, J.C. and Cambien, F (1992) "A case control study of lipoprotein particles in two populations at contrasting risk for coronary heart disease : the ECTIM study", Arteriosclerosis and Thromb. accepted for publication.

11   Bard, J.M., Parra, H.J., Luc, G., Camare, R., Ziegler, O., Dachet, C., Bruckert, E., Douste-Blazy, P., Drouin, P., Jacotot, B., De Gennes, J.L., Keller, U. and Fruchart, J.C. (1991) "Lipoprotein particle analysis comparing simvastatin and fenofibrate", Atherosclerosis 91, S29-S34.

FIBRINOGEN:
PATHOGENETICAL AND THERAPEUTICAL IMPLICATIONS IN ATHEROSCLEROSIS

Matthias **LESCHKE**, MD, Mathias M. **Borst**, MD, Oliver **Rabenau**, MD,
Frank C. **Schoebel**, MD, Bodo E. **Strauer**, MD, FESC

ABSTRACT

In the pathogenesis of atherosclerosis, fibrinogen as the predominant
clotting factor exerts its atherogenous effects through hemostatic and
additional effects of blood flow. According to several epidemiologic
studies fibrinogen has to be considered as a primary coronary risk
factor comparable with other established risk factors, such as
arterial hypertension and cholesterol. In patients with coronary
artery disease, significantly elevated fibrinogen levels are found.
Hyperfibrinogenemia can critically limit coronary blood flow in
microcirculation due to fibrinogen-dependent increase in plasma
viscosity and red-blood-cell aggregation. The importance of fibrinogen
in microcirculatory blood flow can be demonstrated by the benefits of
a reduction of plasma fibrinogen by fibrate therapy, e.g. fenofibrate
treatment, LDL-cholesterol apheresis and a "chronically intermittent
i/v urokinase therapy" in therapy-refractory patients with severe
coronary artery disease.

A. L. Catapano et al. (eds.), Drugs Affecting Lipid Metabolism, 391–398.
© 1993 Kluwer Academic Publishers and Fondazione Giovanni Lorenzini.

INTRODUCTION

It is a well-established fact that apart from other factors, blood
flow, clotting factors and lipid infiltration are important in the
pathogenesis of atherosclerosis and its clinical complications.
Fibrinogen exerts its atherogenous effects as a predominant clotting
factor as well as a limiting factor in rheological blood flow
characteristics. Furthermore, fibrinogen is involved in acute and
chronic phase reactions which contribute to the development of
atherosclerosis [17]. By focussing on the pathogenetic role of
fibrinogen in the development of coronary artery disease, it is shown
in the first part of this paper by which acute and chronic mechanisms
fibrinogen is thought to contribute to atherogenesis. Interestingly,
the effect of fibrinogen on microcirculatory blood flow in myocardial
ischemia has been realized only after successful treatment of
hyperfibrinogenemia. Therefore, in the second part currently available
therapeutical options of influencing elevated levels of fibrinogen are
discussed.

Fibrinogen as coronary risk factor

Like other measurable variables associated with an increased incidence
of coronary artery disease plasma fibrinogen levels vary from time to
time even in healthy subjects. It responds to physiological changes

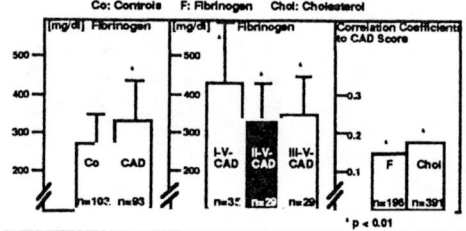

Figure 1: Fibrinogen levels in coronary artery disease (CAD) classified
          into I-vessel, II-vessel, and III-vessel CAD

(pregnancy, stress and varying thyroid activity) and also to injury,
inflammation, malignant disease and acute as well as chronic phase
reactions [17]. As demonstrated in Figure 1 patients with
angiographically documented coronary artery disease have significantly
increased fibrinogen levels as compared to normal controls. Using the
coronary score system of the American Heart Association [1] to
quantify the severity of atherosclerotic lesions in the coronary
system we found nearly almost identical correlation coefficients for
plasma fibrinogen and total serum cholesterol in relationship to the
severity of coronary artery disease [8]. However, it remained to be
established, whether elevated fibrinogen levels are a primary
pathogenetic factor or represent an phenomenon secondary to the
atherosclerotic process in coronary artery disease.

Epidemiological evidence for the role of fibrinogen as a primary risk
factor was provided by the Framingham Study [6]. Data collected
prospectively over a period of 12 years demonstrate a fourfold higher
risk of cardiovascular events in patients with the highest plasma
fibrinogen levels independently of age and other coronary risk
factors. Similar results were obtained by **Meade** et al. [12] in the
"Northwick Park Heart Study", where high fibrinogen levels at the time
of study recruitment correlate with the incidence of cardiovascular
death.

There is strong biochemical evidence for the pathogenetic role of
fibrinogen in the early stages of atherosclerosis. Fibrinogen
facilitates the migration of smooth muscle cells from the media to the
intima of the arterial wall and tends to induce smooth muscle cell
proliferation int he subendothelial layer [13].

Apart from the evidence for hyperfibrinogenemia as a primary coronary
risk factor it is well known that fibrinogen is elevated in states of
chronic inflammation [17]. States of inflammation are triggered by
leucocyte activation, release of mediator substances such als
interleukines, and prostaglandines. These pathogenetic mechanisms of
chronic inflammation are also effective in atherosclerosis [5] and
appear to be activated in chronic cigarette smoking and diabetes [17].
Both are established as primary risk factors for atherosclerosis [2].
Therefore, the hyperfibrinogenemia could be partly a process secondary
to smoking and diabetes mellitus as well as a primary risk factor.

Fibrinogen and blood viscosity

Fibrinogen is one of the main determinants of blood rheology apart
from other acute-phase proteins and high levels of lipoproteins [11].
High levels of fibrinogen lead to elevated plasma viscosity and an
increased tendency of red blood cell to aggregate (Fig. 2). Both of
these factors may result in microcirculatory flow retardation. As a
result of a vicious circle of flow retardation, increased
red-blood-cell aggregation and increased blood viscosity
microcirculatory flow is markedly impaired [15].

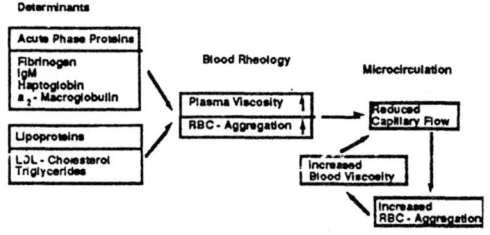

Figure 2: Fibrinogen and blood viscosity

The underlying pathogenetic concept of this mechanism is explained by the law of **Hagen-Poiseuille**. This equation describes the relation of coronary resistance, vessel geometry and blood viscosity. Since an inverse relationship exists for coronary resistance and for the fourth power of the vessel radius, blood viscosity is the limiting factor for blood flow in stenosing coronary artery disease. The pathogenetic concept of hyperfibrinogenemia and its role in elevated blood viscosity in the manifestation of myocardial ischemia is supported by a new therapeutic approach to improve myocardial perfusion by decreasing fibrinogen levels in coronary artery disease [7, 9, 10].

Therapeutical options of lowering fibrinogen levels

In contrast to hyperlipidemia, where diet is efficient in normalizing lipid disorders, dietary efforts have no long-term effect on elevated fibrinogen levels. This may be a reason of the limited benefit of diet modification with regard to the incidence of CAD in the population. The therapeutical goal of treating hyperfibrinogenemia in coronary artery disease is to improve myocardial blood flow acutely and to prevent further progression of CAD or possibly to achieve a regression of atherosclerotic lesions. However, there is only a limited number of pharmacological options to decrease elevated fibrinogen levels.

(1) The oral therapy with certain lipid reducing substance, e.g., fibrate derivates, (2) the "chronically intermittent urokinase therapy" in patients with severe coronary artery disease, therapy-refractory angina and (3) the HELP-therapy (heparin-induced extracorporal precipitation of fibrinogen and cholesterol) in hyperlipidemia and severe atherosclerosis [16].

Fibrate derivates

A number of different agents modify plasma fibrinogen levels in humans. All these agents also lower free fatty acid levels. Evaluation of agents - especially the fibrate derivates - has focussed primarily on their antilipidemic properties, while their fibrinogen-lowering activity has been recognized later. The ability of many fibrate derivates to reduce plasma fibrinogen levels by about 15-20% has been confirmed in many clinical studies in the last years [3, 14].

The principal difficulty in interpreting these drug effects is due to the fact that plasma fibrinogen reductions were often small, the intraindividual fluctuations of plasma fibrinogen levels are often rather high, and the patient collectives were inhomogeneous. Furthermore, it could not be discovered whether the observed effects on fibrinogen were secondary to some other drug effects, e.g. on inflammatory processes or on the underlying disease.

In our study with fenofibrate, 35 patients with coronary artery
disease, hyperfibrinogenemia and hyperlipidemia were enrolled [9]. All
patients received 250 mg fenofibrate per day in a retarded form for
the duration of eight weeks. During treatment antianginal therapy and
diet habits remained unchanged. Secondary to a decrease of fibrinogen
levels by about 17%, plasma viscosity and red-blood-cell aggregation
were significantly reduced (Fig. 3). In 12 of the patients, a
myocardial perfusion scan before and after fenofibrate therapy was
performed.

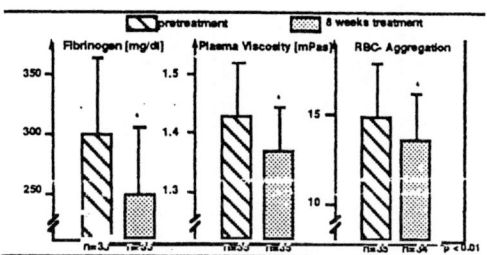

Figure 3:   Fibrinogen, plasma viscosity and red blood cell
            (RBC)-aggregation under fenofibrate

In two patients, we observed a significant global improvement, in six
patients, a regional improvement of myocardial perfusion. The four
patients without demonstrable perfusion improvement presented no
changes in their rheological parameters and in their exercise
tolerance after fenofibrate therapy. These data show that a lipid
lowering therapy with an effect on fibrinogen levels can improve
myocardial ischemia in coronary artery disease with disturbed
microcirculation due to hyperfibrinogenemia and hyperlipoproteinemia.

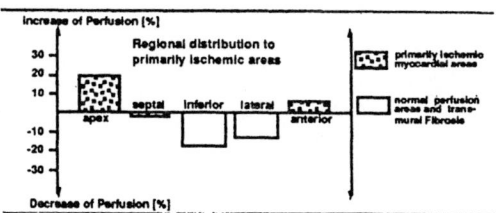

Figure 4:   Percentage changes of regional myocardial perfusion after
            8 weeks fenofibrate therapy (n=12)

This seems to be a further therapeutical effect of fibrate derivate
therapy, which should generally be considered in patients with
clinically manifest atherosclerosis, ischemia and hyperfibrinogenemia.
On the other hand, this therapeutical recommendation must be proven in

further prospective studies especially regarding the efficiency of
long-term therapy.

Intermittent urokinase therapy

As a further therapeutical option taking advantage of a reduction in
fibrinogen levels we introduced the "chronically intermittent i/v
urokinase therapy" in patients with end-stage coronary artery disease
refractory to conventional antianginal therapy and not suitable
anatomy for percutaneous coronary angioplasty or coronary bypass
grafting [10]. The consequences of this therapy are a reduction of
serum fibrinogen and possibly the fibrinolysis of microclots, thus
improving myocardial perfusion. Urokinase therapy was initiated in
highly selected patients during a hospital stay with daily i/v
administration of 500.000 U urokinase until fibrinogen plasma levels
of 150-200 mg/dl were reached. The maintenance therapy with three
times 500.000 U urokinase per week was administered. Due to this
treatment, the frequency of angina pectoris attacks in these patients,
who were severely symptomatic, could be markedly reduced. In some
patients, angina symptoms nearly entirely disappeared as long as
fibrinogen levels were in the desired range.

Complications, e.g. bleeding problems, were seen in only 2 of nearly
90 patients, probably induced by the concomitant acetylsalicylate
therapy, which was added in a daily dose of 50 mg to prevent latent
platelet hyperreactivity due to cleavage products of fibrinogen. No
critical fibrinogen reduction could be observed in none of our
patientes including the two with bleeding problems. The effect of this
low dosage long-term urokinase therapy on overall coagulation
parameters was very small resulting only in a 10-15% prolongation of
prothrombin time. Fibrinogen levels were lowered by about 40%. Apart
from symptomatic improvement of angina pectoris the efficiency of
intermittent urokinase therapy could be documented by a 20%
improvement of global perfusion in standardized quantitative
myocardial scintigraphy and by a significant increase of exercise
tolerance in standardized ergometry.

HELP-therapy

Only in a small group of patients with familial hypercholesterolemia
and severe manifestation of atherosclerosis with symptomatic coronary
artery disease the extracorporal lipid elimination has been applied.
HELP (heparin-induced extracorporal lipid precipitation of fibrinogen
and LDL-cholesterol) therapy eliminates fibrinogen as well as
cholesterol due to a heparin-induced precipitation, thus resulting in
a marked improvement of blood viscosity. The benefitial effects of a
single HELP treatment on microcirculation due to elimination of
cholesterol and fibrinogen, in three patients with coronary artery
disease and familial hypercholesterolemia are demonstrated in Figure
4; the fibrinogen level was reduced by 45%, the LDL-cholesterol by

about 65%. Plasma viscosity decreased by 15% resulting in an increase
of percutaneous oxygen partial pressure by about 45% [7]. This very
impressive increase of percutaneous oxygen partial pressure measured
in primarily normal regions of microcirculatory flow, indicates that
the underlying mechanism of symptomatic relief of angina pectoris
observed in patients treated with HELP therapy is an improved oxygen
transport and release with a higher tissue oxygen uptake due to
decreased fibrinogen levels and, thus, decreased blood viscosity.

CONCLUSIONS

Fibrinogen directly mediates the initial lesions of atherosclerosis by
its subendothelial accumulation and the proliferation tendency of
smooth muscle cells induced by fibrinogen. Its indirect effect include
an augmentation of the atherogenous lesions caused by smoking,
diabetes and hypertension. When the stage of manifest atherosclerosis
is reached, elevated fibrinogen levels result in deterioration of
microcirculatory blood flow, predisposing to thrombus formation and
ischemia. The fact that therapeutical approaches of decreased
fibrinogen levels result in an improvement of myocardial perfusion on
the level of microcirculation should intensify further investigation
of fibrinogen lowering concepts.

REFERENCES

1   Austen WG, Edwards JE, Frye RL, et al (1976) A reporting system
     on patients evaluated for coronary artery disease. Report on
     othe Ad Hoc Committee for Grading of Coronary Artery Disease.
     Council on Cardiovascular Surgery, American Heart Association.
     Circulation 51 [suppl] : 5-0

2   Castelli WP (1984) Epidemiology of coronary heart disease: The
     Framingham Study. Am J Med 76 : 4-12

3   Chakrabarti R, Fearnley GR (1968) Effects of clofibrate on
     fibrinolysis, platelet stickiness, plasmafibrinogen, and serum
     cholesterol. Lancet ii : 1007-1009

4   Gordon RI, Snyder GK, Tritel H, Taylor WJ (1974) Potential
     significance of plasma viscosity and hematocrit variations in
     myocardial infarction. Am Heart J 87 : 175-182

5   Kampschmidt RF, Upchurch HF (1974) Effect of leucocytic
     endogenous mediator on plasma fibrinogen and haptoglobin. Proc
     Soc Exp Bio Med 146 : 904-907

6   Kannel WB, Wolf PA, Castelli WP, D'Agostino RB (1987)
     Fibrinogen and risk of cardiovascular disease. The Framingham
     Study. J Am Med Assoc 258 : 1183-1186

7   Kleophas W, Leschke M, Tschöpe D, Martin J, Schauseil S,
     Schottenfeld Y, Strauer BE, Gries FA (1990) Akute Wirkungen der
     extrakorporalen LDL-Cholesterin- und Fibrinogen-Elimination auf
     Blutrheologie und Mikrozirkulation. Dtsch Med Wschr 115 : 3-7

8   Leschke M, Motz W, Blanke H, Meier M, Kaffarnik H, Strauer BE
     (1987) Die Wertigkeit rheologischer Parameter als Indikatoren
     der koronaren Herzkrankheit im Vergleich zu Lipidparametern.
     In: Strauer BE et al. (eds): Fortschritte in der
     kardiovaskulären Hämorheologie. Münchener Wissenschaftliche
     Publikationen pp 39-44

9   Leschke M, Höffken H, Schmidtsdorff A, Blanke H, Egbring R,
     Joseph K, Strauer BE (1989) Einfluß von Fenofibrat auf
     Fibrinogen- konzentration und Blutfluidität. Dtsch Med Wschr
     114 : 939-944

10   Leschke M, Höffken H, Vogt M, Motz W, Strauer BE (1989)
     Intermittent urokinase therapy as a new strategy concept in
     untractable angina pectoris. J Am Coll Cardiol 13 : 16
     [abstract]

11   Leschke M, Strauer BE (1990) Die Bedeutung rheologischer
     Mechanismen in der Atherogenese. Arzneim Forsch (Drug Res)
     40 : 356-362

12   Meade TW, Chakrabarti R, Haines AP, North WRS, Stirling Y,
     Thompson SG (1980) Hemostatic function and cardiovascular
     death: early results of a prospective study. Lancet i :
     1050-1055

13   Naito M, Hayaski T, Kuzuya M, Funaki C, Asai K, Kuzuya F (1990)
     Effects of fibrinogen and fibrin on the migration of vascular
     smooth muscle cell in vitro. Atherosclerosis 83 : 9-14

14   Niort G, Bulgarelli A, Lanader M, Pagano G (1988) Effect of
     short-term treatment with bezafibrate on plasma fibrinogen,
     fibrinopeptide A, platelet activation and blood filterability
     in atherosclerosis hyperfibrinogenemic patients.
     Atherosclerosis 71 : 113-119

15   Schmid-Schönbein H, Rieger H, Fischer T (1980) Blood fluidity
     as a consequence of red cell fluidity: flow properties of blood
     and flow behaviour of blood vascular diseases. Angiology 31 :
     301-319

16   Seidel D, Wieland H (1982) Ein neues Verfahren zur selektiven
     Messung und extrakorporalen Elimination von
     Low-Density-Lipoproteinen. J Clin Chem Clin Biochem 20 : 684-685

17   Stuart J, George AJ, Davies AJ, Aukland A, Hurlow RA (1981)
     Hematological stress syndrome in atherosclerosis. J Clin Pathol
     34 : 464-467

REGRESSION AND DECREASE IN PROGRESSION OF CORONARY ARTERY DISEASE THROUGH LIPID-LOWERING THERAPY

H. W.· HAHMANN

ABSTRACT. Today there exists a sequence of variously designed studies in which the effect of lipid-lowering intervention on serial angiographies of the coronary arteries and other vessels has been investigated. The aim of our own prospective intervention study was to examine the effect of fenofibrate on the progress of minor coronary narrowings in hypercholesterolemic patients. We compared the angiographic follow-up (average angiographic interval: 21 ± 6 months) of an intervention group treated with 200–400 mg/day of fenofibrate (21 patients, 98 narrowings) with those of an untreated comparison group (21 patients, 93 narrowings) by means of quantitative coronary angiography with computer-assisted contour detection. The low density lipoprotein-cholesterol (LDL) levels of the intervention group (checked every six weeks) were lowered from 229 ± 30 mg/dl by an average of 19.5%, while those of the comparison group were 241 ± 53 mg/dl and remained almost completely unchanged. The distribution of the parameter "Change in Percent Plaque Area" (%PA-change) (classified in patient-related regressions, stillstands and progressions on the basis of the reproducibility of the measuring method) shifted significantly toward regressions (p=0.032) in the intervention group: 33% progressions (comparison group: 67%), 48% stillstands (comparison group: 33%), 19% regressions (comparison group: 0%). The changes in percent diameter reduction and percent plaque area correlated positively to mean intervention cholesterol and LDL levels.
The results indicate the beneficial effect of fenofibrate on minor coronary narrowings, and correspond to the other angiographically controlled lipid-lowering intervention studies which show the benefit of lipid therapy, particularly the lowering of elevated LDL levels in secondary prevention of coronary artery disease.

1. INTRODUCTION

Back in 1979 Blankenhorn recommended evaluating sequential angiographic examinations in order to validate forms of preventive treatments of atherosclerosis [1]. In the meantime the results of a series of such lipid lowering intervention studies have been published.
The study presented here, whose most important results have already been published elsewhere [2, 3], pursues the goal of investigating for the first time the effect of a lipid-lowering therapy with fenofibrate on the progress of minor and moderate coronary stenoses by means of quantitative angiography.

A. L. Catapano et al. (eds.), Drugs Affecting Lipid Metabolism, 399–406.
© 1993 Kluwer Academic Publishers and Fondazione Giovanni Lorenzini. .

2. PATIENTS AND METHODS

2.1. Study Design:

44 patients with angiographically documented coronary heart disease and high blood cholesterol levels were treated with a diet corresponding to the AHA Phase 1 Diet [4] and fenofibrate
(200 to 400 mg/die) in the framework of a prospective intervention study over a period of 3
years. The patients were re-examined every 6 weeks on an outpatient basis, whereby a physical
examination as well as a stress ECG were performed in addition to the determination of the lipoprotein status and the recording of other risk factors. Twenty-one patients underwent a follow-up angiography for clinical reasons after a mean interval of 21 ± 6 months. The time of the
follow-up angiography was determined during the study according to clinical considerations.
The angiographic progress of the minor stenoses was evaluated using digital image processing
and contour finding, and compared with that of a non-randomized comparison group of similar
composition with persistently high blood cholesterol values.

2.2. Inclusion and Exclusion Criteria

The inclusion criteria consisted of a total cholesterol level > 265 mg/dl, successful or unsuccessful PTCA without serious complications, at least one minor or moderate lesion in addition
to a dilated narrowing. Exclusion criteria were a manifest diabetes mellitus, a valvular heart
defect, additional accompanying illnesses which decreased life expectancy, (e.g. malignant
tumors), severely impaired left ventricular function (ejection fraction < 30%), early PTCA in
the subacute infarct phase (particularly after lysis therapy) as well as previous aortocoronary
bypass operations.

2.3. Comparison Group

Before the beginning of the study, patients who had been registered who could not participate
in the study for various reasons, but who had fulfilled the inclusion criteria after the first angiography and for whom no lipid-lowering therapy had been done between the two angiograms
were used as a comparison group. In the second angiography this group showed a risk profile
no different from that in the first angiography, had the same age and sex distribution (16 men, 5
women), and the mean angiography interval was 20 ± 7 months. Concerning the accompanying
medication there were none significant differences between the two groups: In the intervention
group, 13 patients took calcium antagonists, (comparison group: 18), 18 patients took nitrate
(comparison group: 18), 10 patients took beta-blockers (comparison group: 9), 15 patients
took thrombocyte aggregation inhibitors (comparison group: 13) and 14 patients took other
medications (comparison group: 10). The composition of both groups is given in Table 1.

2.4. Lipoprotein Levels

Within the framework of the coronary angiography examinations, blood was taken from the
patients after a minimum 12-hour fast for laboratory lipid determination. Tot cholesterol
was determined by the CHOD-PAP method [5], using an enzymatic color test, while the
triglycerides were determined by a fully enzymatic test (BOEHRINGER MANNHEIM). The
HDL-Chol was measured after precipitation with phosphor-wolfram acid, and magnesium
ions in the excess solutions were measured by means of the CHOD-PAP method. The
LDL-Chol was precipitated out with polyvinylsulfate and calculated from the difference of the
cholesterol values in the blood and in the precipitate excess. Lipid diagnosis in the outpatient
examinations was performed using the same methods in the same laboratory.

Table 1. Composition and severity of the coronary artery disease
in the intervention and comparison groups.

	INTERVENTION GROUP	COMPARISON GROUP
Total	21	21
Male/Female	16/ 5	16/ 5
Age (Years)	56 ± 7	56 ± 8
Gensini Score	22 ±21	21 ±19
Ejection Fraction (%)	65 ± 12	60 ± 16
1-vessel disease	11	7
2-vessel disease	7	11
3-vessel disease	3	3
Post-AMI	7	8
Post-PMI	9	8
Angina Pectoris ≤ Stage 2*	12	8
Angina Pectoris > Stage 2*	9	13
Heart Failure Stage 1 *	15	17
Heart Failure Stage 2 *	6	4
Re-PTCA +	3	4
PTCA elsewhere +	4	4
Bypass ++	1	3
Reinfarction ++	0	2

* = Canadian Cardiovascular Society, ** = New York Heart Association,
+ = during intervention period, ++ = after intervention period,
AMI = anterior myocardial infarct, PMI = posterior myocardial infarct,
PTCA = percutaneous transluminal coronary angioplasty.

2.5. Coronary Angiography

The angiograms of the left and right coronary arteries were prepared in several projections under standardized conditions in our heart catheterization laboratory. The projection angles were documented; the cardiologist performing the second angiography made a particular effort to set the angle of the first angiography very exactly. A few minutes before each angiography, the patient was given 1.2 mg glyceroltrinitrate perlingual. The same contrast medium was used in all cases. The angiographies were documented on 35-mm cinefilm.

2.6. Stenosis Quantification

The scope of a narrowing had to be at least 13.0% (%DR) or 10.0% (%PA) in at least one angiography in order to be included in the evaluation. Only changes in which the proximal or distal vessel segment was clearly not involved were taken into account, and were then used for the determination of the reference diameter in both angiographies. Severe stenoses, obstructions and vessel segments treated with PTCA, as well as vessel segments distal to occlusions were excluded. The best projection was selected on the basis of the least projection- related shortening of the vessel segment to be examined, the fewest overlays and the best possible image quality.
The measurement of stenoses was performed using one method. The selected images were projected and recorded with a video camera. Digitization, further processing and stenosis measurement were done with a KONTRON image analysis system. The algorithm corresponds to the stenosis quantification program described and validated by Reiber et al. [6].

Computed parameter was the percentual diameter reduction (%DR), that is, the diameter reduction at the narrowest point of the stenosis related to a neighboring vessel area which is held to be unchanged. In addition we used the percentual plaque area (%PA) as a measured variable, which was calculated as the integral of the percentual diameter shortening over the total length of the stenosis, and which corresponds to the plaque area in relation to the nominal area in the respective projection. The calculation of these relative values does not require contour finding on the catheter as a standard scale, which is advantageous with respect to the measuring accuracy [7].

The reproducibility of the measuring methods was determined in a preliminary investigation [2]. This variability lies within the scope of comparable investigations [6, 8, 9, 10]. The double value of the standard deviation was used in the definition of stenosis as well as in the definitions of progression and regression of a stenosis. This resulted in a threshold of 13.0% for %DR and a threshold of 10.0% for %PA.

A patient was classified as "progression" if more stenoses showed progressions than regressions. If there were more regressions than progressions, the patient was classified as "regression". If a patient showed no progressions or regressions, or the same number of both, the patient was classified as "stillstand".

2.7. Statistical Methods

Since a patient had an average of 4.7 stenoses, patient–related mean values were calculated for the change in degree of stenosis and for the initial degree of stenosis.

The statistical analyses were carried out with the aid of the SPSSx software package using chi–square test, Wilcoxon–Mann–Whitney–U test, Kruskal–Wallis–H test and Wilcoxon matched–pairs–signed–ranks test.

3. RESULTS

3.1. Risk Factors

Table 2.   Intervention results concerning lipid and lipoprotein levels:
Initial values and changes during observation period.

[mg/dl]	INTERVENTION GROUP		COMPARISON GROUP	
	Initial	Changes	Initial	Changes
Chol	310 ± 36	−19 ± 8 % **	311 ± 61	−3 ± 7 % ns
LDL	229 ± 30	−20 ± 14 % **	241 ± 53	−3 ± 7 % ns
HDL	40 ± 15	+19 ± 44 % ns	43 ± 15	+4 ± 11 % ns
Trigl.	271 ±179	−30 ± 31 % **	211 ±103	+1 ± 18 % ns
	‖———— ns ————‖			

Chol = cholesterol, HDL = high density lipoprotein–cholesterol, LDL = low density lipoprotein–cholesterol, Trigl. = triglycerides.
** Level of significance $p < 0.01$, ns = not significant

The intervention led to statistically significant decreases in Chol–, LDL– and TG levels. The initial lipoprotein values and the mean percentual changes in the intervention and comparison groups are compared in Table 2. Mean values were calculated from the lipid and lipoprotein values of the individual patients over the entire intervention period. Blood pressure values and smoking behavior showed no significant changes in the framework of the intervention and did not differ significantly in the two groups.

3.2. Angiographic Progress

For the evaluation of the angiographic progress an average of 4.7 stenoses per patient was used (intervention group: 98 stenoses, comparison group: 93 stenoses). The change in both angiographic parameters (patient–related mean values) correlated with the mean Chol achieved through the intervention as well as with the LDL levels (%DR change with LDL: r=0.67, p=0.0005; %DR change with Chol: r=0.38, p=0.044), while for HDL and triglycerides no influence on the angiographic progress could be demonstrated (Figure 1).

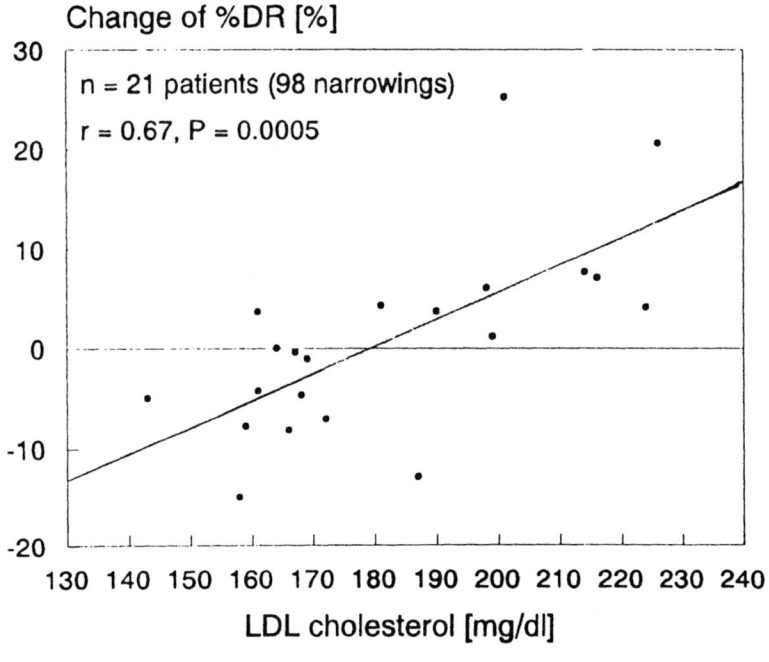

Figure 1. Dependence of the angiographic progress (percent diameter reduction, mean values from an average of 4.7 narrowings per patient) on the mean LDL–cholesterol levels in the intervention period.

After the patients had been classified in the categories regression, stillstand and progression, it was shown that in the intervention group, the entire distribution with regard to the parameter "%PA change" had shifted toward regression: in the intervention group 7 patients were classified as "progression" (comparison group: 14), 10 as "stillstand" (comparison group: 7) and 4 as "regression" (comparison group: 0) (Figure 2). The difference between both groups was statistically significant (p = 0.032). In the case of the parameter "%DR change" the entire distribution had not shifted, but in the intervention group 8 (38%) patients were classified as "regression" (comparison group: 2 (10%)). This difference was also statistically significant (p = 0.030).

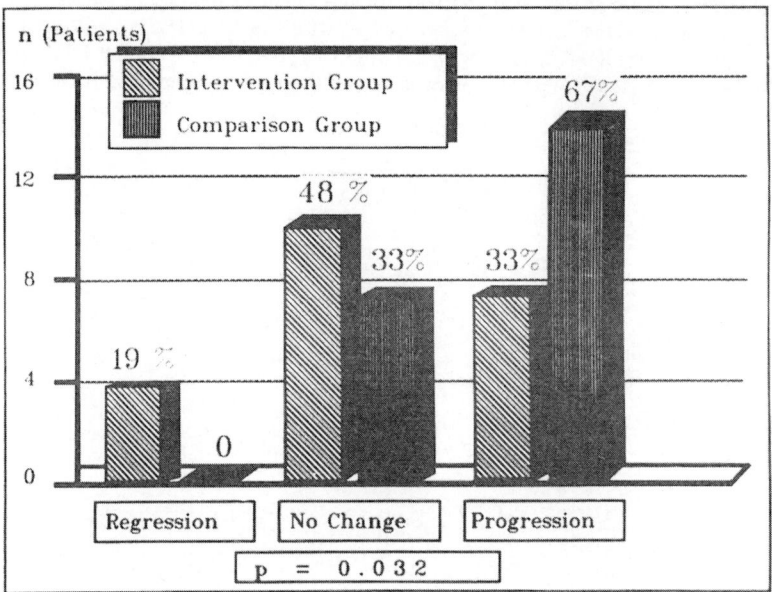

Figure 2.   Comparison of the angiographic follow-ups (%PA change) of the intervention and the comparison groups, classified on the basis of the reproducibility of the measuring method. The patients of the intervention group show a significant shift toward regressions.

4. DISCUSSION

The main result of the study, shown in Figure 2, is related to the parameter %PA change, a halving of the patient-related progressions from 2/3 to 1/3 as well as the occurrence of regressions in the intervention with fenofibrate.

The factor most clearly influencing the progression or regression was LDL, while HDL and triglycerides, as well as other factors, played no role in our study. A further factor influencing the development of coronary stenoses in our study was the initial degree of stenosis, whereby minor stenoses tended toward progressions and more severe stenoses toward regressions. This finding was presented in a similar manner in the INTACT study [11] as well.

Recently a series of studies has been published which, within the framework of secondary prevention of coronary heart disease, verifies the possibility of inhibiting progression and even of regression of arteriosclerotic lesions. The placebo–controlled Cholesterol Lowering Atherosclerosis Study (CLAS) [12–14] showed a significant advantage of the group treated with niacin and colestipol in the angiographic progress, which in comparison to the placebo group was shifted toward regression. The difference between the two groups was even more pronounced after 4 years than after 2 years. In the placebo group, the possibility of preventing a recurrence of arteriosclerotic lesions by means of a low-fat diet was proven. The results of the Familiar Atherosclerosis Treatment Study (FATS) [8], which were published in 1990, showed a reduction in the frequency of progressions and an increase in frequency of regressions of coronary narrowings as well as a reduction in the incidence of cardiovascular events in men with coronary heart disease. These successes were achieved with an intensive lipid–lowering therapy using niacin and colestipol or lovastatin plus colestipol in comparison to a conventionally treated group. The placebo–controlled INTACT study [9, 15], likewise published in 1990, in which the cardiovascular risk factors were left uninfluenced, demonstrated a significant decrease in the frequency of new lesions in the group treated with nifedipine. The results of the Lifestyle Heart Trial [16], published in the same year, indicate the possibility of regression of coronary sclerosis by means of a consistent change in lifestyle. The angiographic progress of these studies was, with the exception of the CLAS study, documented using coronary angiography by means of digital image processing.

These and previous intervention studies [17, 18] taken together show the influence of of elevated LDL levels in progression of coronary stenoses and – with the exception of the otherwise designed INTACT study [9] – the benefit of lipid lowering intervention in secondary prevention of coronary artery disease.

5. Acknowledgement

The author thanks the members of his study group, Thomas Bunte, Nicola Hellwig, Udo Hau, Dieter Becker, Jan Dyckmans, Hans E. Keller, and Hermann J. Schieffer for their friendly and productive cooperation , and Monique Simmer for her excellent editorial assistance. I am particularly indebted to Dr. Ilse Lelieur for her unfailing support.

6. References

1. Blankenhorn DH, Sanmarco ME (1979) `Angiography for study of lipid–lowering therapy`, Circulation 59, 212–214.
2. Hahmann HW, Bunte T, Hellwig N, Hau U, Becker D, Dyckmans J, Keller H–E, and Schieffer H (1991) `Progression and regression of minor coronary arterial narrowings by quantitative angiography after fenofibrate therapy`, Am J Cardiol 67, 957–961.
3. Hahmann, H., Bunte, T., Hellwig, N., Hau, U., Becker, D., Dyckmans, J., Keller, H.E., Schieffer, H. (1991) `Quantitative Koronarangiographie: Progression und Regression von Koronarstenosen – Eine Interventionsstudie mit Fenofibrat`, Z Kardiol 80, 589–594.
4. AHA Special Report (1984) `Recommendations for treatment of hyperlipidemia in adults`, Circulation 69, 1065A–1090A.
5. Kattermann R, Kupke IR, and Borner K (1983) `Vorläufig ausgewählte Methode für die Bestimmung des Gesamt–Cholesterins im Serum`, J Clin Chem Clin Biochem 21, 347–355.

6. Reiber JHC, Serruys PW, Kooijman CJ, Wuns W, Slager CJ, Gerbrands JJ, Schuur-
    biers JCH, den Boer A, and Hugenholtz PG (1985) `Assessment of short-, medium-,
    and long-term variations in arterial dimensions from computer-assisted quantitation
    of coronary cineangiograms`, Circulation 71, 280.

7. Reiber JH, Kooijman CJ, den Boer A, and Serruys PW (1985) `Assessment of dimen-
    sions and image quality of coronary contrast catheters from cineangiograms`, Cathet
    Cardiovasc Diagn 11, 521-531.

8. Brown G, Albers JJ, Fisher LD, Schaefer SM, Lin J-T, Kaplan C, Zhao X-Q, Bisson
    BD, Fitzpatrick VF, and Dodge HT (1990) `Regression of coronary artery disease as
    a result of intensive lipid-lowering therapy in men with high levels of apolipoprotein
    B`, N Engl J Med 323, 1289-1298.

9. Lichtlen PR, Rafflenbeul W, Jost S, Hugenholtz PG, Hecker H, and Deckers JW
    (1990) `Retardation of angiographic progression of coronary artery disease by
    nifedipine`, Lancet 335, 1109-1113.

10. Ellis S, Sanders W, Goulet C, Miller R, Cain KC, Lesperance J, Bourassa MG, and
    Alderman EL (1986) `Optimal detection of the progression of coronary artery disease:
    comparison of methods suitable for risk factor intervention trials`, Circulation 74,
    1235-1242.

11. Jost S, Rafflenbeul W, Nikutta P, Wiese B, Hecker H, Lichtlen PR, and
    INTACT-Gruppe (1991) `Einfluß des Schweregrades von Koronarstenosen auf die
    Entwicklung von Progression oder Regression – Ergebnisse einer prospektiven
    Studie (INTACT)`, Z Kardiol 80 (Suppl.3) P418.

12. Blankenhorn DH, Nessim SA, Johnson RL, Sanmarco ME, Azen SP, and Cashin-
    Hemphill L (1987) `Beneficial effects of combined colestipol-niacin therapy on coro-
    nary atherosclerosis and coronary venous bypass grafts`, JAMA 257, 3233-3240.

13. Blankenhorn DH, Johnson RL, Mack WJ, El Zein HA, and Vailas LI (1990) `The
    influence of diet on the appearance of new lesions in human coronary arteries`, JAMA
    263, 1646-1652.

14. Cashin-Hemphill L, Mack WL, Pogoda JM, Sanmarco ME, Azen SP, and Blanken-
    horn DH (1990) `Beneficial effects of colestipol-niacin on coronary atherosclerosis.
    A 4-year follow-up`, JAMA 264, 3013-3017.

15. Jost S, Deckers J, Nellessen U, Rafflenbeul W, Hecker H, Reiber JHC, Lippolt
    P, Hugenholtz PG, Lichtlen PR, and INTACT-Studiengruppe (1989) `Computer-
    gestützte geometrische Meßtechnik in koronarangiographischen Intervallstudien:
    Ergebnisse bei Erstangiogrammen der INTACT-Studie`, Z Kardiol 78, 23-32.

16. Ornish D, Brown SE, Scherwitz LW, Billings JH, Armstrong WT, Ports TA, McLa-
    nahan SM, Kirkeeide RL, Brand RJ, and Gould KL (1990) `Can lifestyle changes
    reverse coronary heart disease? The Lifestyle Heart Trial`, Lancet 336, 129-133.

17. Brensike JF, Levy RI, Kelsey SF, Passmani ER, Richardson JM, Loh IK, Stone
    NJ, Aldrich RF, Battaglini JW, Moriarty DJ, Fisher ML, Friedman L, Friedewald
    W, Detre KM, and Epstein SE (1984) `Effects of therapy with cholestyramine on
    progression of coronary arteriosclerosis: results of the NHLBI Type II Coronary
    Intervention Study` Circulation 69, 313-324.

18. Arntzenius A, Kromhout D, Barth JD, Reiber JHC, Bruschke AVG, Buis B, van
    Gent CM, Kempen-Voogd N, Strikwerda S, and van der Velde EA (1985) `Diet,
    lipoproteins and the progression of coronary atherosclerosis: the Leiden Intervention
    Trial`, N Engl J Med 312, 805-811.

GLYCATION AND OXIDATION OF PROTEINS: A ROLE IN THE PATHOGENESIS OF ATHEROSCLEROSIS?

Timothy   J. Lyons MD, MRCP

Abstract

Glycation affects any protein exposed to glucose. In long-lived proteins, further reactions lead to unreactive advanced glycation end-products (AGE). Although numerous, the structures of only two AGE products, carboxymethyllysine (CML) and pentosidine, are known. AGE formation involves sequential glycation and free radical oxidation reactions: thus these products may be termed "glycoxidation products". Both glycation and glycoxidation may be important in the development of atherosclerosis, and an increase in either glycative or oxidative stress may promote this disease. Glycation of LDL impairs its recognition by the LDL receptor, stimulates cholesteryl ester (CE) synthesis in macrophages (promoting hyperlipidemia and foam cell formation), and enhances platelet aggregation. Glycation enhances covalent binding of lipoproteins to vascular wall proteins, promoting sequestration. Glycation may cause free radical release, and hence oxidative damage to lipids, apolipoproteins, and any nearby macromolecules. Patients with significant atherosclerosis, whether diabetic or not, tend to have increased peroxidation of plasma lipids. Even if a result, not a cause, of initial vascular injury, plasma lipid peroxides may promote further damage to vessel walls through cytotoxicity to endothelial and smooth muscle cells.
Glycated and glycoxidized lipoproteins may be immunogenic, and lipoprotein- immune complexes may promote arterial injury. Glycation of antithrombin III may impair its function and increase thrombotic tendency. Glycoxidation is of greatest importance in long-lived proteins such as collagen. Collagen CML and pentosidine are functions of patient age, the presence or absence of diabetes, and individual variation in resistance to oxidative stress. Increased glycoxidation of vascular collagens may increase arterial stiffness and alter flow dynamics, may enhance the binding of plasma lipoproteins in vessel walls, and may have a chemotactic effect on macrophages, which possess an "AGE-receptor". It may also promote renal damage, causing proteinuria and hypertension. This suggests that glycoxidation of vascular connective tissue proteins may promote the development of atherosclerosis in patients who are under increased glycative and/or oxidative stress. It may be possible to moderate these stresses using dietary and pharmacologic measures.

Glycation and Glycoxidation

Glycation of proteins involves the covalent binding of glucose to reactive amino-groups, usually located on lysine side-chains and N-terminal amino-acid residues. Subsequently, a complex series of reactions takes place, leading to the formation of a

A. L. Catapano et al. (eds.), Drugs Affecting Lipid Metabolism, 407–420.

wide variety of stable end-products. These reactions are collectively termed "the browning reaction" or "the Maillard Reaction", and the final products are termed "browning products", "Maillard Reaction products", or "Advanced Glycation End-products" (AGE). The chemistry of the initial stage of glycation, and the subsequent formation of the known products of the browning reaction, are shown in the figure 1.

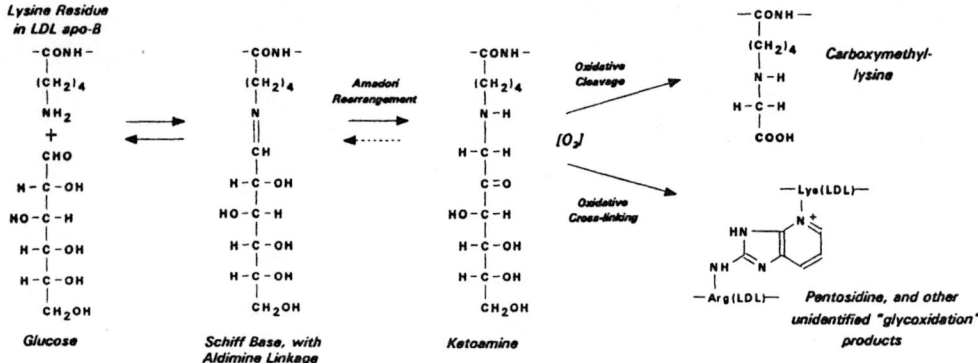

In humans, FL is thought not to accumulate with age, even in long-lived proteins, but rather exists in a steady-state relationship with ambient glucose concentration (1). Metabolic alterations directly attributable to FL are perhaps most likely to affect short-lived proteins, since these do not exist long enough to accumulate high levels of browning products, whose effects might otherwise predominate. The consequences of FL formation in plasma low density lipoproteins (LDL) in atherogenesis will be considered in this article.

Current knowledge concerning the browning process has been reviewed recently by several authors (2-4). Since structural proteins tend to be the longest-lived in the body, they are thought to be the most affected by browning reactions, which are slow but irreversible (5). Browning products, all of which are derived from FL are numerous, and include species which are colored, fluorescent, and which constitute cross-links.

However, only two have been identified conclusively (Figure 1): N^{ε}-carboxymethyllysine (CML) (6) (and the closely related species N^{ε}-carboxymethylhydroxylysine and 3-(N^{ε}-lysino)-lactic acid (7) and pentosidine (8) .

CML is formed by oxidative cleavage of FL. It is not fluorescent, is stable and unreactive, and is not involved in cross-link formation *in vivo*. While it is now known that CML can be formed from species other than glucose (including other sugars and ascorbate) (9), its formation always involves free-radical-mediated oxidation.

Pentosidine is a lysine-arginine cross-link. Originally thought to be derived exclusively from pentoses, it is now known that pentosidine, like CML, can also be formed during interactions between proteins and other species, including glucose (10). Also like CML, pentosidine formation involves oxidation reactions. Unlike CML, pentosidine is intensely fluorescent (8,11,12), contributing about 30% of total Maillard-type fluorescence in collagen. It may be considered a "biomarker" for the extent of browning of proteins (12).

Both CML and pentosidine are formed by combined glycation and oxidation reactions, and it is now known that browning and crosslinking of proteins does not occur in an anti-oxidant environment (13). To emphasize the close inter-relationship of glycation and oxidation, the final products have been collectively termed "glycoxidation products" (14). In long-lived proteins these accumulate with age in a linear fashion, and, like rust on a car, their formation is thought to be irreversible (5).

Increased glycation (15), and subsequent glycoxidation (14) of proteins may, by inducing structural changes, may lead to functional abnormalities of both circulating and tissue proteins. As discussed below, glycation, oxidation and glycoxidation may all contribute, in inter-related ways, to the development of atherosclerosis, and to its acceleration in diabetes. The initial glycation reaction product, FL, may play its most significant and direct role by causing alterations in the metabolism of short-lived plasma constituents, particularly lipoproteins. Free radical-mediated oxidation, perhaps enhanced by glycation, also affects lipoproteins, but is also important in longer-lived structural proteins. Glycoxidation is probably of most significance in long-lived structural proteins in vessel walls.

LDL Glycation and Atherogenesis

It is well established that lipoproteins are implicated in the development of atherosclerosis, and that diabetes, for reasons not fully understood, is an independent risk factor for the development of this condition (16). The possibility that increased glycation of lipoproteins may contribute to the problem of macrovascular disease in diabetes, first suggested by Schleicher et al. in 1981 (17), has therefore been the subject of extensive research.

Binding and degradation of glycated compared to control LDL by human fibroblasts, which possess the classical LDL receptor, was shown to be impaired in proportion to the extent of LDL glycation (18-20). This effect was detectable with degrees of LDL modification observed *in vivo* in diabetic patients (21). Also, when radio-labelled LDL was injected into guinea-pigs and rabbits, the its fractional catabolic rate was found to be significantly lower than that of control LDL. These studies suggested that impaired recognition of glycated LDL by the classical LDL receptor may contribute to the elevation of plasma LDL cholesterol levels and accelerated atherogenesis in diabetic patients, particularly those in poor glycemic control. In contrast to the findings with fibroblasts, however, murine peritoneal macrophages failed to distinguish between control and glycated LDL (18,19).

Subsequent studies by our group demonstrated that in diabetes, the extent of glycation of LDL correlates well with other short- and medium-term indicators of glycemic control (mean plasma glucose, plasma protein glycation and HbA$_{1c}$), and that increased LDL glycation is present even in normolipidemic diabetic patients in satisfactory glycemic control (22). The increase in apo-B glycation in diabetic compared to control patients (1.6 fold higher) was of the same order as that for hemoglobin (1.5 fold) and total plasma proteins (2.2 fold) (22). We confirmed the impaired recognition of LDL from diabetic patients by human fibroblasts (23), and of direct relevance to the development of atherosclerosis, we investigated the interactions of LDL isolated from diabetic patients with human plasma- derived monocyte-macrophages, the main precursors of foam cells in atherosclerosis (24). LDL from Type I diabetic patients stimulated more cholesteryl ester (CE) synthesis and accumulation in human monocyte/macrophages than LDL from non-diabetic control subjects. The composition of LDL was similar in the two groups, and the particles appeared to differ only in the extent of apoprotein glycation, and CE synthesis in the macrophages correlated with LDL glycation. In a later study (25), we investigated human monocyte- macrophage interactions with LDL isolated from patients with Type 2 diabetes and corresponding control subjects. Here, no difference was found in the rate of CE synthesis by macrophages exposed to LDL from the two groups. However, our Type 2 patients were in excellent glycemic control: their mean LDL glycation was increased to a lesser extent (1.2-fold over the control value) than in the Type 1 diabetic patients (1.4 fold increase). In experiments using LDL glycated *in vitro* in anti-oxidant conditions (26), the levels of glycation obtained (4-fold increase) were much greater than those observed *in vivo* (24). This highly glycated LDL stimulated much more CE synthesis and accumulation in macrophages, and receptor-mediated intracellular degradation was also increased.

Since recognition of glycated LDL by the classical LDL receptor in macrophages was diminished, the increased uptake and degradation of the particle was considered to be mediated through a different pathway. Competition studies clearly showed that the scavenger receptor pathway, a putative non-specific FL receptor pathway, and the macrophage glycoprotein receptor pathway were not involved (26). A separate, low affinity, high capacity pathway recognizing glycated LDL was therefore proposed.

Recent studies in our laboratory, as yet unpublished, further support the enhanced atherogenicity of glycated LDL in diabetes. In these studies, we isolated two fractions, "bound" and "unbound" (ie glycated and non-glycated), of intact LDL using boronate affinity chromatography (27). We isolated these LDL fractions from both non-diabetic control subjects and Type 1 diabetic patients. Glycation of the bound and non-bound LDL fractions from each group of patients was measured. In the non-bound fractions glycation was low, and almost identical between control and diabetic samples. In the bound fraction, glycation, corrected for amino-acid content, was increased compared to non-bound in both control subjects (2 fold increase) and diabetic patients (3 fold increase). The fact that the increase in glycation, effectively per LDL particle, was greater in the diabetic patients suggests that a higher proportion of the lysine residues in each particle had been glycated. This may imply that lysine residues other than those which, when glycated, primarily determine binding to the affinity column were glycated in the high ambient glucose concentrations present in diabetes. When the compositions of the bound and non-bound fractions of the diabetic LDL particles were determined, we found that the bound particles were significantly enriched in core constituents (esterified cholesterol and triglycerides), and were correspondingly depleted in the surface constituents (free cholesterol and phospholipids). Similar studies analyzing the composition of the LDL fractions from non-diabetic controls have not yet been performed due to the scarcity of bound material obtainable from this group.

We studied the metabolic behavior of both fractions using human fibroblasts and human monocyte-derived macrophages. With fibroblasts and LDL from non-diabetic control subjects, LDL receptor-mediated degradation was markedly impaired for the bound compared to the non-bound LDL fraction. Non-LDL receptor-mediated degradation was low in both bound and non-bound fractions, and did not differ significantly between them. Similar observations were made for fibroblasts with LDL from diabetic patients. Again, LDL receptor-mediated degradation was markedly depressed for the bound LDL, the effect being similar in magnitude to that seen with bound LDL from non-diabetic subjects. This confirms previous studies where impaired recognition of glycated LDL by LDL receptors on fibroblasts was observed, and again the impairment was directly related to the degree of glycation of the particle. Non-LDL receptor-mediated degradation was low, and similar, in the bound and non-bound fractions.

In human monocyte-macrophages, LDL receptor-mediated degradation of the bound and non-bound LDL fractions isolated from non-diabetic control subjects was similar, in keeping with the conclusion that very mild degrees of glycation will not impair the recognition of LDL by the LDL receptor (25). However, non-LDL receptor-mediated degradation was increased two-fold for the bound, compared to the non-bound, fraction. LDL receptor-mediated degradation of the bound LDL isolated from diabetic patients was somewhat impaired, although not to the same extent as was seen with fibroblasts. Again, non-LDL receptor-mediated degradation was significantly increased in the bound compared to the non-bound fractions, as expected. Thus the increased glycation in the bound LDL particles from diabetic patients seemed to impair their recognition by the macrophage LDL receptor, but stimulates their recognition by non-LDL receptor-mediated mechanisms.

Studies have recently been performed to assess the effect of LDL glycation on platelet aggregation. Watanabe et al. (28) isolated LDL from young Type 1 diabetic patients in good or fair glycemic control, and also from a group of age- and sex-matched non-diabetic controls. Glycation of LDL from the diabetic patients was increased, but its lipoprotein composition was similar in the two groups. Compared to LDL from control subjects, LDL from diabetic patients was a more potent stimulator of thromboxane B2 release and thrombin-induced platelet aggregation. In addition, LDL was glycated *in vitro*, and was found to cause a marked enhancement in thrombin-, collagen-, and ADP-induced platelet aggregation. However, it was noted that in general, the enhancement was seen irrespective of the concentration of glucose used in the incubation - the lowest concentration of glucose (10 mmol/l) being almost as effective as the highest (150 mmol/l). Thus it appeared that the effect was not linearly related to the extent of LDL glycation. It was suggested that subtle alterations in the composition of platelet membranes induced by interaction with glycated LDL may underlie the effects on platelet behavior. Finally, when LDL from Type 1 diabetic patients was subfractionated by affinity chromatography into bound and non-bound fractions, using the method described above (27), platelet aggregation was enhanced to a significantly greater extent by the bound (highly-glycated) fraction (29).

Lipoprotein Glycation and Oxidation

Lipoproteins, containing unsaturated fatty acids in their cores, are particularly vulnerable to oxidative damage, and the role of oxidized lipoproteins in the pathogenesis of atherosclerosis has been reviewed recently (30). The role of oxidized LDL specifically in atherosclerosis in diabetes has also been reviewed (31). Oxidized LDL is a potent stimulator of foam cell formation by macrophages. There are theoretical reasons to believe that the processes of oxidation and glycation may be linked (32), and therefore it is thought that glycation of lipoproteins may enhance the likelihood of oxidative damage. Despite this, there is little evidence to suggest that oxidation of plasma lipoproteins is increased in uncomplicated diabetes, whereas glycation clearly is. Also there are no studies demonstrating a correlation between lipoprotein oxidation and glycemic control in diabetic patients. Nevertheless, the situation may well be different for lipoproteins which have become extravasated, and are sequestered in the vessel wall. Here the processes of glycation, oxidation and browning may be closely interwoven, causing vicious cycles of vascular injury. As discussed below, glycation and browning of vascular connective tissue proteins may increase covalent glucose-mediated binding of lipoproteins, trapping them in the vessel wall, and allowing greater degrees of glycation and oxidation than could otherwise occur. This covalent binding is further enhanced by modifications to the lipoproteins themselves.

Lipoprotein Glycation and the Immune System

Modification of proteins, such as glycation and oxidation, may alter their structure sufficiently to render them immunogenic. Curtiss & Witztum (33) performed studies to investigate the possible immunogenic properties of glycated LDL They injected guinea pigs with homologous LDL which had been subjected to *in vitro* glycation. Heavily glycated particles were potent immunogens, stimulating the production of antibodies which did not interact with unmodified LDL. When the particles were more lightly glycated, as would occur *in vivo*, the resulting LDL was a much less potent immunogen. The existence of even low levels of antibodies against the less modified, FL-containing glycated LDL may have pathophysiologic relevance, since it may imply the presence of circulating antigen-antibody complexes, which, as discussed below, have been found to be potentially atherogenic. In addition, the more severely modified ("glycoxidized") lipoproteins which may be present in vessel walls may behave as much more potent antigens than the less modified particles found in the plasma, stimulating the in situ formation of immune complexes (34).

It has been shown by us (35,36) and by others (37) that LDL/anti-LDL immune complexes (LDL-IC) are potent inducers of foam cell formation. Subendothelial LDL deposits are likely to include LDL-IC formed in situ, and these are probably large, insoluble aggregates. Soluble LDL-IC present in circulation, however, are likely to be formed in antigen excess, and they will tend to be adsorbed to RBC via C3b receptors and other non-specific interactions. In vitro, both insoluble and soluble (RBC adsorbed) LDL-IC induce profound alterations in lipoprotein metabolism and cholesterol homeostasis of monocyte-derived macrophages (35,36).

The rapid transformation of human monocyte-derived macrophages into foam cells is one of the most striking abnormalities induced by either insoluble or RBC-bound LDL-IC. Relatively low concentrations of LDL-IC can induce this response, particularly when RBC-bound LDL-IC are involved: they are IS-fold more potent than insoluble LD-IC. Surprisingly, while inducing foam cell formation, the LDL-IC also stimulates a considerable increase (approximately 20 fold) in LDL receptor activity. The uptake of the LDL,immune complexes by macrophages also leads to activation of the cells, and to the release of Tumor Necrosis Factor α (TNF-α) and Interleukin-1 (IL-1), both of which have potentially atherogenic effects (38-46).

Glycation and Antithrombin III Activity

Brownlee et al (47) showed that increased glycation of antithrombin III impairs in thrombin-inhibiting activity, and suggested that a resulting defect in inhibition of the coagulation cascade could contribute to the accumulation of fibrin in diabetic tissues. Later, Ceriello et al (48) described an inverse correlation between antithrombin III activity and both HbAIc and plasma glucose, independent of plasma concentrations of antithrombin III. They proposed that antithrombin III activity was probably influenced by glycation. In contrast, in vitro glycation of fibrinogen was not found to influence its function, and therefore does not appear to promote thrombosis (49).

Browning of Vascular Structural Proteins

Among the long-lived structural proteins of the body, collagen in its various forms has been the most widely studied. In diabetes, most studies have utilized skin and tendon collagen, but the non-enzymatic nature of the glycation and browning reactions make it reasonable to extrapolate the physico-chemical alterations observed in these collagens to those in other sites, including those in the arterial wall. With advancing age, collagen becomes increasingly insoluble, thermally stable and resistant to enzymatic attack (50). Some of these changes are sufficiently predictable to allow determination of the age of the donor of a collagen sample with considerable accuracy (51). The changes are accompanied by, and are thought to be caused by, the formation of stable cross-links. Evidence is accumulating that many of the cross-links are derived from glucose via glycoxidative reactions of the browning process, in which case the changes in physical properties of collagen with age should be exaggerated in the presence of diabetes. Studies over the past twenty years have demonstrated that this is indeed so (52-55).

Increased glycation of collagen from a variety of sites has been reported in diabetes (56-62). Glycation (FL content) of insoluble skin collagen in diabetes correlates closely with HbAI (59), and falls promptly after a relatively short (4 month) period of improved glycemic control (5). In non-diabetic subjects, collagen glycation increases only very slightly between the ages of 20 and 80 years (1). These findings suggest that collagen glycation is in a steady- state relationship with ambient glucose concentrations.

In contrast to FL glycoxidation (browning) products in insoluble collagen accumulate continuously from birth to death (1,11,52). In diabetic patients, the rate of accumulation is accelerated (63-65). The degree of excess accumulation in diabetes may depend on duration of diabetes, average glycemic control, and individual susceptibility to oxidative damage. The accumulation of glycoxidation products in collagen, like rust on a car, appears to be an irreversible process (5).

Mechanisms by which Glycation and Browning of Vascular Wall Structural Proteins May Accelerate Atherosclerosis

(i) *Increased Vessel Wall Stiffness.*   Monnier et al (63) showed that increased collagen fluorescence is associated with increased arterial stiffness (assessed *in vivo*), and with elevated systolic and diastolic blood pressures. Increased aortic stiffness in autopsy studies of patients with Type 1 diabetes was confirmed by Oxlund et al (66), but the level of glycoxidation products was not determined. It is probable that loss of the normal elasticity and compliance of arteries and arterioles in diabetes is at least partially due to increased glucose-mediated cross-linking. This may contribute directly to the development of hypertension, while arterial stiffness and hypertension together may result in abnormal shear stresses on the endothelium, predisposing it to injury and the development of atherosclerosis.

(ii) *Covalent Binding of Plasma Constituents*   Endothelial injury allows increased permeation of plasma constituents into the vessel wall, where, in diabetic patients, they come into contact with elevated levels of connective tissue glycoxidation products. Also in diabetes the plasma constituents themselves will have undergone increased modification. Brownlee et al (67) demonstrated there is increased LDH-collagen cross-linking when the lipoprotein was exposed to modified collagen (containing browning products), compared to control collagen. In diabetic compared to non-diabetic animals cross-linking of LDL to aortic collagen was increased 2.5 fold. Trapped in a high-glucose environment in the vessel wall, the LDL particles will undergo extensive glycative and oxidative modification, with further increases in particle atherogenicity. Free radical chain reactions in the trapped LDL may damage not only the lipids within the particle, but also neighboring structural proteins and cells, thus propagating injury to the vascular intima and media, and in situ formation of lipoprotein-immune complexes may further enhance foam cell formation.

(iii) *"Autoxidative Glycation"*   Both simple monosaccharides and FL "auto-oxidize" under physiologic conditions, in the presence of traces of metal ions, generating superoxide radicals (32,68,69). Thus, the presence of glucose or glycated collagen (70), catalyzes lipid peroxidation. Conversely, cross-linking of collagen is stimulated by the products of lipid peroxidation, which themselves generate free radicals (71). In diabetes, these inter-related mechanisms are likely to result in a vicious cycle, propagating direct damage to the arterial wall, as well as enhancing lipid peroxidation.

(iv) *The Macrophage "AGE-Receptor"*   As discussed earlier in this chapter, monocyte/macrophages are intimately involved in the development of atherosclerotic lesions. It is now established that these cells possess a specific receptor (72) which recognizes glycoxidation products: this has been termed the "AGE receptor", and has been shown to be distinct from other scavenger receptors (73). Macrophages expressing this receptor are capable of engulfing not just protein molecules, but also entire cells which have glycoxidation products on their surface (74). The presence of glycoxidation (or "AGE") products in vessel walls is chemotactic to circulating monocyte/macrophages, inducing them to migrate through the vascular endothelium (75). Also, the interaction of AGE-proteins with the AGE-receptor has been shown to be accompanied by release of cytokines, TNF-cr and IL-l (76,77), which are known to mediate growth and remodelling processes, and which, as discussed above, may accelerate the atherosclerotic process.

(v) Effects on Vascular Cells   Connective tissue glycoxidation products may influence the growth of neighboring vascular cells. Renal mesangial cell growth, as determined by tritiated thymidine uptake, is inhibited by the presence of glycated collagen (78). Similar effects have been observed with bovine retinal mural cells (pericytes) (79), human umbilical vein endothelial cells (80), all of which fail to thrive *in vitro* on glycated collagen or laminin. Similar effects *in vivo* in human arterial walls may promote atherosclerosis.

(vi) Renal Impairment   Accumulating glycoxidation products may contribute to the development of renal impairment in diabetes (63,81). Recently a correlation between skin collagen browning and microalburninuria, the earliest manifestation of renal disease, was found (unpublished observations). This suggests that a generalized collagen abnormality may underlie the development of microalbuminuria, and this may partly explain the identification of microalbuminuria as a risk factor for macrovascular disease. The mild hypertension and lipid abnormalities associated with renal impairment may further contribute to the development of atherosclerosis.

(vii) Nitric Oxide   Finally, recent evidence suggests that the presence of collagen glycoxidation products quenches the activity of nitric oxide (endothelium-derived relaxing factor, EDRF) both *in vitro* and *in vivo* (82). This quenching leads to an impairment of endothelium-mediated vasodilatation, and therefore may cause abnormalities in vascular tone. It is possible that local abnormalities of flow, perfusion and blood pressure may result, and these may be injurious to arteries and arterioles.

Is it Possible to Inhibit the Glycation and Browning of Vascular Structural Proteins?

If the gradual, and irreversible, accumulation of glycoxidation products in vascular structural proteins is indeed harmful, it would clearly be desirable to inhibit the process, particularly in diabetic patients. Ways to inhibit the "glycosylative" and "oxidative" arms of the process may be considered separately.

Reducing "Glycative" Stress   The most obvious measure is to optimize glycemic control in order to minimize FL formation. Also, the existing levels of FL may be reduced: even a short-term improvement in glycemic control can reduce the FL content of insoluble skin collagen (5) and presumably of arterial collagens as well. This should decrease the subsequent formation of glycoxidation products. In the future, pharmacologic intervention may be possible. Aminoguanidine, a hydrazine which binds to reactive carbonyl groups, has been the subject of intensive study by Brownlee and co-workers (83). It is thought to act by blocking the open-chain form of glucose, and/or reactive dicarbonyl browning intermediates which are derived from the dissociation of FL (84). Aminoguanidine has been successful in preventing the browning process both *in vitro* and *in vivo* (83).

Reducing Oxidative Stress   Currently there is little evidence concerning the efficacy of any treatment aimed to reduce oxidative damage to proteins in diabetes. Probucol may be effective in reducing lipid peroxidation (85), and may therefore have a protective effect in the vessel wall. Another approach involves the supplementation of free radical scavengers. Of these, ascorbate is believed to be the most important (86), and plasma levels of this, and platelet levels of Vitamin E, another free radical scavenger, tend to be abnormally low in diabetic patients (87-89). However, no studies exist to demonstrate that supplementation of these vitamins will affect the progress of atherosclerosis in diabetic patients.

Conclusions

The processes of glycation and browning, or "glycoxidation", are thought to play a significant role in the acceleration of atherosclerosis in diabetes. The initial glycation reaction increases the atherogenicity of lipoproteins, and diminishes the activity of antithrombin III. Glycation is also thought to enhance the propensity of vessel wall structural proteins to bind extravasated plasma proteins, including lipoproteins. In the longer-lived vascular structural proteins, and in trapped, extravasated plasma proteins, browning, or "glycoxidation", reactions ensue. These involve free-radical oxidation, and multiple vicious cycles of damage to the vessel wall may be set in motion: protein cross-linking, lipid peroxidation, foam cell formation, and free-radical mediated cytotoxicity are all inter-related. Finally, the generation of severely modified proteins and lipoproteins may stimulate immune-complex formation. All of these factors combine to accelerate the atherosclerotic process in diabetes.

References

1. Dunn JA, McCance DR, Thorpe SR, Lyons TJ, Baynes JW. Age-dependent accumulation of N^ε–(carboxymethyl)lysine and N^ε-(carboxymethyl)hydroxylysine in human skin collagen. Biochemistry 30:1205-10, 1991.
2. Ledl F, Schleicher E. New aspects of the Maillard reaction in foods and in the human body. Angew Chem (Int Ed Engl) 29:565-94, 1990.
3. Njoroge FG, Monnier VM. The chemistry of the Maillard reaction under physiological conditions: a review. Prog Clin Biol Res 304:85-107, 1989.
4. The Maillard Reaction in Aging, Diabetes and Nutrition. Baynes JW and Monnier VM, eds., Alan R Liss, Inc, New York, 1989.
5. Lyons TJ, Bailie K, Dunn JA, Dyer DG, Thorpe SR, Baynes JW. Decrease in skin collagen glycation with improved glycemic control in patients with insulin-dependent diabetes mellitus. J Clin Invest 87:1910-1915,1991.
6. Ahmed MU, Thorpe SR, Baynes JW. Identification of carboxymethyllysine as a degradation product of fructose-lysine in glycated protein. J Biol Chem 261:4889-4994, 1986.
7. Ahmed MU, Dunn JA, Walla MD, Thorpe SR, Baynes JW. Oxidative degradation of glucose adducts to protein. Formation of 3-(N epsilon-lysino)-lactic acid from model compounds and glycated proteins. J Biol Chem 263:8816-21, 1988.
8. Sell DR, Monnier VM. Structure elucidation of a senescence cross-link from human extracellular matrix. Implication of pentoses in the aging process. J Biol Chem 264:21597-602, 1989.
9. Dunn JA, Ahmed MU, Murtiashaw MH, Richardson JM, Walla MD, Thorpe SR, Baynes JW. Reaction of ascorbate with lysine and protein under autoxidizing conditions: formation of N~-(carboxymethyl)lysine by reaction between lysine and products of autoxidation of ascorbate. Biochemistry 29:10964-70, 1990.
10. Grandhee SK, Monnier VM. Mechanism of formation of the Maillard protein cross-link pentosidine. Glucose, fructose and ascorbate as pentosidine precursors. J Biol Chem 266:11649-53, 1991.

11. Sell DR, Monnier VM. End-stage renal disease and diabetes catalyze the formation of a pentose-derived crosslink from aging human collagen. J Clin Invest 85:380-4, 1990.

12. Dyer DG, Blackledge JA, Thorpe SR, Baynes JW. Formation of pentosidine during nonenzymatic browning of proteins by glucose. Identification of glucose and other carbohydrates as possible precursors of pentosidine in vivo. J Biol Chem 266:11654-60, 1991.

13. Fu M-X, Knecht KJ, Thorpe SR, Baynes JW. Role of oxygen in the cross-linking and chemical modification of collagen by glucose. Proceedings of IDF Satellite Symposium, Diabetes, in press.

14. Baynes JW. Role of oxidative stress in development of complications in diabetes. Diabetes 40:405-412, 1991.

15. Kennedy L, Baynes JW: Non-enzymatic glycation and the chronic complications of diabetes: an overview. Diabetologia 26:93-98, 1984.

16. Stamler J. Epidemiology, established major risk factors, and the primary prevention of coronary heart disease. In: Cardiology. Parmley W, Chatterjee K, Eds. Philadelphia, PA Lippincott 1987, pp 1-41.

17. Schleicher E, Deufel T, Wieland OH. Non-enzymatic glycation of human serum lipoproteins. FEBS Lett 129: 1-4, 1981.

18. Gonen B, Baenziger J, Schonfeld G, Jacobsen D, Farrar P. Non-enzymatic glycation of low-density lipoproteins in vitro. Diabetes 30:875-878, 1981.

19. Witztum JL Mahoney EM, Branks MJ, Fisher M, Elam R, Steinberg D: Nonenzymatic glucosylation of low-density lipoprotein alters its biologic activity. Diabetes 31:283-291, 1982.

20. Sasaki J, Cottam GL. Glycation of LDL decreases its ability to interact with high-affinity receptors of human fibroblasts in vitro and decreases its clearance from rabbit plasma in vivo. Biochem Biophys Acta 713:199-207, 1982.

21. Steinbrecher UP, Witztum JL. Glucosylation of low density lipoproteins to an extent comparable to that seen in diabetes slows their catabolism. Diabetes 33:130-134, 1984.

22. Lyons TJ, Patrick JS, Baynes JW, Colwell JA, Lopes-Virella. Glycation of low density lipoprotein in patients with Type 1 diabetes: Correlatiom with other parameters of glycaemic control. Diabetologia 29:685-689, 1986.

23. Lopes-Virella MF, Sherer GK, Lees AM, Wohltmann H, Mayfield R, Sagel J, Leroy EC, Colwell JA. Surface binding, internalization and degradation by cultured human fibroblasts of low density lipoproteins isolated from type I (insulin-dependent) diabetic patients: changes with metabolic control. Diabetologia 22:430-436, 1982.

24. Lyons TJ, Klein RL Baynes JW, Stevenson HC, Lopes-Virella MF. Stimulation of cholesteryl ester synthesis in human monocyte-derived macrophages by low-density lipoproteins from type I (insulin-dependent) diabetic patients: the influence of non-enzymatic glycation of low-density lipoprotein. Diabetologia 30:916-923, 1987.

25. Klein RL Lyons TJ, Lopes-Virella MF. Metabolism of very low- and low density lipoproteins isolated from normolipidaemic Type 2 (non-insulin-dependent) diabetic patients by human monocyte-derived macrophages. Diabetologia 33:299-305, 1990.

26. Lopes-Virella MF, Klein RL Lyons TJ, Stevenson HC, Witztum JL. Glycation of low-density lipoprotein enhances cholesteryl ester synthesis in human monocyte-derived macrophages. Diabetes 37:550-557,1988.

27. Jack CM, Sheridan B, Kennedy L, Stout RW. Non-enzymatic glycation of low-density lipoprotein. Results of an affinity chromatography method. Diabetologia 31- 126-128, 1988.

28. Watanabe J, Wohltmann HJ, Klein RL Colwell JA, Lopes-Virella MF. Enhancement of platelet aggregation by low density lipoproteins from IDDM patients. Diabetes 37:1652-1657, 1988.
29. Klein RL Lopes-Virella MF, Colwell JA. Enhancement of platelet aggregation by the glycated subfraction of low density lipoprotein (LDL) isolated from patients with insulin-dependent diabetes mellitus (IDDM). Diabetes 39 (Suppl 1): 173a, 1990.
30. Steinberg D, Parthasarathy S, Carew TE, Khoo JC, Witztum JL. Beyond Cholesterol. N Engl J Med 1989; 320:915-924.
31. Lyons TJ. Oxidized Low Density Lipoproteins - A role in the pathogenesis of atherosclerosis in diabetes? Diabetic Medicine:8:411-419, 1991.
32. Wolff SP, Dean RT. Glucose autoxidation and protein modification: the potential role of "autoxidative glycation" in diabetes mellitus. Biochem J 245:243-250, 1987.
33. Curtiss LK, Witztum JL. Plasma apo-lipoproteins A-I, A-II, B, C-I and E are glucosylated in hyperglycemic diabetic subjects. Diabetes 34:452-461, 1985.
34. Brownlee M, Pongor S, Cerami A. Covalent attachment of soluble proteins by non-enzymatically glycated collagen: role in the in situ formation of immune complexes. J Exp Med 158:1739-44, 1983.
35. Griffith RL, Virella GT, Stevenson HC et al. LDL metabolism by macrophages activated with LDL immune complexes: A possible mechanism of foam cell formation. J Exp Med, 168: 1041-1059,1988.
36. Gisinger C, Virella GT, Lopes-Virella MF. Erythrocyte-bound low density lipoprotein (LDL) immune complexes lead to cholesteryl ester accumulation in human monocyte derived macrophages. Clin Immunol Immunopath 59: 37-52, 1991.
37. Klimov AN, Denisenko AD, Popov AV et al. Lipoprotein-antibody immune complexes: Their catabolism and role in foam cell formation. Atherosclerosis 58:1-15, 1985.
38. Luscimkas FW, Brock AF, Arnaout MA, et al. Endothelial-leukocyte adhesion molecule-1-dependent and leukocyte (CD11/CD18)-dependent mechanisms contribute to polymorphonuclear leukocyte adhesion to cytokine-activated human vascular endothelium. J Immunol 142:2257-2263, 1989.
39. Bevilacqua MP, Pober JS, Majeau GR, et al. Interleukin-1 induces biosynthesis and cell surface expression of procoagulant activity in human vascular endothelial cells. J Exp Med 160:618-622,1984.
40. Martin S, Maruta K, Burkart V et al. IL-1 and INF-g increase vascular permeability. Immunology 64:301-305, 1988.
41. Warner SJC, Auger KR, Libby P. Interleukin-1 induces interleukin-1. II. Recombinant human interleukin-1 induces interleukin-1 production by adult human vascular endothelial cells. J Immunol 139:1911-1917,1987.
42. Breviario F, Bertocchi F, Dejana E et al. IL-1 induced adhesion of polymorphonuclear leukocytes to cultured human endothelial cells. Role of platelet-activating factor. J Immunol 141:3391-3397, 1988.
43. Pohlman TH, Staness KA, Beatty PG et al. An endothelial cell surface factor(s) induced in vitro by lipopolysaccharide, interleukin-1 and tumor necrosis factor α increases neutrophil adherence by a CDw18-dependent mechanism. J Immunol 136:4548-4553, 1986.
44. Kilpatrick JM, Hyman B, Virella G. Human endothelial cell damage induced by interactions between polymorphonuclear leukocytes and immune complex-coated erythrocytes. Clin Immunol Immunopath 44:335-347, 1987.
45. Raines EW, Dower SK, Ross R. Interleukin-1 mitogenic activity for fibroblasts and smooth muscle cells is due to PDGF-AA. Science 243:393-396,1989.
46. Nawroth PP, Bank I, Hadley D et al. Tumor necrosis factor/ cachectin interacts with endothelial cell receptors to induce release of interleukin-1. J Exp Med 165:1363-1375, 1986.

47. Brownlee M, Vlassara H, Cerami A. Inhibition of heparin-catalyzed antithrombin III activity by non-enzymatic glycation: possible role in fibrin deposition in diabetes. Diabetes 33: 532-535,1984.

48. Ceriello A, Guigliano D, Quatraro A, Stante A, Concoli G, Dello Russo P, D'Onofrio F. Daily rapid blood glucose variations may condition antithrombin biological activity but not its plasma concentration in insulin dependent diabetes: a possible role for labile non-enzymatic glycation. Diab Metab 13:16-19, 1987.

49. McVerry VA, Thorpe S, Gaffney JP, Huehns ER. Non-enzymatic glycation of fibrinogen. Haemostasis 10: 261-270, 1981.

50. Hamlin CR, Kohn RR. Evidence for progressive, age-related structural changes in post-mature human collagen. Biochim Biophys Acta 236:458-67, 1971.

51. Hamlin CR, Kohn RR. Determination of human chronological age by study of a collagen sample. Exp Gerontol 7:377-9, 1972.

52. Hamlin CR, Kohn RR, Luschin JH. Apparent accelerated aging of human collagen in diabetes mellitus. Diabetes 24:902-4,1975.

53. Yue DK, McLennan S, Delbridge L, Handelsman DJ, Reeve T, Turtle JR. The thermal stability of collagen in diabetic rats: correlation with severity of diabetes and non-enzymatic glycation. Diabetologia 24:282-5, 1983.

54. Monnier VM, Cerami A. Non-enzymatic browning in vivo. Possible process for aging of long-lived proteins. Science 211:491-3, 1981.

55. Bailey AJ, Kent MJC. Non-enzymatic glycation of fibrous and basement membrane collagens. In: The Maillard Reaction in Aging, Diabetes and Nutrition. Baynes JW and Monnier VM, eds., Alan R Liss, Inc, New York, 1989, ppl09-22.

56. Rosenberg H, Modrak JB, Hassing JM, Al-Turk WA, Stohs SJ. Glycated collagen. Biochem Biophys Res Comm 91:498-501, 1979.

57. Cohen MP, Urdanivia E, Surma M, Wu V-Y. Increased glycation of glomerular basement membrane collagen in diabetes. Biochem Biophys Res Comm 95:765-69, 1980.

58. Schneider SL, Kohn RR. Glycation of human collagen in aging and diabetes mellitus. J Clin Invest 66:1179-81, 1980.

59. Lyons TJ, Kennedy L Non-enzymatic glycation of skin collagen in patients with limited joint mobility. Diabetologia 1985; 28:2-5.

60. Vishwanath V, Frank KE, Elmets CA, Dauchot PJ, Monnier VM. Glycation of skin collagen in Type I diabetes mellitus: correlations with long-term complications. Diabetes 35:916-21, 1986.

61. Vogt BW, Schleicher ED, Wieland OH. -amino-lysine-bound glucose in human tissues obtained at autopsy. Diabetes 31:1123-7,1982.

62. Garlick RL, Bunn HF, Spiro RG. Non-enzymatic glycation of basement membranes from human glomeruli and bovine sources. Diabetes 37:1144-50, 1988.

63. Monnier VM, Vishwanath V, Frank KE, Elmets CA, Dauchot P, Kohn RR. Relations between complications to Type I diabetes mellitus and collagen-linked fluorescence. N Engl J Med 314:403-408, 1986.

64. Monnier VM, Sell DR, Abdul-Karim FW, Emancipator SN. Collagen browning and cross-linking are increased in chronic experimental hyperglycernia. Relevance to diabetes and aging. Diabetes 37:867-72,1988.

65. Baynes JW, Dyer DG, Dunn JA, Thorpe SR, Lyons TJ, McCance DR. Accumulation of Maillard reaction products in skin collagen in diabetes and aging. Diabetologia 34(Suppl 2):A7, 1991.

66. Oxlund H, Rasmussen LM, Andreassen TI, Heickendorff L. Increased aortic stiffness in patients with type 1 (insulin-dependent) diabetes mellitus. Diabetologia 32:748-52, 1989.

67. Brownlee M, Vlassara H, Cerami A. Nonenzymatic glycation products on collagen covalently trap low-density lipoprotein. Diabetes 34:938-41, 1985.

68. Gillery P, Monboisse JC, Maquart FX, Borel JP. Glycation of proteins as a source of superoxide. Diab Metab 14:25-30, 1988.

69. Mullarkey CJ, Edelstein D, Brownlee M. Free radical generation by early glycation products: a mechanism for accelerated atherogenesis in diabetes. Biochem Biophys Res Cornmun 173:932-9, 1990.
70. Hicks M, Delbridge L Yue DK, Reeve TS. Catalysis of lipid peroxidation by glucose and glycated collagen. Biochem Biophys Res Commun 151:649-55, 1988.
71. Hicks M, Delbridge L Yue, DK, Reeve TS. Increase in crosslinking of nonenzymatically glycated collagen induced by products of lipid peroxidation. Arch Biochem Biophys 268:249-54, 1989.
72. Vlassara H, Brownlee M, Cerami A. Accumulation of diabetic rat peripheral nerve myelin by macrophages increases with extent and duration of nonenzymatic glycation. J Exp Med 160:197-207, 1984.
73. Vlassara H, Brownlee M, Cerami A. Novel macrophage receptor for glucose-modified proteins is distinct from previously described scavenger receptors. J Exp Med 164:1301-9, 1986.
74. Vlassara H, Valinsky J, Brownlee M, Cerarni C, Nishimoto S, Cerami A. Advanced glycation end products on erythrocyte cell surface induce receptor-mediated phagocytosis by macrophages. A model for turnover of aging cells. J Exp Med 166:539-49, 1987.
75. Kirstein M, Brett J, Radoff S, Ogawa S, Stern D, Vlassara H. Advanced protein glycation induces transendothelial human monocyte chemotaxis and secretion of platelet-derived growth factor: role in vascular disease of diabetes and aging. Proc Natl Acad Sci USA 87:9010-4,1990.
76. Vlassara H, Brownlee M, Manogue KR, Dinarello CA, Pasagian A. Cachectin/TNF and ILrl induced by glucose-modified proteins: role in normal tissue remodeling. Science 240:1546-8, 1988.
77. Vlassara H, Brownlee M, Cerami A. Macrophage receptor-mediated processing and regulation of advanced glycation end product (AGE)-modified proteins: role in diabetes and aging. Prog Clin Biol Res 304:205-18, 1989.
78. Crowley ST, Brownlee M, Edelstein D, Satriano JA, Mori T, Singhal PC, Schlondorff DO. Effects of nonenzymatic glycation of mesangial matrix on proliferation of mesangial cells. Diabetes 40:540-7,1991.
79. Tsilibary EC, Charonis AS, Gerritsen AE, Reger LA. Retinal mural cell response to non-enzymatically glucosylated basement membrane components. Diabetes 40(suppl1):A1206.
80. Takeda H, Watanabe K, Suzuki D, Miyano R, Tanaka K, Machimura H, Yagame M, Watanabe S, Inoue W, Kaneshige H, Sakai H. Functional changes of cultured endothelial cells induced by glycated extracellular matrix. Diabetes 40(suppll):A492, 1991.
81. Makita Z, Radoff S, Rayfield EJ, Yang Z, Skolnik E, Delaney V, Friedman EA, Cerami A, Vlassara H. Advanced glycation end products in patients with diabetic nephropathy. N Engl J Med 325:836-42, 1991.
82. Bucala R, Tracey KJ, Cerami A. Advanced glycation products quench nitric oxide and mediate defective endothelium-dependent vasodilatation in experimental diabetes. J Clin Invest 87:432-8, 1991.
83. Brownlee M, Vlassara H, Kooney A, Ulrich P, Cerami A. Aminoguanidine prevents diabetes-induced arterial wall protein cross-linking. Science 232:1629-32, 1986.
84. Requena JR. The main mechanism of action of aminoguanidine. Diabetologia 34(suppl2):A162, 1991.
85. Parthasarathy S, Young SG, Witztum JL, Pittman RC, Steinberg D. Probucol inhibits oxidative modification of low density lipoprotein. J Clin Invest 77:641-4, 1986.
86. Frei B, England L Ames BN. Ascorbate is an outstanding antioxidant in human plasma. Proc Natl Acad Sci USA 86:6377-81, 1989.

87. Som S, Basu S, Mukherjee D, Deb S, Choudhury PR, Mukherjee S, Chatterjee SN,
     Chatterjee IB. Ascorbic acid metabolism in diabetes mellitus. Metabolism 30:572-
     577, 1981.
88. Jennings PE, Chirico S, Jones AF, Lunec J, Barnett AH. Vitamin C metabolites
     and microangiopathy in diabetes mellitus. Diabetes Res 6:151-154,1987.
89. Karpen CW, Cataland S, O'Dorisio TM, Panganamala RV. Production of 12 HETE
     and vitamin E status in platelets from type 1 human diabetic subjects. Diabetes
     34:526-531, 1985.

A Modern View of Atherogenesis

Colin J. Schwartz

Recent years have seen the conceptually restrictive unifocal hypotheses of atherogenesis abandoned in favor of a more unified approach to pathogenesis. In essence, there is now a consensus that atherosclerosis is an inflammatory process involving complex interactive cascades of inflammatory mediators, along with the reparative responses of the arterial wall, all occurring in a hyperlipidemic and dyslipoproteinemic environment. Key players in these cascades and currently the subject of intense investigation, are the monocyte-derived macrophage, and the net oxidative stress status of the arterial intima. Lipoproteins, particularly those of the low density family are essential participants in the atherogenic scenario.

Roles of the Endogenous Cells of the Arterial Wall.
This category includes endothelial (EC) and smooth muscle (SMC) cells, of which more than one type may exist. Selected roles of these two cell types of particular relevance to atherogenic mechanisms are summarized in Table 1. The endothelium clearly plays a major role in macromolecular transport, including the transcytosis of plasma lipoproteins. It is important to emphasize that lipoprotein influx to the arterial intima is not dependent upon endothelial cell denudation. Both EC and SMC express and synthesize MCP-1, a monocyte-specific chemoattractant, the synthesis of which is augmented by oxidatively modified low density lipoproteins (Ox-LDL). Endothelial cells also play a key role in blood monocyte recruitment to the arterial intima, an essential element in atherogenesis. Specifically both EC-derived 1L-1ß and VCAM-1 are likely key players in monocyte attachment to the endothelium, an important prelude to intimal monocyte recruitment.

The intimal generation of reactive oxygen species (ROS) or free radicals is another important facet of atherogenesis. Both EC and SMC, along with activated intimal monocyte-derived macrophages contribute to the oxidative stress status (OSS) of the intima. Many other aspects of endothelial biology are of interest and potential importance, including its thromboresistant qualities and the synthesis of endothelial derived relaxing factors (EDRF) or nitric oxide, likely responsible for the regulation of vascular tone and the development of arterial spasm.

A. L. Catapano et al. (eds.), Drugs Affecting Lipid Metabolism, 421–425.

Smooth muscle cells contribute in a major way to the growth and maturation of the atherosclerotic plaque, not as significant progenitors of foam cells, but as the source of fibrillary and non-fibrillary connective tissue elements. The factors regulating smooth muscle cell migration to the intima, and their subsequent proliferation have yet to be fully characterized, but likely involve both the platelet derived growth factor (PDFGF) and fibroblast growth factor (FGF) families. Intimal proteoglycans and fibrillary connective tissue elements are thought to trap lipoproteins in microdomains facilitating their oxidative modification.

Table I

Selected Cellular Roles of Particular Relevance to Atherogenesis

		Endothelial Cells (EC)	Smooth Muscle Cells (SMC)
1)	Lipoprotein Transcytosis	+	-
2)	Synthesis of MCP-1	+	+
3)	Generation of Free Radicals	+	+
4)	Synthesis of IL-ß	+	+
5)	Synthesis of ELAMS (VCAM-1)	+	-
6)	Functional LDL (B/E) Receptors	+	+
7)	Functional Scavenger Receptors	+	-*
8)	Collagen and Elastin Synthesis	-**	+
9)	Proteoglycan Synthesis	-	+
10)	Thromboresistance	+	-
11)	Synthesis of EDRF	+	-

*Scavenger receptor function can be demonstrated in SMC only under special circumstances.
**Collagen synthesis by EC is minimal except for synthesis of basement membrane.   IL-1ß = Interleukin 1ß;   ELAM = endothelial leukocyte adhesion mole-cule;   V-CAM = Vascular cell adhesion molecule; EDRF = endothelial derived relaxing factor (nitric oxide).

Exogenous (Blood) Components Participating in the Atherogenic Process. The formed elements of particular importance include peripheral blood monocytes, T-lymphocytes, and platelets. Non-cellular participants include a spectrum of plasma proteins including lipoproteins, fibrinonectins, and fibrinogen. Fibrinogen is becoming increasingly prominent on the horizon, because of the role of hyperfibrinogenemia as an independent predictor of CHD risk. Of the diverse and heterogeneous lipoprotein family, low density lipoprotein (LDL) including the small dense LDL phenotype (LDL-B), and lipoprotein (a) (Lp(a)) are of particular importance. Lp(a) likely provides a functional link between abnormal lipid metabolism and hemostasis via the inhibition of fibrinolysis. It is also of interest that the small dense LDL particles (LDL-B) more readily enter the arterial intima and are more susceptible to oxidative modification.

When one adds to these multiple and diverse cellular and non-cellular factors the roles of inflammatory cytokines such as 1L-1ß, mitogens including FGF and PDGF, and chemoattractants such as MCP-1, a complex pathogenic arena emerges. Moreover, all of these phenomena interact at differing stages in the atherogenic sequence.

Early lesion Development.
In Table 2 we summarize the quintet of determinants of early lesion development. Let us commence by examining the subject of monocyte recruitment. Attachment of monocytes to the arterial endothelium is a prelude to their migration to the subendothelial space (SES). Attachment can be enhanced by endothelial activation which itself can be induced experimentally by tumor necrosis factor (TNFα) and bacterial lipopolysaccharide (LPS). A variety of endothelial leukocyte adhesion molecules and adhesive cytokines such as 1L-1ß participate actively in this process.

The mechanisms and routes of monocyte transendothelial migration are not fully established and, in fact, it has not been determined whether all monocytes migrate between endothelial cells; some might pass directly through the cell much as some cancer cells can, possibly involving the secretion of selected metalloproteases.

The net intimal accumulation of monocytes at specific sites suggests that monocyte migration is under the control of a chemical guidance system. One identified chemoattractant for monocytes has been called "monocyte chemotactic protein 1" (MCP-1). Another, as described by Steinberg, is "oxidatively modified LDL or Ox-LDL. MCP-1 is monocyte-specific and active at approximately 10^{-9} molar concentrations. Lymphocytes and neutrophils lack receptors for MCP-1" and each monocyte has approximately 2-3,000 MCP-1 receptors. When minimally modified LDL is introduced into the system the

Table II
The Determinants of Early Lesion Development

A. Focal Intimal Influx and Accumulation of Plasma Lipoproteins (LDL, LDL-B, Lp (a))
B. Low Hemodynamic Shear Stress with Areas of Reversing Blood Flow.
C. An Augmented Net Oxidative Stress Status (OSS).
D. Oxidative Modification of Intimal Lipoproteins.
E. Focal Blood Monocyte Recruitment to the Arterial Intima.

expression of the message for MCP-1 and its synthesis increases in a dose-dependent manner. Our presumption for now is that the minimally modified LDL has undergone mild oxidation.

Once the monocytes have entered the subendothelial space they undergo a process of activation and differentiation and evolve into macrophages. Macrophage activation is associated with an increased generation of free radicals, secretion of many hydrolytic and proteolytic enzymes and numerous other functional changes. If migration-inhibition factors are present, such as Ox-LDL, a prolonged intimal residence time occurs. These monocyte-derived macrophages have many actual or potential roles in atherogenesis. Because of their phagocytic capacity, the phagocytosis of LDL aggregates may provide one pathway for the non-receptor-mediated uptake of lipoproteins. Macrophages secrete mitogens, including those that stimulate smooth muscle proliferation. They also generate reactive oxygen species, (ROS) which result in lipoprotein oxidation, membrane injury, and cytotoxicity. The uptake of oxidatively modified lipoproteins by the non-down-regulating macrophage scavenger receptor leads to intracellular cholesterol and cholesteryl ester accumulation and foam cell formation, pathognomonic of the early atherosclerotic lesion. While oxidative modification appears to be particularly important in this process, non enzymatic glycation, such as occurs in diabetes mellitus, may also play a significant role, particularly when it occurs in conjunction with oxidation.

Net Oxidative Stress Status (OSS) and Intimal Lipoprotein Oxidation.
As indicated in Table 2, these are both important determinants of early lesion development. The net oxidative stress status of the arterial intima reflects the relative balance among the mechanisms generating oxidants, and the amounts and efficiencies of both the intra-and-extra-cellular antioxidant defense systems. As described above, the sites of intimal free radical generation are both endothelial and smooth muscle cells, and activated macrophages.
In terms of intimal lipoprotein oxidation, the precise nature of the chemical and structural changes occurring in both the lipid and protein moieties after exposure to oxidant stress is poorly documented. Once initiated, however, peroxy radicals can themselves give rise to a propagated lipid oxidative reaction.
LDL oxidation can lead to a number of biologic sequelae, including diminished B/E receptor recognition, increased scavenger receptor recognition, and increased MCP-1 expression and secretion. Ox-LDL is also chemotactic and augments interleukin-1 expression and synthesis, which plays an important role in monocyte attachment. Furthermore, it acts as a migration inhibition factor, inactivates EDRF, is antigenic, and augments the expression of macrophage colony-stimulating factors. Oxidized LDL is remarkably cytotoxic, probably due to the aldehyde 2,4 - decadienal.
Plaque Formation and Progression.
Atherosclerotic lesions do not occur at random, but consistently exhibit a focal topographic distribution, providing evidence for the role of the focal hemodynamic environment in lesion initiation or progression. There is now considerable evidence that atherosclerosis develops preferentially in areas of low hemodynamic shear stress with domains of reversing flow, where the residence times of molecules such a lipoproteins, and cells such as monocytes are prolonged.
The fatty streak is probably the earliest identifiable stage in lesion formation and is probably reversible. If the process is not reversed at this point, however, the lesions grow with a continuing recruitment monocytes, intimal lipoproteins influx and accumulation and lipoprotein oxidation. Further, smooth muscle cells migrate from the media into the subendothelial space presumably under the guidance of PDGF, and proliferate as a result of stimulation by fibroblast growth factors (FGFs). Three pivotal changes take place next: the formation of an extracellular lipid core from foam cells, probably caused by the cytoxicity of oxidized LDL molecules; smooth-muscle cell proliferation, which is probably under FGF regulation; and connective tissue synthesis. Thus the lesion is converted from a fatty streak to a

progressing atheromatous plaque. The plaque contains lymphocytes likely indicating an autoimmune process. Thrombosis, although it does not initiate atherogenesis, certainly adds significantly to the later stages of plaque growth.

Therapeutic Implications:
While strategies to lower LDL-C remain important, the emerging importance of lipoprotein oxidation as a pivotal mechanism in atherogenesis highlights the likely therapeutic value of both pharmacologic (eg. Probucol) and natural (Vitamin E, C, ß carotenes) antioxidants.

Suggested reading

Steinberg D, Parthasarathy S, Carew TE, Khoo JC, and Witztum JL (1989). Beyond Cholesterol: Modifications of Low-Density Lipoprotein that Increase Its Atherogenicity. New England J Med, 320 pp. 915-924.

Meade TW, Mellows S, Borozovic M, Miller GJ, Chakrabarti RR, North WRS, Haines AP, Stirling Y, Imeson JD, and Thompson SG (1986). Haemostatic function and ischaemic heart disease: Principle results of the Northwick Park Heart Study. Lancet, 2 pp. 533-537.

Brown MS, Goldstein JL (1983). Lipoprotein metabolism in the macrophage: Implications for cholesterol deposition in atherosclerosis. Ann Rev Biochem, 52 pp. 223.

Hessler JR, Morel DW, Lewis LJ, Chisolm GM (1983). Lipoprotein oxidation and lipoprotein-induced cytotoxicity. Arteriosclerosis, 3 pp. 215.

Schwartz CJ, Valente AJ, Sprague EA, Kelley JL, and Nerem RM (1991). The Pathogenesis of Atherosclerosis: An Overview. Clinical Cardiology, 14 pp. 1-16.

Schwartz CJ, Valente AJ, Sprague EA, Kelley JL, Cayatte AJ, and Rozek MM (1992). Pathogenesis of the Atherosclerotic Lesion: Implications for Diabetes Mellitus. Diabetes Care, 15 pp. 1156-1167.

Schwartz CJ, Valente AJ, Sprague EA, Kelley JL, Cayatte AJ, and Mowery J (1992). Atherosclerosis: Potential Targets for Stabilization and Regression. Circulation, 86 Suppl. III, pp. 117-123.

Schwartz CJ and Sprague EA (1992). Vascular Endothelium and Hemodynamic Stress. Nutr Metab Cardiovasc Dis, pp.

DEFECTIVE CATABOLISM OF OXIDIZED LDL BY J774 MURINE MACROPHAGES

Paola Roma, Franco Bernini, Roberta Fogliatto, Stefano M. Bertulli, Simonetta Negri, Remo Fumagalli and Alberico L. Catapano

A number of in vitro (2-4) and ex vivo (5-9) data support the hypothesis that a modified form of LDL, namely oxidized LDL (OxLDL), is a physiological ligand for the scavenger receptor (10,11), and may lead to the massive deposition of intracellular esterified cholesterol, thus sustaining the genesis and progression of atherosclerotic lesions. This hypothesis may result controversial, since recent findings indicate that, in murine macrophages, OxLDL are not efficiently degraded intracellularly (12,13) and poorly stimulate ACAT activity. The following experiments were designed to verify the extent of OxLDL internalization and to study their cellular localization. The possibility for an intracellular accumulation of degradation products of OxLDL was also considered.

METHODS

Cells.
J774 murine macrophages, an established cell line (16), were used to study the metabolism of oxidized LDL. EAhy-926, a permanent human hybrid cell line expressing factor VIII-related antigen (17), a model for human endothelial cells, was used for biological oxidation of lipoproteins.

Lipoproteins.
LDL (1.019-1.063 g/ml) were isolated from human plasma by sequential ultracentrifugation (18). Acetylation was performed according to Basu et al. (19). Chemical oxidation was performed under sterile conditions, by incubating LDL at 37° C for 24 hours, at 0.2 mg protein/ml in PBS + 20 μM CuSO$_4$, and blocked in ice, with the addition of BHT 40 μM. Biological oxidation was performed, under sterile conditions, by incubating LDL in the presence of EAhy-926 cells at 37° C for 24 hours, at the concentration of 0.07-0.1 mg protein/ml, in serum-free medium containing 12 μM CuSO$_4$ (20), and blocked as above. LDL incubated in the same conditions but in the absence of cells were used as control lipoproteins for BioOxLDL. Oxidized LDL and BioOxLDL were concentrated by ultrafiltration under N$_2$ pressure, desalted in PBS and sterile filtered. Modification of lipoproteins was routinely tested by non denaturing gel electrophoresis in 0.8% agarose in 0.1 M TRIS, pH 8.6, at 200 V (22).

A. L. Catapano et al. (eds.), Drugs Affecting Lipid Metabolism, 427–439.
© 1993 Kluwer Academic Publishers and Fondazione Giovanni Lorenzini.

Iodination.
Lipoproteins were labelled with ^{125}I-NaI according to Bilheimer et al. (25), desalted
by gel filtration of Sephadex G-25 eluted with PBS and sterile filtered.

Cholesterol loading of cells and cholesterol determination.
J774 cells were incubated at 37° C in MEM + 0.2% FAF-BSA (medium A), alone
or containing modified lipoproteins at increasing concentrations, for 18 hours.
At the end of the incubation lipids were extracted from washed cells with
hexane:isopropylic alchool 3:2 (v:v). Lipid extracts were dried under a N_2 stream
and redissolved in hexane: one third of the extract was used for the determination of
total cholesterol by an enzymatic colorimetric assay (26). Thin layer
chromatography (TLC) was performed on the remaining portion of the extract in
petroleum ether:diethyl ether:acetic acid 70:30:1 (v:v:v). The percentages of free
and esterified cholesterol were determined by enzymatic colorimetric assay on
extracts of the corresponding areas scraped from the plates.
Cellular proteins were dissolved in 1 N NaOH and quantitated according to Lowry
(27).

ACAT assay.
Cell monolayers were washed overnight in medium A, then incubated for 2, 6 or 9
hours in medium A alone or containing OxLDL, BioOxLDL (40 μg cholesterol/ml)
or AcLDL (30 μg cholesterol/ml). Cells were then incubated with ^{14}C-oleate-
albumin complex (0.1 mM) for 2 hours and ACAT activity determined as described
(28).

Uptake and degradation of lipoproteins.
J774 cells were incubated for 18 hours in medium A with or without chloroquine
100 μM, washed and incubated for 5 hours at 37°C in medium A containing [125]I-
OxLDL or ^{125}I-AcLDL (10 μg/ml). Total uptake and degradation were determined
as described (29).
J774 macrophages were incubated at 37°C for 4 hours in medium A containing one
of the following lipoproteins: ^{125}I-AcLDL, ^{125}I-OxLDL, ^{125}I-LDL incubated in
MEM + 12 μM $CuSo_4$ in the absence of cells, and ^{125}I-BioOxLDL (7 and 14
μg/ml). Non specific uptake and degradation were evaluated in the presence of a 30
fold excess of the unlabelled ligand.
Intracellular degraded ligand was quantitated after incubating cell pellets in Kyro
EOB, according to Brown et al. (29).

Binding and internalization of lipoproteins.
In this experiment two sets of conditions were used: a) cells were incubated at 4°C
for 2 hours in HCO_3^- free medium A, 10 mM HEPES, containing I-OxLDL (10
μg/ml); b) cells were incubated at 37°C for 5 hours in medium A, containing the
radioactive lipoproteins as above.
Cells from a) and b) were washed and incubated in medium A at 37°C for 10' with
trypsin (0.05%) or pronase (0.25%), or at 4°C for 1 hour in the presence of an
excess of unlabelled ligand (1 mg/ml). Radioactivity released into the medium by
these treatments was taken as the binding component of total uptake, whereas the
remaining, cell associated, radioactivity was taken as internalization.

Filipin stain.
J774 cells were incubated at 37°C for 5 or 18 hours in medium A alone or with the addition of AcLDL or OxLDL (50 μg cholesterol/ml). At the end of the incubation the cells were washed, fixed, incubated in PBS containing filipin 0.005% (30) and viewed with a fluorescence microscope (Zeiss Octivert) at 630 x magnification.

Subcellular fractionation.
J774 cells were grown in 100 mm Petri dishes and incubated at 37°C for 18 hours in medium A alone or containing OxLDL or AcLDL (50 μg cholesterol/ml). At the end of the incubation washed cells were homogenized and subcellular fractions were obtained by density gradient centrifugation in Percoll 7.8% (31). Protein content and the activity of two marker enzymes (N-acetyl ß-glucosaminidase and 5' nucleotidase) (31) was determined on eleven fractions (1 ml) collected from the gradient. Cholesterol was quantitated on lipid extracts of the same fractions.

Degradation of lipoproteins by partially purified lysosomal enzymes.
J774 cells were homogenized. The lysate was centrifuged at 750 x g (10') and the supernatant at 10.000 x g (20'). The pellet was resuspended in water and freeze-thawed six times to disrupt the lysosomes (33); 25 μg of protein were then mixed with increasing amounts of ^{125}I-LDL, ^{125}I-AcLDL or ^{125}I-OxLDL (0.20 to 1.95 μg/ml) in a final volume of 0.1 ml of either citrate-buffered MEM, pH 4.5, or TRIS-buffered MEM, pH 9, and incubated for 4 h at 37°C. The degradation of the radioactive substrate was measured as TCA non precipitable, non iodide radioactivity, as above.

RESULTS

Initially, a comparison between chemically oxidized LDL (OxLDL) and biologically oxidized LDL (BioOxLDL) was performed.
Their electrophoretic mobilities were, respectively, 1.8 times and 1.5 times that of native LDL. In J774 macrophages both OxLDL and, although less efficiently, BioOxLDL caused a concentration dependent accumulation of cholesterol, which was mainly unesterified. Even at the highest loading esterified cholesterol did not exceed 21% of total cholesterol (fig. 1). Consistent with this observation both lipoproteins activated ACAT very poorly (880 and 754 pmoles ^{14}C-cholesteryl oleate/mg cell protein in OxLDL- and BioOxLDL-incubated cells, respectively, versus 425 and 7070 pmoles ^{14}C-cholesteryl oleate/mg cell protein in control and AcLDL-incubated cells, respectively) (fig. 2).
Figure 3 illustrates the specific uptake and degradation of radioactively labelled AcLDL, OxLDL, BioOxLDL and sham-incubated LDL by J774 macrophages. LDL incubated in MEM without cells neither were taken up by macrophages nor were degraded, indicating that cells are required to induce LDL modification. Specific uptakes of iodinated OxLDL, BioOxLDL and AcLDL were comparable. While ^{125}I-AcLDL were efficiently degraded (4,231 and 7,426 ng/mg cell protein at 7 and 14 μg/ml) both ^{125}I-OxLDL and ^{125}I-BioOxLDL underwent a relatively poor degradation (respectively 840 and 1,250 ng/mg cell protein, at 7 and 14 μg/ml, 539 and 883 ng/mg cell protein, at the same concentrations). Altogether these data indicate that the behaviour of OxLDL and BioOxLDL is very similar, if not

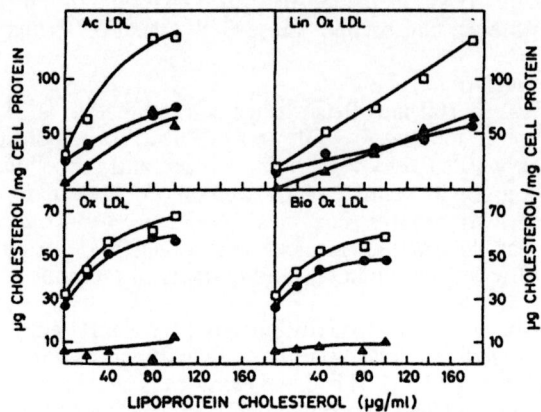

Figure 1. Effect of modified LDL on the cholesterol content of J774 macrophages. Cells were washed and incubated at 37°C for 18 hours in medium A alone or containing AcLDL, OxLDL or BioOxLDL at the indicated concentrations of lipoprotein cholesterol. At the end of the incubation lipids were extracted from washed cells and total (□), free (●) and esterified (▲) cholesterol were quantitated as described in Methods.

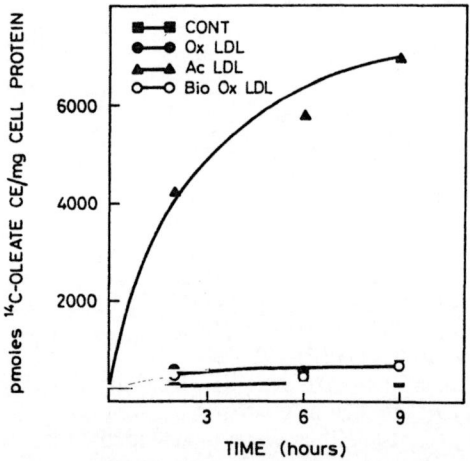

Figure 2. Effect of modified LDL on ACAT activity in J774 macrophages. Cells were washed in medium A, then incubated at 37°C for the indicated times in medium A alone or containing OxLDL, BioOxLDL (50 μg lipoprotein cholesterol/ml) or AcLDL (30 μg lipoprotein cholesterol/ml). Cells were then incubated in medium A containing ^{14}C-oleate-albumin complex (0.1 mM) for 2 hours. Lipids were extracted from washed cells and the radioactivity in esterified cholesterol was determined as described in Methods.

identical. Since OxLDL and BioOxLDL displayed similar metabolic behaviours the former were used as a model to investigate the cellular processing of oxidatively modified LDL.

The hypothesis that the poor degradation of OxLDL may depend upon the blockade of a chloroquine-sensitive pathway was tested. In cells treated with chloroquine 100 μM the degradation of both iodinated AcLDL and OxLDL dropped to 27-28% of the degradation in untreated cells (table 1). Uptake of ^{125}I-AcLDL was most

Table 1. Effect of chloroquine (Chl) on uptake and degradation of ^{125}I-OxLDL and ^{125}I-AcLDL in J774 macrophages.

^{125}I LP	Chl	Uptake	Degradation
		(μg/mg cell protein)	
OxLDL	-	2263 $\pm$ 28*	1027 $\pm$ 75*
OxLDL	+	3086 $\pm$509	282 $\pm$ 15
AcLDL	-	1289 $\pm$ 34	3069 $\pm$117
AcLDL	+	4380 $\pm$376	855 $\pm$140

Cells were incubated for 18 hours in medium A with (+) or without (-) chloroquine 100 μM, washed and incubated for 4 hours at 37°C in medium A containing ^{125}I-OxLDL or ^{125}I-AcLDL (10 μg/ml). Total uptake and degradation were quantitated described in Methods.

* Data are the mean $\pm$ S.D. of three determinations.

sensitive to chloroquine, with a 3.4 fold increase over control values, versus 1.4 fold for OxLDL (table 1). The observation that, although scarce, the degradation of OxLDL is sensitive to chloroquine (table 1) suggests that this takes places within an acidic compartment; furthermore, these data indicate that the cellular processing of OxLDL is partially blocked, or extremely slow. The possibility for an intracellular accumulation of products of apoB hydrolysis, which would lead to underestimate lipoprotein degradation, was also evaluated. With two different concentrations of ^{125}I-OxLDL the amount of intracellular degraded ligand did not exceed 8.5% of total intracellular lipoprotein. An explanation to these findings could be that, once bound to the cellular surface, OxLDL are poorly internalized. Binding and internalization of ^{125}I-OxLDL at 4°C and 37°C were quantitated by mean of three alternative methods. Binding of ^{125}I-OxLDL to J774 cells, determined as the amount of lipoprotein displaced by a 100 fold excess unlabelled ligand, was the same at 4°C

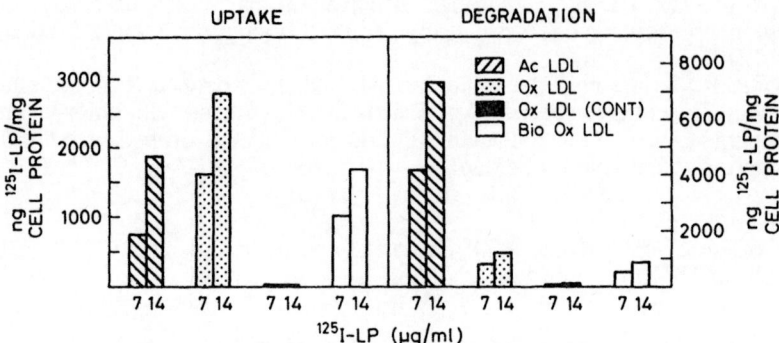

Figure 3. Uptake and degradation of modified LDL by J774 macrophages. J774 macrophages were incubated at 37°C for 4 hours in medium A containing one of the following lipoproteins: ^{125}I-AcLDL, ^{125}I-OxLDL, ^{125}I-LDL incubated in MEM + 12 μM CuSo$_4$ in the absence of cells, and ^{125}I-BioOxLDL (7 and 14 μg/ml). Non specific uptake and degradation were evaluated in the presence of a 30 fold excess of the unlabeled ligand. Specific uptake and degradation were quantitated as described in Methods.

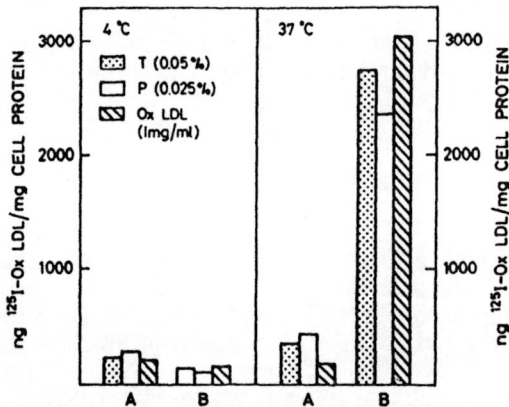

Figure 4. Binding and internalization of ^{125}I-OxLDL by J774 macrophages. Cells were incubated for 2 hours at 4°C or for 5 hours at 37°C in medium A containing ^{125}I-OxLDL (10 μg/ml), washed and incubated for 10' at 37°C in medium A with the addition of 0.05% trypsin (T), 0.025% pronase (P), or 1 hour at 4°C in medium A containing OxLDL (1.0 mg/ml). Binding (A) was quantitated as the radioactivity released into the medium by the above treatments; internalization (B) as the radioactivity which remained associated to the cells after extensive washing.

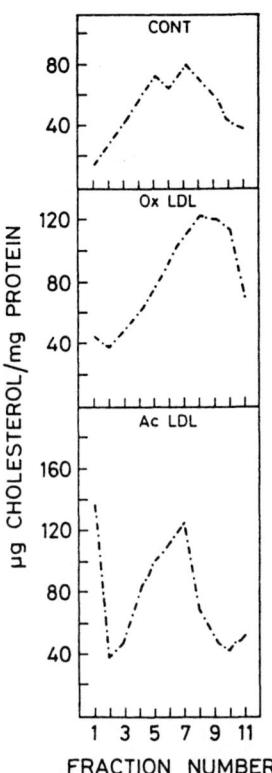

Figure 5. Effect of modified LDL on the cholesterol/protein ratio in subcellular fractions of J774 macrophages. Cells were incubated at 37°C for 18 hours in medium A alone or containing AcLDL or OxLDL (50 lipoprotein cholesterol/ml). Washed cells were homogenized in solution C and spun at 2000 x g twice. Pooled supernatants (1 ml) were loaded onto 11 Percoll 7.8% in solution C and spun at 20000 x g for 40'. Eleven fractions were collected from the gradient and protein and cholesterol were quantitated as described in Methods.

and 37°C similarly, only minor differences were observed after trypsin or pronase treatment of the cells. With all treatments internalization was scarce at 4°C and increased 20-26 fold at 37°C (fig. 4), indicating that OxLDL are bound and subsequently internalized. Internalization of bound OxLDL was confirmed by localization of cellular free cholesterol. In both control and AcLDL-incubated cells, probing with filipin revealed the diffuse presence of free cholesterol on the plasma membrane and within the cells. With OxLDL, besides what seen in control cells, a punctuated intracellular fluorescence pattern was evident both after 5 hours and, more markedly, after 24 hours of incubation. To gain further insight into the distribution of cholesterol within cells exposed to OxLDL cellular membranes and organelles were fractionated on density gradients and the cholesterol/protein ratio was calculated for each fraction (fig. 5). In control cells this ratio peaked

DEGRADATION OF ^{125} I–LP BY LYSOSOME–
ENRICHED CELL SUBFRACTIONS

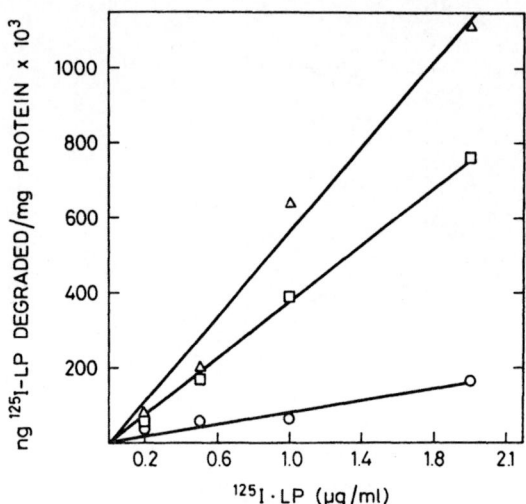

Figure 6. Degradation of native and modified LDL by lysosomal enzymes. A lysosome-enriched cell subfraction was obtained from J774 macrophages as described in Methods. Lysosomes were lysed by repeated freeze-thawing and 25 μg/protein were incubated at 37°C for 4 hours in citrate-buffered MEM, pH 4.5 (final volume 100 μl), containing the indicated concentrations of ^{125}I-LDL (□), ^{125}I-AcLDL (△) or ^{125}I-OxLDL (○). Degradation of lipoproteins was quantitated as TCA non precipitable, non iodide radioactivity present in the medium, as described in Methods.

between light membranes and dense lysosomes. In AcLDL-loaded cell, besides this peak, a very high cholesterol/protein ratio was detected at the top of the gradient, presumably due to floating cholesteryl ester droplets. In cells incubated with OxLDL only a major peak was observed in the bottom fractions of the gradient, thus suggesting different localizations for OxLDL- and AcLDL-derived cholesterol.

The accumulation of OxLDL within the cell could result either from an inhibitory effect of these lipoprotein on proteolytic enzymes or from a lack of activity of these enzymes on OxLDL.

To investigate this aspect in further detail the susceptibility of OxLDL, AcLDL and native LDL to hydrolysis by lysosomal enzymes was evaluated by direct incubation of the iodinated lipoproteins with cellular fractions enriched in lysosomes. Fig. 6 illustrates the results of this experiment. At pH 4.5 degradation was linear in the concentration range utilized: for ^{125}I-OxLDL, though, it was markedly lower than for the other substrates (0.166 ng/mg protein versus 1.13 ng/mg protein for ^{125}I-AcLDL and 0.76 ng/mg protein for ^{125}I-LDL at 2 μg lipoprotein protein/ml; fig. 6). Degradation of any of the lipoprotein was not detectable either at pH 9 or in the absence of cellular protein (not shown).

DISCUSSION

Recently two relevant features of the in vitro metabolism of OxLDL by murine macrophages have been outlined: i) OxLDL load the cells with high amounts of cholesterol, largely unesterified, and ii) the protein moiety of OxLDL is relatively poorly degraded, thus resulting in a disproportion between degradation and uptake by the cells.

Aim of our study was to elucidate the pathway that OxLDL follow after binding to the cell membrane. Several lines of evidence indicate that OxLDL are bound and subsequently internalized by macrophages: i) a high percentage of ^{125}I-OxLDL that associated to the cells during an incubation at 37°C was not displaced by treatments which selectively remove membrane-bound ligands; furthermore, only a minor percentage of cell-associated OxLDL-radioactivity was not precipitable with trichloroacetic acid; ii) when cells were incubated with OxLDL and then fractionated on density gradients, dense, lysosome-containing membranes, were enriched in cholesterol; iii) fluorescence microscopy, using filipin as a probe to localize free cholesterol, indicated, as expected on the basis of parallel biochemical determinations, a much higher content of free cholesterol in cells preincubated with OxLDL. The intracellular perinuclear distribution of cholesterol was also suggestive of a lysosomal localization.

That different lipoproteins may follow different pathways and may be degraded within lysosomes to various extents has recently been proposed by Ellsworth (32) and Tabas (33), who also observed differences in the ability to stimulate ACAT activity. Our data on OxLDL could be explained either by the presence of a cellular pathway specific to oxidized LDL, not leading to significant degradation of the internalized ligand, or by a defective action of lysosomal enzymes on OxLDL. The data on the degradation of OxLDL by partially purified lysosomal enzymes favour the latter possibility. We cannot exclude, however, that OxLDL may follow a specific intracellular pathway leading to their accumulation in organelles containing little enzymatic activity.

From these observations one could speculate that, as far as OxLDL are concerned, cells are in a "chloroquine-like" state: lysosomal proteolysis is almost blocked, and chloroquine treatment of cells cannot cause further accumulation of undegraded ligand. On the other hand, because a treatment with chloroquine abolishes the little degradation that OxLDL undergo, the latter is likely to take place in an acidic endo/lysosomal compartment. This is in agreement with the observations made with partially purified lysosomes. These data confirm the observed resistance of OxLDL to cathepsins (34) and suggest a resistance to other lysosomal proteolytic enzymes.

Further investigation is required to assess the relevance of the above findings in the development of atheroscletic lesions, provided that OxLDL are an adequate model for in vivo oxidized lipoproteins. However, some speculations are suggested by the present results. Cells may overload with free cholesterol as an acute response to high local concentrations of oxidized lipoproteins; only at later times may ACAT be activated to yeld the massive amounts of esterified cholesterol generally observed in lesion areas. Though, the observation of free cholesterol in lesion is not an uncommon finding (35,36). Moreover, even a temporary accumulation of free cholesterol, by altering the cellular pools of the lipid, may elicit regulatory as well as inflammatory responses. Modified lipoproteins can stimulate the transcription of the genes for apoE (37), TNF (38), and growth factors (39).

Further knowledge on the effect of OxLDL on the transcription of other genes, both directly and undirectly (i.e. genes of the immune system), involved in lipid metabolism may help to gain a boader understanding of the complexity of atherosclerosis.

ACKNOWLEDGEMENTS

The Authors wish to thank Miss Maddalena Marazzini for typing the manuscript. This work was supported, in part, by a grant from Progetto Finalizzato Invecchiamento from CNR (Publication No. 923188), and an educational grant from Bayer Italy to ALC.

BIBLIOGRAPHY

1)   Ross, R. (1986) 'The pathogenesis of atherosclerosis. An update', New Engl. J. Med. 314, 488-500.
2)   Cathcart, M.K., Morel, D.W., Di Corleto, P.E., and Chisolm, G.M. III. (1984) 'Monocytes and neutrophils oxidize low density lipoprotein making it cytotoxic', J. Leukocyte Biol. 38, 341-350.
3)   Morel, D.W., Di Corleto, P.E., and Chisolm. G.M. (1984) 'Endothelial and smooth muscle cells alter low density lipoprotein in vitro by free radical oxidation', Arteriosclerosis 4, 357-364.
4)   Heinecke, J.W., Baker, L., and Chait, A. (1986) 'Superoxide-mediated modification of low density lipoprotein by arterial smooth muscle cells', J. Clin. Invest. 77, 757-761.
5)   Parthasarathy, S., Wieland, E., and Steinberg, D.A. (1989) 'Role for endothelial cell lipoxygenase in the oxidative modification of low density lipoprotein', Proc. Natl. Acad. Sci. USA. 86, 1046-1050.
6)   Ylä-Herttuala, S., Palinski, W., Rosenfeld, M.E., Parthasarathy, S., Carew, T.E., Butler, S., Witztum, J.L., and Steinberg, D. (1989) 'Evidence for the presence of oxidatively modified low density lipoprotein in atherosclerotic lesions of rabbit and man', J. Clin. Invest. 84, 1086-1095.
7)   Palinski, W., Rosenfeld, M.E., Ylä-Herttuala, S., Gurtner, G.C., Socher, S.S., Butler, S.W., Parthasarathy, S., Carew, T.E., Steinberg, D., and Witztum, J.L. (1989) 'Low density lipoprotein undergoes oxidative modification in vivo', Proc. Natl. Acad. Sci. USA. 86, 1372-1376.
8)   Rosenfeld, M.E., Khoo, J.C., Miller, E., Parthasarathy, S., Palinski, W., and Witztum, J.L. (1991) 'Macrophage-derived foam cells freshly isolated from rabbit atherosclerotic lesions degrade modified lipoproteins, promote oxidation of low-density lipoproteins, and contain oxidation-specific lipid-protein adducts', J. Clin. Invest. 87, 90-99.
9)   Rosenfeld, M.E., Palinski, S., Ylä-Herttuala, S., Butler, S., and Witztum, J.L. (1990) 'Distribution of oxidation specific lipid-protein adducts and apolipoprotein B in atherosclerotic lesions of varying severity from WHHL rabbits', Arteriosclerosis 10, 336-349.

10)   Brown, M.S. and Goldstein, J.L. (1983) 'Lipoprotein metabolism in the macrophage: implication for cholesterol deposition in atherosclerosis', Annu. Rev. Biochem. 52, 223-261.

11)   Matsumoto, A., Naito, M., Itakura, H., Ikemoto, S., H. Asaoka, Hayakawa, I., Kanamori, H., Aburatani, H., Takaku, F., Suzuki, H., Kobari, Y., Miyai, T., Takahashi, K., Cohen, E., Wydro, R., Housman, D.E., and Kodama, T. (1990) 'Human macrophages scavenger receptors: primary structure, expression and localization in atherosclerotic lesions', Proc. Natl. Acad. Sci. USA. 87, 9133-9137.

12)   Sparrow, C.P., Parthasarathy, S., and Steinberg, D.A. (1989) 'A macrophage receptor that recognizes oxidized low density lipoprotein but not acetylated low density lipoprotein', J. Biol. Chem. 264, 2599-2604.

13)   Roma, P., Catapano, A.L., Bertulli, S.M., Varesi, L., Fumagalli, R., and Bernini, F. (1990) 'Oxidized LDL increase free cholesterol content and fail to stimulate cholesterol esterification in murine macrophages', Biochem. Biophys. Res. Comm. 171, 123-131.

14)   Yokode, M., Kita, T., Kikawa, Y., Ogorochi, T., Narumiya, S., and Kawai, C. (1988) 'Stimulated arachidonate metabolism during foam cell transformation of mouse peritoneal macrophages with oxidized low density lipoprotein', J. Clin. Invest. 81, 720-729.

15)   Jialal, I. and Chait, A. (1989) 'Differences in the metabolism of oxidatively modified low density lipoprotein and acetylated low density lipoprotein by human endothelial cells: inhibition of cholesterol esterification by oxidatively modified low density lipoprotein', J. Lipid Res. 30, 1561-1568.

16)   Ralph, P., Prichard, J., and Cohn, M. (1975) 'Reticulum sarcoma: an effector cell in antibody-dependent cell-mediated immunity', J. Immunol. 114, 898-905.

17)   Edgell, C.J.S., Mc Donald, C.C., and Graham, J.B. (1983) 'Permanent cell line expressing human factor VIII-related antigen established by hybridization' Proc. Natl. Acad. Sci. USA 80, 3734-3737.

18)   Havel, R.J., Eder, H.A., and Bragdon, J.H. (1955) 'The distribution and chemical composition of ultracentrifugally separated lipoproteins in human serum', J. Clin. Invest. 34, 1345-1353.

19)   Basu, S.K., Goldstein, J.L., Anderson, R.G.W., and Brown, M.S. (1976) 'Degradation of cationized low density lipoprotein and regulation of cholesterol metabolism in homozygous familial hypercholesterolemia fibroblasts', Proc. Natl. Acad. Sci. USA 73, 3178-3182.

20)   Bernini, F., Bertulli, S.M., Roma, P., Fumagalli, R., and Catapano, A.L. 'Biological modification of LDL by the permanent human endothelial cell line EAhy 926: evidence for a defective processing by macrophages' 17-19/5/1990 Brugge; 55th Meeting of the European Atherosclerosis Society.

21)   Steinbrecher, U.P., Lougheed, M., Kwan, W.C., and Dirks, M. (1990) 'Recognition of oxidized low density lipoprotein by the scavenger receptor of macrophages results from derivatization of apolipoprotein B by products of fatty acid peroxidation', J. Biol. Chem. 264, 15216-15223.

22)   Noble, R.P. (1968) 'Electrophoretic separation of plasma lipoproteins in agarose gel', J. Lipid Res. 9, 693-700.

23)   Heinecke, J.W., Rosen, H., Suzuki, L., and Chait, A. (1987) 'The role of sulphur-containing amino acids in superoxide production and modification of low density lipoprotein by arterial smooth muscle cells', J. Biol. Chem.

262, 10098-10103.
24) Weber, K. and Osborn, M. (1969), 'The reliability of molecular weight determination by sodium dodecyl sulfate polyacrylamide gel electrophoresis', J. Biol. Chem. 244, 4406-4412.
25) Bilheimer, D.W., Eisenberg, S., and Levy, R.I. (1973) 'The metabolism of very low density lipoprotein proteins. I. Preliminary in vitro and in vivo observations', Biochim. Biophys. Acta. 250, 212-221.
26) Trinder, P. (1969) 'Determination of glucose in blood using glucose oxidase with an alternative oxigen acceptor', Ann. Clin. Biochem. 6, 24-27.
27) Lowry, O.H., Rosebrough, N.J., Farr, A.L., and Randall, R.J. (1951) 'Protein measurement with the Folin phenol reagent', J. Biol. Chem. 193, 265-275.
28) Goldstein, J.L., Ho, Y.K., Basu, S.K., and Brown, M.S. (1979) 'Binding site on macrophages that mediates the uptake and degradation of acetylated low density lipoprotein, producing massive cholesterol deposition', Proc. Natl. Acad. Sci. USA. 76, 333-337.
29) Brown, M.S., Dana, S.E., and Goldstein, J.L. (1974) 'Regulation of 3-hydroxy-3-methylglutaryl coenzyme A reductase activity in cultured human fibroblasts. Comparison of cells from a normal subject and from a patient with homozygous familial hypercholesterolemia', J. Biol. Chem. 249, 789-796.
30) Kruth, H.S., Comly, M.E., Butler, J.D., Vanier, M.T., Fink, J.K., Wenger, D.A., Patel, S., and Pentchev, P.J. (1986) 'Type C Niemann-Pick disease. Abnormal metabolism of low density lipoprotein in homozygous and heterozygous fibroblasts', J. Biol. Chem. 261, 16769-16774.
31) Liscum, L., Ruggiero, R.M., and Faust, J.R. (1989) 'The intracellular transport of low density lipoprotein-derived cholesterol is defective in Niemann-Pick type C fibroblasts', J. Cell Biol. 108, 1625-1636.
32) Ellsworth, J.L., Fong, L.G., Kreamer, F.B., and Cooper, A.D. (1990) 'Differences in the processing of chylomicron remnants and ß-VLDL by macrophages', J. Lipid Res. 31, 1399-1411.
33) Tabas, I., Lim, S., Xu, X.X., and Maxfield, F.R. (1990) 'Endocytosed ß-VLDL and LDL are delivered to different intracellular vesicles in mouse peritoneal macrophages' J. Cell Biol. 111, 929-940.
34) Lougheed, M., Zhang, H., and Steinbrecher, U.P. (1991) 'Oxidized low density lipoprotein is resistant to cathepsins and accumulates within macrophages', J. Biol. Chem. 266, 14519-14525.
35) Lupu, F., Danaricu, I., and Simionescu, N. (1987) 'Development of intracellular lipid deposits in the lipid-laden cells of atherosclerotic lesions', Atherosclerosis. 67, 127-142.
36) Johnson, W.J., Mahlberg, F.M., Rothblat, G.H., and Phillips, M.C. (1991) 'Cholesterol transport between cells and high density lipoproteins', Biochim. Biophys. Acta. 1045, 291-298.
37) Mazzone, T., Gump, M., Diller, P., and Getz, G. (1987) 'Macrophage free cholesterol content regulates apolipoprotein E synthesis', J. Biol. Chem. 262, 11657-11662.
38) Hamilton, T.A., Ma, G.P., and Chisolm, G.H. (1990) 'Oxidized low density lipoprotein suppresses the expression of tumor necrosis factor-alpha

mRNA in stimulated murine peritoneal macrophages', J. Immunol. 144, 2343-2350.

39) Rajavashisth, T.B., Andalibi, A., Territo, M.C., Berliner, J.A., Navab, M., Fogelman, A.M., and Lusis, A.J. (1990) 'Induction of endothelial cell expression of granulocyte and macrophage colony-stimulating factors by modified low-density lipoproteins', Nature. 344, 254-257.

Abbreviations: LDL, low density lipoproteins; OxLDL, oxidatively modified low density lipoproteins; BioOxLDL, low density lipoproteins oxidatively modified by incubation with endothelial cells; AcLDL, acetylated low density lipoproteins; ACAT, acyl CoA: cholesterol acyltransferase; FAF-BSA, fatty acid free-bovine serum albumin.

ANALYSIS OF LIPID VS. NON-LIPID EFFECT ON ATHEROSCLEROSIS DEVELOPMENT

J. REGNSTRÖM[1], J. NILSSON[1], A. G. OLSSON[2], L. A. CARLSON[1], U. ERIKSON[3] AND G. WALLDIUS[1]

ABSTRACT. The Probucol Quantitative Regression Swedish Trial (PQRST) investigates to what extent the addition of the drug probucol to a conventional treatment of hypercholesterolaemia with diet and cholestyramine can influence the development of femoral atherosclerosis. The study comprises 303 hypercholesterolaemic men and women with angiographically visible atherosclerosis and treatment continues for three years. Atherosclerosis development is determined with yearly arteriograms, which are subjected to computer estimation of atherosclerosis. The last angiogram will be performed in December 1992. In a prerandomization treatment period the effects of the drug on plasma cholesterol was evaluated and a decrease of at least 8 percent was needed for both cholestyramine alone and for the subsequent addition of probucol to allow inclusion in the randomized study. During the prerandomization diet, cholestyramine+placebo and cholestyramine+probucol periods it was tested to what extent treatment could affect patient low density lipoprotein (LDL) binding to fibroblast LDL receptors, degradation by macrophages and LDL TBARS content with and without previous in vitro Cu^{2+} oxidation of LDL. Diet, cholestyramine and cholestyramine+probucol decreased total cholesterol from baseline by 4 and 3, 23 and 23 and 37 and 36 percent in active and placebo groups, respectively. High density lipoprotein (HDL) cholesterol increased slightly on cholestyramine but decreased by 31 and 27 percent in active and placebo groups, respectively, when probucol was added to diet+cholestyramine. No treatment affected fibroblast binding, macrophage degradation or TBARS in native LDL. However, if patient LDL was oxidized fibroblast binding was only about 50 percent during diet and cholestyramine treatment. Macrophage degradation and TBARS of LDL was greatly enhanced by oxidation during both treatments. Probucol treatment abolished the decreased fibroblast binding and to a great extent also macrophage degradation and TBARS production Thus probucol prevented LDL from deleterious oxidative effects. The PQRST will answer whether probucol treatment will influence atherosclerosis development. If so, subgroup analysis will hopefully indicate what effect may be the mechanism of action of probucol, its plasma cholesterol lowering effect or its antioxidant effect, or both.

A. L. Catapano et al. (eds.), Drugs Affecting Lipid Metabolism, 441–446.
© 1993 Kluwer Academic Publishers and Fondazione Giovanni Lorenzini.

1. Aim of study

The Probucol Quantitative Regression Swedish Trial (PQRST) [1] is an ongoing double blind controlled study testing whether the addition of probucol 1 g daily to a conventional treatment for hypercholesterolaemia with diet and cholestyramine in the dose of 16 g daily could influence the development of atherosclerosis.

2. Patients

Males and females not above 70 years old with or without symptom-giving peripheral artery disease (PAD) and a serum total cholesterol >6.86 mmol/l (265 mg/dl), a low density lipoprotein (LDL) cholesterol >4.53 mmol/l (175 mg/dl), and a total triglyceride <4mmol/l (350 mg/dl) were included in the study in Linköping and in Stockholm. PAD was verified initially by non-invasive means. Of referred patients 303 (146 males) were randomized to the controlled study.

3. Design of study

The trial consists of a prerandomization phase and a randomization phase. It is described in detail elsewhere [1], As the study is ongoing results will be given from the prerandomization phase of the study only.

3.1. PRERANDOMIZATION PHASE. This is performed to test eligibility and drug effects. After diet advice patients are given cholestyramine 16 g daily plus probucol placebo for two months. The placebo is switched to probucol verum for another two months. Total plasma cholesterol should decrease by at least 8 percent from previous treatment on the two drug regimes to allow inclusion of the patient.

3.2. RANDOMIZATION PHASE. This continues for three years during which half of the patients receives cholestyramine+probucol verum and half cholestyramine+probucol placebo. Femoral angiography is performed yearly. The last angiography is scheduled to December 1992.

4. Methods

4.1. LIPOPROTEIN ANALYSIS. Serum lipoproteins were determined according to Carlson [2]. Cholesterol and triglyceride concentrations in the different lipoprotein fractions were determined according to the laboratory routine [2].

4.2. OXIDATION OF LDL. Iodinated (^{125}I) LDL [3] was dialysed against phosphate buffered saline containing $CuSO_4$ for 18 h at 4°C. Lipid peroxidation was measured as thiobarbituric acid reactive substances (TBARS) and was expressed as malondialdehyde (MDA) equivalents according to Yagi [4].

4.3. BINDING TO LDL RECEPTORS. Analysis of LDL receptor binding was performed according to Goldstein & Brown [5]. Human lung embryo fibroblasts were incubated with ^{125}I LDL or ^{125}I-oxidatively modified LDL. After incubation and washing the cells were incubated with heparin. The released radioactivity measures the binding of LDL to receptors. The protein content of the cells was determined and the LDL receptor binding expressed as ng heparin-releasable LDL per mg cell protein.

4.4. MACROPHAGE LDL DEGRADATION. Mouse peritoneal macrophages were incubated with ^{125}I LDL or ^{125}I-oxidatively modified LDL for 5 h at 37°C. The degradation was measured as the trichloroacetic acid-soluble ^{125}I in the medium supernatant after precipitation of protein and free iodide. It was related to the cellular protein content.

5. Results

5.1. SERUM LIPOPROTEIN CONCENTRATIONS. In Table 1 is given the serum lipid and lipoprotein concentrations at baseline, on diet on cholestyramine and on the combination of cholestyramine and probucol.

Table 1. Serum lipid and lipoprotein concentrations at baseline and at the end of each treatment period in a subsample (n=143) of responders to cholestyramine and probucol during the prerandomization phase of the PQRST, mmol/l. mean±SEM.

	Total chol.	Total TG	VLDL chol.	LDL chol	HDL chol
Baseline	9.11	2.04	0.89	6.68	1.47
Diet	8.81	1.94	0.84	6.38	1.45
C+PL	7.03	2.24	0.93	4.47	1.51
C+PB	5.81	1.91	0.74	3.95	1.05

chol.=cholesterol, TG=triglycerides, VLDL=very low density lipoprotein, LDL=low density lipoprotein, HDL=high density lipoprotein, C=cholestyramine, PL=placebo, PB=probucol

Dietary treatment decreased total and LDL cholesterol and total triglycerides by about 3 to 4 percent. Treatment with cholestyramine decreased total and LDL cholesterol by 20 and 30 percent, respectively, while total triglycerides increased by 15 percent. Probucol decreased total cholesterol by little more than 1 mmol/l. A little less than half of this decrease was due to the HDL cholesterol decreasing effect of probucol and the rest to an LDL effect.

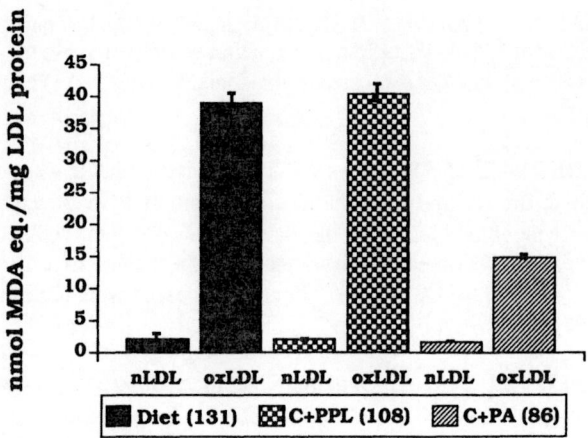

Fig. 1. Effect of oxidation on TBARS content of LDL expressed as nmol MDA eq./mg LDL
protein. nLDL and oxLDL stand for native and oxidized LDL, respectively. Treatments were diet,
cholestyramine + probucol placebo (C+PPL) and cholestyramin+probucol active (C+PA). Means
and standard errors are given.

5.2. LIPID PEROXIDATION. In figure 1 is given the LDL oxidation as expressed in MDA
equivalents per mg LDL protein.in patient native and oxidized LDL. During all three treatments only
a small amount of TBARS were present in native LDL. During dietary and cholestyramine
treatments oxidation resulted in a tenfold increase in TBARS content of LDL. Probucol addition to
treatment attenuated this effect of oxidation significantly.

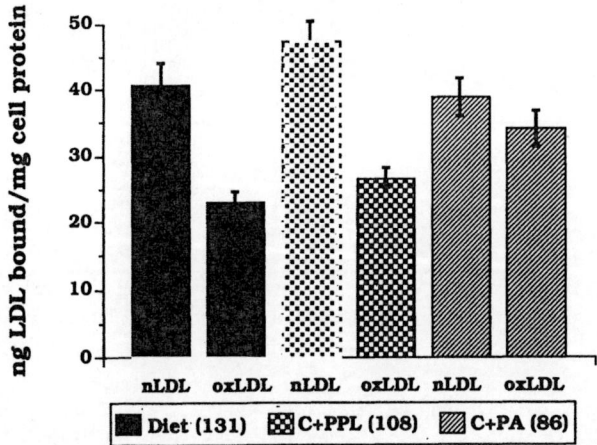

Fig. 2. Effects of oxidation of LDL on its binding to B,E receptors on fibroblasts. The decreased
binding after oxidation on diet and on diet + cholestyramine is essentially abolished during the
additional treatment with probucol. Means and standard errors are given.

5.2. LDL BINDING. Figure 2 shows the LDL binding to fibroblasts. Native LDL bound to fibroblasts during all treatments about equally and with between 40 and 50 ng LDL per mg cell protein. Oxidation decreased binding both during diet and cholestyramine by about half. Probucol treatment abolished this decrease almost completely.

5.3. MACROPHAGE DEGRADATION OF LDL The effect on macrophage degradation is given in Figure 3. Macrophages degraded some LDL during all three treatments. The degradation was markedly increased if LDL was oxidized, indicating an enhanced uptake of the modified LDL by these cells. Probucol treatment almost completely abolished this uptake.

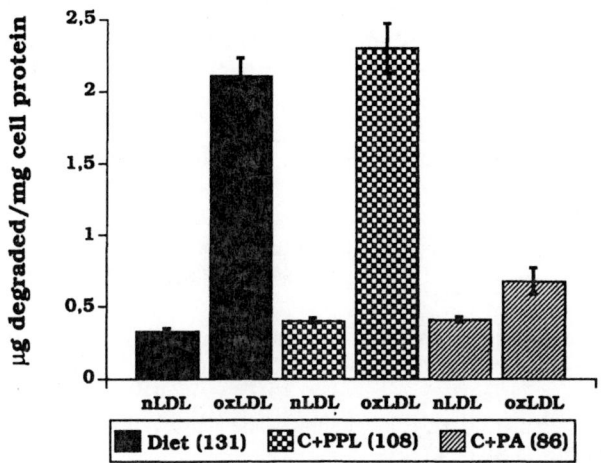

Fig. 3. Effect of LDL oxidation on macrophage degradation Degradation was greatly enhanced after oxidation during diet and diet + cholestyramine treatment. During probucol treatment this increase was very small. Means and standard errors are given.

6. Discussion

The present study demonstrates a fundamental difference in the effect of two serum cholesterol lowering drugs, cholestyramine and probucol, on the response of LDL to oxidation. While treatment with the former drug did not influence significantly the production of TBARS, the binding of LDL to its receptor, or the LDL uptake by macrophages as induced by copper oxidation, probucol treatment was able to abolish most of these effects. As LDL oxidation is regarded as an important step in the atherogenic process [6], these effects of probucol are of potentially great importance.

The PQRST investigates if treatment with probucol can retard the development of femoral atherosclerosis in hypercholesterolaemia. Its design included a serum cholesterol criterion of 8 percent decrease. Therefore the PQRST is a test of the serum lipid lowering effect of the drug. However by subgroup analysis we hope that it will be possible to test what effects are the most important for the femoral atherosclerosis development, the LDL cholesterol lowering effect or any of the antioxidant effects, or both.

7. References

1.   Walldius G, Carlson LA, Erikson U, Olsson AG, Johansson J, Mölgaard J, Nilsson S, Stenport G, Kaijser L, Lassvik C and Holme I. (1988) 'Development of femoral atherosclerosis in hypercholesterolemic patients during treatment with cholestyramine and probucol/placebo: Probucol Quantitative Regression Swedish Trial (PQRST): A Status Report', The Am J of Cardiol 62, 37B-43B.

2.   Carlson K. (1973) 'Lipoprotein fractionation', Ass Clin Pathol 5, 32.

3.   Regnström J, Walldius G, Carlson LA, Nilsson J. (1990) 'Effect of probucol treatment on the susceptibility of low density lipoprotein isolated from hypercholesterolemic patients to become oxidatively modified in vitro', Atherosclerosis 82, 43-51.

2.   Yagi K. (1976) 'A simple fluorometric assay for lipoperoxide in blood plasma', Biochem. Med, 15, 212.

5.   Brown MS, Goldstein JL. (1975) 'Regulation of the activity of the low density lipoprotein in human fibroblast', Cell 6, 307.

6.   Witztum JL, Steinberg D. (1991) 'Role of oxidized low density lipoprotein in atherogenesis', J Clin Invest 88, 1785-1792.

ATHEROGENICITY OF TRIGLYCERIDE-RICH LIPOPROTEINS: CELLULAR ASPECTS

Sandra H. Gianturco, Francois M. Booyse, and William A. Bradley

ABSTRACT

Abnormal triglyceride-rich lipoproteins (TGRLP) are found in many fasting hypertriglyceridemic (HTG) subjects and postprandially in subjects with profiles associated with cardiovascular risk (elevated plasma triglyceride or cholesterol levels or low HDL levels). Both fasting and postprandial abnormal TGRLP, but not normal VLDL or LDL, bind to an unregulated receptor expressed on reticuloendothelial cells that is distinct from the LDL or the acetyl-LDL receptor. Binding of abnormal TGRLP to this receptor is associated with macrophage lipid engorgement and endothelial cell dysfunction in vitro (impaired fibrinolysis and release of t-PA, phenotypic switching to multinucleated giant cells as observed over atherosclerotic lesions). Normal TGRLP or LDL do not bind to this receptor and do not have these potentially atherogenic cellular effects. Uptake of abnormal TGRLP by this receptor pathway may be involved in atherogenesis if similar phenomena occur in vivo.

RESULTS AND DISCUSSION

One of the factors thought to be involved in the initiation of atherosclerosis is abnormal cellular uptake of atherogenic lipoproteins. Abnormal or excessive uptake of certain lipoproteins can convert macrophages into foam cells and also may cause endothelial cell dysfunction. Many studies have shown that native LDL do not have these potentially atherogenic characteristics in vitro, however, without extensive chemical modification [1]. In contrast, some abnormal native triglyceride-rich lipoproteins (TGRLP) exhibit atherogenic potential without in vitro modification, since these TGRLP can cause massive lipid accumulation in macrophages and perturb endothelial cell function in vitro. Generally, the abnormal TGRLP are from subjects with hypertriglyceridemia, although some, but not all, postprandial TGRLP subspecies also appear to be atherogenic, as described below. A characteristic of TGRLP relevant to foam cell formation and atherosclerosis is that each large TGRLP particle carries much more cholesterol and cholesteryl ester than does each LDL particle. Each chylomicron has approximately 60,000 molecules of cholesterol plus cholesteryl ester, each

447

A. L. Catapano et al. (eds.), Drugs Affecting Lipid Metabolism, 447–451.
© 1993 Kluwer Academic Publishers and Fondazione Giovanni Lorenzini.

VLDL S_f 100-400 ~ 10,000, and each LDL only ~2000 total sterol molecules per particle [2]. In addition, each TGRLP carries an enormous number of triglyceride molecules (~24,000 in VLDL S_f 100-400 and ~500,000 in chylomicrons and only 300 in LDL). Moreover, in hypertriglyceridemic subjects, large VLDL are enriched in cholesteryl esters relative to comparable normal VLDL subspecies [3]. Thus TGRLP could be atherogenic (i.e. deliver excess cholesterol to monocyte-macrophages or cells of the artery wall) if they are avidly taken up by the cells. One chylomicron could deliver 30 times as much cholesterol as could one LDL particle. Triglycerides, when hydrolyzed intracellularly, could produce potentially toxic levels of fatty acids and perturb cellular functions, participating in atherogenesis.

Since large TGRLP have a short half life in plasma compared to LDL, it is reasonable to hypothesize that only those TGRLP that have rapid access to cells, i.e., receptor-mediated mechanisms, might be atherogenic. Fortunately, not all TGRLP bind specifically to cellular receptors. Large VLDL (S_f 60-400) from fasting normal subjects do not bind to the LDL receptor [4-6] and do not cause rapid, receptor-mediated lipid engorgement in macrophages [7]. Small normal VLDL S_f 20-60 can bind to the LDL receptor [5,6] but do not cause lipid loading in macrophages [7].

TGRLP from hypertriglyceridemic subjects are abnormal in composition, distribution, and cellular interactions, and are potentially atherogenic. Large HTG-VLDL (S_f 60-400) isolated from fasting HTG subjects contain extra apoE of a conformation different from that in comparable normal VLDL and this apoE mediates binding to the LDL receptor (R) [8,9], an ability that VLDL S_f 60-400 from fasting subjects with normal plasma triglyceride levels lack [4-6]. HTG-VLDL from some, but not all, hypertriglyceridemic subjects are taken up by a distinct, unregulated macrophage receptor pathway we have identified and termed the "abnormal TGRLP receptor" [10]. Macrophage uptake of chylomicrons and abnormal TGRLP appears to be mediated primarily by this receptor, which is distinct from both the LDL R and the acetyl LDL R in apparent molecular weight, ligand specificity, and expression during differentiation. The abnormal TGRLP receptor appears to be restricted to cells of reticuloendothelial origin, since it is present on murine and human monocytes and macrophages as well as on endothelial cells, but is not detectable in fibroblasts or hepatoma cells. The macrophage membrane binding proteins (MBP) that are likely receptor candidates have an apparent molecular weight of 190 kilodaltons in murine P388D1 macrophages [10]. There are two MBPs in human monocyte-macrophage plasma membranes [10] and THP-1 monocytes with identical ligand specificities, of 200 and 235 kilodalton apparent molecular weights. Although apoE is both necessary and sufficient for binding of TGRLP of S_f 100-400 to the LDL receptor [11], apoE is not required for binding to the distinct macrophage receptor [10]. The TGRLP which bind to the receptor candidate proteins on ligand blots and promote macrophage lipid accumulation are enriched in apoB-48 or fragmented apoB-100 [8], and these apoB species appear to mediate binding to the receptor, as indicated by increased binding of TGRLP upon proteolysis of the apoprotein.

Chylomicrons and HTG-VLDL also have the abnormal ability to cause a phenotypic switching of certain endothelial cells to a multinucleate "giant cell" morphology in vitro (unpublished results). This may be relevant to atherosclerosis since giant cells are reported to comprise up to 50% of the endothelial cells over atherosclerotic lesions [12,13]. HTG-VLDL and chylomicrons, but not normal VLDL or LDL, cause giant cell formation in growing cultures of porcine coronary endothelial cells. Few giant cells were induced by TGRLP in human umbilical vein or aortic endothelial cells or in porcine aortic, pulmonary, or umbilical vein cells, indicating vascular bed specificity. Cultures containing giant cells exhibited impaired fibrinolysis, and HTG-VLDL specifically inhibited surface localized plasmin generation by normal endothelial cell cultures. Thus TGRLP may be mechanistically linked to the impaired fibrinolysis and increased atherosclerosis associated with hypertriglyceridemia and may be induced by postprandial TGRLP abnormalities.

We have begun studies to test the hypothesis that subjects with fasting profiles associated with increased atherosclerosis risk have one or more atherogenic TGRLP subspecies postprandially, whereas "atherogenic" postprandial TGRLP occur in normal subjects with a protective fasting lipoprotein profile only transitorily, if at all. To identify potentially atherogenic changes in postprandial TGRLP, subjects consumed a standardized test meal composed of eggs, cheese, toast, and a milkshake and isolated TGRLP subspecies before and every 2 h after the meal. Our preliminary studies indicate that in the postprandial state, large TGRLP subspecies (S_f 60-400) from normal subjects acquire extra apoE and, consequently, the ability to bind to LDL receptors. These normal postprandial TGRLP, however, do not induce macrophage lipid accumulation. In subjects with normal fasting lipoprotein profiles, only the S_f >400 fraction causes significant lipid accumulation in a standardized 4 h incubation with human THP-1 monocyte-macrophages. In subjects with abnormal fasting lipoprotein profiles, however, smaller postprandial TGRLP show enhanced binding to the macrophage abnormal TGRLP receptor and up to a ten-fold increased ability to cause macrophage lipid loading relative to postprandial TGRLP from normal subjects of the same relative size and lipid composition. The enhanced macrophage uptake is most pronounced in the S_f 100-400 subfraction, peaks at 2-4 hours postprandially, and declines by 6 to 8 hours. Both the S_f >400 fraction and the S_f 100-400 fraction from abnormal subjects at 4 hours postprandially caused a 7-fold greater cholesteryl ester accumulation in human macrophages than did modified LDL (both oxidized LDL and acetyl LDL). In some subjects, even smaller TGRLP subspecies acquire the ability to cause massive lipid accumulation late in the postprandial period (6-8 h postprandially).

These studies in vitro demonstrate abnormal cellular uptake of HTG-VLDL and postprandial TGRLP from subjects with certain lipoprotein profiles associated with increased risk. The abnormal uptake appears to be mediated primarily by a distinct, unregulated macrophage receptor and leads to massive lipid accumulation in macrophages. Abnormal TGRLP also interact with receptors on endothelial cells and impair surface localized plasmin generation by endothelial cells and cause phenotypic switching of coronary artery endothelial cells to functionally deficient giant cells. These abnormal interactions are potentially atherogenic and may be causally related to the increased cardiovascular disease associated with these disorders.

ACKNOWLEDGEMENTS

This work was supported in part by National Institutes of Health grants HL43373, HL44480, HL46304, and HL17667.

REFERENCES

1. Brown, M.S., and Goldstein, J.L. (1983) 'Lipoprotein metabolism in the macrophage: Implications for cholesterol deposition in atherosclerosis', Ann Rev Biochem 52, 223-261.
2. Shen, B.W., Scanu, A.M., and Kezdy, F.J. (1977) 'Structure of human serum lipoproteins inferred from compositional analysis', Proc Natl Acad Sci USA 74, 837-841
3. Eisenberg, S., Gavish, D., Oschry, Y., Fainaru, M., Deckelbaum, R.J. (1984) 'Abnormalities in very low, low, and high density lipoproteins in hypertriglyceridemia Reversal toward normal with bezafibrate treatment', J Clin Invest 74, 470-482
4. Gianturco, S.H., Gotto, A.M. Jr, Jackson, R.L., Patsch, J.R., Taunton, O.D., Sybers, H.D., Yeshurun, D.L., and Smith, L.C. (1978) 'Control of 3-hydroxy-3-methylglutaryl-CoA reductase activity in cultured human fibroblasts by very low density lipoproteins of subjects with hypertriglyceridemia', J Clin Invest 61, 320-328.
5. Gianturco, S.H., Packard, C.J., Shepherd, J., Smith, L.C., Catapano, A.L., Sybers, H.D., Gotto, A.M. Jr. (1980) 'Abnormal suppression of 3-hydroxy-3-methylglutaryl-CoA reductase activity in cultured human fibroblasts by hypertriglyceridemic very low density lipoprotein subclasses', Lipids 15, 456-463.
6. Gianturco, S.H., Brown, F.B., Gotto, A.M. Jr, and Bradley, W.A. (1982)'Receptor-mediated uptake of hypertriglyceridemic very low density lipoproteins by normal human fibroblasts', J Lipid Res 23, 984-993.
7. Gianturco, S.H., Bradley, W.A., Gotto, A.M. Jr, Morrisett, J.D., and Peavy, D.L. (1982) 'Hypertriglyceridemic very low density lipoproteins enhance triglyceride synthesis and accumulation in mouse peritoneal macrophages', J Clin Invest 70, 168-178.
8. Gianturco, S.H., Gotto, A.M. Jr, Hwang, S-L.C., Karlin, J.B., Lin, A.H.Y., Prasad, S.C., and Bradley, W.A. (1983) 'Apolipoprotein E mediates uptake of Sf 100-400 hypertriglyceridemic very low density lipoproteins by the low density lipoprotein receptor pathway in normal human fibroblasts', J Biol Chem 258, 4526-4533.
9. Bradley, W.A., Hwang, S-L-C., Karlin, J.B., Lin, A.H-Y., Prasad, S.C., Gotto, A.M. Jr, and Gianturco, S.H. (1984) 'Low density lipoprotein (LDL) receptor binding determinants switch from apolipoprotein E (apoE) to apoB during conversion of hypertriglyceridemic very low density lipoprotein (HTG-VLDL) to LDL', J Biol Chem 259, 14728-14735.
10. Gianturco, S.H., Lin, A.H-Y., Hwang, S-L.C., Young, J., Brown, S.A., Via, D.P., and Bradley, W.A. (1988) 'A distinct murine macrophage receptor for human triglyceride-rich lipoproteins', J Clin Invest 82(5), 1633-1643.
11. Bradley, W.A. and Gianturco, S.H. (1986) 'ApoE is necessary and

sufficient for the binding of large triglyceride-rich lipoproteins to the LDL receptor; apoB is unnecessary', J Lipid Res 27, 40-48.

12. Repin, V.S., Dolgov, V.V., Zaikina, O.E., Novikov, I.D., Antonov, A.S., Nikolaeva, M.A., and Smirnov, (1984) 'Heterogenicity of endothelium in human aorta: A quantitative analysis by scanning electron microscopy', Atherosclerosis, 50, 35.

13. Bürrig, K-F. (1991) 'The endothelium of advanced arteriosclerotic plaques in humans', Art & Thromb 11, 1678-1689.

ATHEROGENICITY OF TRIGLYCERIDE-RICH LIPOPROTEINS: CLINICAL ASPECTS

JAMES SHEPHERD, MURIEL CASLAKE, ALLAN GAW, BRUCE GRIFFIN, GRACE LINDSAY AND CHRISTOPHER PACKARD

ABSTRACT. A growing body of evidence suggests that triglyceride-rich particles in the plasma contribute to the process of atherogenesis. Some may do so directly while others operate by proxy through their influence on circulating cholesterol-rich lipoproteins. Here we describe recent studies which assessed the influence of triglyceride on low density lipoprotein structure and metabolism. Our observations are consistent with the view that the shrinkage in LDL size which occurs with increasing plasma triglyceride is associated with defective binding of the lipoprotein to its receptor and channelling of its catabolism into potentially atherogenic receptor-independent pathways. Fibrate therapy, which lowers plasma triglyceride, reverses these phenomena and redirects the clearance of LDL towards the receptor route.

Introduction

Chylomicra and very low density lipoproteins (VLDL) are responsible for transporting more than 95% of the triglycerides which circulate in the human bloodstream. Each species is subject to the same lipolytic degradation process which has a profound influence on the structure, metabolism and function of cholesterol-enriched low and high density lipoproteins (LDL and HDL). As our understanding of these metabolic interrelationships grows it is becoming increasingly clear that the epidemiologic association between triglyceride levels in the plasma and coronary heart disease risk may be, at least in part, dependent on LDL and HDL modification. Here we review recent studies which assess (A) the impact of plasma triacylglycerols on LDL turnover and (B) the effects of fibrate therapy on this process.

(A) Plasma triglyceride and low density lipoprotein metabolism

Low density lipoprotein, the major cholesterol transporter in human

A. L. Catapano et al. (eds.), Drugs Affecting Lipid Metabolism, 453–466.

plasma, is generated by the stepwise delipidation of very low density
lipoprotein.   Apolipoprotein B_{100} (apoB), common to both lipoprotein
species, is conserved in the remodelling process, and constitutes a
useful marker of its progress.   Early studies of the metabolism of
trace-labelled VLDL established its precursor relationship to LDL in
both normal (1) and dyslipidaemic subjects (2). However subsequent
detailed investigations indicated that the link is   imprecise.   That
is, not all VLDL apoB is converted to LDL apoB, nor is it the sole
source of the latter (3).
Metabolic studies (4) have failed to demonstrate a significant
association between VLDL triglyceride transport and plasma LDL
levels. However it is possible to observe in epidemiological surveys
a   positive   association   between plasma   triglyceride and LDL
cholesterol   levels within the "normal" range for these lipid
parameters (5). This relationship persists after correction for the
confounding effects of age and weight. Our ability to confirm this
finding in a local coronary risk factor screening program (Figure 1)
prompted us to examine more closely the link between LDL metabolism
and plasma triglyceride levels.

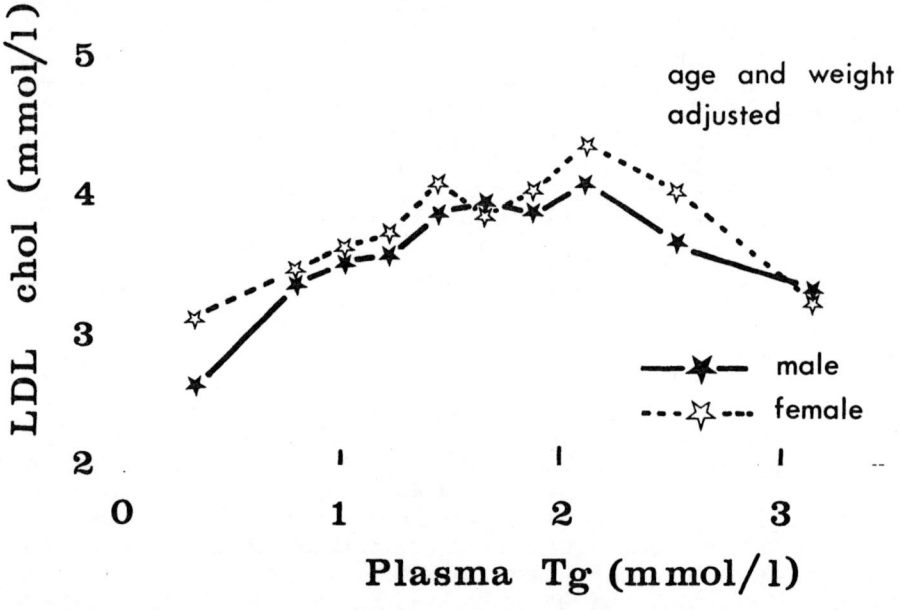

Figure 1.
The relationship between LDL cholesterol and plasma triglyceride in
1843 men and 1881 women.   LDL cholesterol was calculated by the
Friedewald equation.

The association, particularly strong in young adults, led us to
recruit a group of 25 subjects aged 19–39 years to test the

possibility that the rate of LDL apo B synthesis or catabolism might be influenced by variations in plasma triglyceride.

Although early investigations of LDL metabolism in normolipaemic subjects (6,7) assumed structural and metabolic homogeneity within this lipoprotein class, we now know that it consists of three to four discrete components, each of which makes a contribution to its overall catabolism (8,9). In the studies described here we have adopted a previously defined multicompartmental modelling procedure which takes account of LDL catabolism from the plasma and the appearance of its degradation products in urine (10). The results demonstrate that LDL in normolipaemic subjects is heterogeneous and can be modelled as two distinct species. The behaviour of one of these is closely linked to the level of triglyceride in the plasma.

Subjects and methods

21 male and 4 female healthy volunteers were recruited from a local coronary screening program and examined on an outpatient basis, an arrangement which provides appropriate steady-state conditions for kinetic analysis (7). Low density lipoprotein was prepared from the plasma of each individual and divided into two aliquots which were labelled separately with ^{125}I and ^{131}I. The ^{131}I-LDL preparation was then treated with 1, 2 cyclohexanedione to block its recognition by LDL receptors and restrict its catabolism to pathways which operate independently of the receptor mechanism. Ten minutes after simultaneous reinjection of the tracers into their respective donor a baseline blood sample was drawn and thereafter fasting samples were collected daily for the next 14 days. Continuous 24 hour urine collections were also initiated at the time of tracer injection and continued for the remaining 14 days of the study. Details of all procedures used are reported elsewhere (11).

Plasma ^{125}I and ^{131}I radioactivities data were analysed by the procedure of Matthews (12), as adapted in this laboratory (13) to determine fractional catabolic rates (FCR) for total, receptor-dependent and receptor-independent apo LDL catabolism. The rate of elimination of ^{125}I labelled native apo LDL represents total catabolism of this fraction while that of the ^{131}I CHD-modified tracer is used as a measure of receptor-independent activity. The difference between these two FCR's (native - CHD) therefore provides an index of the activity of the receptor pathway. The urine/plasma radioactivity ratios for both native and CHD-modified apo LDL were calculated from the urinary output of ^{125}I or ^{131}I in a 24 hour period and the plasma radioactivity at the beginning of the period. Since there is approximately a half-day delay between the clearance of radioactivity from the plasma and its appearance in urine (10, 14) the latter value represents the relevant mean plasma radioactivity for the 24 hour urine collection. The synthetic rate for apo LDL was calculated as the product of the apo LDL circulating mass and the fractional catabolic rate.

As an alternative to the above analytical procedure, plasma and urine radioactivities were also analysed by multicompartmental modelling

using the SAAM 29 computer program (14). With this approach we noted
as reported earlier by Boston et al (10) and Foster et al (14), that
LDL could not be treated as a single homogeneous entity, but required
the presence of two plasma pools to allow for simultaneous fitting of
the plasma and urine radioactivities.

Results

(a) Curve peeling (Matthews) analysis
In these young healthy adults the plasma concentration of apo LDL
rose 50% across the quintiles of triglyceride, the total circulating
mass of apoprotein in quintile 5 (highest triglyceride) being double
that in quintile 1 (Table 1). The rate of apo LDL production as
calculated by the curve peeling procedure of Matthews (12, 13) was
similar to that observed in earlier studies (7, 15) and varied little
between the quintiles.

Table 1   Plasma Triglyceride and apo LDL metabolism

   Kinetic analysis by curve peeling (Matthews) procedure.

Apo LDL Quintile	Circulating apo LDL mass (mg)	Apo LDL Synthesis (mg/kg/d)	Apo LDL fractional catabolism (pools/d)	Plasma Triglyceride (mmol/l)
1	1670±167[+]	12.4±2.0	0.45±0.03	0.82±0.33
2	2035±210	12.7±2.5	0.38±0.04	1.14±0.32
3	2477±78	12.3±3.0	0.36±0.05	1.10±0.16
4	2640±80	13.1±1.6	0.35±0.05	1.22±0.18
5	3371±611	13.4±2.2	0.32±0.04	1.54±0.40

* ranked in quintiles according to apo LDL mass
+ Mean ± 1.SD

Thus the increase in apo LDL mass in quintiles 1 through 5 derived
from a reduction in its total fractional catabolic rate which fell by
30% across the groups. Use of the CHD-modified LDL tracer allowed us
to calculate the contribution of both the receptor-mediated and
receptor-independent catabolic mechanisms. This approach showed that
the increase in the circulating mass of apo LDL was strongly related
to a reduction in its receptor-mediated FCR ($r=-0.55$, $p<0.01$) and not
to any change in the FCR via receptor-independent pathway(s)
($r=-0.30$, $p=0.143$).

(b) Multicompartmental analysis

Examination of the urinary radioactivity excretion data and calculation of the daily urine/plasma clearance rate (U/P ratio) indicated that the kinetics of apo LDL metabolism were more complex than the Matthews analytical approach had first suggested. In virtually all subjects the U/P ratio for native LDL, which acts as a daily index of the catabolic potential of apo LDL, fell from a peak value at 2–4 days post injection to a much lower value by days 10–12 (Figure 2). The fall off was steeper for subjects with lower apo LDL mass. The U/P ratio observed for cyclohexanedione modified LDL on the other hand was constant over the 14 day period (Figure 2) indicating that the increased catabolism of the native LDL in the early stages of the turnover was due to a receptor–mediated process.

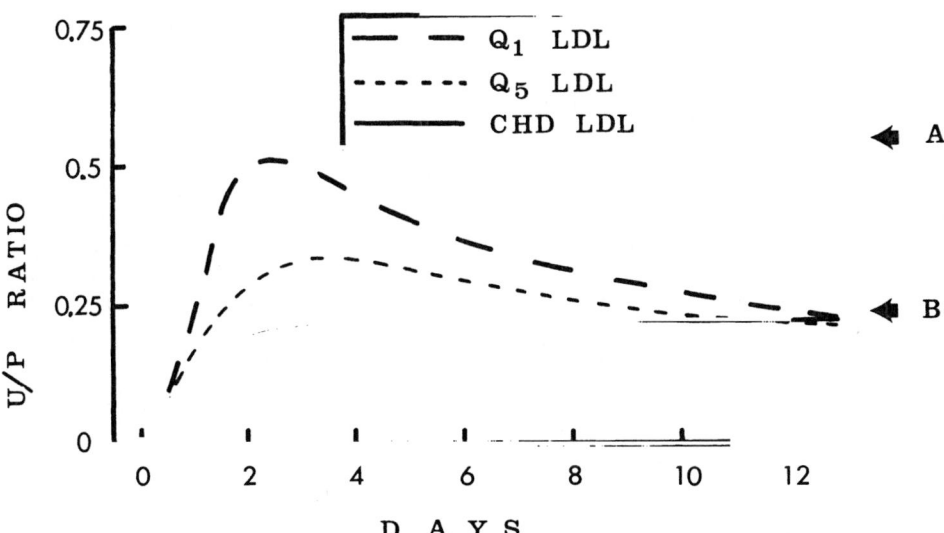

Figure 2.
Mean urine/plasma radioactivity ratios for native and CHD – modified LDL in subjects from quintiles 1 and 5. A and B represent the ratios observed for pools A and B respectively in the model discribed in Figure 3.

These data are incompatible with a simple one–compartment model in which apo LDL has a constant catabolic rate. They point to the presence of metabolic heterogeneity and when urine and plasma radioactivities are combined using multicompartmental modelling procedures two plasma apo LDL compartments are required to provide a satisfactory fit (Figure 3).

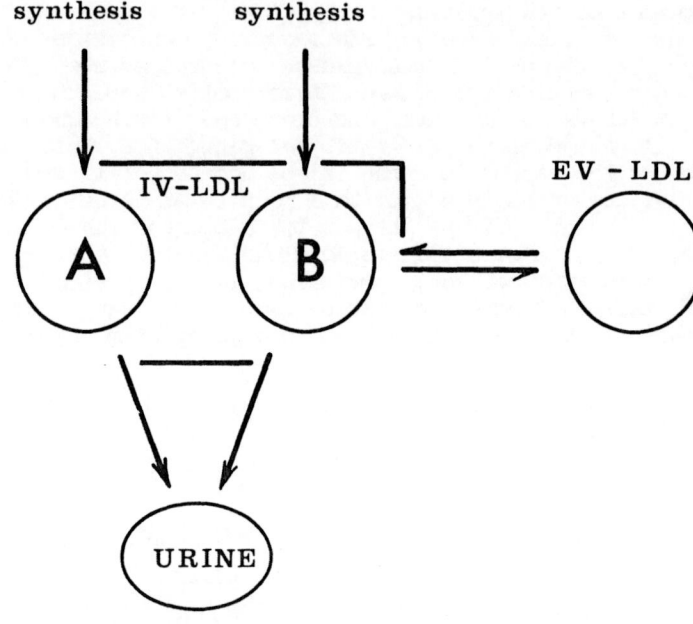

Figure 3.
Multicompartmental model used to describe apo LDL kinetics. Pools A
and B are two plasma compartments invoked to produce a satisfactory
fit to urinary radioactivity excretion data. ^{125}I – CHD LDL plasma
and urine data were used simultaneously to derive kinetic parameters·

One represents LDL with a rapid catabolic rate and high affinity for
the receptor (pool A, Figure 3) while the other defines a lipoprotein
which is more slowly catabolised (pool B) by mechanisms featuring a
reduced level of receptor activity. Using this model it is now
possible to make a different interpretation of the results presented
in Figure 2. If plasma apo LDL were limited entirely to pool A then
a constant daily U/P ratio of about 0.55 would pertain throughout the
turnover. Likewise, if all material were in pool B, the U/P ratio
would be about 0.23. The fall-off in U/P ratios from day 2 to day 12
reflects the heterogeneous mix of LDL present in the plasma.
Individuals with lower apo LDL mass show a high proportion of pool A
to pool B. As the more rapidly catabolised pool A species is cleared
from the plasma over the first 10 days, the U/P ratio decreases until
all subjects achieve approximately the same terminal U/P value which
is determined by slowly metabolised pool B apo LDL.
Kinetic parameters and pool sizes for apo LDL pools A and B, based on
compartmental analysis, are given in Table 2.

Table 2   Plasma triglyceride and apo LDL metabolism

Multicompartmental kinetic analysis

(a) apo LDL, pool A

			Fractional	Catabolic Rate
Quintile	Mass (mg)	Synthesis (mg/kg/d)	Total (pools/d)	Receptor (pools/d)
1	1058±150*	10.0±2.1	0.57±0.06	0.30±0.08
2	936±195	12.2±1.9	0.69±0.06	0.35±0.04
3	1552±337	12.1±3.9	0.53±0.04	0.25±0.04
4	1400±345	9.6±2.7	0.48±0.09	0.26±0.08
5	1491±424	8.4±3.4	0.45±0.15	0.21±0.11

(b) apo LDL, pool B

			Fractional	Catabolic Rate
Quintile	Mass (mg)	Synthesis (mg/kg/d)	Total (pools/d)	Receptor (pools/d)
1	510±213	2.6±0.5	0.25±0.02	0.12±0.03
2	1044±247	4.1±1.1	0.23±0.03	0.10±0.02
3	924±324	2.7±1.2	0.21±0.02	0.12±0.01
4	1239±364	4.2±1.8	0.23±0.03	0.10±0.03
5	1880+438	6.3±1.7	0.26±0.04	0.12±0.03

* Mean ±1.0 SD

Data for both the native and CHD-modified tracers were used in the
analysis.   In these normal subjects, the amount of apo LDL in pool A
was approximately 50% higher in quintiles 4 and 5 compared to
quintiles 1 and 2. This was due to a reduction in the fractional
catabolic   rate from this compartment   which was significantly
inversely related to apo LDL pool A mass (r=-0.55, p<0.01).
Synthesis of apo LDL into pool A was relatively constant in these
subjects.
Much greater changes were apparent in the circulating mass of pool B
apo LDL. It rose more than threefold between quintiles 1 and 5 as a
result of an increase in synthesis (the correlation coefficient

between pool B apo LDL mass and pool B synthesis was 0.89, p<0.001). The fractional catabolic rate from this compartment did not change with increasing apo LDL mass in line with the observation that the U/P ratio fell to the same limiting value in all subjects (Figure 2). Thus as total apo LDL mass increased in these normal subjects the ratio of pool A/pool B material fell from 2.1 (quintile 1) to 0.79 (quintile 5). A stronger relationship was observed between the total apo LDL mass and pool B mass (r=0.83, p<0.0001) than between the former and pool A mass (r=0.61, p<0.01).

Discussion

The results of our kinetic studies were analysed first by the curve-peeling method (12) used previously by ourselves and others (6, 7) and secondly by multicompartmental modelling taking into account urinary excretion rates of degraded apo LDL. The standard Matthews approach (12) showed that the rise in apo LDL was associated with a fall in its fractional rate of catabolism. Without a knowledge of the urine data we would therefore have concluded that in some way an increase in plasma triglyceride was associated with a reduction in the efficiency of LDL catabolism, the favoured explanation for this being that LDL receptors were downregulated. However, the urine data showed that reality was much more complex. If our initial conclusions had been correct, the daily average urine/plasma ratios in all subjects would have been constant over the 14 day turnover and the average for each quintile would have shown a progressive fall with increasing LDL mass. The curves which were observed reflect the earlier findings of Boston et al (10) who first postulated on the basis of a falling urine/plasma ratio over time that LDL was metabolically heterogeneous. Matthews analysis fails in this situation since it assumes that the kinetics describe clearance of a homogeneous tracer by a single catabolic mechanism (12, 14). In the face of tracer heterogeneity, the Matthews procedure cannot identify whether the activity of the removal mechanism is altered or the relative proportions of subcomponents in the tracer are changed. Multicompartmental modelling taking urine excretion data into account suggest in the present study that the latter scenario applies. The minimal computer model required to satisfy both the urine and plasma radioactivity curves necessitated the presence of two circulating LDL pools with differing kinetic characteristics. This model is identical to those described earlier by Boston et al (10) and Foster et al (14). When LDL levels are low the majority of the lipoprotein is associated with pool A and is metabolised rapidly by a receptor-mediated process. As the LDL mass rises, more of this material is found in the slowly catabolised pool B. The overall fall in total apo LDL clearance identified by Matthews analysis results from accumulation of material in pool B. In these young normolipidaemic individuals fractional catabolism of apo LDL from pool A fell modestly as the apo LDL concentration rose. In contrast the FCR for pool B was insensitive to mass. The rate of production of apo LDL in pool B was the principal determinant of the circulating lipoprotein concentration and this parameter was strongly and positively linked to the plasma triglyceride level.

It is likely that the metabolic heterogeneity observed in our subjects is caused by underlying structural heterogeneity. Recent work by Austin el al (16) has shown that in the general population LDL structure is strongly influenced by the level of plasma triglyceride. They found that individuals with plasma triglyceride levels above about 1.1 mmol/l (100 mg/dl) were more likely to express what they called the "Pattern B" phenotype for LDL which is associated with a predominance of smaller particles and higher apoB concentrations (above 85 mg/dl). "Pattern A" (in which larger LDL particles are predominant) is seen below this triglyceride level. If we examine our subjects in light of these values, quintiles 1 and 2 would represent subjects with "pattern A" while the top two quintiles fall into the "pattern B" category.

(B) Fibrate-induced triglyceride reduction: Effects on LDL metabolism

The fibrates are a family of hypolipidaemic drugs which lower plasma triglyceride primarily by promoting the lipolysis of triglyceride-rich particles through activation of lipoprotein lipase (17). Their actions on LDL are variable and depend on the initial plasma triglyceride level. In severely hypertriglyceridaemic individuals, LDL particles are small and dense and the low level of LDL in this condition is due to its hypercatabolism possibly by receptor-independent pathways (17). Fibrate treatment suppresses this high rate of clearance and redirects LDL catabolism into the receptor route (17). The overall effect of these changes is to increase the initially low levels of plasma LDL cholesterol, alter LDL composition and increase the average LDL particle size. Conversely, in hypercholesterolaemic, normotriglyceridaemic subjects, initially elevated LDL cholesterol levels are decreased by fibrate therapy. In a previous investigation of the mechanism of action of bezafibrate (18) we ascribed this effect to increased clearance of LDL through the receptor pathway. At the time we surmised that the drug was operating to suppress hepatic cholesterol synthesis and so activate clearance of LDL by receptors. However, in the light of present knowledge of the heterogeneity of LDL it is pertinent to ask whether it was the receptor or the ligand itself that changed during fibrate therapy. It is arguable that the drug, by altering LDL composition and size, increases the propensity of the particles for degradation by the receptor mechanism. This we examined using fenofibrate as a hypolipidaemic agent in a group of hypercholesterolaemic, normotriglyceridaemic subjects. The results are consistent with the view that the nature of the lipoprotein ligand was affected by therapy.

Methods and Results

Eight hypercholesterolaemic subjects (1 male, 7 female) volunteered

for the study. Despite a three months sterol lowering diet their
plasma cholesterol values persisted above 7.0 mmol/l. In each case,
plasma triglyceride was less than 2.3 mmol/l (Table 3).

Table 3   Effects on fenofibrate on apo LDL metabolism

            Kinetic analysis by curve peeling (Matthews) procedure

Parameter	Control	Fenofibrate	Significance
Plasma cholesterol (mmol/l)	8.01±0.39 *	5.71±0.27	<0.001
Plasma triglyceride (mmol/l)	1.63±0.12	1.06±0.09	<0.001
Apo LDL (mg/dl)	128±8	90±6	<0.005
Apo LDL Synthesis (mg/kg/d)	11.35±1.03	13.3±1.3	NS
Apo LDL Fractional Catabolism (pools/d)	0.255±0.015	0.422±0.031	<0.0005
Apo LDL Absolute Catabolism via receptors (mg/kg/d)	5.67±0.54	8.12±0.85	<0.02

* Mean ± SEM

The study was carried out in two phases. In the first, subjects
underwent serial measurements of plasma lipids and lipoproteins and
determination of native and cyclohexanedione-treated radiolabelled
LDL turnover using the procedures indicated earlier and including
continuous 24 hour urine collections. These measurements were
repeated in the second phase after eight weeks of therapy with
fenofibrate at 300mg/day (given as 100mg t.i.d.).

Discussion

Treatment with the drug (Table 3) reduced plasma cholesterol and
triglyceride by lowering the circulating mass of VLDL and LDL.
Matthews (12) curve peeling analysis showed that therapy was
associated with a 65% increase in the fractional catabolic rate (FCR)
of apo LDL. This change was apparently responsible for the 30%
decrease in the concentration of apo LDL in the plasma since there
was no significant effect of the drug on total apo LDL synthesis.

When LDL catabolism was divided into receptor-dependent versus receptor-independent pathways, it was observed that the FCR for the former was increased by 105%. Furthermore the amount apo LDL degraded by the receptor route rose by 43% (P<0.02, Table 3) while that removed by the receptor-independent pathway was unchanged. These results are virtually the same as data from a previous study (18) which examined the effects of bezafibrate on apo LDL turnover. However when we combined the analysis of urine and plasma data using the two pool model described above (Figure 3) it became clear that fenofibrate had produced its effects on LDL metabolism not primarily by altering the activity of the receptors but rather by making the circulating LDL particles better ligands. (Figure 4).

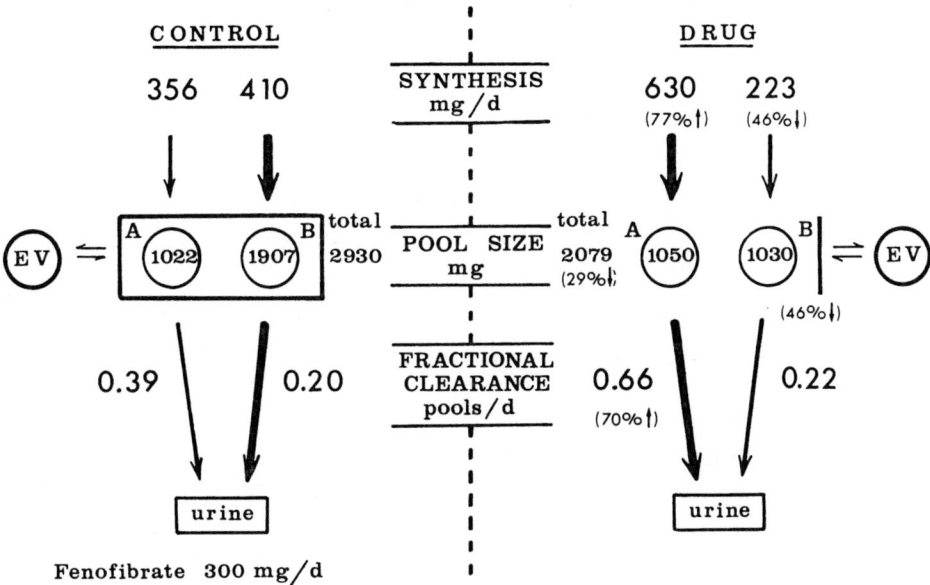

Figure 4.
Multicompartmental kinetic analysis of plasma and urinary radioactivity decay data for native and CHD modified LDL before and during treatment with fenofibrate. Modelling was performed using the procedures outlined in section (A) of this article.

In the control situation, approximately 3gm of LDL apoB circulated in the bloodstream. Two thirds existed in a form (Figure 4, pool B) which was cleared slowly (with a fractional removal rate of 20% per day) while the catabolism of the remainder (pool A) was approximately twice as fast. Treatment with fenofibrate halved the mass of the slowly cleared material in pool B, not by increasing its rate of catabolism but rather by limiting its synthesis. Conversely, input into pool A increased by more than 70% as did the rate of clearance

from this pool so that its overall mass remained the same.
These changes in LDL metabolism were associated with an alteration in
its structure, the average particle size increasing during fibrate
therapy (Figure 5).

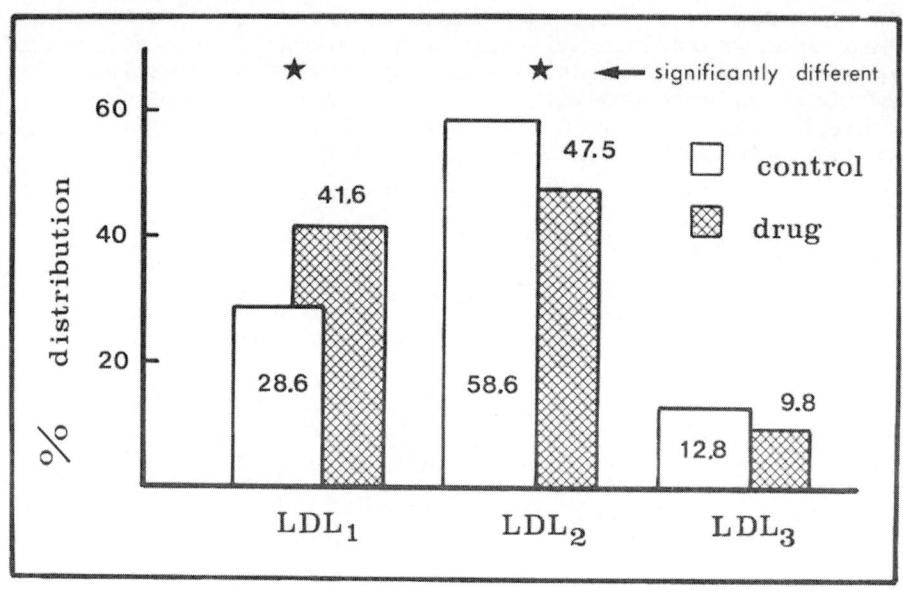

Figure 5.
Effects of fenofibrate (300 mg/d) on LDL subfraction distributions in
the plasma. Treatment increased the average size of LDL in the
circulation by reducing the number of circulating small dense LDL
particles.

We speculate that either the reduction in plasma triglyceride
circulating mass induced by the fibrate led to decreased neutral
lipid exchange and a compositional change in LDL so that on treatment
it became larger, more lipid-rich and had an increased affinity for
receptors (19) or that increased lipoprotein lipase activity promoted
the formation of receptor-active LDL regardless of the size and lipid
content of the VLDL precursor.
On the basis of our studies in normal and hypercholesterolaemic
subjects we conclude that the kinetics of LDL are strongly influenced
by plasma VLDL (triglyceride) levels. In hypercholesterolaemia
fenofibrate lowers plasma triglyceride and corrects the underlying
metabolic abnormality in LDL turnover. This may well improve the
atherogenic profile of the plasma lipids, a premise which still
requires to be tested in a prospective intervention study.

Acknowledgements

We acknowledge the excellent secretarial assistance of Sandra Hammond. This work was supported by grants from the British Heart Foundation (87/101 and 89/107).

References

1. Sigurdsson, G., Nicoll, A. and Lewis, B. (1975) 'Conversion of very low density lipoprotein to low density lipoprotein', J. Clin. Invest. 56, 1481–1490.
2. Reardon, M.F., Fidge, N.H. and Nestel, P.J. (1978) 'Catabolism of very low density lipoprotein in man' J. Clin. Invest. 61, 850–860.
3. Shepherd, J. and Packard, C.J. (1987) 'Metabolic heterogeneity in very low density lipoproteins' Am. Heart J. 113, 503–508.
4. Grundy, S.M., Mok, H.Y.I., Zech, L., Steinberg, D. and Berman, M.(1979) 'Transport of very low density lipoprotein triglycerides in varying degrees of obesity and hypertriglyceridaemia' J. Clin. Invest. 63, 1274–1283.
5. Phillips, N.R., Havel, R.J. and Kane, J.P. (1981) 'Levels and interrelationships of serum and lipoprotein cholesterol and triglycerides' Arteriosclerosis, 1, 13–24.
6. Langer, T. Strober, W. and Levy, R.I. (1972) 'The metabolism of low density lipoprotein in familial type II hyperlipoproteinaemia' J. Clin. Invest. 51, 1528–1536.
7. Packard, C.J., Third, J.L.H.C., Shepherd, J., Lorimer, A.R., Morgan, H.G. and Lawrie, T.D.V. (1976) 'Low density lipoprotein metabolism in a family of familial hypercholesterolaemic patients' Metab. Clin. Exp., 25, 995–1006.
8. Krauss, R.M. and Burke, D.J. (1981) 'Identification of multiple subclasses of plasma lipoproteins in normal humans' J. Lipid Res., 23, 97–104.
9. Griffin, B.A., Caslake, M.J., Yip, B., Tait, G.W., Packard, C.J. and Shepherd, J. (1990) 'Rapid isolation of low density lipoprotein subfractions from plasma by density gradient ultracentrifugation' Atherosclerosis, 83, 59–67.
10. Boston, R.C., Grief, P.C. and Berman, M. (1982) In 'Lipoprotein Kinetics and Modeling' Academic Press Inc, New York, NY, 437–460.
11. Caslake, M.J., Packard, C.J., Series, J.J., Yip, B., Dagen, M.M. and Shepherd, J. (1992) 'Plasma triglyceride and low density lipoprotein metabolism' Europ. J. Clin Invest., 22, 96–104.
12. Matthews, C.M.E. (1957) 'The theory of tracer experiments with 131$_I$-labelled plasma proteins. Phys. Med. Biol., 2, 36–53.
13. Shepherd, J., Bicker, S., Lorimer, A.R. and Packard, C.J. (1979) 'Receptor-mediated low density lipoprotein catabolism' J. Lipid Res., 20, 999–1006.

14. Foster, D.M., Chait, A., Albers, J.J., Failor, R.A., Harris, C.
    and Brunzell, J.D. (1986) 'Evidence for kinetic heterogeneity
    among low density lipoproteins' Metab. Clin. Exp., 35, 685–
    696.
15. Packard, D.J., McKinney, L., Carr, K. and Shepherd, J. (1983)
    'Cholesterol   feeding   increases   low   density   lipoprotein
    synthesis' J. Clin. Invest., 72, 45–51.
16. Austin, M.A., King, M.C., Vranizan, K.M. and Krauss, R.M. (1990)
    'Atherogenic lipoprotein phenotype. A proposed genetic marker
    for coronary heart disease risk.' Circulation, 82, 495–506.
17. Shepherd, J., Caslake, M.J., Lorimer, A.R., Vallance, B.D.,
    Packard,   C.J.   (1985)   'Fenofibrate   reduces   low   density
    lipoprotein   catabolism   in   hypertriglyceridaemic   subjects'
    Arteriosclerosis, 5, 162–168.
18. Stewart, J.M., Packard, C.J. Lorimer, A.R., Boag, D.E. and
    Shepherd, J. (1982) 'Effects of bezafibrate on receptor-
    mediated and receptor-independent low density lipoprotein
    catabolism   in   type   II   hyperlipoproteinaemic   subjects'
    Atherosclerosis, 44, 355–365.
19. Kleinman, Y., Oschry, Y. and Eisenberg, S. (1987) 'Abnormal
    regulation of LDL receptor activity and abnormal cellular
    metabolism of hypertriglyceridaemic low density lipoprotein :
    normalization with bezafibrate therapy' Eur. J. Clin. Invest.,
    17, 538–543.

FACTORS INFLUENCING THE ALTERED LIPOPROTEIN SYSTEM IN HYPERTRIGLYCERIDEMIA

M-R Taskinen

INTRODUCTION

Plasma concentration of triglycerides is determined by the balance between the production of triglyceride rich particles (chylomicrons and VLDL) and their catabolism through VLDL–IDL–LDL delipidation cascade. Both processes are influenced by a number of genetic and environmental factors. Overall hypertriglyceridemias are commonly associated with multiple defects of VLDL metabolism which also are reflected in IDL and LDL. In addition metabolism of high density lipoproteins (HDL) is closely linked to that of VLDL particles as evidenced by the tight inverse correlation found between VLDL triglycerides and HDL cholesterol in general population. Consequently hypertriglyceridemia is accompanied by multiple metabolic consequences which include increased postprandial lipemia, compositional changes of VLDL, lowering of HDL cholesterol, preponderance of small dense LDL and changes of clotting system. At least some if not all of these changes are potentially atherogenic and may explain the association of triglycerides with coronary artery disease (CAD). Growing evidence indicate that hypertriglyceridemia is commonly found in patients with CAD (1–4) although the role of VLDL per se has been disputed. Since triglyceride rich particles are highly heterogenic precise identification of atherogenic and anti–atherogenic fractions is needed to define targets for intervention.

Insulin resistance and hypertriglyceridemia

Hypertriglyceridemia and low HDL cholesterol are members in the clustering of metabolic abnormalities in the syndrome X (5) or insulin resistance syndrome (IRS)(6). The concentrations of both triglycerides and HDL cholesterol are closely related to insulin resistance measured by using euglycemic clamp technique, in normal subjects as well as in subjects with impaired glucose tolerance and NIDDM (7, 8). Hyperinsulinism is also common in endogenous hypertriglyceridemia. We have recently reported that even

467

A. L. Catapano et al. (eds.), Drugs Affecting Lipid Metabolism, 467–475.
© 1993 Kluwer Academic Publishers and Fondazione Giovanni Lorenzini.

hypertriglyceridemic patients with normal oral glucose tolerance test are resistant to the glucoregulatory actions of insulin (9). These observations have raised the question whether insulin resistance is a primary defect underlying hypertriglyceridemia and/or lowering of HDL. Familial clustering of hypertriglyceridemia low HDL cholesterol and hypertension has been recently described and the subjects also have markers of insulin resistance (10). Recent data also suggest that dyslipidemia is preceeded by hyperinsulinism (6). Family members of hypertriglyceridemic subjects represent a target group to test if serum triglycerides represent an early marker of insulin resistance. During ten years follow–up of 47 siblings from six pedigrees with familial hypertriglyceridemia the prevalence of IGT and NIDDM were 49 % and 21 % which is markedly higher than in general population (11). When the subjects were grouped according to baseline serum triglyceride tertiles there was a significant difference of fasting serum insulin concentration between the highest and lowest tertile. At follow–up of 10 yrs 76 % of the subjects belonging to the highest triglyceride tertile at baseline were glucose intolerant compared to only 20 % of the subjects in the lowest triglyceride tertile. When the discriminant power of baseline metabolic variables was analyzed by employing stepwise discriminant analyses baseline serum triglycerides turned out to be the most powerful predictor of future IGT and NIDDM. Taken together these observations suggest that hypertriglyceridemia in these families is an early marker of insulin resistant state and increases susceptibility to develope NIDDM.

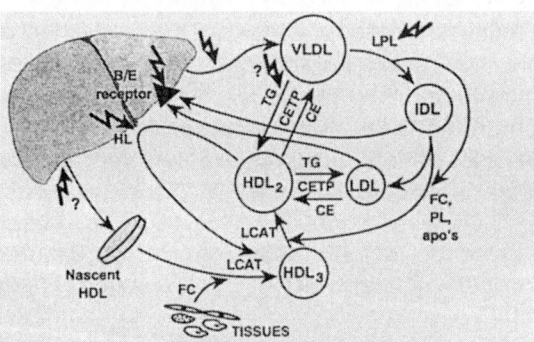

Fig 1. Schematic outline of VLDL–IDL–LDL cascade and the metabolism of HDL. The arrows indicate possible sites of insulin action in the cascade.

It should be recognized that insulin has several sites of action on lipoprotein metabolism (Fig 1). Insulin influences VLDL metabolism in the liver and plays a critical role in the regulation of lipoprotein lipase (LPL) which is the rate limiting enzyme in the lipolysis of triglyceride rich particles. Recent evidence indicate that insulin may also regulate hepatic lipase which participates in the conversion of IDL into LDL (12, 13). Hyperinsulinism can influence LDL metabolism via increasing LDL receptor activity and consequently cellular cholesterol uptake (14). Whether insulin modulates synthesis of apo A–I and A–II or nascent HDL particles is open as well as possible action of insulin on intravascular remodelling of lipoproteins via action of cholesteryl ester transfer protein (CETP). Considering the relationships between insulin resistance and hypertriglyceridemia several questions can be raised; 1. Does insulin resistance enhance VLDL production and release 2. Does insulin resistance influence the lipolytic enzymes involved in the delipidation cascade 3. Does insulin resistance interfere with triglyceride metabolism in skeletal muscle where the primary defect of insulin action on glucose metabolism is considered to reside (15, 16).

Regulation of VLDL metabolism in the liver

The production of VLDL particles consists of the synthesis of triglycerides and apo B–100 and their assembly to VLDL particles which are secreted into the circulation (Fig 2)(17, 18). Assembly of VLDL takes place in the endoplasmic reticulum and Golgi body. Hormonal and metabolic control of both apo B and triglyceride synthesis occur at several steps which are not well understood. Interesting questions relate to: 1. interference of hormones with the synthesis and trafficing of apo B or its assembly with triglycerides 2. mechanisms by which substrate availability (free fatty acids) modulates the synthesis of triglycerides and apo B. 3. whether the synthesis of apo B and triglycerides always is co–ordinated or can it be disrupted at some regulatory step 4. intracellular trafficking of apo B and its regulation. The fact that insulin resistance is closely related to VLDL production raises the question how insulin and free fatty acids might influence VLDL metabolism.

Fig 2. Schematic outline of VLDL triglyceride and apo B metabolism in the liver. The figures indicate regulatory sites of insulin action in synthesis and secretion of VLDL. TGFAs indicates storage pool of triglycerides in liver. TGFA$_R$ indicate the release pool of triglycerides in liver.

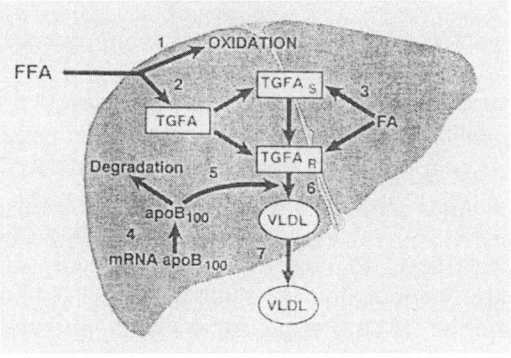

Insulin and VLDL metabolism. The general hypothesis has been that the sequence of events leading to hypertriglyceridemia is as follows: insulin resistance, hyperinsulinemia, increased hepatic VLDL production and hypertriglyceridemia (5). This concept is based on the conjecture that insulin directly stimulates VLDL production and secretion. However, it should be recognized that insulin has multiple sites of action on both triglyceride and apo B metabolism in the liver (Fig 2). Although the action of insulin on triglyceride synthesis is well documented its effects on the metabolism of apo B seem to be more complex (17, 18). Notably only a small fraction of newly synthesized apo B is assemblied with triglycerides and secreted (18). Interestingly insulin seems to increase apo B mRNA (19). Insulin has been reported to inhibit in vitro apo B secretion by increasing intracellular degradation of apo B (20-22). It has been suggested that the trafficking of apo B may co-ordinate the distribution of VLDL between storage and release pools (21). Notably acute vs chronic effects of insulin seem to be different (23, 24).

Although substantial amount of evidence indicate that hyperinsulinism is accompanied by increased VLDL production in man the exact mechanisms of action at different regulatory sites is so far unclear. To evaluate the action of insulin in vivo on the VLDL-IDL-LDL cascade we followed the metabolism of apo B-containing particles in NIDDM patients with poor metabolic control and repeated the studies after amelioration of glycemic control on intensive insulin therapy employing radioisotopic VLDL turnover methodology (25). These kinetic studies demonstrated that although insulin therapy induced multiple changes in the processing of apo B it had no effect on total apo B production. In NIDDM patients with poor control the major output of VLDL particles consisted of large VLDL (Sf 60-400) while NIDDM patients treated with insulin produced preferentially small VLDL (Sf 20-60). Note that intensive insulin therapy doubled the plasma insulin concentration. The data does not support the concept that hyperinsulinism per se is accompanied by increase of apo B production.

FFA and VLDL metabolism. A key component in VLDL synthesis is the flux of FFA into the liver. Increased flux of FFA into liver results in enhanced synthesis of triglycerides (26). Since one major action of insulin is to suppress lipolysis in peripheral tissues insulin also regulates the flux of FFA into the liver. Growing evidence suggest that FFA regulates apo B metabolism in the liver although the data are partly controversial. Dixon et al. (27) reported that FFA may protect against intracellular degradation of apo B. Recently we demonstrated that the plasma concentration of FFA is elevated in both NIDDM and endogenous hypertriglyceridemia. In hypertriglyceridemia patients FFA suppression during euglycemic clamp was significantly less than in normolipidemic controls matched for age and body weight (9). The slope of FFA suppression during insulin infusion and fasting FFA concentration explained together 81 % of the variation in the plasma triglyceride concentration.

Fig 3. Lipid oxidation rates (μmol/kg·min) in basal state (■) and during euglycemic clamp (rate of insulin infusion 320 pmol/m²·min)(□) in hypertriglyceridemic patients (HTG) with normal glucose tolerance, in NIDDM patients and in matched normolipidemic subjects (Saloranta C. et al., unpublished data).

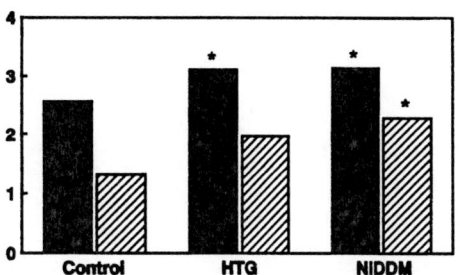

Since plasma FFA oxidation is primarily determined by the plasma FFA concentration (28), FFA oxidation is expected to be increased not only in NIDDM but also in endogenous hypertriglyceridemia. Indeed we observed that the basal lipid oxidation is increased to the same extent in hypertriglyceridemic subjects than in NIDDM patients (Fig 3). Further the suppression of lipid oxidation during insulin infusion is clearly impaired. The physiological relevance of these findings is that increased flux of FFA to liver may be the major factor leading to hypertriglyceridemia in insulin resistant states. On the other hand exposure of skeletal muscle to elevations of plasma FFA can induce further deterioration of glucose utilization in skeletal muscle (29, 30).

Catabolism of triglyceride rich particles.

Although the basis for elevation of triglyceride rich particles in insulin resistant states is overproduction of these lipoproteins the question raises whether insulin resistance with hyperinsulinism can alter the activity of lipolytic enzymes i.e. lipoprotein lipase (LPL) and hepatic lipase (HL). Insulin plays a role in the regulation of lipoprotein lipase and the enzyme activity is low in insulin deficient states (31). It should be recognized that the individual variation of LPL and HL activites are high in general population. In both endogenous hypertriglyceridemia and NIDDM LPL activity is commonly within the low normal range (31). Therefore a reduced lipolytic capacity may contribute to development of hypertriglyceridemia in the presence of VLDL overproduction. Family studies also indicate that genetic factors induce variability of lipolytic capacity (32). Whether heterozygous forms of functional LPL deficiencies due to mutated LPL genes are underlying the expression of dyslipidemias in insulin resistant states remains to be established.

Fig 4. LPL and HL activities
in lean and obese hypertriglyceridemia patients (□) and
in normolipidemic control
subjects (■) matched for age
and BMI. From Sane et al.
(32) with permission.

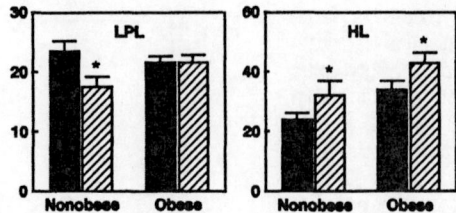

There is evidence suggesting that hepatic lipase is increased in NIDDM (33). This raises the question whether portal concentration of insulin regulates hepatic lipase activity. In endogenous hypertriglyceridemia HL activity is increased in both lean and obese subjects compared to normolipidemic controls (Fig 4). When we subgrouped the siblings of hypertriglyceridemia subjects by tertiles of fasting insulin hepatic lipase activity was significantly higher in the highest tertile compared to the lowest one. This preliminary data support the concept that hepatic lipase is regulated by insulin and is elevated in insulin resistant states with portal hyperinsulinism. High hepatic lipase could account, at least partly, for the lowering of HDL.

Summary

Hypertriglyceridemia is accompanied by multiple metabolic consequences which are potentially atherogenic. Although the relationship between hypertri-glyceridemia and insulin resistance is not fully understood we suggest that hypertriglyceridemia is an early marker of insulin resistance. The clinical expression of the metabolic disorder will be determined by the presence of genetic background predisposing to other metabolic abnormalities included in insulin resistance syndrome.

References

1.   Castelli, W.P. (1986) 'The triglyceride issue: A view from Framingham', Am. Heart. J. 112, 432–437.

2.   Austin, M.A. (1991) 'Plasma triglyceride and coronary heart disease', Arterio-scler. Thromb. 11, 2–14.

3.   Assmann, G. and Schulte, H. (1991) 'Triglycerides and atherosclerosis: Results from the prospective cardiovascular Münster study', Atheroscler. Reviews 22, 51–57.

4.   Manninen, V., Tenkanen, L., Koskinen, P., Huttunen, J.K., Mänttäri, M., Heinonen, O.P., and Frick, M.H. (1992) 'Joint effects of serum triglyceride and LDL cholesterol and HDL cholesterol concentrations on coronary heart disease risk in the Helsinki Heart Study', Circulation 85, 37–45.

5. Reaven, G.M. (1988) 'Role of insulin resistance in human disease', Diabetes 37, 1595-1607.

6. Haffner, S.M., Valdez, R.A., Hazuda, H.P., Mitchell, B.D., Morales, P.A., and Stern, M.P. (1992) 'Prospective analysis of the insulin-resistance syndrome (Syndrome X)', Diabetes 41, 715-722.

7. Abbott, W.G.H., Lillioja, S., Young, A.A., Zawadzki, J.K., Yki-Järvinen, H., Christin, L., and Howard, B.V. (1987) 'Relationships between plasma lipoprotein concentrations and insulin action in an obese hyperinsulinemic population', Diabetes 36, 897-904.

8. Laakso, M., Sarlund, H., and Mykkänen, L. (1990) 'Insulin resistance is associated with lipid and lipoprotein abnormalities in subjects with varying degrees of glucose tolerance', Arterioscler. 10, 223-231.

9. Yki-Järvinen, H., and Taskinen, M-R. (1988) 'Interrelationships among insulin's antilipolytic and glucoregulatory effects and plasma triglycerides in nondiabetic and diabetic patients with endogenous hypertriglyceridemia', Diabetes 37, 1271-1278.

10. Williams, R.R., Hunt, S.C., Hopkins, P.N., Stults, B.M., Wu, L.L., Hasstedt, S.J., Barlow, G.K., Stephenson, S.H., Lalouel, J.M., and Kuida, H. (1988) 'Familial dyslipidemic hypertension: evidence from 58 Utah families for a syndrome present approximately 12 % of patients with essential hypertension', JAMA 259, 3579-3586.

11. Sane, T., and Taskinen, M-R. (1991) 'Familial hypertriglyceridemia predicts development of impaired glucose tolerance and NIDDM', Diabetes 40, suppl 1, 551A:2199.

12. Baynes, C., Henderson, A.D., Anyaoku, V., Richmond, W., Hughes, C.L., Johnston, D.G., and Elkeles, R.S. (1991) 'The role of insulin insensitivity and hepatic lipase in the dyslipidaemia of Type 2 diabetes', Diab. Med. 8, 560-566.

13. Demant, T., Carlson, L.A., Holmquist, L., Karpe, F., Nilsson-Ehle, P., Packard, C.J., and Shepherd, J (1988) 'Lipoprotein metabolism in hepatic lipase deficiency: studies on the turnover of apolipoprotein B and on the effect of hepatic lipase on high density lipoprotein' J. Lipid. Res. 29, 1603-1611.

14. Bierman, E.L. (1992) 'George Lyman Duff Memorial Lecture: Atherogenesis in diabetes', Arterioscler. Thromb. 12, 647-656.

15. Eriksson, J., Franssila-Kallunki, A., Ekstrand, A., Saloranta, C., Widén, E., Schalin, C., and Groop, L. (1989) 'Early metabolic defects in persons at increased risk for non-insulin-dependent diabetes mellitus', N. Engl. J. Med. 321, 337-343.

16.   Vaag, A., Henriksen, J.E., and Beck–Nielsen, H. (1992) 'Decreased insulin activation of glycogen synthase in skeletal muscle in young nonobese caucasian first–degree relatives of patients with non–insulin–dependent diabetes mellitus', J. Clin. Invest. 89, 782–788.

17.   Gibbons, G.F. (1990) 'Assembly and secretion of hepatic very–low–density lipoprotein', Biochem. J. 268, 1–13.

18.   Borén, J., Wettesten, M., Sjöberg, A., Thorlin, T., Bondjers, G., Wiklund, O., and Olofsson, S–O. (1990) 'The assembly and secretion of apoB 100 containing lipoproteins in Hep G2 cells', J. Biol. Chem. 265, 10556–10564.

19.   Sparks, J.D., Zolfaghari, R., Sparks, C.E., Smith, H.C. and Fisher, E.A. (1992) 'Impaired hepatic apolipoprotein B and E translation in streptozotocin diabetic rats', J. Clin. Invest. 89, 1418–1430.

20.   Sparks, J.D., and Sparks, C.E. (1990) 'Insulin modulation of hepatic synthesis and secretion of apolipoprotein B by rat hepatocytes', J. Biol. Chem. 265, 8854–8862.

21.   Jackson, T.K., Salhanick, A.I., Elovson, J., Deichman, M.L., and Amatruda, J.M. (1990) 'Insulin regulates apolipoprotein B turnover and phosphorylation in rat hepatocytes', J. Clin. Invest. 86, 1746–1751.

22.   Salhanick, A., Schwartz, S.I., and Amatruda, J.M. (1991) 'Insulin inhibits apolipoprotein B secretion in isolated human hepatocytes', Metabolism 40, 275–279.

23.   Salhanick, A.I., Deichman, M.L., and Amatruda, J.M. (1992) 'Chronic (in vivo) and acute (in vitro) effects of insulin on apolipoprotein B (apo B) synthesis and secretion in rat hepatocytes', Diabetes 41, suppl 1, 17A:65.

24.   Lewis, G., Uffelman, K., and Steiner, G. (1992) 'Acute hyperinsulinemia (HI) decreases VLDL triglyceride (TG) and VLDL apo B production in vivo in humans', Diabetes 41, suppl 1, 25A:97.

25.   Taskinen, M.R., Packard, C.J., and Shepherd, J. (1990) 'Effect of insulin therapy on metabolic fate of apolipoprotein B–containing lipoproteins in NIDDM', Diabetes 39, 1017–1027.

26.   Havel, R.J., Kane, J.P., Balasse, E.O., Segel, N., and Basso, L.V. (1970) 'Splanchnic metabolism of free fatty acids and production of triglycerides of very low density lipoproteins in normotriglyceridemic and hypertriglyceridemic humans', J. Clin. Invest. 49, 2017–2035.

27.   Dixon, J.L., Furukawa, S., and Ginsberg, H.N. (1991) 'Oleate stimulates secretion of apolipoprotein B–containing lipoproteins from Hep G2 cells by

inhibiting early intracellular degradation of apolipoprotein B', J. Biol. Chem. 266, 5080–5086.

28. Groop, L.C., Bonadonna, R.C., Shank, M., Petrides, A.S., and DeFronzo, R.A. (1991) 'Role of free fatty acids and insulin in determining free fatty acid and lipid oxidation in man', J. Clin. Invest. 87, 83–89.

29. Nuutila, P., Koivisto, V.A., Knuuti, J., Ruotsalainen, U., Teräs, M., Haaparanta, M., Bergman, B., Solin, O., Voipio-Pulkki, L-M., Wegelius, U., and Yki-Järvinen, H. (1992) 'Glucose-free fatty acid cycle operates in human heart and skeletal muscle in vivo', J. Clin. Invest. 89, 1767–1774.

30. Nurjhan, N., Consoli, A., and Gerich, J. (1992) 'Increased lipolysis and its consequences on gluconeogenesis in non-insulin-dependent diabetes mellitus', J. Clin. Invest. 89, 169–175.

31. Taskinen, M-R., and Kuusi, T. (1987) 'Enzymes involved in triglyceride hydrolysis', in J. Shepherd and C. Packard (eds.), Lipoprotein Metabolism, W.B. Saunders Company, Eastbourne, pp. 639–666.

32. Sane, T., and Nikkilä, E.A. (1988) 'Very low density lipoprotein triglyceride metabolism in relatives of hypertriglyceridemic probands', Arterioscler. 8, 217–226.

33. Kasim, S., Tseng, K., Jen, K-L., and Khilnani, S. (1987) 'Significance of hepatic triglyceride lipase activity in the regulation of serum high density lipoproteins in type II diabetes mellitus', J. Clin. Endocrinol. Metab. 65, 183–187.

EFFECTS OF FIBRATES ON THE ALTERED LIPOPROTEIN SYSTEM IN HYPERTRIGLYCERIDEMIA

Shlomo Eisenberg, M.D., Professor of Medicine, Lipid Research Laboratory

Fibric acid derivatives are being used for treatment of hyperlipidemia syndromes for more than 25 years. The drugs markedly lower plasma triglyceride levels, increase HDL cholesterol and have a variable effect on the LDL system. Accordingly, fibrates are considered among the first drugs of choice for patients with type III and type IV hyperlipidemia, are also effective in patients with type V and decrease LDL in some but not all patients with hyperlipidemia types IIA and IIB. The mechanisms responsible for the lipid lowering effects of fibrates are increase of low lipoprotein lipase activity, stimulation of LDL catabolism via receptor-dependent pathway and decreased catabolism of apo A-I the major apoprotein of high density lipoproteins (1). The drugs may also have a direct effect on hepatic lipid metabolism.

Studies carried out in our laboratory during recent years have focused on the effects of one fibric acid analogue - bezafibrate - on the structure, composition and metabolism of lipoproteins in patients with various forms of hyperlipidemia. In addition to the known effects of fibrates on lipoprotein and apoprotein levels, our studies have also elucidated another facet of lipid lowering therapy: correction of abnormal structure and cell metabolism of lipoprotein particles. These data are summarized below, according to the lipoproteins investigated.

Chylomicrons and very low density lipoproteins (VLDL)

The effect of fibrates on chylomicrons and chylomicron remnants has been examined in only a few studies. In a recently published investigation, chylomicron and chylomicron remnants response after a vitamin A-fatty meal challenge was determined in patients with type IV hyperlipidemia before and during gemfibrozil therapy (2). A greatly exaggerated response was observed in the patients before initiation of therapy which reverted towards normal during therapy. As chylomicrons and their remnants are potentially atherogenic lipoprotein particles, the effect was regarded beneficial.

Fibrates effectively reduce plasma VLDL levels in most patients with hypertriglyceridemia (1). In our study of 16 patients, bezafibrate reduced mean VLDL levels by more than 50% but the individual response varied between 20-80% (3). In another study (4), patients with hypercholesterolemia without (type IIA) or with (type IIB) hypertriglyceridemia were studied. The hypotriglyceridemic response in patients with type IIB was similar to that observed in type IV, and an effect was also found in patients with type IIA. Postheparin plasma lipoprotein lipase was measured in the two studies. Bezafibrate therapy increased the activity of lipoprotein lipase in all patients and this effect is presumably responsible for the hypotriglyceridemic effect of the drug.

A. L. Catapano et al. (eds.), Drugs Affecting Lipid Metabolism, 477–481.
© 1993 Kluwer Academic Publishers and Fondazione Giovanni Lorenzini.

VLDL was isolated and characterized in the two studies. Abnormal structure and composition was found in the patients with hypertriglyceridemia. The HTG-VLDL was enriched with free and esterified cholesterol but contained relatively less triglycerides and apoproteins. These abnormalities reflect an exaggerated lipid (cholesteryl ester and triglyceride) transfer between the large mass of plasma VLDL and the low and high density lipoproteins (3). Indeed, a strong positive relationship between the degrees of VLDL abnormalities and plasma triglyceride levels was found. The best indicator for VLDL abnormality was the cholesteryl ester to protein ratio, presumably because of the effects of the lipid transfer reaction on the former and of the changing VLDL particle distribution profile on the latter. Bezafibrate caused reversal towards normal of all compositional abnormalities (3).

More recently, the effects of bezafibrate therapy on the cellular metabolism of HTG-VLDL by receptors was investigated (5,6). These studies were carried out after fractionation of the VLDL to 3 density fractions - VLDL-I, VLDL-II and VLDL-III and with and without the addition of exogenous recombinant apo E-3 (5). Normolipidemic VLDL (N-VLDL) exhibited a typical behavior with minimal metabolic activity without exogenous apo E-3 and a many-fold enhancement of its cellular reactivity after the addition of exogenous apo E-3 (5). The metabolic activity of N-VLDL-I was the lowest, of VLDL-III the highest, and that of N-VLDL-II intermediate. Abnormal metabolism of HTG-VLDL populations was found (6). First, the HTG-VLDLs exhibited a pronounced metabolic activity even without addition of exogenous apo E-3. Second, addition of apo E-3 markedly enhanced the cellular metabolism of the HTG-VLDLs to levels higher than those observed for N-VLDL. Third, the metabolic activity of HTG-VLDL-I was higher than that of HTG-VLDL-III and was 2-3 folds higher than that of N-VLDL-I. Of particular importance was the observation that the cell metabolism of the different VLDL fractions was strongly related to the cholesteryl ester to protein ratio and reversed towards normal when bezafibrate therapy was initiated. Fourth, HTG- VLDLs were able to downregulate cellular cholesterol synthesis in excess of their rate of degradation, especially when exogenous apo E-3 was not added. This finding indicated ability of HTG-VLDL to donate cholesterol - especially cholesteryl esters - to the cells by a process distinctly different from receptor-dependent pathways. Fifth, all these abnormalities were normalized when the VLDL was obtained from the patients 2 weeks after initiation of bezafibrate therapy. Thus, bezafibrate therapy not only reduced high VLDL levels but also corrected abnormal composition, structure and cell metabolism of the HTG-VLDL.

Low density lipoproteins (LDL)

Fibrates are used in patients with high LDL plasma levels without (type IIA) or with (type IIB) elevated triglycerides. All preparations are effective in reducing high LDL cholesterol and apo B levels, although differences between preparations may exist. Individual responses however may vary markedly. In some hypercholesterolemic patients, fibrate therapy reduces LDL levels by as much as 20-40%. In others, it is not effective. The reason for this remarkable variation in response is not known. Therapy of patients with hypertriglyceridemia and normal or low LDL levels (type IV) in contrast is often associated with an increase of the LDL cholesterol levels. In such patients fibrate therapy reduces VLDL levels but increases LDL. It should however be noted that the absolute levels of LDL cholesterol in the treated type IV patients seldom exceeds the normal recommended level. We suggested that the LDL response to bezafibrate is related to the initial plasma triglyceride levels and reflects effects of an interaction of several metabolic pathways (4). These include correction of abnormal LDL composition (see below), increased conversion of VLDL to LDL (due to correction of the abnormal composition of HTG-VLDL) and effects on LDL clearance by LDL receptors. The first two mechanisms are predicted to cause an increase of LDL cholesterol levels in type IV patients, while the third is responsible for the reduction of LDL cholesterol levels in patients with type IIA. Patients with type IIB should exhibit intermediate behavior, and that is indeed what has been observed (4).

Abnormalities of the LDL system in hypertriglyceridemica were studied in detail in our laboratory (3). We noted several abnormalities of HTG-LDL preparations: higher density, smaller size, high protein and triglyceride content, and low free and esterified cholesterol. All six abnormalities reverted towards normal when bezafibrate therapy was initiated. Next, we investigated the cell metabolism of HTG-LDL (7,8). The cholesterol-poor LDL particle was relatively inefficient in regulating sterol and LDL receptor protein synthesis. Unexpectedly, we also observed decreased affinity of the abnormal HTG-LDL particle towards LDL receptors in fibroblasts. That was found to be due to reversible conformational alteration of the apo B-100 of the lipoprotein (9). Yet in spite of the low affinity of the HTG-LDL towards the receptor, LDL uptake in cells that have been down-regulated after 48h incubation with the abnormal HTG-LDL was either normal or even higher than normal (8). These metabolic abnormalities also reverted towards normal after initiation of bezafibrate therapy.

The observations summarized above demonstrate clearly the ability of fibrate therapy to normalize an abnormal LDL system. We believe that the abnormal LDL system may directly or indirectly be responsible for accelerated atherosclerosis found in patients with hypertriglyceridemia (1). Therapy that causes correction of the LDL abnormalities therefore may be beneficial even if associated with an increase of the LDL cholesterol to levels that are currently considered below those associated with increased risk for developing atherosclerosis.

High Density Lipoproteins (HDL)

Fibrate therapy consistently causes an increase of high density lipoprotein cholesterol and apo A-I levels in all different forms of hyperlipidemia (3,4). In normotriglyceridemic type IIA patients, fibrates cause an average increase of HDL-C of about 10%. In hypertriglyceridemic subjects especially those with low HDL cholesterol levels, the response is more pronounced and elevation of HDL levels of 40-50% are commonly observed.   One mechanism responsible for the increase of HDL cholesterol level is undoubtedly the reduction of plasma triglyceride levels and the increase of the low plasma lipoprotein lipase activity (10). A direct effect of fibrates on the HDL system may also exist but has not so far been carefully investigated. Of interest, bezafibrate therapy is associated with an especially good response in patients with type IIB although their initial plasma triglyceride concentration is less than that of type IV patients.

Bezafibrate corrects abnormal structure and composition of HDL in patients with hypertriglyceridemia either with or without elevated LDL levels. In these patients, HDL is found exclusively in the dense HDL_3 populations (3,4). $HTG-HDL_3$ is denser than normal HDL_3 (implying a high protein contribution and a smaller diameter of the particles), is enriched with triglycerides and contains substantially less cholesteryl ester molecules than normal HDL_3. All these abnormalities are related to the plasma triglyceride levels and revert towards normal when bezafibrate therapy is initiated. The mechanism by which HDL exerts its effect on the prevention of atherosclerotic diseases is not clear (10). Hence, whether $HTG-HDL_3$ is as effective as or less effective than normal HDL in this process, is unknown. Many studies have demonstrated that HDL apoprotein catabolism is accelerated in subjects with hypertriglyceridemia (for a review, see ref. 10). The mechanism behind the accelerated apoprotein catabolism in HTG-states was recently elucidated and found to reflect a general phenomenon: increased apo A-I and apo A-II fractional catabolic rate in smaller and denser HDL particles as compared to larger and less dense particles (11). Bezafibrate corrects the abnormal structure and composition of HDL and that in turn reduces HDL apoprotein catabolism. Thus, it is possible that fibrates will play a role in preventing the development of atherosclerosis not only by raising HDL levels but also by normalizing abnormal structure, composition and metabolism of the lipoprotein. Indeed, data from the Helsinki Heart Study tend to support this notion (12,13).

Conclusions

The data discussed above indicate that fibrates may play a dual role in the treatment of the hyperlipidemic patient. First, a reduction of the levels of the atherogenic lipoproteins VLDL and LDL, and elevation of the levels of the antiatherogenic lipoprotein, HDL. Second, correction of abnormal structure, composition and metabolism of all lipoproteins, an effect especially pronounced in patients with hypertriglyceridemia with or without elevated LDL. With regard to the first mechanism it is interesting to note the effects of bezafibrate therapy on an atherogenic index - for example, the LDL cholesterol to HDL cholesterol ratio. A dramatic reduction of this ratio is seen in patients with type IIA and type IIB who exhibit a very high ratio before therapy is initiated. In type IV patients, whose LDL to HDL ratio is low, there is no worsening of this ratio in spite of the increase of LDL cholesterol. In these patients however, another atherogenic ratio, that of VLDL to HDL cholesterol, decreases dramatically, from 5.3 to 1.7. With respect to the second effect of bezafibrate on the lipoprotein system - i.e., normalization of abnormal structure, composition and metabolism - we can only speculate. Abnormal lipoproteins have repeatedly been shown to be associated with accelerated atherosclerosis and tendency to form foam cells in tissue culture experiments (14,15). One of the outstanding examples is B-VLDL in type III patients; other examples are abnormal IDL in similar patients, HTG-VLDL in hypertriglyceridemia and the proteinrich, dense and small LDL in patients with hyperapobetalipoproteinemia. As discussed above, most if not all these lipoprotein abnormalities respond to fibrate therapy. An anti-atherogenic effect of fibrate therapy was indeed convincingly demonstrated in the Helsinki Heart Study, employing gemfibrozil (12,13) and this effect was especially pronounced in patients with high plasma triglyceride levels, low HDL cholesterol and high LDL to HDL ratio (16). Yet, further studies are needed to continue to clarify the role of fibrate therapy as a first line of defence against atherosclerosis in susceptible subjects, especially those with low HDL cholesterol and with or without high triglyceride levels.

References

1. Eisenberg S, Gavish D, Kleinman Y.: Bezafibrate. In: Levy RI, Shepherd J, Packard CJ, Miller NE. (eds.). Pharmacological Control of Hyperlipidemia. AR Prous, Barcelona 1986, pp. 145-169.
2. Weintraub M, Eisenberg S, Breslow JL.: Different patterns of post prandial lipoprotein metabolism in normal, Type IIA, Type III and Type IV hyperlipoproteinemic individuals. Effects of treatment with cholestyramine and gemfibrozil. J Clin Invest 1987;79:1110-1119.
3. Eisenberg S, Gavish D, Oschry Y, et al.: Abnormalities in very low, low and high density lipoproteins in hypertriglyceridemia. Reversal towards normal with bezafibrate treatment. J Clin Invest 1984;74: 470-482.
4. Gavish D, Oschry Y, Fainaru M, et al.: Change in very low-, low- and high-density lipoproteins during lipid lowering (Bezafibrate) therapy. Studies in Type IIA and Type IIB hyperlipoproteinemia. Eur J Clin Invest 1986;16:61-68.
5. Eisenberg S, Friedman G, Vogel T.: Enhanced metabolism of normolipidemic human plasma very low density lipoprotein in cultured cells by exogenous apolipoprotein E-3. Arteriosclerosis 1988;8:480-487.

6.   Sehayek E, Eisenberg S.: Abnormal composition of hypertriglyceridemic very low density lipoprotein determines abnormal cell metabolism. Arterosclerosis 1988;10:1088-1095.
7.   Kleinman Y, Eisenberg S, Oschry Y, et al.: Defective metabolism of hypertriglyceridemic low density lipoprotein in cultured human skin fibroblasts. J Clin Invest 1985;75:1796-1803.
8.   Kleinman Y, Oschry Y, Eisenberg S.: Abnormal regulation of LDL receptor activity and abnormal cellular metabolism of hypertriglyceridaemic low density lipoprotein. Normalization with bezafibrate therapy. Eur J Clin Invest 1987;17:538-543.
9.   Kleinman Y, Schonfeld G, Gavish D, et al.: Hypolipidemic therapy modulates expression of apolipoprotein B epitopes on low density lipoproteins. Studies in mild to moderate hypertriglyceridemic patients. J Lipid Res 1987;28:540-548.
10.   Eisenberg S.: High density lipoprotein metabolism (JLR Review). J Lipid Res 1984;25:1017-1058.
11.   Brinton EA, Eisenberg S, Breslow JL.: Increased apo A-I and apo A-II fractional catabolic rate in patients with low HDL-cholesterol levels with or without hypertriglyceridemia. J Clin Invest 1991;87: 536-544.
12.   Frick MM, Elo O, Haapa K, et al.: Helsinki Heart Study. Primary prevention trial with gemfibrozil in middle-aged men with dyslipidemia. N Engl J Med 1987;317:1237-1245.
13.   Manninen V, Elo O, Frick MH, et al.: Lipid alternations and decline in the incidence of coronary heart disease in the Helsinki Heart Study. JAMA 1988;260:641-651.
14.   Mahley R, Angelin B.: Type III hyperlipoproteinemia. Recent insights into the genetic defect of familial dysbetalipoproteinemia. Adv Intern Med 1984;29:385-411.
15.   Eisenberg S.: Dyslipoproteinemia and Atherosclerosis. In: Ollson AG (ed). Atherosclerosis, Biology and Clinical Science. Churchill Livingston, 1987 pp. 281-290.
16.   Manninen V, Tekkanen L, Koskinen P, et al.: Joint effects of serum triglyceride and LDL cholesterol and HDL cholesterol concentrations on coronary heart disease risk in the Helsinki Heart Study: Impli cations for treatment. Circulation 1992;85:37-45.

TRIGLYCERIDE-RICH LIPOPROTEINS: ROLE IN ATHEROGENESIS AND HAEMOSTASIS

C. R. SIRTORI and M. R. LOVATI

ABSTRACT. Triglyceride-rich lipoproteins, particularly very low density lipoproteins (VLDL), are now recognized as a crucial factor in atherogenesis and thrombosis (Consensus-Hypertriglyceridemia as a vascular risk factor, Eur. Heart J., 11 Suppl. H: 44-48, 1990). Epidemiological data suggest that hypertriglyceridemia (HTG) may lead to arterial disease within a complex syndrome, associated to reduced high density lipoprotein (HDL) cholesterol and, possibly, to increased insulin resistance. Animal models proving the atherogenicity of VLDL are not numerous: the best has been developed in rabbits, receiving a single non lethal dose of tetrachloro-dibenzodioxin (TCDD) (Lovati et al., 1984, Toxicol. Appl. Pharmacol., 75, 91-97,). This leads to a stable HTG, associated to the development of arterial lesions, characteristically enriched with TG.
In humans, increasing interest has been focused on the reduced fibrinolysis, characteristic of HTG. Reduced fibrinolysis has been recently attributed to increased levels of an endogenous inhibitor (PAI-1), produced both by endothelial cells and by hepatocytes. In addition, fibrinogenemia is frequently elevated in hypertriglyceridemic patients, although the mechanism is far from clear.
In an attempt to modify some of the major risk factors associated to HTG, fibric acids offer a potential therapeutic tool. They can improve clearance of VLDL and also reduce (not all) fibrinogen levels; the activity on insulin resistance is variable. Bezafibrate administration is definitely associated with reduced VLDL and increased HDL, as well as reduced fibrinogenemia, most clearly in patients with elevated levels. In addition, it can reduce platelet aggregability, particularly after collagen induction, by a mechanism not linked to cyclooxygenase inhibition.

1. Introduction

Triglyceride-rich lipoproteins, in particular very low density lipoproteins (VLDL) are being increasingly recognized as a crucial risk factor for atherogenesis and thrombosis (1, 2). This recognition is based upon epidemiological data (in particular from Northern European countries), upon studies on the clotting system in hypertriglyceridemic patients and also upon the linkage between hypertriglyceridemia (HTG) and the polymetabolic syndrome (syndrome X), characterized, in addition to HTG, by reduced HDL cholesterol, impaired carbohydrate tolerance and insulin resistance (3). A shortcoming in the evaluation of HTG as an atherogenic syndrome is the apparent lack of animal models reproducing the disorder. This review will attempt to summarize available data in animal models, supporting the atherogenicity of HTG, and will also describe changes in TG metabolism

A. L. Catapano et al. (eds.), Drugs Affecting Lipid Metabolism, 483–491.
© 1993 Kluwer Academic Publishers and Fondazione Giovanni Lorenzini.

related to environmental contaminants. In addition, the major alterations of clotting, particularly as relates to fibrinogen and fibrinolysis, possibly consequent to HTG, will be reviewed, also examining the effects of drug treatments.

2. Atherogenicity of triglyceride rich lipoproteins

The potential of TG rich lipoproteins, both VLDL and IDL, to enhance lipid deposition in arterial macrophages, has been well characterized in in vitro models (4), as also reported in this Symposium by Gianturco et al. VLDL from HTG patients may lead to the accumulation of TG and also of CE in macrophages and they may also exert clearcut toxic effects, similar to those of oxidized low density lipoproteins (LDL).

However, the most frequent objection to the hypothesis of HTG as an atherogenic syndrome is related to the supposed lack of adequate animal models, demonstrating a correlation between elevated triglyceridemia and arterial disease. This is actually not so. We were the first to describe a model, clearly showing that the acute administration of a low dose of tetrachloro-p-dibenzodioxin (**TCDD**) can lead to a significant hypertriglyceridemia, associated with the development of arterial lesions (5). These lesions in the aorta are typically enriched with TG.

Brewster et al. (6) more recently reported that, in rabbits on a normolipidemic regimen, the administration of 1 or 50 µg/kg of TCDD ip caused, within 10 days, a significant HTG with a dose dependent decrease of the adipose tissue lipoprotein lipase (LPL) activity and of hepatic LDL binding. The electron microscopic examination of aortic arches 20 d after a single ip administration of 50 µg/TCDD/kg (Fig. 1) revealed ruffling, denudation, and sloughing off of the cell surface with the appearance of macrophage-like structures in the intima and media of the endothelium. These alterations resemble pre-atherosclerotic lesions, typical of animals with hyperlipidemia (7).

The reason why other models of dietary or drug induced HTG fail to elicit similar overt changes is probably that, in these cases, eg ethanol, high-carbohydrate diets, etc., the HTG is not sufficiently sustained. This condition is instead satisfied in the TCDD induced metabolic disorder, where the prolonged inhibition of LPL activity allows the maintenance of a significant hyperlipidemia, with mild alterations of plasma cholesterol and insulin levels (6).

The case of TCDD has drawn attention to other possible environmental contaminants leading to clearcut plasma lipid disorders. Possibly the best characterized, in the opposite direction, is the case of **ozone** that, when given at relatively high concentrations (3 ppm) to rats can instead lead to reduced triglyceridemia (Table 1) as well as to a dose dependent rise of HDL levels (8). These observations have never been substantiated in larger animal models. Another well known contaminant, instead, carbone disulphide (CS_2) leads to oxidative changes in lipoproteins, with a consequently increased

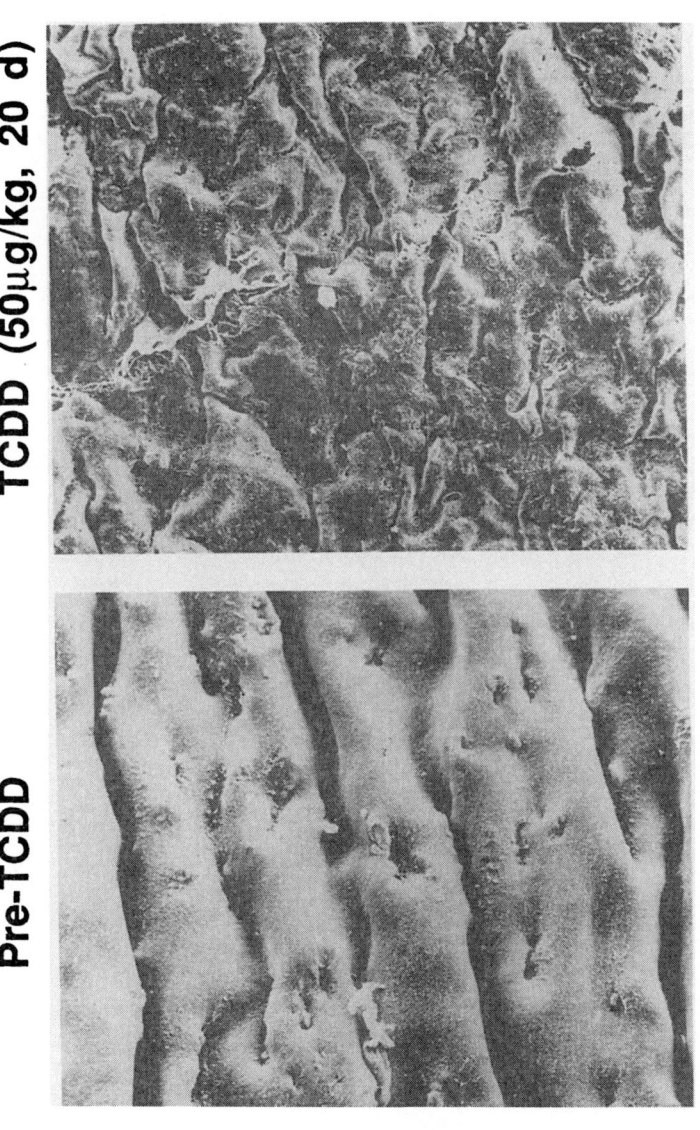

RABBITS: *Internal surface of the aortic arch*

Pre-TCDD   TCDD (50µg/kg, 20 d)

Figure 1. Scanning electron micrograph of internal surface of the aortic arch in normal rabbits either untreated (left) or treated 20 days before with a single, non toxic dose of TCDD (50 µg/kg). Significant endothelial denudation with surface ruffling is visible, together with the enrichment of triglycerides in the aortic wall (see text) (from 6, with kind permission).

atherogenic potential (9). Effects on lipoproteins of other widely diffused environmental chemicals (NO_2, SO_2 or others) await clarification.

Table 1. Ozone, effect on plasma lipids in rats (from 8)

Concentrations :	0, 1, 1.75, 3 ppm	
Exposure time:	5 h/day, 10 days	

	0 ppm	3 ppm
	mg/dl	
Chol	6 8	7 3
TG	4 6	22**
HDL-Chol	5 4	60**

3. *Hypertriglyceridemia leads to major defects in the coagulative/fibrinolytic system*

An enhanced risk of thrombosis is the most feared complication of hyperlipoproteinemias. In hypercholesterolemias, the major mechanism explaining the enhanced thrombotic risk is platelet hyperaggregability, probably consequent to the increased cholesterol content of platelet membranes (10). Platelets from type II patients release increased amounts of thromboxane B_2, thus indicating a stimulated eicosanoid production (11).

In the case of type IV hyperlipoproteinemia, although some authors similarly suggest a raised platelet aggregability (12), this has not been a consistent finding, also in view of the difficulty in establishing hyperaggregability in lipemic sera. In HTG, the major defect has been repeatedly shown to lie in the **fibrinolytic system.** Already 20 years ago Epstein et al. (13) showed that after exercise fibrinolytic activity is raised to a lesser extent in type IV patients vs controls. More recently, Simpson et al. (2) could demonstrate a reduction of circadian fibrinolysis in type IV patients vs controls; treatment with diet and/or fibric acids may reduce triglyceridemia and raise fibrinolysis.

A new opening in the understanding of the mechanism/s whereby elevated TG may impair fibrinolysis has come from studies in young coronary patients, establishing the association between increased plasma levels of a potent inhibitor of fibrinolytic activity and HTG (14). The so called plasminogen activator inhibitor type 1 (PAI-1), is a serine protease inhibitor (serpin) secreted by endothelial and liver cells (15). It is a protein of 379 aminoacids, whose gene is located on chromosome 7. More recent investigations have clearly shown that the increased levels of circulating PAI-1 are directly correlated with plasma TG, as well as with insulin (16). The in vitro incubation of VLDL, particularly from HTG patients, with both endothelial and liver cells, induces a prompt and sustained release of PAI-1 (17). Interestingly, this serpin may represent as much as 12.5% of all proteins, secreted by the endothelial cells (15).

At present, only scant data support the possible pharmacological correction of elevated PAI-1 levels. Only two drugs have been clearly shown to reduce PAI-1 levels. One is stanazolol, an anabolic steroid (18) and the other is metformin, an antidiabetic biguanide (19). The case of metformin is of particular interest, since this drug may affect insulin resistance, thus exerting a primary activity in the insulin resistance/polymetabolic syndrome (syndrome X), characterized, in addition, by hypertension, hypertriglyceridemia and carbohydrate intolerance (3). In our hands, the activity of metformin was clearly substantiated in patients with peripheral arterial disease, where there was a progressive reduction of this thrombotic index during prolonged treatment (Table 2) (20).

TABLE 2. Fibrinolysis after low dose metformin in patients with peripheral vascular disease (PVD) (from 20)

	9 PVD pts, Met 500 mg bid			
	Basal	1 mo	4 mo	P
Fibrinolytic act	13.8	13.9	13.0	n.s.
PAI-1 act (AU/ml)	17.2	10.3	12.8	n.s.
t-PA ag (ng/ml)	17.2	14.6	11.2	<0.01
PAI-1 ag (ng/ml)	13.2	8.9	7.7	<0.01

A thrombotic index frequently associated with HTG is **increased plasma fibrinogen.** The basis of this correlation is far from clear. Animal data showing a parallel rise of TG and fibrinogen in rats treated with Triton WR 1339 (21). There is also evidence that aged Watanabe rabbits with an inherited hyperlipidemia, develop significant rises of plasma fibrinogen (22). Interestingly some, not all, fibric acids are capable of significantly reducing elevated fibrinogen levels. The exception is that of gemfibrozil, never shown to reduce this thrombotic index.

Among fibric acids, bezafibrate seems to be the most effective. It has been shown to effectively reduced fibrinogenemia in patients with elevated levels of this parameter (23). In a controlled study in our clinical center, fibrinogenemia was significantly reduced in the bezafibrate arm of a cross-over investigation (24). In addition, there was clear evidence of a significant correlation between the fall of fibrinogenemia and the pre-treatment levels, thus suggesting that the activity of the drug may also be part of a "normalization" phenomenon, although certainly the mechanism of this correction is far from clear.

Although the correlation between HTG and increased plasma **platelet aggregability**, if any, is still unclear (12) also because of the above described technical difficulties, still some data support a significant activity both on aggregation and on platelet turnover by, e.g. clofibrate (25). In two studies evaluating gemfibrozil we only could show, in one a small not statistically significantly reduction of thromboxane B_2 (TXB_2) release by platelets after collagen induced aggregation (26). More recently, within the above quoted bezafibrate study (24), it was noted that after drug treatment platelets show a reduced responsiveness, in particular to collagen (Fig. 2), but this change in aggregability is apparently not related to eicosanoid metabolism, since TXB_2 release was not reduced by drug treatment.

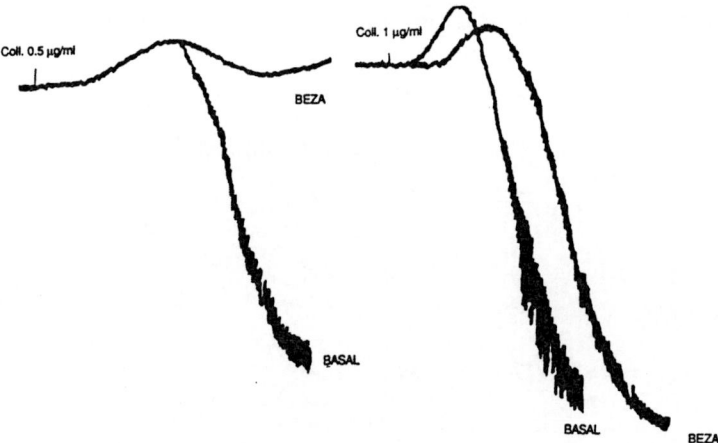

Figure 2. Threshold aggregatory concentrations of collagen increase after bezafibrate in type IV. AC_{50}s rise from 0.50 to 0.85 µg/ml (p< 0.001) (from 24).

4. Conclusions

Hypertriglyceridemias and, in general, elevations in blood of triglyceride rich lipoproteins is, per se a major risk factor for arterial disease. This is substantiated by at least one major animal model in rabbits, after a single, not overtly toxic dose of TCDD. In this model, the arterial lesions are typically TG enriched, whereas it appears that even in clinical hypertriglyceridemic conditions, CE enrichment in the artery may be the major finding. In addition to the typical atheromatous changes occurring in HTG, this condition is accompanied by other alterations of the clotting system, in particular of fibrinolysis and fibrinogen, possibly affecting in an indirect way the plasma fibrinogen/platelet interaction. Although raised PAI-1 levels seem to be rather weakly responsive to pharmacological treatment, other parameters of increased coagulability may well respond to drugs, in particular to bezafibrate. This type of approach offers, therefore, an interesting insight into the pathogenesis of arterial disease in hypertriglyceridemia and provides the ground for developing preventive treatments for this frequent metabolic disorder.

5. References

1. Böttiger, L.E. and Carlson, L.A. (1980) Risk factors for ischaemic vascular death for men in the Stockholm Prospective Study, Atherosclerosis 36, 389-409.
2. Simpson, H.C.R., Mann, Y.I., Meade, J.W., Chakrabarti, R., Stirling, Y. and Woolf, L. (1983) Hypertriglyceridemia and hypercoagulability, Lancet i, 786-789.
3. Reaven, G.M. (1988) Role of insulin resistance in human disease, Diabetes 37, 1595-1607.
4. Gianturco, S.H., Bradley, W.A., Gotto, A.M. jr, Morrisett, J.D. and Peavy, D.L. (1982) Hypetriglyceridemic very low density lipoproteins induce triglyceride synthesis and accumulation in mouse peritoneal macrophages, J. Clin. Invest. 70, 168-178.
5. Lovati, M.R., Galbussera, M., Franceschini, G., Weber, G., Resi, L., Tanganelli, P. and Sirtori, C.R. (1984) Increased plasma and aortic triglycerides in rabbits after acute administration of 2,3,7,8-tetrachlorodibenzo-p-dioxin, Toxicol. Appl. Pharmacol. 75, 91-97.
6. Brewster, D.W., Bombick, D.W., Matsumura, F. (1988) Rabbit serum hypertriglyceridemia after administration of 2,3,7,8-tetrachlorodibenzo-p-dioxin (TCDD), J. Toxicol. Environ. Health 25, 495-507.
7. Shio, H., Haley, N.Y., Flower, S. (1979) Characterization of lipid-laden aortic cells from cholesterol-fed rabbits. III. Intracellular localization of cholesterol and cholesteryl ester, Lab. Invest. 41, 160-167.
8. Mole, M.L., Stead, A.G., Gardner, D.E., Miller, F.J. and Graham, J.A. (1985) Effect of ozone on serum lipids and lipoproteins in the rat, Toxicol. Appl. Pharmacol. 80, 367-376.

9.Laurman, W., Salmon, S., Maziere, C., Maziere, J.C., Auclair, M., Theron, L. and Santus, R. (1989) Carbon disulfide modification and impaired catabolism of low density lipoprotein, Atherosclerosis 78, 211-218.
10.Stuart, M.J., Gerrard, J.M. and White, J.F. (1980) Effect of cholesterol on production of thromboxane B2 by platelets in vitro, N. Engl. J. Med. 302, 6-10.
11.Eynard, A.R., Tremoli, E., Caruso, D., Magni, F., Sirtori, C.R. and Galli, G. (1986) Platelet formation of 12-hydroxyeicosatetraenoic acid and thromboxane B2 is increased in type IIa hypercholesterolemic subjects, Atherosclerosis 60, 61-66.
12.Joist, J.H., Baker, K. and Schonfeld, G. (1979) Increased in-vivo and in-vitro platelet function in type II and type IV hyperlipoproteinemia, Thromb. Res. 15, 95-108.
13.Epstein, S.E., Rosing, D.R., Brakman, D.R., Redwood, D.R. and Astrup, T. (1970) Impaired fibrinolytic response to exercise in patients with type-IV hyperlipoproteinaemia, Lancet ii, 631-634.
14.Hamsten, A., Wiman, B., De Faire, U. and Blombäck, M. (1985) Increased plasma levels of a rapid inhibitor of tissue plasminogen activator in young survivors of myocardial infarction, N. Engl. J. Med. 313, 1557-1563.
15.Andreasen, P.A., Georg, B., Lund, L.R., Riccio, A. and Stacey, S.N. (1990) Plasminogen activator inhibitors: hormonally regulated serpins, Mol. Cell. Endocrinol., 68: 1-19.
16.Juhan-Vague, I., Alessi, M.C., Holy, P., Thirion, X., Vague, P., Declerck, P.J., Serradimigni, A. and Collen, D. (1989) Plasma plasminogen activator inhibitor-1 in angina pectoris. Influence of plasma insulin and acute-phase response, Arteriosclerosis 9, 362-367.
17.Mussoni, L., Maderna, P., Camera, M., Bernini, F., Sironi, L., Sirtori, M. and Tremoli, E. (1990) Atherogenic lipoproteins and release of plasminogen activator inhibitor (PAI-1) by endothelial cells, Fibrinolysis 4, 79-81.
18.Verheijen, J.H., Rijken, D.C., Chang, G.T.G., Preston, F.E. and Kluft, C. (1984) Modulation of rapid plasminogen activator inhibitor in plasma by stanazolol, Thromb. Haemostas. 51, 396-397.
19.Vague, P., Juhan-Bague, I., Alessi, M.C., Badier, C. and Valadier, J. (1987) Metformin decreases the high plasminogen activator inhibition capacity, plasma insulin and triglyceride levels in non-diabetic obese subjects, Thromb. Haemostas. 57, 326-328.
20.Montanari, G., Bondioli, A., Rizzato, G., Puttini, M., Tremoli, E., Mussoni, L., Mannucci, L., Pazzucconi, F. and Sirtori, C. R. (1992) Treatment with low dose metformin in patients with peripheral vascular disease. Pharmacol. Res. 25, 63-73.
21.Obazaki, M., Suzuki, M. and Oguchi, K. (1990) Changes in coagulative and fibrinolytic activities in Triton WR 1339-induced hyperlipidemia in rats, Jpn. J. Pharmacol. 52, 353-361.
22.Mori, Y., Wada, H., Nagano, Y, Deguchi, K., Kita, T. and Shirakawa, S. (1989) Hypercoagulable state in the Watanabe heritable hyperlipidemic

rabbit, an animal model for the progression of atherosclerosis - effect of probucol on coagulation, Thromb. Haemostas. 61, 140-143.

23. Durrington, P.N., Winocur, P.M. and Bhatnagar, D. (1990) Bezafibrate retard in patients with insulin-dependent diabetes. Effects on serum lipoproteins, fibrinogen and glycemic control. J. Cardiovasc. Pharmacol. 16 (Suppl. 9), S30-S34.

24. Pazzucconi, F., Mannucci, L., Mussoni, L., Gianfranceschi, G., Maderna, P., Franceschini, G., Sirtori, C.R. and Tremoli, E. Bezafibrate lowers plasma lipids, fibrinogen and platelet aggregability in hypertriglyceridemic patients, Eur.J. Clin. Pharmacol., in press.

25. Harker, A.L. and Hazzard, W. (1979) Platelet kinetic studies in patients with hyperlipoproteinemia: effects of clofibrate therapy, Circulation 60, 492-496.

26. Sirtori, C.R., Franceschini, G., Gianfranceschi, G., Sirtori, M., Montanari, G., Tremoli, E., Maderna, P., Colli, S. and F. Zoppi (1987) Effects of gemfibrozil on plasma lipoprotein-apolipoprotein distribution and platelet reactivity in patients with hypertriglyceridemia, J. Lab. Clin. Med. 110, 279-286.

The Role of Plasma Membrane Cholesterol Pools in the Regulation of Cellular Cholesterol Efflux

Florence Mahlberg , Sean Davidson , David Bernard and George Rothblat

Abstract

Analysis of the kinetics of cholesterol efflux from a number of different cell types has demonstrated the presence of slow and fast pools of cholesterol. The half-times (t½) for cholesterol efflux from these pools was similar with all cell types, however, the distribution of the cholesterol between these pools differs considerably, depending on cell type. The contribution of the fast pool to cholesterol efflux ranged from approximately 50% in Fu5AH rat hepatoma cells to essentially no fast pool in rabbit smooth muscle cells. These observations led us to propose a model for the mechanism and regulation of cholesterol efflux based on the interaction of the amphipathic helices of apolipoproteins with membrane domains of cholesterol.

Results and Discussion

Reverse cholesterol transport is a process by which excess cholesterol is transported from peripheral cells to the liver for excretion. The first step of this pathway involves the transfer of cholesterol molecules from the plasma membrane of the donor cell to the acceptor lipoprotein particle. HDL, or subfractions of HDL, are believed to be the physiological acceptors. The most generally accepted mechanism for this process involves the movement of cholesterol molecules through an aqueous phase (for a review, see [1,2]). A variety of studies have demonstrated that this transfer is influenced by the physical and compositional characteristics of the acceptor particle, such as the size [3], the lipid composition, particularly the cholesterol to phospholipid mass ratio [4,5] and in some cases, the apolipoprotein composition [6,7]. Early investigations demonstrated that the addition of apolipoproteins to phospholipid liposomes enhances the efficiency of the phospholipid in stimulating cholesterol release. Part of this increased efficiency was attributed to the ability of apolipoproteins to convert liposomes to smaller apolipoprotein-phospholipid structures and, hence, increasing the relative surface area of the particles [3]. However, additional investigations have demonstrated that factors other than increased surface area must be invoked to explain the increased cholesterol release provoked by some apolipoproteins. For instance, when acceptor particles are reconstituted with phosphatidylcholine (PC) and purified apolipoproteins so that the complexes are similar in lipid to protein ratio and in size, it is observed that acceptors containing apoAI are consistently more efficient in removing cellular cholesterol than particles containing apoAII or apoC's [8].

A. L. Catapano et al. (eds.), Drugs Affecting Lipid Metabolism, 493–498.

In more recent investigations we have conducted detailed studies on the efflux of cho
lesterol from a variety of different cell types. Efflux of cholesterol from pre-labeled cells was
studied over a 12 hr period and the kinetic data derived from this type of experiment was ana
lyzed using nonlinear regression analysis [9]. Our initial studies used J774 mouse macrophage
cells exposed to apoAI/PC discs and computer analysis of the data indicated that cholesterol
efflux was consistently best fitted to a line describing the release from two kinetic compartments [9]. Additional studies on the J774 cells established that these pools are not a reflection
of bidirectional flux of cholesterol between cells and acceptor particles, and that plasma mem
brane fractions isolated from the J774 cells exhibited kinetics similar to that of whole cells
[9].

We had previously observed that the rate of release of cholesterol from various cell
types differed considerably, with t½ for efflux ranging from a low of approximately 2 hr with
Fu5AH rat hepatoma cells to greater than 24 hr with a number of cell types including smooth
muscle cells and fibroblasts [10]. To determine if these large differences in the efficiency by
which cells release cholesterol to exogenous acceptors is linked to the presence of plasma
membrane cholesterol pools, we have screened a number of cell types by quantitating the re
lease of labeled cholesterol to apoAI/PC particles that served as a common cholesterol acceptor. The data are presented in the Table and demonstrate that there are extensive differences
in the distribution of fast and slow kinetic pools of cholesterol among cell types and these
differences can generally be linked to the overall rate of release of cholesterol from the cells.

KINETIC POOLS OF CHOLESTEROL IN CELLS

| Cell | FAST POOL | | SLOW POOL | |
	t½	%	t½	%
Fu5AH	1.8	53	15	47
L-Cells	2.0	27	13	73
CHO	1.5	19	14	81
J774	1.9	10	20	90
MPM[1]	1.2	7	27	93
3T3-L1	1.2	5	26	95
FIBRO[2]	1.1	5	29	95
SMC[3]	ND	ND	20	100

ApoAI/PC acceptor particle added at 400 ug PC/ml. ND = none detected
[1] mouse elicited peritoneal macrophages, [2] human skin fibroblasts
[3] rabbit aortic smooth muscle cells

As can be seen from the Table, the contribution of the fast pool to the efflux of cholesterol ranged from more then 50% with the Fu5AH at one extreme to essentially no fast pool in the case of the smooth muscle cells. It is also apparent that the t½ for efflux from the fast pool does not differ greatly among the cell types, with the t½ for cholesterol efflux from the fast pool ranging between 1.2 to 2.0 hr. The t½ for efflux from the slow pool exhibits somewhat greater variation ranging from 13 to 29 hr. Thus, the major determinants influencing the overall efflux of cholesterol from cells are the size of the fast pool and the rate of release from the slow pool.

Our studies on the efflux of cholesterol from cells demonstrated that: 1) cholesterol is released from 2 kinetic pools in cells 2) the size of the fast and slow pools differ among cell types, and 3) the apolipoprotein composition of the acceptor particle can modulate cholesterol efflux by changing the size of the pools [9]. These observations have led us to propose a new model to explain the mechanism and regulation of cholesterol efflux from cells.

The central premise of this model is the existence of heterogeneous domains of cholesterol within plasma membranes. We propose that cholesterol efflux from cell membranes is influenced by three factors, 1) the distribution of cholesterol between cholesterol-rich and cholesterol-poor membrane domains, 2) the diffusion of cholesterol molecules through the unstirred water layer and 3) the transient interaction of segments of the amphipathic helix of the HDL apolipoproteins with the cholesterol-poor membrane domains, resulting in enhanced cholesterol efflux.

The packing of cholesterol within domains is governed by a variety of factors including cholesterol to phospholipid ratios, phospholipid composition and the presence of membrane proteins [11-14]. In addition, lipid lateral packing density within the domains would differ and packing defects would be present at domain boundaries [15,16]. Since the rate of desorption of cholesterol from a membrane into the aqueous phase is, in large part, a function of the strength of the interaction of the cholesterol molecule with adjacent phospholipid molecules [1], the individual domains might be expected to exhibit differences in the rate constant for cholesterol desorption. The rate of efflux from sterol-poor domains is predicted to be faster than that from sterol-rich domains since the cholesterol molecules in the sterol-poor domains would probably be less tightly packed and thus more likely to undergo desorption into the aqueous phase [11]. Thus, the presence of domains would result in the appearance of different kinetic pools of cholesterol within the membrane. Although these kinetic pools may sometimes be a reflection of the transbilayer distribution of cholesterol between the two leaflets of the membrane [13], the lateral domains of cholesterol within a leaflet are postulated to be of primary importance in the present model.

It is now possible to formulate a working hypothesis in which the association of amphipathic helixes of the apolipoproteins with specific lipid domains in membranes would result in the modulation of cholesterol efflux from these membranes. One of the most efficient acceptors of cellular cholesterol has been shown to be small HDL particles that are enriched in both phospholipid and protein and relatively depleted in cholesterol [17]. The physicochemical characteristics of these particles are consistent with the nascent HDL discs that arise from the synthesis of HDL by the liver and intestine and from lipolysis of triglyceride-rich lipoproteins [18]. The results from the studies of Segrest, et al. [19] would predict that on such a small disc the hinged region of the apoAI would be in the "open" configuration, i.e. removed from the surface of the disc and extended into the aqueous phase. It could be this extended hinge region that would interact with specific lipid domains in the plasma membrane. Because of the reduced packing pressure that would be present in the cholesterol-poor domains it can be suggested that it would be these domains that would exhibit the greatest interaction with the apolipoprotein. Thus, the acceptor lipoprotein particle would be loosely and transiently anchored to particular areas of the plasma membrane through the association of amphipathic helixes with membrane lipids. This type of lipoprotein-membrane interaction would be considerably less stringent than ligand-receptor reactions and would be more consistent with the mechanism of association of HDL with cells that was suggested by Tabas and Tall [20] and more recently by Leblond and Marcel [21].

If the events described above occurred, one would anticipate that the association of the acceptor lipoprotein with the membrane would serve to enhance the removal of cellular cholesterol by either changing the size and/or rate of removal of cholesterol from these domains. According to the aqueous diffusion model, when excess acceptor is present the rate-limiting step in the efflux of cell cholesterol is the desorption of cholesterol from the membrane into the aqueous phase. However, when acceptor concentration is not in excess, the movement of the desorbed cholesterol molecule through the unstirred water layer becomes an additional rate limiting step (cf. [1]). Under these conditions, the increased local concentration resulting from the anchoring of the acceptor particles to the cholesterol-poor membrane domains would increase efflux of cholesterol from these domains. Depending on the depth to which the hinged region of apoAI was spread or embedded into the membrane, the distance between the lipoprotein acceptor and the membrane donor would be in the range of 5 to 30A. Since the length of a cholesterol molecule is about 17 A [22], the need to traverse an unstirred water layer would be largely eliminated. Although we have focused this discussion on the hinged region of apoAI, amphipathic helixes of other apolipoproteins may behave in a similar manner.

The greater lipid lateral packing density within the cholesterol-rich domains would result in the affinity of the amphipathic helixes being reduced or eliminated in these regions. Because of the reduced thermal motions of the cholesterol molecules in these domains, the desorption from the membrane would be slower and the rate constant would not be readily influenced by the apolipoprotein composition of the acceptor. The primary factors regulating flux from these membrane domains would then be the physicochemical characteristics of the acceptor particle, such as phospholipid composition and surface area [3,23].

The amphipathic helix anchor model that we have proposed for the efflux of cholesterol can explain much of the diverse data that is available in the scientific literature. More importantly, it is a model that can be tested using a number of different experimental approaches. It can be anticipated that the use of isolated plasma membrane preparations, monoclonal antibodies to specific epitopes on apolipoproteins and synthetic polypeptides having amphipathic helixes will provide the experimental systems necessary to test this model.

Acknowledgments

The studies reported in this paper were supported by Program Project Grant HL 22633 and Training Grant HL 07443 from the National Heart, Lung and Blood Institute of the National Institute of Health, and a postdoctoral fellowship from the American Heart Association, Southeastern Pennsylvania affiliate (FM).

References

1. Phillips, M.C., Johnson, W.J. and Rothblat, G.H. (1987) `Mechanisms and consequences of cellular cholesterol exchange and transfer'. Biochim. Biophys. Acta 906, 223-276.

2. Johnson, W.J., Mahlberg, F.H., Rothblat, G.H. and Phillips, M.C. (1991) `Cholesterol transport between cells and high density lipoproteins'. Biochim. Biophys. Acta 1085, 273-298.

3. DeLamatre, J., Wolfbauer, G., Phillips, M.C. and Rothblat, G.H. (1986) `Role of apolipoproteins in cellular cholesterol efflux'. Biochim. Biophys. Acta 875, 419-428.

4. Bamberger, M.J., Glick, J.M. and Rothblat, G.H. (1983) `Hepatic lipase stimulates the uptake of high density lipoprotein cholesterol by hepatoma cells'. J. Lipid Res. 24, 869-876.

5. Picardo, M., Massey, J.B., Kuhn, D.E., Gotto, Jr.,A.M., Gianturco, S.H. and Pownall, H.J. (1986) `Partially reassembled high density lipoproteins. Effects on cholesterol flux, synthesis, and esterification in normal human skin fibroblasts'. Arteriosclerosis 6, 434-441.

6. Stein, O., Stein, Y., Lefevre, M. and Roheim, P.S. (1986) `The role of apolipoprotein A-IV in reverse cholesterol transport studied with cultured cells and liposomes derived from an ether analog of phosphatidylcholine'. Biochim. Biophys. Acta 878, 7-13.

7. Barbaras, R., Puchois, P., Fruchart, J.-C. and Ailhaud, G. (1987) `Cholesterol efflux from cultured adipose cells is mediated by LpAI particles but not by LpAI:AII particles'. Biochem. Biophys. Res. Comm. 142, 63-69.

8. Mahlberg, F.H., Glick, J.M., Lund-Katz, S. and Rothblat, G.H. (1991) `Influence of apolipoproteins AI, AII and C on the metabolism of membrane and lysosomal cholesterol in macrophages'. J. Biol. Chem. 266, 19930-19937.

9. Mahlberg, F.H. and Rothblat, G.H. (1992) `Cellular cholesterol efflux: role of cell membrane kinetic pools and interaction with apolipoproteins AI, AII, and Cs'. J. Biol. Chem. 267, 4541-4550.

10. Rothblat, G.H., M. Bamberger and M.C. Phillips. 1986. Reverse cholesterol transport. In: Methods in Enzymology, Vol. 129. J. Albers and J. Segrest, editors. Academic Press, New York. 628-644.

11. Schroeder, F., Jefferson, J.R., Kier, A.B., Knittel, J., Scallen, T.J., Wood, W.G. and Hapala, I. (1991) `Membrane cholesterol dynamics: cholesterol domains and kinetic pools'. Proc. Soc. Exp. Biol. Med. 195, 235-252.

12. Hui, S.W. 1988. The spatial distribution of cholesterol in membranes. In: Biology of Cholesterol. P.L. Yeagle, editor. CRC Press, Boca Raton, FL. 213-231.

13. Bittman, R. 1988. Sterol exchange between Mycoplasma membranes and vesicles. In: Biology of Cholesterol. P.L. Yeagle, editor. CRC Press Inc., Boca Raton, FL. 173-195.

14. Jefferson, J.R., Slotte, J.P., Nemecz, G., Pastuszyn, A., Scallen, T.J. and Schroeder, F. (1991) `Intracellular sterol distribution in transfected mouse L-cell fibroblasts expressing rat liver fatty acid-binding protein'. J. Biol. Chem. 266, 5486-5496.

15. Linden, C.D., Wright, ,K.L., McConnell, H.M. and Fox, C.F. (1973) `Lateral phase separations in membrane lipids and the mechanism of sugar transport in Escherichia coli'. Proc. Natl. Acad. Sci. USA 70, 2271-2275.

16. Phillips, M.C., Graham, D.E. and Hauser, H. (1975) `Lateral compressibility and pentration into phospholipid monolayers and bilayer membranes'. Nature 254, 154-156.

17. Castro, G.R. and Fielding, C.J. (1988) `Early incorporation of cell-derived cholesterol into pre-B-migrating high-density lipoprotein'. Biochemistry 27, 25-29.

18. Eisenberg, S. (1984) `High density lipoprotein metabolism'. J. Lipid Res. 25, 1017-1058.

19. Segrest, J.P., Jones, M.K., DeLoff, H., Brouillette, C.G., Venkatachalapathi, Y.V. and Anantharamaiah, G.M. (1992) `The amphipathic helix in the exchangeable apolipoproteins: A review of secondary structure and function'. J. Lipid Res. 33, 141-165.

20. Tabas, I. and Tall, A.R. (1984) `Mechanism of the association of HDL 3 with endothelial cells, smooth muscle cells, and fibroblasts'. J. Biol. Chem. 259, 13897-13905.

21. Leblond, L. and Marcel, Y.L. (1991) `The amphipathic α-helical repeats of apolipoprotein A-I are responsible for binding of high density lipoproteins to HepG2 cells'. J. Biol. Chem. 266, 6058-6067.

22. Craven, B.M. (1976) `Crystal structure of cholesterol monohydrate'. Nature 260, 727-729.

23. Rothblat, G.H. and Phillips, M.C. (1982) `Mechanism of cholesterol efflux from cells. Effects of acceptor structure and concentration'. J. Biol. Chem. 257, 4775-4782.

KINETICS OF EXOGENOUS DI-LINOLEYL PHOSPHATIDYLCHOLINE AND INCORPORATION IN PLASMA AND RBC LIPIDS IN MAN

C. GALLI, C. MOSCONI, F. MARANGONI, M. GIANFRANCESCHI,
M.T. ANGELI and C.R. SIRTORI

ABSTRACT. The plasma kinetics and the incorporation in plasma and red blood cell lipids of di-linoleyl phosphatidyl choline (DLPC), labeled with ^3H in the choline moiety and with ^{14}C linoleic acid ony in position 2, were studied in normal volunteers. The peaks of activity were at around 24 h for ^3H and at around 8-16 h for ^{14}C. The $^3H/^{14}C$ ratio progressively increased in total plasma lipids. The ^3H label was mainly incorporated in HDL, but radioactivity was retained longer and with the same $^3H/^{14}C$ ratio as in the administered compound in LDL. Incorporation of both labels in red blood cell lipids was slower than in plasma lipids, but they were retained much longer. Unlabeled DLPC (4g/day, four weeks) was also administered to moderately hyper-cholesterolemic women. At the end of treatment, significant elevation of plasma PC (concentration and percentage of phospholipids) and of linoleic acid in PC and cholesterol esters were observed. These findings indicate that exogenous DLPC is retained in plasma (unmodified in the LDL fraction) and in circulating cells, and significantly raises plasma PC and linoleic acid in selected lipid pools.

1. INTRODUCTION.

The administration of phosphatidylcholine (PC) is considered an interesting approach in the general preventive management of arterial disease [1,2]. In particular, the di-linoleyl moiety (DLPC) of the compound has been used for human treatment. Studies in experimental animals [3,4] have shown that this compound given p.o. is hydrolyzed in the intestinal mucosa and partly resynthesized into a complete PC molecule. Only limited information is available on the metabolic fate of exogenous PC in humans, obtained from studies carried out using a DLPC labeled either in the choline or in the acyl moieties [5-7]. Studies on the distribution of orally administered DLPC, labeled in the choline and in both the acyl moieties in position 1 and 2, have shown a preferential incorporation in HDL vs LDL and have provided data on

499

A. L. Catapano et al. (eds.), Drugs Affecting Lipid Metabolism, 499–505.
© 1993 Kluwer Academic Publishers and Fondazione Giovanni Lorenzini.

the plasma elimination kinetics for the choline and especially for the fatty acids [7], which are difficult to interprete, since both fatty acids were labeled.

The use of PC selectively labeled in the 2 position, where the fatty acid may only be cleaved by phospholipase A_2, allows a better evaluation of the fate of the acyl moiety. This type of substrate was used in the investigation carried out in healthy volunteers [8], reported in summary in this chapter.

An additional aspect which we have investigated concerns the contribution of the linoleic acid associated with the administered DLPC, to the levels of linoleic acid in plasma lipids, in a study carried out in moderately hyper-cholesterolemic female patients. The different kinetics for the absorption and transport of PC *vs* that of triglycerides may in fact lead to incorporations in lipids which could be different from those expected when linoleic acid is supplied as a triglyceride.

2. EXPERIMENTAL DESIGN AND METHODS

2. 1. Fate of doubly labeled DLPC.

DLPC, selectively labeled with ^{3}H-choline (in the three methyl groups) and ^{14}C linoleic acid in the 2- position was prepared by the group of Prof. C.Scolastico, at the Institute of Organic Chemistry of the University of Milano. The selective labeling of the 2-position of PC with ^{14}C linoleic acid in the preparation, and subsequently in the PC isolated from plasma, was checked with the use of a specific PLase A2. Six healthy subjects (3 males and 3 females), fully informed of the modalities and end points of the study, in fasting conditions, received 750 mg of a DLPC preparation containing 90 µCi of ^{3}H choline and 30 µCi of ^{4}C fatty acid. Blood samples were drawn at various time intervals, up to 144 h after administration. Plasma and red blood cells (RBC) were separated. S elected samples up to 120 h were used for lipid and lipoprotein analysis. Lipids were extracted from plasma and RBC and radioactivity was measured in total lipid extract as well as, after chromato-graphic separation, in single lipid classes. Plasma aliquots were used for separation of lipoproteins by ultracentrifugation, and ^{3}H and ^{14}C radioactivity was measured in single lipoprotein fractions.

2.2. Administration of DLPC to hypercholesterolemic subjects and plasma PC and linoleic acid levels in plasma lipid pools.

Three capsules/day of DLPC (4.05 g/day) were given to six moderately hyper-cholesterolemic female subjects (289 ± 44 mg/dl) for a period of 4 weeks. No modification of the diet was made during the treatment. Levels of plasma cholesterol, total phospholipids (PL) and phosphatidyl-choline (PC), and of linoleic and arachidonic acids in plasma lipids (total, PL, PC, LPC, CE and TG) were measured before and at the end of treatment.

3. RESULTS

3.1. Fate of exogenous doubly labeled DLPC.

The peaks of plasma concentrations of ^{3}H choline and of ^{14}C linoleic acid associated to total lipids were reached at around 24 h for the ^{3}H and between 8 and 16 h for the ^{14}C isotope (Fig. 1). At 120 h still about 7% of the ^{3}H isotope and about 3% of the ^{14}C isotope (% of the dose) were found in plasma lipids. The half-lives of decay of radioactivity in the β phase was 172 h for ^{3}H and 70 for ^{14}C. The Isotopic ratio ^{3}H/^{14}C (not shown) remained close to that of the administered compound (3:1 ratio) until around 24 h, and increased progressively later on reaching a value of about 10:1 at 120 h.

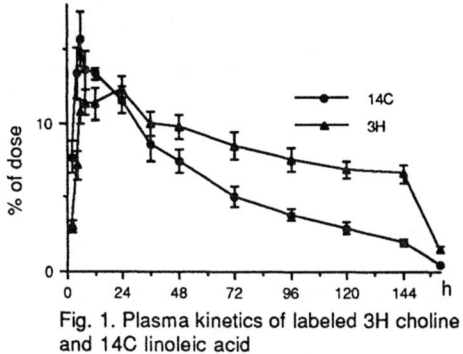

Fig. 1. Plasma kinetics of labeled 3H choline and 14C linoleic acid

The incorporation of ^{3}H and ^{14}C radioactivities in lipoproteins followed different time course as shown in Fig. 2 (percentages of total radioactivity). At 4 h, the highest percentage of ^{3}H radioactivity was in HDL, followed by LDL and VLDL. There was an increase in the relative proportion of radioactivity in HDL, up to 16 h, in association with a decline in VLDL, whereas changes in

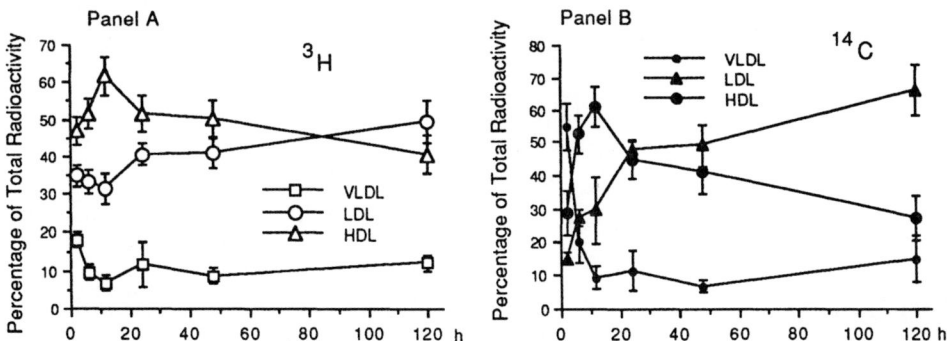

Fig. 2. Percentage distribution of total ^{3}H (Panel A) and ^{14}C (Panel B) radioactivities in lipoproteins

LDL were limited. The ^{14}C radioactivity at 4 h was associated with VLDL for about 60 % and decreased markedly to about 10 % in this fraction at 16 h, whereas in HDL there was a marked elevation, with a peak at 16 h, followed by slow decline later on, and in LDL there was elevation up to 24 h, followed by a slower rise up to 120 h. The 3H/ 14 C ratio in lipoproteins (Fig. 3)

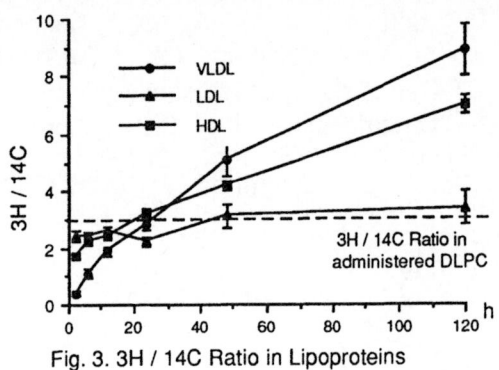

Fig. 3. 3H / 14C Ratio in Lipoproteins

remained constant and very close to that in the administered compound (i.e. around 3) only in LDL. In HDL the ratio remained close to 3 only in the first 24 h, and increased later on, whereas in VLDL the ratio was very low at 4 h (due to the high incorporation of the ^{14}C fatty acid in this fraction), and kept increasing to very high values up to 120 h, reflecting the progressive loss of labeled fatty acid from this lipoprotein. The incorporation of the two labels in plasma and red blood cell lipids followed quite different patterns as shown in Fig.4, which presents the time course of the incorporation of ^{3}H and ^{14}C in the choline-glycerophospholipids (PC and lyso PC). The ^{3}H label was associated for over 90 % with choline-glycerophospholipids, with minimal incorporation in sphingomyelin. The proportion of ^{3}H radioactivity associated with PC was in the order of 80 % of total, initially, with progressive decline to about 60 %, in concomitance with the accumulation in LPC. Comparison of the accumulation

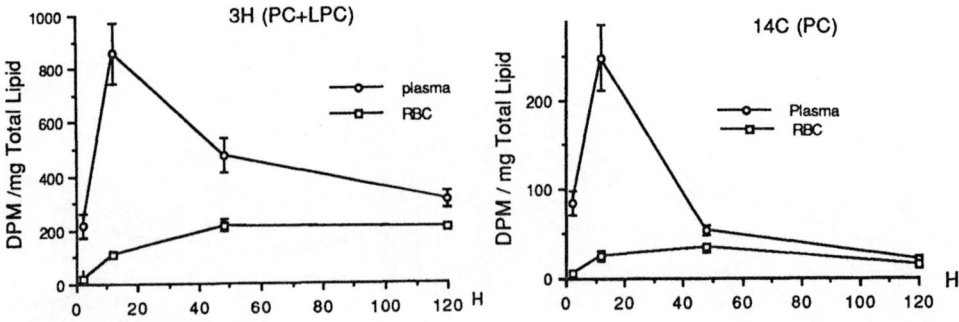

Fig.4. Specific activities of labeling of plasma and RBC choline-glycero phospholipids: ^{3}H in PC + LPC (Panel A) and ^{14}C in PC (Panel B).

curves for ^{3}H in plasma and RBC lipids (dpm/mg total lipids) shows, as expected, a marked rise of in plasma, peaking at 16 h, followed by progressive decline, whereas in RBC there was a slow increase up to about 44 h, followed by a plateau maintained up to 120 h. At this time interval the incorporations in plasma and in RBC were within the same range. The ^{14}C radioactivity in the choline phospholipids was detectable only in PC, where was retained in the position 2 of glycerol as assessed by the use of phospholipase A_2, whereas no radioactivity was found in LPC. These two observations confirm the presence of the ^{14}C labeled fatty acid only in position 2 of PC and indicate that this position was retained *in vivo*. The incorporation of the isotope in plasma and RBC PC followed a pattern similar to that observed for the ^{3}H radioactivity, i.e. the incorporation in RBC was slow but was retained longer, and at 120 h identical levels were reached in plasma and RBC PC.

3.2. Effects of exogenous DLPC on plasma cholesterol and PL and on the linoleic acid levels in selected lipid pools, in hypercholesterolemic subjects.

The administration of 3 capsules/day of DLPC (1.35 g / each capsule) for a period of four weeks resulted in a statistically significant reduction of plasma total cholesterol from the initial value of 288 ± 44 mg/dl (x ± SD) to 248 ± 17, but tnere was no change of HDL levels. In addition there were significant elevations of the levels of plasma PC and total phospholipids (PL), as well as of those of PC as % of total PL (Fig. 5A and B). The fatty acid patterns of plasma lipid classes were analyzed, and the levels of selected fatty acids, before and after treatment, in those plasma lipid fractions in which differences occurred, are reported in Tab. 1. There were significant elevations of linoleic acid in total lipids, PC and cholesterol esters, associated with a reduction of palmitic. As a consequence, total polyunsaturates and the unsaturation index of the various fractions were enhanced, and saturates were reduced.

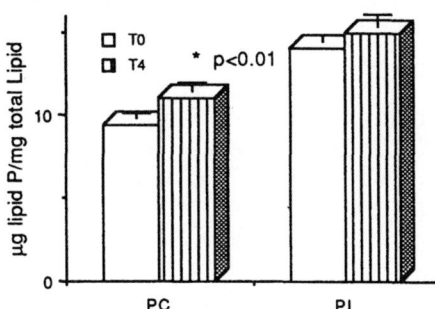

Fig. 5A. Levels of plasma PC and total PL before (T0) and 4 weeks after (T4) treatment

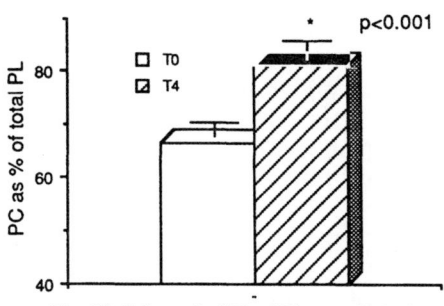

Fig. 5B. PC as % of Total Plasma PL before (T0) and 4 weeks after (T4) treatment

Tab. 1. Levels of selected fatty acids in plasma lipids before and after treatment with DLPC

FA	TL		PC		CE	
	Before	After	Before	After	Before	After
16:0	25.4±0.7	21.9±1.3*	40.5±0.8	33.9±0.9*	16.5±0.8	15.41.0
18:2	27.1±1.0	31.2±1.0*	17.0±0.7	22.0±0.7*	42.9±1.3	47.2±1.5*
SAT	31.8±1.1	27.6±1.5*	56.1±1.0	50.2±1.0*	18.6±0.9	18.0±1.4
PUFA	39.9±0.7	45.5±1.0*	32.7±1.5	37.3±1.2*	52.3±1.4	56.3±1.4
U.I.	136.7±1.7	150.5±3.5*	106.9±4.6	120.0±4	153.6±2.3	157.8±2.4

FA, Fatty Acid; TL, Total Lipids, PC, phosphatidylcholine; CE, cholesterol esters; Sat, saturates; PUFA, poly-unsaturated fatty acids; U.I. , Unsaturation index (sum of products of % of each fatty acid x number of double bonds).

4. DISCUSSION AND CONCLUSIONS.

The fate of orally administered PC has been studied in experimental animals and humans and the general conclusions are that a large proportion of the molecule is hydrolyzed at the intestinal mucosa and that up to 50 % of the formed LPC may be reesterified after absorption (3). Studies in man have been carried out with the oral administration of doubly labeled DLPC, labeled with ^{3}H in the choline, and with ^{14}C in the fatty acids, which were both in the 1 and 2 positions (7). These studies have shown that most of the choline radioactivity was linked to PC, whereas the ^{14}C activity was distributed also in non polar lipids. The peak of ^{14}C in plasma was reached earlier than that of ^{3}H, but declined faster. The half-life of decay of radioactivity was around 65 h for ^{3}H and around 32 for [14]C. The ^{3}H/^{14}C ratio at the peak of activity was twice that in the administered compound and the ratio continued to rise later on. The choline radioactivity was incorporated more readily and preferentially in HDL. Our data, obtained with the use of a DLPC in which the ^{14}C labeled linoleic acid was esclusively in the 2 position, substantially confirmed some of the previous findings, but provided new iinformation on the kinetics of the DLPC molecule. The major point is that the 2 position appeared to be better preserved from hydrolysis since the isotopic ratio at the time of peak activity was substantially the same as in the administered molecule, and remained in the same range up to 24 h. As a consequence of the relative stability of the molecule, the plasma half life for ^{14}C activity was longer than previously observed. An additional observation is that the doubly labeled PC in LDL remained intact throughout the whole period at study and was removed very slowly. This may be relevant for the effects of the incorporated PC on the properties of this lipoprotein. Finally the incorporation of both isotopes in RBC was slow but was retained without significant decay up to 120 H.

The data obtained with the administration of 4 g/day of DLPC for a period of 4 weeks to hypercolesterolemic women indicate that, in spite of the large endogenous pool of PC, which is also biosynthesized, relatively low doses of the compound significantly raise the levels of circulating PL and especially the proportion of PC over total PL. The increment of circulating PC was calculated in the order of 25 mg/dl. In addition, there was a significant accumulation of 18:2 in various lipid fractions, especially in PC and in the cholesterol esters. Since the supply of this fatty acid with the product was relatively small (about 2 g/day), it would appear that linoleic acid is retained in circulating PC and then is selectively transferred to CE, possibly through the activity of the LCAT. In our experiment there was also a significant reduction of total cholesterol, but the limited number of subjects and the design of the experiment do not allow definite conclusions on this effect. The data in the literature, in this respect, are also not conclusive.

In conclusion our studies show that exogenous PC is incorporated, to a significant extent in non modified form, in circulating lipoproteins, and is retained for a very long period of time, especially in LDL. It accumulates also in red blood cells, and the long residence in this cells may represent a form of lipid store. The administered PC provides also a supply of linoleic acid to selected lipid pools, resulting in the modifications of characteristics, such as the degree of unsaturation, which may affect physico-chemical and functional properties. These influences appear relevant to the effects of exogenous PC on lipid and lipoprotein metabolism, which have been observed in animal and human studies.

Acknowledgements. These studies were supported by contracts of Nattermann Gmbh, Köln, Germany, and Rhone Poulenc, Pharma,l.

5. REFERENCES

1. Adams, CWM, Abdullah, YH, Bayliss, OB, and Morgan, RS (1967) J.Pathol. Bacteriol.94, 77-87
2. Williams, KJ, Werth, VP, and Wolff, JA (1984) Persp. Biol. Med. 27, 417-431
3. Lekim, D, and Betzing, H (1976) Hoppe Seyler's Z. Physiol. Chem. 357, 1321-1331
4. Partasarathy,S, Subbaiah, PV, and Ganguly, J (1974) Biochem J,140, 503-508
5. Wagener, H (1972) in Phospholipide (G.Schettler, Ed.) pp. 59-69, G. Thieme Verlag, Stuttgart, Germany
6. Beil, FU, and Grundy, SM (1980) J Lipid Res 21, 525-536
7. Zierenberg, O, and Grundy, SM (1982) J Lipid Res 23,1136-1142
8. Galli, C, Sirtori, CR, Mosconi, C, Medini, L, Gianfranceschi, G, Vaccarino, V, and Scolastico, C, Lipids, in press

ALIMENTARY LIPEMIA AND PHOSPHOLIPIDS

G. SALVIOLI, R. PANINI, R. LUGLI, J.M. PRADELLI
University of Modena,Chair of Geriatrics and Gerontology,
Ospedale Estense, Viale Vittorio Veneto,9
41100 Modena
Italy

ABSTRACT. The ability of purified soybean phosphatidylcholine (PPC) to influence alimentary lipemia was investigated in a cross over study on ten healthy subjects receiving a constant diet over two periods (A and B) each lasting 10 days. At the end of each period a fat-rich semisolid meal containing 1 g of fat/Kg body weight was given and alimentary lipemia evaluated as the composition of triglyceride-rich lipoprotein (TRL). During period B, subjects were administered 3 g/day of PPC and 4 g of the same compound was added to the fatty meal. The maximum peaks of postprandial plasma triglycerides (TG) were higher and appeared faster at the end of period B even though the area under the TG curve was smaller. Supplementation with PPC induced both an increase of phosphatidylcholine (PC) containing linoleic acid and the appearance of dilinoleoyl lecithin in TRL; this molecular species is largely represented in soybean PC but normally absent in human plasma.

1. INTRODUCTION

Serum TG levels after a fat-rich meal vary greatly [1], as a consequence of both the rate of intestinal absorption and clearance of postprandial triglyceride-rich lipoproteins (TRL) [2]. Clearance of TRL from the serum depends to a great extent on the precise composition [3] and size [4] of these particles. The lipid moiety of TRL (chylomicrons, CM, and very low lipoproteins, VLDL) is largely represented by a core of TG surrounded by free cholesterol (Chol) and phospholipids (PL) (above all phosphatidylcholine). The composition of dietary TG significantly influences the molecular species of PC in chylomicrons [2]. Moreover, the acyl chain composition of PC influences the clearance of CM, which is significantly faster with molecular species of greater hydrophilicity [5][6]. Since high density lipoproteins are formed during TRL hydrolysis, the concentration of these lipoproteins increases in the postprandial period [1], especially when the fatty meal contains large amounts of phospholipids [7].

Whereas animal PC bears almost exclusively palmitic acid (16:0) in the sn-1 position and an unsaturated fatty acid in the sn-2 position, purified soybean PC (PPC) contains some molecular species with linoleic acid in the sn-1 position [8].

Postprandial events have been shown to play a crucial role in atherogenesis via remnant particles [9], which have significant circulating levels for at least 12-24 hours after a meal; thus, modification of the composition of these particles may have therapeutic significance. Therefore, it is of interest to study whether the amount of phospholipids (PL) in a fat meal induces variations of

A. L. Catapano et al. (eds.), Drugs Affecting Lipid Metabolism, 507–513.
© 1993 Kluwer Academic Publishers and Fondazione Giovanni Lorenzini.

alimentary lipemia. Accordingly, the aim of this study was to determine if PPC administration affects, a) the postprandial response to a fatty meal, and b) the composition of PC molecular species in tryglyceride-rich lipoproteins.

2. MATERIALS AND METHODS

2.1 Subjects.

Ten healthy male subjects ranging in age from 28 to 70 years were admitted to the study. The subjects gave informed content for the investigation, which consisted of two periods (A and B) each of 10 day duration with a 2 week free interval.

A constant diet of 40 Cal/Kg was administered containing 55% of calories as carbohydrates and 28% as fat, with a polyunsaturated to saturated fatty acid ratio of 0.8. The subjects received 3 g/day of oil mixture during period A and 3 g of purified soybean lecithin (PPC, Rhône Poulenc Rorer, Milan) during period B; feeding sequence was A-B in subjects 1, 3, 5, 7 and 9, and B-A in the others. Table 1 reports the fatty acid compositions of the soybean product and oil mixture. At the end of each period the subjects were fed a fat-rich semisolid meal containing 1 g of fat/Kg body weight; the lipid composition (by weight) of the meal was 98.7% TG, 0.6% PL and 0.7% Chol. Four grams of oil mixture or PPC were added to the meal in period A and B, respectively.

Table 1. Percentage fatty acid composition of PPC and oil mixture added to test the meal

Fatty acid	PPC (**)			oil mixture*
	1-position	2-position	total	
16:0	24	2	12	8
16:1	-	-	1	1
18:0	8	1	4	4
18:1	11	10	10	20
18:2	52	80	67	62
18:3	5	7	6	5

(*) Contains 20% soy, 20% corn and 60% safflower oils; (**) from Lekim[8].

The fat load was ingested in a single dose within 20 minutes after, a 12 hour overnight fast. Blood samples were collected before and 3, 4, 5, 6, 8 and 10 hours after the test meal. Postprandial lipemia was quantitated from the plasma response curves: we evaluated the maximum peak of both total plasma TG and TRL-TG and the time of appearance of the maximum TG-peak.

2.2 Lipid Analysis.

Blood was collected in tubes containing EDTA (0.1% final concentration). Plasma samples (6 ml), obtained at the times indicated above, were subjected to a single centrifugation at a density of 1.006 g/ml in a Beckman 65 rotor (39,000 rpm for 18 h, at 4°C); the fraction containing

TRL was aspirated and stored at -30°C until analysis.

Plasma (and lipoproteins) were assayed for lipids TG using Boehringer Kits. Plasma and TRL fraction were extracted with chloroform:methanol 2:1 containing 0.01% BHT; the chloroform phase was run on 20 cm silica gel plates with chloroform/methanol/water/acetic acid (130:90:10:1 by vol) containing 0.1% BHT. The PC spot was scrapped off, eluted and then hydrolyzed with phospholipase C (from *Bacillus Cereus*). The resultant 1,2 diradylglycerols were transformed into diradylglycerobenzoates [10] and purified on silica gel G plates [10]. Diacylglycerobenzoates were separated by HPLC on a Licrospher R18 column (25x0.4 cm, 5μ particle size) using acetonitrile:propan-2-ol (80:20 v/v) as isocratic solvent. Peaks were detected at 230 nm; the retention times and areas of the peaks were measured with a Hewlett-Packard recording integrator and recognized by referencing against the retention time of 16:0-18:1 PC. The various molecular species were identified by GLC analysis.

Statistical analysis was run on a computer program for paired and non-paired t-test.

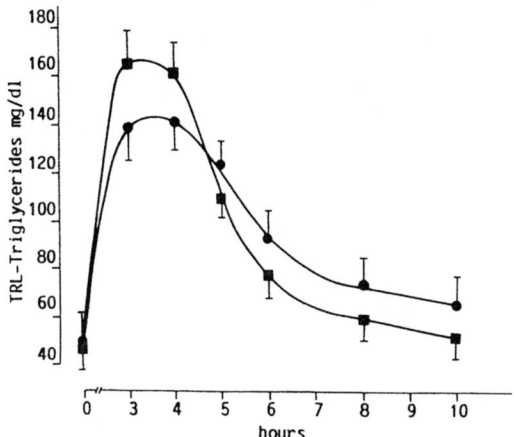

Fig. 1. Alimentary lipemia. Variations of TRL-triglycerides. Fat load with PPC (■) or oil mixture(●).

3. RESULTS

Figures 1 and 2 illustrate the overall triglyceride and phospholipid responses. PPC supplementation of the fatty meal decreased the time of appearance of the maximum TG peak and led to a greater increase of circulating TG and PL; the same behaviour was observed for total TG (Fig 3). TG increased 91.6% in period B and 83.4% in period A. However, the total areas under the TG curves were lower when the subjects received PPC: one explanation may be that TRL clearance was faster in period B, as indicated by the downward slope of the curves.

Table 2 reports the lipid composition of TRL during the fatty meal: treatment with PPC (period B) increased the PL content of TRL over that in period A, with a consequent rise in the PL to Chol ratio. The fatty acid composition of TRL-PLs during the meal had a higher 18:2 concentration when PPC was given, as compared to period A (Table 3).

Table 4 lists the molecular species of TRL-PC found after the fat-rich meals. PPC administration raised the percentage of 16:0-18:2 and 18:0-18:2 in the lecithin fraction. Moreover, 2.6%

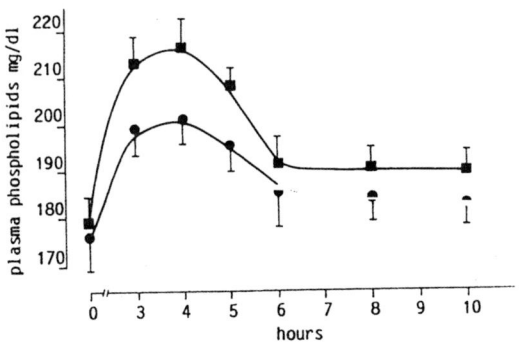

Fig. 2. Alimentary lipemia. Variations of plasma PL. Fat load with PPC (■) or oil mixture (●).

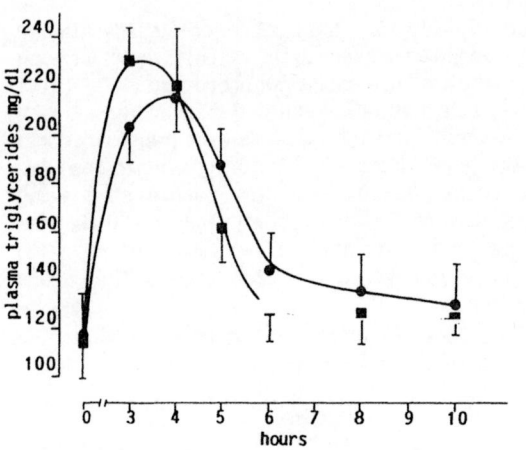

Fig.3. Alimentary lipemia. Variations of total TG. Fat load with PPC (■) or oil mixture (●).

of the PC fraction was represented by 18:2-18:2 PC; this species could not be detected in TRL four hours after administration of a fatty meal not containing PPC but enriched with oils whose fatty acid content is similar to PPC.

4. DISCUSSION

Our study showed that short term administration of PPC and its incorporation into a test meal (period B) induced a faster appearance of alimentary lipemia with higher peaks followed by a faster clearance of plasma triglycerides. Other papers have demonstrated that administration of PPC affects the intestinal phase of lipid metabolism [11], facilitating the lymphatic output of triglycerides during the absorption of high fat loads [12]. Fat absorption increases PL turnover in the enterocytes [12], where lysolecithin, formed by the action of phospholipase A2 on biliary and dietary PC, is incorporated into CM after reacylation in the mucosal cells [13]. The intake of exogenous lecithin is usually limited (2-4 g per day), whereas about 8-10 g are exported in the lymph when a fatty diet is ingested [14]: biliary PC, rich in 16:0-18:2 and 16:0-18:2 species, could be an important source of luminal lecithin above all when fat intake is low [15][16], as when 4 grams of PPC were added to the fatty meal (period B).

PL content can modulate both the transformation of CM into other particles and hepatic recognition of post alimentary lipoprotein particles [17][18]. When the dietary intake of PC is high, its hydrolysis in the intestine may be incomplete; indeed, the activity of phospholipase A2 is much lower than that of triglyceride lipase [19]. Therefore, a prolonged presence of intact PC molecules occurs in the distal segments of the small intestine [16].

Table 2. Lipid composition of triglyceride-rich lipoproteins.

	basal period		post fat-rich meal (maximum peak)	
	A	B	A	B
triglyceride	50.2±7.3	46.2±5.5	144.7± 28.3	165.2± 29.8
cholesterol	21.5±2.7	19.5±1.9	46.9± 3.4	45.7± 4.2
phospholipid	16.8±1.7	18.0±2.0	39.5± 3.6	44.3± 4.8

Values are means ±SD, expressed in mg/dl.   Period B: PPC administration.

Table 3. Fatty acid composition of phospolipids in TRLs.

fatty acid		peak post-alimentary lipemia		
	basal	without PPC	with PPC	
16:0	28.8±3.4	29.1±3.0	26.5±3.2	
16:1	1.7±0.2	1.8±0.3	1.7±0.2	
18:0	16.4±2.4	16.3±2.0	14.8±2.1	
18:1	19.2±2.0	18.2±1.9	18.7±1.8	
18:2	21.3±2.7	21.9±2.3	25.8±2.5	(*)
18:3	2.7±0.2	2.6±0.2	2.5±0.3	
20:4	2.6±0.3	2.9±0.3	2.9±0.3	
20:6	3.3±0.5	3.2±0.4	3.1±0.3	

Values represent percentage means±SD. (*) $p < 0.05$ between basal and period B.

Table 4. Species of TRL-PC after a fat-rich meal with and without PPC.

molecular species	period A	period B
16:0-22:6	4.5±0.8	3.8±0.5
16:0-20:4	2.2±0.4	1.9±0.2
16:0-18:2	34.6±3.2	35.1±2.4
16:0-18:1	20.4±2.6	16.1±2.4
18:0-20:4	6.4±1.0	6.9±0.8
18:0-18:2	16.5±1.8	18.1±1.7
18:0-18:1	2.5±0.4	1.3±0.2
18:1-18:2	4.2±1.0	5.2±0.9
18:1-18:1	1.4±0.3	1.5±0.3
18:2-18:2	--	2.6±0.4

The values are percentage means±SD of recognized molecular species of PC.
Period B: PPC administration.

The lysolecithin produced by hydrolysis of PPC may be resynthesized into lecithin in the intestinal cell, with probable formation of 18:2-18:2 PC [20]. TRL enrichment with PC containing 18:2 molecular species could facilitate their transfer to HDL formed during CM clearance [1]; their high hydrophilicity increases the exchange rate with other lipoprotein particles [6].

In our study PPC feeding influenced alimentary lipemia and the lipid composition of postprandial lipoprotein particles, increasing the PL to Chol ratio of TRL (Table 2). Simonsson et al. [21] reports that supplementation of a fatty meal with egg lecithin has no influence on both PL content and fatty acid composition of plasma and lipoprotein lipids; they conclude that PL can be substituted by an equivalent amount of dietary TG with similar fatty acid composition. In the guinea pig dietary soybean and egg PC with contrasting fatty acid composition have a different effect on plasma lipids, suggesting a dietary phospholipid effect modulated by the fatty acid composition of ingested PL [22]. Contrasting effects of dietary soybean lecithin and corn oil on lipoprotein lipids have been reported by Childs et al. [23].

In our study ten male subjects received a similar substitution: only the administration of PPC (3 g/day for 10 days and 4 g with the fatty meal] influenced both the phospholipid composition and fatty acid pattern of TRL and the time-curve of alimentary lipemia. No variations were observed when a mixture of oils having the same fatty acid composition as PPC was given.

An interesting point is the appearance of 18:2-18:2 PC molecular species in TRL (Table 4): this observation can be explained by resynthesis of dilinoleoyl lecithin from an unsaturated lysolecithin or by intestinal absorption of the intact molecule, as suggested above.

The enrichment of TRL with PC molecular species containing linoleic acid could play a role in the control of the postprandial events of lipoprotein metabolism: *in vitro* polyunsaturated fatty acid-containing CM are more susceptible to lipolysis [4]. *In vivo,* clearance of CM and remnants are accelerated by a polyunsaturated-rich diet [24], probably due to increased activity of lipoproteinlipase [25]. The finding is important since postprandial lipemia is limited by clearance rather than absorption of TG [26]. We conclude that PPC feeding induces important variations of alimentary lipemia; this result should be viewed in light of the observation that the clearance of CM and their remnants is impaired in coronary atherosclerosis [27].

5. REFERENCES

1) Tall, A.R. (1986) 'Metabolism of postprandial lipoproteins', Methods Enzymol. 129, 469-482.
2) Robins, S.J., Fasulo, J.M., Robins, V.F., and Patton, G.M. (1985) 'Response of serum triglycerides of endogenous origin to the administration of triglyceride-rich lipid particles', Am. J. Physiol. 257, E469-E482.
3) Weintraub, M.S., Zechner, R., Brown, A., Eisenberg, S., and Breslow, J.L. (1988) 'Dietary polyunsaturated fats of the ω-6 and ω-3 series reduce postprandial lipoprotein levels', J. Clin. Invest. 82, 1884-1893.
4) Weintraub, M.S., Eisenberg, S., and Breslow, J.L. (1987) 'Dietary fat clearance in normal subjects is regulated by genetic variations in apolipoproteins E', J. Clin. Invest. 80, 1571-1577.
5) Patton, G.M., Clark, S.B., Fasulo, J.M., and Robins, S.J. (1984) 'Utilization of individual lecithins in intestinal lipoprotein formations in the rat', J. Clin. Invest. 73, 231-240.
6) Patton, G.M., Robins, S.J., Fasulo, J.M., and Bennet Clark, S. (1985) 'Influence of lecithin acyl chain compostion on the kinetics of exchange between chylomicrons and high density lipoproteins', J. Lipid Res., 26, 1285-1293.
7) Taskinen, M.R. and Kuusi, T. (1986) 'High density lipoproteins in postprandial lipemia. Relation to sex and lipoprotein lipase activity', Atherosclerosis 59, 121-130.
8) Lekim, D. and Betzing, H. (1974) 'Der Einbau von EPL-Sustanz in Organe von gesunden und durch Galaktosamine geschadigten Ratten', Arzneim. Forsch. 24, 1217-1221.
9) Zilversmit, D.B. (1974) 'Atherogenesis: a postprandial phenomenon', Circulation 60, 473-483.
10) Blank, M.L., Robinson, M., Fitzgerard, V., and Snyder, F. (1984) 'Novel quantitative methods for determination of molecular species of phospholipids and diglycerides', J. Chromatography 298, 473-483.

11) Beil, F.U. and Grundy, S.M., (1980) 'Studies on plasma lipoproteins during absorption of exogenous lecithin in man', J. Lipid Res. 21, 525-536.

12) Parlier, R.D., Frase, S., and Mansbach, C.M. (1989) 'Intraenterocyte distribution of absorbed lipid and effects of phosphatidylcholine', Am. J. Physiol. 256, G349-G355.

13) Nilsson, A. (1968) 'Intestinal absorption of lecithin and lysolecithin by lymph fistula in rats', Biochim. Biophy. Acta. 152, 379-390.

14) Börgstrom, B. (1976) 'Phospholipid absorption', in K. Rommel, H. Goebel and R. Bohmer (eds.), Lipid Absorption: Biochemical and Chemical Aspects, University Park Press, Baltimore, pp. 65-70.

15) Tsao, P., Balint, J.A., and Simmonds, W.J., (1976) 'Role of biliary lecithin in lymphatic transport of fat'. Gastroenterology 13, 1362-1367.

16) Carey, M.C., Small, D.M., and Bliss, C.M. 'Lipid digestion and absorption', Ann. Rev. Physiol. 45, 661-677.

17) Barenstajn, J. and Kotlar, T.J. (1990) 'Phospholipids as modulators of hepatic recognition of chylomicron remnants. Observation with emulsified lipoprotein lipids', Biochem. J. 269, 539-542.

18) Bennet Clark, S.B. and Derksen, A. (1987) 'Phosphatidylcholine composition of emulsion influences triacylglycerol lipolysis and clearance from plasma', Biochim. Biophys. Acta 920, 37-46.

19) Arnesjö, B., Nilsson, A., Barrowman, J., and Börgstrom B. (1969) 'Intestinal digestion and absorption of cholesterol and lecithin in humans', Scand. J. Gastroenterol. 4, 635-665.

20) Zierenberg, O. and Grundy, S.M. (1982) 'Intestinal absorption of polyenephosphatidylcholine', J. Lipid Res. 23, 1136-1142.

21) Simonsson, P., Nilsson, A., and Åkesson, B. (1982) 'Postprandial effects of dietary phospatidylcholine on plasma lipoproteins in man', Amer. J. Clin. Nutr. 35, 36-41.

22) O'Brien, B. and Corrigan, S.M. (1988) 'Influence of dietary soybean and egg lecithin on lipid responses in cholesterol-fed guinea pigs', Lipids 23, 647-650.

23) Child, M.T., Bowlin, J.A., Ogilvie, J.T., Hazzard, W.R., and Albers, J.J. (1981) 'The contrasting effects of a dietary soya lecithin product and corn oil on lipoprotein lipids in normolipidemic and familial hypercholesterolemic subjects', Atherosclerosis 38, 217-228.

24) Demacker, P.N.M., Reijnen I.G.M., Katan M.B., Stuyt P.M.J., and Stalenhoef A.F.H. (1991) 'Increased removal of remnants of triglyceride-rich lipoproteins on a diet rich in polyunsaturated fatty acids', Eur. J. Clin. Invest. 21, 197-203.

25) Harris, W.S., Connor, W.E., Alam, N., and Illingworth D.R. (1988) 'Reduction of postprandial triglyceridemia in humans by dietary n-3 fatty acids', J. Lipid Res. 29, 1451-1460.

26) Cohen, J.C. (1988) 'Chylomicron triglycerides clearance: comparison of three assessment methods', Am. J. Clin. Nutr. 49, 305-313.

27) Simpson, H.S., Williamson, C.M., Olivecrona, T., Pringle, S., Maclean, J., Larimer, A.R., Bonnefons, F., Bogaievsky, Y., Packard, C.J., and Shepard, J. (1990) 'Postprandial lipemia, fenofibrate and coronary artery disease', Atherosclerosis 85, 193-202.

INDEX

Medical Science Symposia Series

KLUWER ACADEMIC PUBLISHERS – DORDRECHT / BOSTON / LONDON